Clinical Handbooks in Neuropsychology

Series Editor
William B. Barr
New York University
New York, NY, USA

For further volumes:
http://www.springer.com/series/8438

Lisa D. Ravdin • Heather L. Katzen
Editors

Handbook on the Neuropsychology of Aging and Dementia

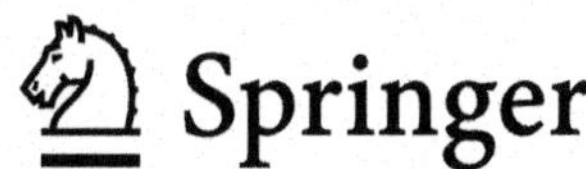

Editors
Lisa D. Ravdin
Department of Neurology
& Neuroscience
Weill Cornell Neuropsychology Service
Weill Medical College of Cornell
University
New York Presbyterian Hospital
New York, NY, USA

Heather L. Katzen
Division of Neuropsychology
Department of Neurology
University of Miami Miller
School of Medicine
Miami, FL, USA

ISBN 978-1-4614-3105-3 (Hardcover)
ISBN 978-1-4614-9140-8 (Softcover)
ISBN 978-1-4614-3106-0 (eBook)
DOI 10.1007/978-1-4614-3106-0
Springer New York Heidelberg Dordrecht London

Library of Congress Control Number: 2012937655

Printed on acid-free paper

Springer is part of Springer Science+Business Media (www.springer.com)

Preface

The *Clinical Handbooks in Neuropsychology* series was designed to be a departure from typical texts by focusing on concrete clinical descriptions and detailed instructions regarding how neuropsychologists evaluate various patient conditions. This particular book was created with the knowledge that older adults are the fastest growing segment of the population, and neuropsychologists are increasingly being called upon to evaluate seniors in a variety of contexts. Many predict that 15–20% of the baby-boomer generation will develop some form of cognitive decline over the course of their lifetime, with estimates escalating to up to 50% in those achieving advanced age. Although much attention has been directed at Alzheimer's disease, the most common form of dementia, it is estimated that nearly one-third of those cases of cognitive decline result from other neuropathological mechanisms.

Handbook on the Neuropsychology of Aging and Dementia is a unique work that provides clinicians with expert guidance and a hands-on approach to neuropsychological practice with older adults. The authors of each chapter are expert practitioners, recognized by their peers as opinion leaders on their chosen chapter topics. The book is divided into two parts: the first addresses special considerations for the evaluation of older adults, and the second focuses on common referral questions likely to be encountered when working with this age group. In many chapters, case examples are provided to highlight common issues that may arise when a particular disorder is considered in the differential diagnosis. Suggested test batteries are also provided in many cases, and each chapter concludes with a user-friendly list of *Clinical Pearls*, items extracted from the text that include expert tips and key take-home messages on each topical area.

The field of neuropsychology has played a critical role in developing methods for early identification of late life cognitive disorders as well as the differential diagnosis of dementia. Each chapter in this work reinforces the notion that neuropsychological measures provide the clinician with sensitive tools to differentiate normal age-related cognitive decline from disease-associated impairment, aid in differential diagnosis of cognitive dysfunction in older adults, as well as identify cognitive deficits most likely to translate into functional impairments in everyday life.

Our contributing authors embraced the approach of providing insightful commentary and useful strategies gained from their clinical experience, and we are grateful to them for generously giving their time and expertise to this project. We appreciate the support of Janice Stern, Springer's senior editor for health and behavior, and Bill Barr, series editor, who together were the driving force behind this project. Finally, a special thanks to Brooke Schiowitz and James Maniscalco, who were extraordinarily helpful with administrative aspects of preparing this work.

New York, NY, USA Lisa D. Ravdin
Miami, FL, USA Heather L. Katzen

Contents

Contributors

Alyssa Arentoft Department of Psychology, Fordham University, New York, NY, USA

Stephanie Assuras Department of Psychiatry, Harvard Medical School, Massachusetts General Hospital, Boston, MA, USA

Department of Neurology, Brigham and Women's Hospital, Boston, MA, USA

Rosemary Bakker Division of Geriatrics, Department of Medicine, Weill Cornell Medical College, New York, NY, USA

Kimberly K. Bares Minneapolis VA Health Care System, Minneapolis, MN, USA

Russell M. Bauer Department of Clinical and Health Psychology, University of Florida, Gainesville, FL, USA

Brian D. Bell Charles Matthews Neuropsychology Laboratory, Department of Neurology, University of Wisconsin School of Medicine and Public Health, Madison, WI, USA

W.S. Middleton Memorial Veterans Hospital, Madison, WI, USA

Linas A. Bieliauskas Neuropsychology Section, Department of Psychiatry, Mental Health Service, Ann Arbor VA Healthcare System, University of Michigan Healthcare System, Ann Arbor, MI, USA

Nina Browner Department of Neurology (CB 7025), University of North Carolina School of Medicine, Chapel Hill, NC, USA

Shane S. Bush VA New York Harbor Healthcare System, New York, NY, USA

Desiree Byrd Departments of Pathology and Psychiatry, The Mount Sinai School of Medicine, New York, NY, USA

Gregg L. Caporaso Division of Neurology, Westchester Health Associates, Yorktown Heights, NY, USA

Gordon J. Chelune Department of Neurology, Center for Alzheimer's Care, Imaging and Research, University of Utah School of Medicine, Salt Lake City, UT, USA

Stephanie Cosentino Cognitive Neuroscience Division of the Gertrude H. Sergievsky Center, Taub Institute for Research on Alzheimer's Disease and the Aging Brain, and Department of Neurology, Columbia University Medical Center, New York, NY, USA

Kelly Coulehan Department of Psychology, Fordham University, New York, NY, USA

George M. Cuesta Burke Rehabilitation Hospital, Weill Cornell Medical College, White Plains, NY, USA

Department of Veterans Affairs, Manhattan Vet Center, Readjustment Counseling Service, Veterans Health Administration, Manhattan, NY, USA

Lauren L. Drag Neuropsychology Section, Department of Psychiatry, University of Michigan Healthcare System, Sunnyvale, CA, USA

Kevin Duff Department of Neurology, Center for Alzheimer's Care, Imaging and Research, University of Utah School of Medicine, Salt Lake City, UT, USA

Matthew R. Ebben Department of Neurology and Neuroscience, Center for Sleep Medicine, New York Presbyterian Hospital, Weill Cornell Medical College, New York, NY, USA

Joseph W. Fink Department of Psychiatry and Behavioral Neuroscience, University of Chicago, Chicago, IL, USA

Anna Rita Giovagnoli Department of Clinical Neurosciences, Neuropsychology Laboratory, Carlo Besta Neurological Institute, Milan, Italy

Chaya B. Gopin Department of Neurology, North Shore University Hospital, Manhasset, NY, USA

Department of Psychiatry, The Zucker Hillside Hospital, Glen Oaks, NY, USA

Jose Gutierrez Department of Neurology, Neurological Institute, Columbia University, New York, NY, USA

Robin C. Hilsabeck Psychology Service, South Texas Veterans Health Care System, San Antonio, TX, USA

Department of Psychiatry, University of Texas Health Science Center at San Antonio, San Antonio, TX, USA

Department of Psychiatry, University of California, San Diego, San Diego, CA, USA

Steven Hoover Department of Psychiatry, Mount Sinai School of Medicine, Elmwood Park, NJ, USA

Karin F. Hoth Division of Psychosocial Medicine, Department of Medicine, National Jewish Health, Denver, CO, USA

Departments of Psychiatry and Neurology, University of Colorado Denver, Aurora, CO, USA

Department of Medicine, National Jewish Health, Denver, CO, USA

Richard S. Isaacson Department of Neurology, University of Miami Miller School of Medicine, Miami, FL, USA

Angela Jefferson Vanderbilt Memory & Alzheimer's Center, Department of Neurology, Vanderbilt University Medical Center, Nashville, TN, USA

Heather L. Katzen Division of Neuropsychology, Department of Neurology, University of Miami Miller School of Medicine, Miami, FL, USA

Dimitris N. Kiosses Department of Psychiatry, Weill Cornell Institute of Geriatric Psychiatry, Weill Medical College of Cornell University, White Plains, New York, NY, USA

Elizabeth Kozora Department of Medicine, National Jewish Health, Denver, CO, USA

Departments of Psychiatry and Neurology, University of Colorado Medical School, Aurora, CO, USA

Joel H. Kramer Memory and Aging Center, University of California, San Francisco, CA, USA

Taylor Kuhn Department of Clinical and Health Psychology, University of Florida, Gainesville, FL, USA

Greg J. Lamberty Minneapolis VA Health Care System, Minneapolis, MN, USA

Amanda K. LaMarre Memory and Aging Center, University of California, San Francisco, CA, USA

Elizabeth Lane Department of Psychology, Division of Behavioral Neurosciences, University of Missouri, St. Louis, MO, USA

Bonnie Levin Division of Neuropsychology, Department of Neurology, University of Miami Miller School of Medicine, Miami, FL, USA

David Loewenstein Department of Psychiatry and Behavioral Sciences, Miller School of Medicine, University of Miami Miller School of Medicine, Miami, FL, USA

Kevin J. Manning Department of Psychology, Drexel University, Philadelphia, PA, USA

Bernice A. Marcopulos Department of Graduate Psychology, James Madison University, Harrisonburg, VA, USA

Paul J. Mattis Center for Neurosciences, The Feinstein Institute for Medical Research, Manhasset, NY, USA

Department of Neurology, North Shore University Hospital, Manhasset, NY, USA

Movement Disorders Center, Great Neck, NY, USA

Monica Rivera Mindt Department of Psychology, Fordham University, New York, NY, USA

Departments of Pathology and Psychiatry, The Mount Sinai School of Medicine, New York, NY, USA

Kathryn Lombardi Mirra Department of Neurology, North Shore University Hospital, Manhasset, NY, USA

Department of Psychiatry, The Zucker Hillside Hospital, Glen Oaks, NY, USA

Joel E. Morgan Department of Neurology and Neurosciences, UMDNJ—New Jersey Medical School, Madison, NJ, USA

Joy M. O'Grady Neuropsychological Services of Virginia Inc,, Richmond, VA, USA

Robert Paul Department of Psychology, Division of Behavioral Neurosciences, University of Missouri, St. Louis, MO, USA

Edward A. Peck III Neuropsychological Services of Virginia Inc,, Richmond, VA, USA

Donna Rasin-Waters VA New York Harbor Healthcare System, New York, NY, USA

Lisa D. Ravdin Department of Neurology & Neuroscience, Weill Cornell Neuropsychology Service, Weill Medical College of Cornell University, New York Presbyterian Hospital, New York, NY, USA

Lucien W. Roberts III Neuropsychological Services of Virginia Inc, Richmond, VA, USA

Lauren A. Rog Illinois Institute of Technology, Chicago, IL, USA

Arthur C. Russo Psychology Department, VA New York Harbor Healthcare System, Brooklyn, NY, USA

Fordham University, New York, NY, USA

Mary Sano Department of Psychiatry, Mount Sinai School of Medicine, New York, NY, USA

James J Peters Veterans Administration Medical Center, Bronx, NY, USA

David J. Schretlen Department of Psychiatry and Behavioral Sciences, Johns Hopkins University School of Medicine, Baltimore, MD, USA

Russell H. Morgan Department of Radiology and Radiological Science, Johns Hopkins University School of Medicine, Baltimore, MD, USA

Maria T. Schultheis Department of Psychology, Drexel University, Philadelphia, PA, USA

Department of Biomedical Engineering, Drexel University, Philadelphia, PA, USA

Yaakov Stern Cognitive Neuroscience Division of the Gertrude H. Sergievsky Center, Taub Institute for Research on Alzheimer's Disease and the Aging Brain, and Department of Neurology, Columbia University Medical Center, New York, NY, USA

Alexander I. Tröster Barrow Neurological Institute, Phoenix, USA

Tracy D. Vannorsdall Department of Psychiatry and Behavioral Sciences, Johns Hopkins University School of Medicine, Baltimore, MD, USA

Amy L. Webb Psychology Service, South Texas Veterans Health Care System, San Antonio, TX, USA

Hepatology Clinic, South Texas Veterans Health Care System, San Antonio, TX, USA

Department of Medicine, University of Texas Health Science Center at San Antonio, San Antonio, TX, USA

Jeffrey S. Wefel Section of Neuropsychology, Department of Neuro-Oncology, University of Texas M.D. Anderson Cancer Center, Houston, TX, USA

Mariana E. Witgert Section of Neuropsychology, Department of Neuro-Oncology, University of Texas M. D. Anderson Cancer Center, Houston, TX, USA

Part I

Assessment of Older Adults: Special Considerations

Special Considerations for the Neuropsychological Interview with Older Adults

1

Stephanie Assuras and Bonnie Levin

Abstract

The clinical interview is an essential part of a neuropsychological evaluation for any age, but particularly among older adults because of the myriad of physical, cognitive, psychological and social changes associated with the normative aging process. This essential data can be used to guide the testing process, assist in formulating a differential diagnosis, and informing recommendations. This chapter provides guidelines for developing an interview designed to provide a level of insight and understanding of a patient's presentation that cannot be obtained from psychometric testing, and is specific to the presenting concerns of older adults.

Keywords

Neuropsychological interview • Cognitive complaints • Somatic/sensory/motor symptoms • Emotional functioning • Activities of daily living • Functional capacity • Collateral information • Medical history • Social history

The neuropsychological interview presents a unique opportunity to gather essential data that can be used to guide the testing process and assist in formulating a differential diagnosis. A comprehensive interview not only provides important background information that cannot be obtained from psychometric testing but it also offers an opportunity for the examiner to gather critical behavioral observations that are often witnessed only in a less-structured setting. Although interviews vary in their focus and depth, they provide a framework from which examiners can assess demographic and referral information, data pertaining to presenting complaints and symptom progression, information regarding activities of daily living, pertinent environmental risk factors, and relevant background information regarding past medical, developmental, educational, and

S. Assuras, Ph.D. (✉)
Department of Psychiatry, Harvard Medical School, Massachusetts General Hospital, One Bowdoin Square, 7th Floor, Boston, MA 02114, USA

Department of Neurology, Brigham and Women's Hospital, Boston, MA, USA
e-mail: sassuras@partners.org

B. Levin, Ph.D.
Division of Neuropsychology, Department of Neurology, University of Miami Miller School of Medicine, 1120 NW 14th Street, Room 1337, Miami, FL 33136, USA
e-mail: blevin@med.miami.edu

L.D. Ravdin and H.L. Katzen (eds.), *Handbook on the Neuropsychology of Aging and Dementia*, Clinical Handbooks in Neuropsychology, DOI 10.1007/978-1-4614-3106-0_1,

psychosocial history. The interview also offers the opportunity to assess the caregiver's perspective of the patient's cognitive status, additional stressors, and available resources that can be used to guide the treatment recommendations.

Demographic and Referral Information

The first questions posed by the examiner will set the tone for the rest of the interview. Asking a patient to provide demographic information can be a good way to begin establishing rapport. In addition to essential information such as one's name, date of birth, handedness, gender, educational level, and living arrangement, patients should also explain in their own words, whenever possible, who referred them for testing and the reason for the referral. This is really the first opportunity that the examiner will have to assess the level of insight and ability to formulate one's thoughts. Other important questions that should be addressed before testing begins are medication regimen, their primary language and, when applicable, secondary language, and whether the patient requires glasses, hearing assistive devices, and/or ambulatory assistance.

Physical, Cognitive, and Emotional Complaints

One goal of the interview is to document the specifics of the complaints and the time course of symptoms to determine the severity level and to assess whether there has been a change from a premorbid condition. There are several different approaches used to evaluate current physical, cognitive, and emotional complaints. These include (1) having the patient or caregiver fill out a structured questionnaire, (2) asking the patient to elaborate on each of his or her concerns and the examiner records the complaints verbatim, or (3) start the interview using a structured format where the examiner systematically reviews a predetermined list of possible symptoms. The best approach usually involves a combination of these interviewing techniques such as having patients verbally describe their chief concerns and then following up with a more structured series of questions or having the examiner administer a formal questionnaire before testing begins and then reviewing each item with the patient and caregiver during the interview.

Physical Symptoms

The most common noncognitive neurologic complaints reported by older adults are headache, dizziness, numbness/tingling, visual changes, and problems with balance. Generally speaking, physical complaints can be grouped into motor, sensory, and somatic functions. Important areas to address with regard to motor changes include weakness, gait and balance difficulties (such as shuffling and smaller steps), motor slowing, the presence of tremor, stiffness, numbness, difficulty pronouncing words clearly, and difficulty with eye movements (e.g., upward gaze). Some motor symptoms such as tremor and motor slowing may be obvious, but others such as weakness or stiffness are more subtle and would be missed unless the patient is directly questioned. It is also important to follow up individual questions with further inquiry. For example, when the patient confirms that he or she has balance difficulties, it is important to ask about a history of falls. Keeping in mind that falls are the most common reason for hospitalization among older adults [1], this line of questioning will not only provide information with regard to a past history of possible traumatic injury or the presence of a movement disorder but it will also alert the clinician to possible safety concerns.

Sensory complaints are subjective and require that patients be able to express their concerns. Typical sensory complaints include pain, visual and auditory changes, appetite change (e.g., increased consumption of sweets), changes in smell and odor detection, dizziness, and heart palpitations. Somatic complaints, which can be difficult to disentangle from sensory symptoms, are frequent and include an array of gastrointestinal problems (bowel and bladder), constipation, headaches and arthritic pain, and sleep disturbances.

Table 1.1 Examples of question topics for interviewing older adults

Cognitive symptoms	Physical symptoms	Emotional symptoms
Difficulty remembering conversations	Difficulty pronouncing words clearly	Lack of interest in activities
Unsure of previous day's activities	Visual or auditory changes	Reduced initiation
Repeating questions	Difficulty with eye movements (e.g., upward gaze)	Apathy
Forgetting why you walked into a room or what you need at the store	Changes in smell and odor detection	Irritability
Difficulty coming up with the right word or remembering people's names	Gait changes (e.g., shuffling, smaller steps, slowing)	Restlessness
Poor attention/concentration when reading or watching television	Reduced balance, increased falls	Depressed mood
Slower thinking and problem solving	Urinary changes (frequency, urgency, incontinence)	Hallucinations (describe content, quality, e.g., if they elicit fear)
Difficulty planning and organizing tasks	Constipation	Inappropriate behavior (e.g., approaching strangers, making inappropriate comments)
Inability to complete multiple steps	Dizziness/heart palpitations	Increased nervousness or worry
Difficulty performing routine tasks, such as making coffee	Numbness, weakness, or tremor	Fatigue or reduced energy
	Appetite changes, increase or decrease (e.g., increased consumption of sweets) Sleep changes	Past or present suicidal ideation

Since sensory complaints have been linked to depression [2], this area should be carefully addressed with older adult patients. Sleep quality plays an important role in alertness, attention, and overall cognitive functioning, and is often a contributing factor to cognitive decline [3]. Given the high prevalence of sleep disorders in this age group, clinicians should be aware of common complaints such as difficulty falling or staying asleep, sleep-disordered breathing, frequent awakening, snoring, awakening to a choking sensation, use of sleep aids, feelings of daytime fatigue and napping. If a family member reports unusual behaviors during sleep such as dream enactment (shouting out loud, punching a bed partner, or other forms of acting out a dream), they should be noted and explored in greater detail for possible REM sleep behavior disorder, a condition associated with parkinsonism. Questions regarding urinary function are important and should extend beyond asking about frank incontinence to include inquiries regarding urinary urgency and frequency, since these may be early features of normal pressure hydrocephalus (NPH) [4]. Additionally, somatic symptoms related to autonomic function, such as impotence and dizziness or hypotension, may be relevant when a movement disorder such as multiple system atrophy or other Parkinson's plus disorder is on the list of differentials (see Table 1.1 for examples to guide questioning of various symptoms) [5].

Cognitive Symptoms

The most common cognitive complaint among older adults is memory [6]. It has been estimated that subjective memory complaints are as high as 56% in community-based samples [7]. Typical memory complaints are difficulty recalling names, faces, and appointments, problems recalling numbers such as phone numbers, repeating questions, word-finding difficulties, misplacing personal items, disorientation while traveling, and losing one's train of thought [8].

It is not uncommon for a patient to report memory difficulties when, in fact, the problem actually stems from a different etiology, but one that impacts memory. For example, upon closer questioning, the clinician may find that the problem is actually difficulty finding words or attending to task demands and may signify deficits in aspects of cognition other than memory, language, or attention. Another common cognitive complaint is executive dysfunction [9], the category of skills involved in sustaining attention, goal setting, problem solving, planning, organization, and decision making. The executive functions have been shown to be a major determinant of one's ability to perform instrumental activities of daily living such as financial decision making and medication management, and they also predict onset and progression of instrumental functional decline [10]. Since patients with executive dysfunction are frequently not aware of their difficulties, examiners should ask directed questions during the interview that relate to specific executive abilities. Topics from which to draw interview questions are listed in Table 1.1.

Emotional Symptoms

Careful questioning regarding mood and personality change is an important part of the interview. First, depression and anxiety complaints, especially at the subsyndromal level, are common among older adults [11]. A recent survey published by the Centers for Disease Control indicated that 16% of suicide deaths were among those 65 years of age and older, higher than the rate of 11 per 100,000 in the general population [12]. Depression in older adults often goes untreated as the symptoms, which may present as somatic or cognitive complaints (e.g., memory problems, confusion, social withdrawal, loss of appetite, weight loss, and irritability), are not recognized as such. Furthermore, symptoms of depression are often mistaken as signs of dementia (see Chap. 8). It is essential that the interviewer take the time to question an individual about past and present suicidal ideation and attempts to self-harm. Any mention of suicidal thoughts or behavior should be carefully followed up with questions aimed at undercovering the seriousness of intent and the necessity for intervention.

Personality changes are often the first symptom of a degenerative disease. In older adults, behavioral symptoms are the presenting feature in frontotemporal lobar degeneration, behavioral variant, various cortical dementias including Alzheimer's disease, early stages of Parkinson's and Parkinson's plus syndromes such as progressive supranuclear palsy, Wilson's disease, Huntington's disease, and myasthenia gravis [13–17]. Symptoms may include inappropriate laughing or crying, apathy, and social withdrawal. Although observed more frequently in younger adults, the effect of autoimmune illnesses such as systemic lupus erythematosus and multiple sclerosis can present with psychiatric symptoms, including psychosis [18, 19]. Furthermore, patients with endocrine and metabolic disorders, such as hypoparathyroidism and hypercortisolism, can present with both cognitive decline and psychosis, as well as personality changes [20]. Third, a careful intake of mood and personality change is especially important in formulating recommendations, which may include pharmacologic treatment, behavioral intervention, or psychotherapy.

Functional Capacity

An individual's ability to perform basic and complex activities of daily living (ADL) is a measure of one's functional status. This is an especially important area to address in the older adult because impairment in social and/or occupational function is a key component to a diagnosis of dementia. A patient's functional capacity should be comprehensively examined, focusing on basic and instrumental ADLs. Basic ADLs include questions pertaining to independence in bathing, dressing, and feeding, whereas instrumental ADLs involve higher-order abilities such as one's ability to pay bills, shop for food and prepare a meal, manage finances, and manage a medication schedule. In some cases, it is hard to tell whether an individual who lives in a supportive

Table 1.2 Assessing functional independence/activities of daily living (ADL)

Basic ADLs
Personal hygiene
Toileting (the ability to use a restroom)
Dressing
Feeding oneself
Instrumental ADLs
Managing finances/paying bills
Looking up phone numbers
Doing housework
Using computer
Shopping
Cooking
Making appointments
Driving/traveling
Medication management

environment (a spouse pays the bills, the staff in the assisted-living facility prepares the meals and makes sure patients take their medication) has actually changed or whether the patient has retained the skill but relies on others as a matter of convenience. In this case, it is important to inquire about specific operational skills such as whether the patient is capable of carrying out emergency procedures if left alone, following a recipe if necessary, balancing a check book to pay bills, using email, etc. (see Table 1.2).

Taking a History

Medical History

Documenting a patient's medical history is necessary in order to formulate a differential diagnosis and to make treatment recommendations. A patient's ability to convey this information can be as informative as the history itself. Commonly reported cardiometabolic risk factors known to impact cognition include hypertension, hypercholesterolemia, type 2 diabetes, and heart disease and vascular conditions associated with ischemia or kidney disease. Clinicians should address past illnesses, surgeries, injuries, and treatments, including metastatic cancer, cardiovascular diseases (e.g., heart disease, stroke), surgeries, especially those involving general anesthesia, alcohol and substance use, prior head trauma, with particular attention to those involving concussion and/or loss of consciousness, periods of confusion, infectious disease (Hepatitis C, HIV), and unusual dietary or sleep patterns. How the patient manages these conditions (e.g., checking blood sugar, compliance with blood pressure medication, dietary practices, exercise regimen, etc.) will provide valuable information with regard to an individual's ability to participate in self-care and manage oneself independently. In addition, specific questions should address patient's medication, prescribed and over-the-counter. Past medication and prior hospitalizations should also be addressed with the patient and/or caregiver. Finally, the patient's family medical history should be carefully assessed in order to understand relevant genetic risk factors. This is likely to become an increasingly important area to address given that family health history reflects inherited genetic susceptibility for a large number of neurologic diseases.

Social History

A comprehensive interview should include a careful assessment of one's past social experiences, educational attainment, and occupation. There are many ways to assess this information, but most of the time, it is best to probe beyond a simple question. For example, questions pertaining to level of education should always be followed up with inquiries pertaining to past history of learning difficulties, school failure, and other issues relating to academic performance, as well as occupational achievement. This can be a challenging area to assess with older adults because societal mores and educational opportunities were different decades ago. Yet, establishing if the patient has a longstanding and developmental vulnerability in cognitive function is critical to understanding if a current level of impairment represents a decline.

Conclusion

The interview is an essential part of a neuropsychological evaluation for any age, but particularly among older adults, because of the myriad of physical, cognitive, psychological, and social changes associated with the normative aging process. These normative changes are further compounded by the onset of a disease. A carefully conducted interview will play a critical role in establishing a diagnosis and generating treatment recommendations. In addition, it provides an opportunity to observe and document information that cannot be obtained from psychometric testing. The interview also creates a forum for establishing rapport with the patient and allows the clinician to verify important demographic and historical information from a caregiver. This chapter has provided guidelines for developing an interview designed to provide a level of insight and understanding of a patient's presentation, which cannot be obtained through other means.

Clinical Pearls

- The clinical interview provides a level of insight and understanding of a patient's presentation, which cannot be obtained through other means.
- A patient's ability to convey his/her history during the interview session can be as informative as the history itself. Observations regarding a patient's expressive and receptive language, level of insight, and ability to formulate thoughts are as valuable as the test data and scores.
- Use of a combination of interviewing techniques, such as verbal description of complaints, a structured series of questions, and a formal review of each item with the patient and caregiver, is ideal. Using a questionnaire to gather background information can be useful, but this information should always be reviewed with the patient and follow-up questions should be asked. Patients typically elaborate and provide much more detailed information when questions are asked verbally.
- Do not rely solely on behavioral observations without further probing. For example, motor symptoms such as tremor or paralysis are visible, but other motor abnormalities such as weakness or stiffness are more subtle and would be missed unless the patient is directly questioned.
- Not all complaints should be taken at face value. It is important to ask the patient to give examples of the type of cognitive problems they are experiencing. While memory complaints are the most common, the deficits may actually be in language (e.g., difficulty finding words) or attention (e.g., attending to task demands).
- Personality changes are often the first symptom of a degenerative disease. Therefore, careful assessment of emotional and behavioral changes is critical. Since patients frequently lack insight into their own behavior, a collateral source should be consulted.
- It can be challenging to determine whether an individual who lives in a supportive environment has experienced a decline in functional independence. Every interview should inquire about specific functional abilities and give examples of instrumental activities of daily living. Knowledge of safety procedures should also be routinely assessed.

References

1. Milat AJ, et al. Prevalence, circumstances and consequences of falls among community-dwelling older people: results of the 2009 NSW Falls Prevention Baseline Survey. N S W Public Health Bull. 2011;22(3–4):43–8.
2. Chakraborty K, et al. Psychological and clinical correlates of functional somatic complaints in depression. Int J Soc Psychiatry. 2012;58(1):87–95.
3. Kronholm E, et al. Self-reported sleep duration and cognitive functioning in the general population. J Sleep Res. 2009;18(4):436–46.
4. Tsakanikas D, Relkin N. Normal pressure hydrocephalus. Semin Neurol. 2007;27(1):58–65.
5. Gilman S, et al. Consensus statement on the diagnosis of multiple system atrophy. J Neurol Sci. 1999;163(1):94–8.
6. Minett TS, et al. Subjective memory complaints in an elderly sample: a cross-sectional study. Int J Geriatr Psychiatry. 2008;23(1):49–54.
7. Reid LM, Maclullich AM. Subjective memory complaints and cognitive impairment in older people. Dement Geriatr Cogn Disord. 2006;22(5–6):471–85.

8. Ahmed S, et al. Memory complaints in mild cognitive impairment, worried well, and semantic dementia patients. Alzheimer Dis Assoc Disord. 2008;22(3):227–35.
9. Hirschman KB, et al. Cognitive impairment among older adults in the emergency department. West J Emerg Med. 2011;12(1):56–62.
10. Carlson MC, et al. Association between executive attention and physical functional performance in community-dwelling older women. J Gerontol B Psychol Sci Soc Sci. 1999;54(5):S262–70.
11. Wilkins CH, Mathews J, Sheline YI. Late life depression with cognitive impairment: evaluation and treatment. Clin Interv Aging. 2009;4:51–7.
12. Centers for Disease Control and Prevention, N.C.f.I.P.a.C. Web-based injury statistics query and reporting system. 2005.
13. Akil M, Brewer GJ. Psychiatric and behavioral abnormalities in Wilson's disease. Adv Neurol. 1995;65:171–8.
14. Cummings JL. Behavioral and psychiatric symptoms associated with Huntington's disease. Adv Neurol. 1995;65:179–86.
15. Aarsland D, Litvan I, Larsen JP. Neuropsychiatric symptoms of patients with progressive supranuclear palsy and Parkinson's disease. J Neuropsychiatry Clin Neurosci. 2001;13(1):42–9.
16. Marchello V, Boczko F, Shelkey M. Progressive dementia: strategies to manage new problem behaviors. Geriatrics. 1995;50(3):40–3. quiz 44–5.
17. Musha M, Tanaka F, Ohuti M. Psychoses in three cases with myasthenia gravis and thymoma—proposal of a paraneoplastic autoimmune neuropsychiatric syndrome. Tohoku J Exp Med. 1993;169(4):335–44.
18. Aggarwal A, et al. Acute psychosis as the initial presentation of MS: a case report. Int MS J. 2011;17(2):54–7.
19. Wright MT. Neuropsychiatric illness in systemic lupus erythematosus: insights from a patient with erotomania and Geschwind's syndrome. Am J Psychiatry. 2010;167(5):502–7.
20. Ghosh A. Endocrine, metabolic, nutritional, and toxic disorders leading to dementia. Ann Indian Acad Neurol. 2010;13 Suppl 2:S63–8.

Consideration of Cognitive Reserve

2

Stephanie Cosentino and Yaakov Stern

Abstract

This chapter reviews the concept of cognitive reserve, including relevant theoretical issues, various means of characterizing this construct, and its clinical implications. We begin with a broad overview of the epidemiological evidence in support of the concept of cognitive reserve, and review neuroimaging studies that contribute to our understanding of this construct. We then review several theoretical issues surrounding the mechanisms by which cognitive reserve confers its benefits, and outline the advantages and disadvantages of various methods of estimating reserve. We conclude by discussing the clinical implications of cognitive reserve and listing several specific recommendations for the application of cognitive reserve in clinical practice.

Keywords

Cognitive reserve • Dementia • Cognition • Aging • Assessment • Diagnosis

Introduction to Cognitive Reserve

The idea of reserve against brain damage stems from the repeated observation that there is not a direct relationship between degree of brain pathology or damage and the clinical manifestation of that damage. For example, Katzman and colleagues described ten cases of cognitively normal elderly women who were discovered to have advanced Alzheimer's disease (AD) pathology in their brains at death [1]. In more recent cohort studies, it has been estimated that approximately 25% of individuals who have postmortem neuropathological evidence of AD are not demented during their lives [2]. This discrepancy raises the question of how brain function and structure become decoupled and whether certain person-specific variables provide reserve against the clinical effects of pathological brain

S. Cosentino, Ph.D. (✉) • Y. Stern, Ph.D.
Cognitive Neuroscience Division of the Gertrude H. Sergievsky Center, Taub Institute for Research on Alzheimer's Disease and the Aging Brain, and Department of Neurology, Columbia University Medical Center, New York, NY, USA
e-mail: sc2460@columbia.edu; ys11@columbia.edu

L.D. Ravdin and H.L. Katzen (eds.), *Handbook on the Neuropsychology of Aging and Dementia*, Clinical Handbooks in Neuropsychology, DOI 10.1007/978-1-4614-3106-0_2,

changes. Several theoretical models have been put forth to address this issue.

The cognitive reserve (CR) model suggests that the brain actively attempts to cope with brain damage by using preexisting cognitive processing approaches or by enlisting compensatory approaches [3, 4]. Individuals with high CR would be more successful at coping with the same amount of brain damage than those with low CR. In this scenario, brain function rather than brain size is the relevant variable. This characteristic distinguishes the CR model from the brain reserve model in which reserve derives from brain size or neuronal count [5]. According to the CR model, the same amount of brain damage or pathology will have different effects on different people, even when brain size is held constant.

Epidemiological studies have helped to shape our understanding of the nature of cognitive reserve and the person-specific variables which appear to enhance reserve. Many studies have demonstrated the beneficial effects of education [6], occupation [7], leisure [8, 9], and intellectual ability [10] on dementia incidence. In 1994, Stern and colleagues reported incident dementia data from a follow-up study of 593 community-based, non-demented individuals aged 60 years or older [7]. After 1–4 years of follow-up, 106 became demented with all but five meeting research criteria for AD. The risk of dementia was increased in subjects with low education, such that the relative risk (RR) of developing dementia over the follow-up period was 2.2 times higher in individuals with less than 8 years of education as compared to those with more years of education. Similarly, risk of incident dementia was increased in those with low lifetime occupational attainment (RR=2.25) and greatest for subjects with both low education and low lifetime occupational attainment (RR=2.87).

To the extent that aspects of educational and occupational attainment reflect lifetime exposures that would increase CR, it would be logical to expect that environmental exposures later in life would also be beneficial. In a subsequent study, the same group assessed participation in a variety of leisure activities characterized as intellectual (e.g., reading, playing games, going to classes) or social (e.g., visiting with friends or relatives) in a population sample of non-demented elderly in New York [9]. During follow-up, subjects who engaged in more of these activities had 38% less risk of developing dementia. Interestingly, specific classifications of leisure activity (such as purely intellectual activities) did not provide better prediction then a simple summation of all the considered activities.

A meta-analysis examining cohort studies of the effects of education, occupation, premorbid IQ, and mental activities on dementia risk over approximately 7 years revealed that 25 of 33 datasets demonstrated a significant protective effect of these variables [11]. The summary overall risk of incident dementia for individuals with high levels of the protective variable as compared to low was 0.54, a decreased risk of 46%. There is also evidence for the role of education in age-related cognitive decline, with many studies of normal aging reporting slower cognitive and functional decline in individuals with higher educational attainment [12–19]. These studies suggest that the same factors that delay the onset of dementia also allow individuals to cope more effectively with brain changes encountered in normal aging. The concept of CR provides a ready explanation for the manner in which intellectual functioning, education, and other life experiences may allow individuals to sustain greater burdens of brain pathology or age-related changes before demonstrating cognitive and functional deficits.

Neuroimaging studies have also provided evidence in support of cognitive reserve and have contributed to our conceptualization of this phenomenon. Our original functional imaging study found that in patients matched for overall severity of dementia (i.e., clinical expression of disease), the parietotemporal cerebral flow deficit was greater in those with more years of education [20]. This observation was confirmed in a later PET study in which higher education correlated negatively with cerebral metabolism in prefrontal, premotor, and left superior parietal association areas after controlling for clinical dementia severity [21]. Similar observations have been made for occupational attainment [22] and leisure activities [23] and across multiple markers of pathology including white matter abnormalities [24] and amyloid deposition [25]. The negative

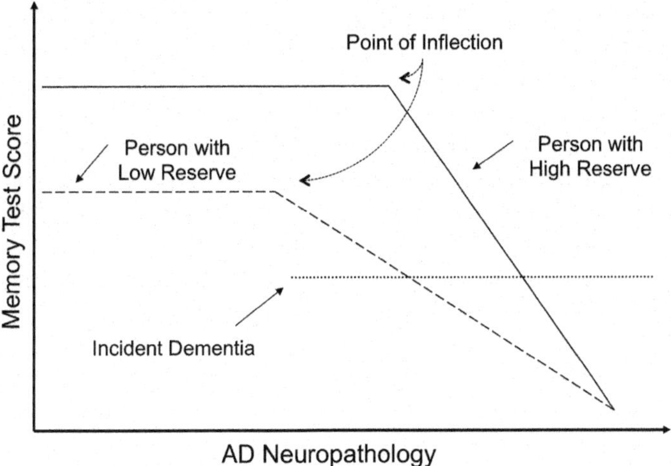

Fig. 2.1 Effect of cognitive reserve on dementia onset and course

Note: Figure 2.1 illustrates the way in which cognitive reserve may mediate the relationship between AD pathology and its clinical expression. We assume that AD pathology slowly increases over time, and this is graphed on the x-axis. The y-axis represents cognitive function, in this case memory performance. AD pathology begins to develop many years before the disease is expressed clinically and slowly becomes more severe. At some point, this developing pathology will begin to produce the initial cognitive changes associated with dementia. This is labeled as the point of inflection in the figure. The pathology will subsequently result in symptoms of sufficient severity to allow the clinical diagnosis of AD (indicated by the dotted line labeled Incident Dementia). The cognitive reserve (CR) model predicts that because there are individual differences in reserve capacity, there will be individual differences in the amount of pathology required for the initial expression of clinical symptoms and the subsequent diagnosis of disease. Because people with higher cognitive reserve can tolerate more AD pathology, memory function will begin to be affected later in time, after more pathology has accumulated, pushing back the "point of inflection." Therefore, all other things being equal, dementia should emerge later in people with higher cognitive reserve. This leads to the prediction that the rate of incident dementia should be lower in individuals with higher cognitive reserve. An assumption of this model is that at some point, AD pathology must become too severe to support the processes that mediate either cognitive reserve or memory function. The timing of this final common endpoint will be the same in all patients, regardless of their level of cognitive reserve. It then follows that the time between the point of inflection and this common endpoint will be shorter in patients with higher cognitive reserve. This leads to the prediction that memory decline after the inflection point must be more rapid in patients with higher cognitive reserve. Although this trajectory might appear counterintuitive at first, its theoretical basis is illustrated in this figure, and it has been supported by multiple epidemiological studies

correlations between the exposures of interest and pathology are consistent with the CR hypothesis' prediction that at any given level of clinical disease severity, those with higher CR should have greater pathology (see Fig. 2.1).

Results and interpretations of these studies have been further supported by prospective projects with subsequent neuropathological analysis. Specifically, education has been found to modify the association between AD pathology and levels of cognitive function. With brain pathology held constant, higher education was associated with better cognitive function [26] and less likelihood of having received a clinical diagnosis of dementia in life [27]. These studies converge nicely with epidemiological evidence that supports that higher levels of education, occupational attainment, and leisure activity reduce dementia incidence, and suggest that these variables influence dementia risk by enhancing cognitive reserve.

Theoretical Issues

Despite the wealth of information that has accumulated in support of the concept of cognitive reserve, there are many aspects of this construct that have yet to be fully elaborated. It is important to highlight these issues prior to discussing the various means of characterizing reserve and considering the clinical implications of cognitive reserve. The intent of the current chapter is not to fully explore these theoretical issues but simply to raise the reader's awareness of the unanswered questions surrounding the construct of cognitive reserve.

First, the precise manner in which cognitive reserve affords protection from pathology is not understood. As discussed above, we know that across individuals, there is a discrepancy between brain changes or pathology and cognitive change such that in some individuals, cognitive function remains relatively preserved in the face of pathological markers. As such, individuals with high cognitive reserve are not necessarily protected from developing pathology, but rather that they are spared the clinical effects of such pathology. Thus, when we refer to the preservation of a cognitive function such as memory in the sections below, we are in fact talking only about memory itself and not the integrity of the brain areas underlying that cognitive function (e.g., hippocampus). Indeed, the concept of cognitive reserve only applies when considering variability in cognitive functioning (i.e., memory) in the face of changes in brain integrity (i.e., hippocampal volume).

This raises one of the puzzling questions surrounding reserve: memory and hippocampal integrity are intimately related and the mechanisms underlying the decoupling of structure and function are not clear. From a strict point of view, the differences in cognitive processing envisioned by the CR model must also have a physiologic basis, in that the brain must ultimately mediate all cognitive function. The difference is in terms of the level of analysis. Presumably, the physiologic variability subsumed by cognitive reserve is at the level of variability in synaptic organization or in relative utilization of specific brain regions. Thus, cognitive reserve implies anatomic variability at the level of brain networks, while brain reserve implies differences in the quantity of available neural substrate.

Moreover, we must acknowledge the possibility that life exposures that are associated with reserve also affect brain structure or brain pathology and not simply cognitive properties. Evidence for this possibility comes from two recent studies, one of which found reduced rate of hippocampal atrophy over 3 years in individuals with higher levels of complex mental activity across the lifespan [28], and the second which found microstructural differences in the hippocampus as a function of education [29]. Additionally, the child developmental literature suggests that not only do individuals with higher IQ have larger brain volume [30, 31] but that cognitively stimulating aspects of life experience may also be associated with increased brain volume. It is also now clear that stimulating environments and exercise promote neurogenesis in the dentate gyrus [32, 33]. Both exercise and cognitive stimulation regulate factors that increase neuronal plasticity (such as brain derived neurotrophic factor) and resistance to cell death. Finally, there is some evidence to suggest that environmental enrichment might act directly to prevent or slow the accumulation of AD pathology [34].

In sum, there appears to be growing evidence that the experiences that provide cognitive reserve may indeed reflect not only a cognitive advantage but a structural advantage as well. Thus, brain reserve and cognitive reserve concepts are not mutually exclusive, and it is likely that both are involved in providing reserve against brain damage. A complete model of cognitive reserve will have to integrate the complex interactions between genetics, the environmental influences on brain reserve and pathology, and the ability to actively compensate for the effects of pathology.

Setting aside the question of brain integrity, and considering cognitive reserve only, we return to the question of why insult to brain structure does not invariably affect cognition. We have observed that individuals with higher cognitive reserve (defined using a literacy measure) have less rapid memory decline over time than those with lower literacy levels [35]. However, the manner in which this memory advantage is conferred is unknown. It may be that preserved memory reflects preservation of the memory networks per se or use of alternative and supportive skills such as enhanced organizational strategies [36]. Stern and colleagues have described these two potential neural implementations of cognitive reserve as *neural reserve* and *neural compensation* [4, 37, 38]. The idea behind *neural reserve* is that there is natural interindividual variability in the brain networks or cognitive processes that underlie the performance of any task. This variability could be in the form of differing efficiency or capacity of these networks, or in greater flexibility in the networks that can be invoked to perform a task. While healthy individuals may invoke these networks when coping with increased task demands, the networks could also help an individual cope with brain pathology. An individual whose networks are more efficient, have greater capacity, or are more flexible might be more capable of coping with the challenges imposed by brain pathology. In contrast, *neural compensation* refers to the process by which individuals suffering from brain pathology use brain structures or networks (and thus cognitive strategies) not normally used by individuals with intact brains in order to compensate for brain damage. The term compensation is reserved for a situation where it can be demonstrated that the more impaired group is using a different network than the unimpaired group.

It is not yet clear whether or when each of these forms of reserve come into play. The answer to this question has several implications, one of which pertains to the applicability of cognitive reserve under various conditions. Specifically, if the benefits of cognitive reserve are attributable to the flexible application of alternative strategies for completing a task (compensation), specific aspects of brain function may receive less assistance from cognitive reserve than others. It may be that a cognitive skill such as verbal recall can be accomplished in a number of ways that differentially employ serial rehearsal, semantic processing, or working memory. In contrast, there may be fewer cognitive routes to reproduce a complex figure or detect a subtle visual detail amid a complex scene. In this scenario, a compensatory reserve mechanism might be less applicable to spatial skills than to verbal memory. However, it is also possible that critical issue is not task specific, but rather, person specific. That is, based on life experience, one person may have multiple ways of approaching a spatial task but less flexibility for a verbal task, whereas the opposite pattern may exist in another individual. If the crux of cognitive reserve is the ability to apply alternative approaches to accomplish tasks, then the benefit of reserve may be linked directly to the flexibility of the task (and corresponding skill) itself or to a person's premorbid cognitive style.

One final question is whether or not deterioration of specific cognitive functions can directly affect cognitive reserve. For example, if cognitive reserve is closely aligned or even overlaps with executive abilities [39], is it the case that cognitive reserve is less able (or unable) to stave off executive deficits as opposed to declines in other domains such as memory or language? That is, is cognitive reserve itself vulnerable to a particular presentation of disease? Or, is cognitive reserve a construct that is "immune" to the regional distribution of pathology, independent of the cognitive abilities that may be affected, functioning universally under a wide variety of lesions? While the answer to this question is not entirely clear, recent studies examining the effects of reserve on information processing efficiency in individuals with multiple sclerosis may shed light on the issue [40–43]. For example, Sumowksi and colleagues showed that the negative effect of brain atrophy on rapid information processing was attenuated in individuals with higher levels of reserve [41], suggesting that reserve confers benefits to cognitive functions whose nature is quite similar to some conceptualizations of reserve. That is, the information processing measure was comprised of the Symbol Digit Modalities Test [44] and the Paced Auditory Serial Addition Test [45], tasks which require mental flexibility and fluidity. Similarly, although speculative, one perspective of cognitive reserve is that it represents the mental flexibility to develop alternative strategies in the face of pathology, and to fluidly apply such strategies to the task at hand. The reported benefits of reserve on information processing and efficiency in the above studies are interesting and raise many questions for future work. For the time being, such studies may offer preliminary evidence either that (1) reserve is immune to the distribution of pathology or (2) reserve is fundamentally different than the cognitive skills assessed in these studies.

Estimating Cognitive Reserve

A practical question for the clinician is how to account for cognitive reserve in the diagnostic process. In this section, we review the advantages and disadvantages of several approaches including the following: (1) measurement of individual characteristics (demographic and lifestyle), (2) consideration of cumulative life experiences, (3) estimation of intellectual functioning, (4) implementation of statistical approaches (use of latent or residual variables), and (5) derivation of brain network patterns. Prior to discussing these approaches, it is also important to consider that although epidemiological work has led to the conceptualization of reserve as a reflection of important lifetime experiences, the cognitive advantage which manifests as reserve might also have played an important role early in life to afford individuals the desire and ability to pursue certain life experiences such as graduate school, for example. Thus, the effects of lifetime experiences are not necessarily separate from early life factors. Although certain work has suggested that reserve is a cumulative process built on both early life and late life experiences [46], the causal pathway of cognitive reserve has not been fully delineated. As the reader considers the clinical implications of cognitive reserve and the various methods for measuring reserve, it is important to be aware of the larger questions surrounding its origins and characteristics.

Individual Characteristics

One of the most commonly used methods of characterizing reserve involves quantifying individual characteristics that have been associated with reduced risk of dementia including education, occupation, intellectual functioning, leisure activity, and social engagement. The advantage of this approach is that these variables are relatively easy to acquire and quantify, and at face value, are generally plausible proxies for reserve. A disadvantage is that these variables may be singular representations of a multidimensional mechanism such that characterization of education in isolation, for example, might account for a relatively small proportion of the variance in overall cognitive reserve. Moreover, these variables are rather agnostic with regard to the source and nature of cognitive reserve and may confound multiple other factors with "true" reserve (e.g., education may impart greater knowledge and access to health care which in turn may promote health-related behaviors and enhance cognitive functioning). As such, use of variables such as those listed above, although convenient, should not be the sole indicators of CR.

Cumulative Life Experiences

A second approach for characterizing cognitive reserve is one in which multiple or cumulative life experiences are synthesized to develop a more comprehensive estimation of an individual's reserve. The purported benefit of this approach is that it synthesizes numerous experiences, all of which have been shown through epidemiological work to confer protection against the development of dementia. The consideration of comprehensive life experiences offers the opportunity to capture a wide array of factors that may uniquely contribute to reserve, if indeed reserve is created through a cumulative process. Valenzuela and Sachdev [47] developed the Lifetime of Experiences Questionnaire (LEQ) as a means of capturing and quantifying various social, academic, occupational, and leisure activities spanning young to late adulthood. The questionnaire showed good reliability and validity and was useful in predicting which individuals would demonstrate cognitive decline over an 18-month period.

While this appears to be a powerful method of capturing a myriad of experiences relevant to the construct of cognitive reserve, there are several issues to consider. It is possible that the summation of experiences within this questionnaire may not be more predictive than any individual variable, and compiling these experiences may even obscure the effect of the most relevant variable. For example, Hall and colleagues found that the effect of education on cognitive decline prior to dementia diagnosis was negligible after accounting for cognitively stimulating leisure activities later in life [48], suggesting one of two possible scenarios raised by the authors. First, it could be that the effects of education were mediated by mental activities late in life or second, that education influenced reserve directly with no additional benefit conferred by later life mental stimulation. Researchers must carefully consider these issues; however, a lifetime approach to characterizing reserve for clinical purposes is certainly useful in that it comprehensively quantifies important experiences that may delay cognitive decline in the face of advancing pathology.

Intellectual Function

A third and very different means of characterizing reserve is the assessment of intellectual functioning, typically via a single-word reading test, such as the Wechsler Test of Adult Reading [49] or the North American Adult Reading Test [50], or a subtest of the Wechsler Adult Intelligence Scales such as Vocabulary or Information [51]. Word reading measures evaluate an individual's ability to pronounce a series of phonologically regular and irregular words ranging in difficulty, and are based on the idea that correct pronunciation of the more difficult items requires previous exposure to such words. Like vocabulary and fund of information, this ability is generally spared early in the course of dementia, reflecting its reliance on long-term, crystallized knowledge versus the more fluid abilities affected early in disease [52–56].

The characterization of IQ is believed to offer a thumbnail sketch of an individual's lifetime intellectual achievement, highly related to, though not necessarily synonymous with, the concept of cognitive reserve. An advantage of using IQ to characterize cognitive reserve is that in contrast to an external exposure variable such as education or occupation, an internal and broadly stable capability such as IQ is presumably more closely associated with the cognitive and neural representation of reserve. Unfortunately, a corresponding disadvantage is that IQ scores do change in the course of disease and therefore can be contaminated by the disease process itself (unlike education or occupation). Moreover, while reading scores are fairly stable in the very early stages of degenerative illnesses, they are certainly not valid estimates of premorbid IQ in a language predominant illness, nor are they valid estimates in non-native English speakers.

Despite the differences in applying IQ versus an exposure variable such as education, there is statistical evidence that both share common statistical variance that is distinct from cognitive functions more broadly [39]. The presence of both convergent and discriminant validity in this context provides support for both of these variables as independent proxies for reserve, as well as evidence for the construct validity of reserve. This is an important finding because the coherence of cognitive reserve as a construct remains under question, leading several groups to argue that latent variables derived through structural equation modeling may be the most appropriate way to capture the essence of reserve [57, 58]. Although the details of these models are beyond the scope of this chapter, the idea is that through statistical data reduction, we can boil down the overgeneralized concept of reserve into its core elements and identify those variables that are central to its construct versus those that may be extraneous. A necessary drawback, however, is that representation of cognitive reserve through shared variance may not reflect aspects of reserve potentially captured selectively by each unique variable.

Statistical Approaches

A statistical approach to identifying reserve has recently been proposed by Reed and colleagues [59] by decomposing the variance of a specific cognitive skill such as episodic memory. Specifically, the authors partitioned the variance explained by demographic variables (education, sex, and ethnicity), structural brain imaging variables, and a third residual component. By definition, this residual component approximates the concept of cognitive reserve as it represents the unexplained variance in cognitive performance after accounting for brain structure, and in this case, demographics. Interestingly, the authors included education as part of the demographics variable to isolate a component that would be uncontaminated by the indirect effects of education on brain integrity (e.g., access to health care and knowledge of health-promoting behaviors). Results showed that residual scores correlated with another measure of reserve (word reading), modified rates of conversion from mild cognitive impairment to dementia over time, and modified rates of decline in executive function. Finally, baseline brain status had less of an effect on cognitive decline over time in individuals with high residual scores than low residual scores.

In addition to providing an operational measure of reserve that is quantitative, continuous, and specific to the individual, the residual approach to characterizing reserve allows the estimate of cognitive reserve to change over time. This fluid characteristic may or may not be appealing to individual researchers and clinicians, depending on the particular question or task at hand. The authors also note that a potential problem with this approach is that, depending on the specific brain and cognitive variables used to define reserve, different measures of reserve will be applicable to a person at any given time. Practically speaking, a primary drawback to using residual scores is that it is currently not feasible for the clinician to apply such scores on an individual basis. This may change in the future with greater access to imaging technologies, and availability of normative or group data with which to derive an individual's residual score.

Brain Network Patterns

A future goal for representing reserve is through an identifiable brain network or series of networks. Such networks might be derived using functional imaging techniques that capture the neural signature of cognitive reserve. For example, Stern and colleagues examined whether or not a common neural network, whose expression varied as a function of cognitive reserve, could be detected across verbal and spatial delayed match-to-sample tasks [60]. Indeed, in the group of young adults, such a network was identified, and expression of this network was entirely independent of task performance. The invocation of this network on divergent tasks was uniquely related to cognitive reserve, as assessed with a composite of vocabulary and word reading, suggesting that the network may represent a generalized neural instantiation of reserve.

The utility of a brain network for capturing cognitive reserve is multifold. First, to the extent that reserve truly has a neural signature, the identification of a brain network that "behaves" like cognitive reserve (e.g., correlates with traditional reserve variables, persists across divergent task demands, and interacts with task performance in the expected way) would be a more direct way to measure the construct. Second, a brain network would be a nonbiased characterization of reserve that could be used universally in a manner that tests such as vocabulary or single-word reading cannot, due to their influences from culture and language. Third, a brain network is malleable in a way that fixed life experiences are not, and thus lends itself to examination in the context of a longitudinal study. For example, interventional studies aimed at increasing reserve could use a brain network to measure reserve both pre- and post-intervention, and unlike cognitive testing, this network would be resistant to practice effects.

Application of Cognitive Reserve in Clinical Practice

While the concept of cognitive reserve is on the one hand intuitive, it is also easily misunderstood and conducive to misapplication in part due to the thorny theoretical and methodological issues discussed above. However, there is nothing magical about the concept of reserve, and most clinicians generally consider the role of reserve in their assessment and case conceptualization (even if not explicitly). In this section, we provide concrete suggestions for the consideration and application of cognitive reserve in clinical practice.

First, when assessing cognition as part of a diagnostic evaluation, it is important to take into account the most appropriate and valid indicator of cognitive reserve for a given patient. In the event that an individual's level of education is not believed to be a good representation of his or her optimal cognitive functioning, assessment of IQ or consideration of occupation may provide a more accurate estimate. Alternatively, in a non-native English speaker, education may be a better representation than single-word reading to estimate IQ. Although, it should be noted that the availability of tests in other languages is increasing, such as Spanish [61], French [62], Japanese [63], and Swedish [64]. Application of a non-English assessment tool would be appropriate only in circumstances when the remainder of the neuropsychological battery can also be validly administered in the same language, as direct comparisons of IQ and neuropsychological scores would be otherwise impossible.

Integration of the most appropriate and valid measure of cognitive reserve into the diagnostic formulation is critical. Individuals with high reserve, by definition, will not demonstrate clinical symptoms as early as individuals with low levels of reserve. On the one hand, this issue could partially be a problem with instrumentation, such that (1) more challenging tests with higher ceilings may better detect changes in individuals with very high levels of functioning, (2) tests that are more pathologically specific (e.g., associative learning tasks for the hippocampus) may have greater sensitivity in high reserve individuals, or (3) better normative data may allow for better detection of impairment in individuals with high levels of intellectual functioning. Indeed, quantitative consideration of IQ scores appears to improve the sensitivity of cognitive testing for detecting pathology. Rentz and colleagues [65] found that when memory scores in a group of cognitively "normal" individuals were adjusted based on IQ, the adjusted memory scores correlated with cerebral perfusion in areas vulnerable to the early stages of AD pathology. That is, those with higher IQ (i.e., reserve) had greater pathology despite similar cognitive performance, and these individuals showed greater cognitive decline over the following 3 years than the individuals whose IQ-adjusted memory scores were intact [65].

In theory, there would still be a period of time during which even the most sensitive measures would fail to detect change in those with high reserve given the apparent "lag" between pathological changes and their cognitive sequelae. Therefore, from a clinical standpoint, neuropsychological testing will be less sensitive to the presence of early pathology in those with high reserve *even when we consider current test scores in the context of a person's optimal level of functioning* (e.g., *IQ*, *education*). As such, the only action to be taken by clinicians is to be aware of this conundrum and to appreciate that intact cognition in individuals with high levels of reserve does not preclude the presence of disease.

The standard and generally useful approach taken by neuropsychologists is to formally adjust cognitive scores for education, a procedure which, in theory, allows for the interpretation of current cognitive performance in the context of an individual's expected performance. For example, we know that there are baseline differences in cognitive performance such that in the absence of pathology, a 70-year-old with 8 years of education might recall fewer words over the course of a list learning test than a 70-year-old with 19 years of education. The corollary of this phenomenon is that the patient with 19 years of education would have had to sustain a greater degree of neuropathology to reach a certain score than the individual with 6 years of education, all other things being equal. However, this observation does not, in and of itself, reflect cognitive reserve. Rather, reserve accounts for the ability of the individual with 19 years of education to maintain baseline cognitive functioning for a longer period of time than the individual with 6 years of education in the face of advancing pathology.

Information regarding brain integrity should be integrated with cognitive data for diagnostic purposes, whenever possible. Of course, this process is done regularly in most clinical settings and adds important information and greater clarity to the overall clinical picture. In this context, however, the focus is on the relevance of neuroimaging as a means to understand the influence of cognitive reserve on the clinical presentation. Neuroimaging tools have the potential, particularly in individuals with high reserve who maintain cognitive functioning for an extended period of time, to detect pathological changes when impairment on neuropsychological testing is absent or subtle. For example, at a given level of clinical severity, AD patients with higher education have a more severe pattern of AD-related changes on PET scan than those with lower education [66, 67].

More recently, the sensitivity of a variety of imaging tools for detecting pathological changes prior to cognitive change has been demonstrated on structural MRI [68] and functional MRI (fMRI) [69], as well as through examination of activity level in the default network on resting fMRI [70]. Moving forward, in vivo amyloid imaging, although not currently used in clinical practice, will certainly play an important role in identifying neuropathological changes in asymptomatic individuals as the field moves toward earlier identification of disease. While these various technologies enable the consideration of cognitive reserve as a factor influencing the clinical presentation and diagnosis of a patient, a current challenge to integrating imaging information is applying results from group studies to individual patients. Ideally, research studies might generate a cutoff value so that performance scores below this cutoff would raise concern for the presence of pathological changes. Such a value would be selected based on its utility in distinguishing between cognitively normal individuals who go on to develop cognitive impairment and other clinical endpoints versus those who remain cognitively healthy. This type of value has been identified for the purposes of distinguishing healthy elders from those diagnosed with AD [71, 72], and future work will aim to make this distinction at earlier time points.

Another recommendation for applying the concept of cognitive reserve to clinical practice is to consider it as a factor that will influence rate of cognitive decline following diagnosis. Although cognitive reserve delays the manifestation of cognitive deficits, symptoms progress fairly rapidly once evident (see Fig. 2.1). In fact, decline is more rapid in individuals with high reserve than those with low reserve, even when accounting for a multitude of other factors that may contribute to disease course [73–75]. This counterintuitive acceleration in rate of change is believed to reflect the increasingly high pathological burden that the brain can no longer tolerate. Certainly, this has practical implications for the patient, family, and health-care providers. It may also have direct relevance for the effectiveness of treatment.

Cognitive reserve may influence an individual's response to treatment with currently available medications as well as future drug therapies. The treatment of degenerative diseases such as Alzheimer's disease is certain to be most effective when done preventatively, when the burden of pathology in the brain is very low or absent altogether. Thus, in order to develop reasonable expectations about a medication's effectiveness, it will be important to have knowledge of three variables: cognitive performance, cognitive reserve, and pathological burden. As we have reinforced throughout this chapter, it is the combination of these three variables that enables an accurate understanding of disease severity. From a clinical standpoint, treatment in an individual with mildly impaired cognition and high cognitive reserve may be more or less effective depending on the status of the third variable, pathological burden. With little to no evidence of pathology, an individual with these characteristics would be an ideal candidate for therapy. In contrast, in the context of significant pathology, disease-delaying agents may be entirely ineffective, and this possibility should be anticipated by the clinician.

A final insight for clinicians is that while a wide range of evidence exists from epidemiological studies linking certain life experiences and individual characteristics to lower rates of dementia, this evidence is not sufficient to determine definitively whether or not such experiences directly prevent or delay dementia. As mentioned earlier, there may be a separate unidentified variable accounting for the observed relationship between specific experiences (e.g., completing crossword puzzles) and dementia risk. As such, intervention studies are needed to firmly establish causal links between life experiences, individual characteristics, and cognitive reserve, and such studies are underway. Therefore, while recommending that patients engage in certain activities such as mental enrichment and physical fitness is likely not to be harmful and may in fact have numerous positive effects, clinicians should be careful not to present these activities as established treatments or fully proven preventative strategies against dementia.

Clinical Pearls

- When formulating clinical impressions, apply the most appropriate and valid indicator of cognitive reserve for each individual patient. This may be an individual characteristic such as level of education; a representation of cumulative life experiences spanning social, academic, occupational, and leisure activities; or a measure of intellectual functioning. Moving forward, statistically and neuroanatomically derived measures of cognitive reserve may also become valuable for clinical purposes.
- Integrate neuroimaging tools to complement cognitive data for diagnostic purposes.
- Consider cognitive reserve as a factor that may affect rate of decline. The apparent yet counterintuitive acceleration of decline associated cognitive reserve may reflect a state of increasingly high pathological burden that the brain can no longer tolerate.
- Appreciate that cognitive reserve may be a factor that influences response to treatment.
- Be aware that epidemiological studies linking life experiences to reduced dementia risk are observational, and intervention studies are needed to determine definitively if specific experiences and activities enhance reserve and lower dementia risk.

Acknowledgments This project was supported by Dr. Cosentino's Beeson Career Development Award in Aging (1K23 AG032899-01) and Dr. Stern's project, "Imaging of Cognition and Memory" (R01 AG26158).

References

1. Katzman R, Aronson M, Fuld P, Kawas C, Brown T, Morgenstern H, et al. Development of dementing illnesses in an 80-year-old volunteer cohort. Ann Neurol. 1989;25:317–24.
2. Ince PG. Pathological correlates of late-onset dementia in a multicenter community-based population in England and Wales. Lancet. 2001;357(9251):169–75.
3. Stern Y. What is cognitive reserve? theory and research application of the reserve concept. J Int Neuropsychol Soc. 2002;8:448–60.
4. Stern Y. Cognitive reserve. Neuropsychologia. 2009; 47:2015–28.
5. Katzman R. Education and the prevalence of dementia and Alzheimer's disease. Neurology. 1993;43:13–20.
6. Qiu C, Backman L, Winblad B, Aguero-Torres H, Fratiglioni L. The influence of education on clinically diagnosed dementia incidence and mortality data from the Kungsholmen Project. Arch Neurol. 2001;58(12):2034–9.
7. Stern Y, Gurland B, Tatemichi TK, Tang MX, Wilder D, Mayeux R. Influence of education and occupation on the incidence of Alzheimer's disease. J Am Med Assoc. 1994;271:1004–10.
8. Akbaraly TN, Portet F, Fustinoni S, Dartigues JF, Artero S, Rouaud O, et al. Leisure activities and the risk of dementia in the elderly: results from the Three-City Study. Neurology. 2009;73(11):854–61.
9. Scarmeas N, Levy G, Tang MX, Manly J, Stern Y. Influence of leisure activity on the incidence of Alzheimer's disease. Neurology. 2001;57(12):2236–42.
10. Schmand B, Smit JH, Geerlings MI, Lindeboom J. The effects of intelligence and education on the development of dementia. A test of the brain reserve hypothesis. Psychol Med. 1997;27(6):1337–44.
11. Valenzuela MJ, Sachdev P. Brain reserve and dementia: a systematic review. Psychol Med. 2005;25:1–14.
12. Albert MS, Jones K, Savage CR, Berkman L, Seeman T, Blazer D, et al. Predictors of cognitive change in older persons: MacArthur studies of successful aging. Psychol Aging. 1995;10:578–89.
13. Butler SM, Ashford JW, Snowdon DA. Age, education, and changes in the Mini-Mental State Exam scores of older women: findings from the Nun Study. J Am Geriatr Soc. 1996;44:675–81.
14. Chodosh J, Reuben DB, Albert MS, Seeman TE. Predicting cognitive impairment in high-functioning community-dwelling older persons: MacArthur Studies of Successful Aging. J Am Geriatr Soc. 2002;50:1051–60.
15. Christensen H, Korten AE, Jorm AF, Henderson AS, Jacomb PA, Rodgers B, et al. Education and decline in cognitive performance: compensatory but not protective. Int J Geriatr Psychiatry. 1997;12:323–30.
16. Colsher PL, Wallace RB. Longitudinal application of cognitive function measures in a defined population of community-dwelling elders. Ann Epidemiol. 1991;1(3):215–30.

17. Farmer ME, Kittner SJ, Rae DS, Bartko JJ, Regier DA. Education and change in cognitive function: the epidemiologic catchment area study. Ann Epidemiol. 1995;5:1–7.
18. Lyketsos CG, Chen L-S, Anthony JC. Cognitive decline in adulthood: an 11.5-year follow-up of the Baltimore Epidemiologic Catchment Area Study. Am J Psychiatr. 1999;156(1):58–65.
19. Snowdon DA, Ostwald SK, Kane RL. Education, survival and independence in elderly Catholic sisters, 1936–1988. Am J Epidemiol. 1989;130:999–1012.
20. Stern Y, Alexander GE, Prohovnik I, Mayeux R. Inverse relationship between education and parietotemporal perfusion deficit in Alzheimer's disease. Ann Neurol. 1992;32:371–5.
21. Alexander GE, Furey ML, Grady CL, Pietrini P, Brady DR, Mentis MJ, et al. Association of premorbid intellectual function with cerebral metabolism in Alzheimer's disease: implications for the cognitive reserve hypothesis. Am J Psychiatry. 1997; 154(2):165–72.
22. Stern Y, Alexander GE, Prohovnik I, Stricks L, Link B, Lennon MC, et al. Relationship between lifetime occupation and parietal flow: implications for a reserve against Alzheimer's disease pathology. Neurology. 1995;45:55–60.
23. Scarmeas N, Zarahn E, Anderson KE, Habeck CG, Hilton J, Flynn J, et al. Association of life activities with cerebral blood flow in Alzheimer disease: implications for the cognitive reserve hypothesis. Arch Neurol. 2003;60:359–65.
24. Brickman AM, Siedlecki KL, Muraskin J, Manly JJ, Luchsinger JA, Yeung LK, et al. White matter hyperintensities and cognition: testing the reserve hypothesis. Neurobiol Aging. 2011;32(9):1588–98.
25. Rentz DM, Locascio JJ, Becker JA, Moran EK, Eng E, Buckner RL, et al. Cognition, reserve, and amyloid deposition in normal aging. Ann Neurol. 2010;67(3):353–64.
26. Bennett DA, Wilson RS, Schneider JA, Evans DA, Mendes De Leon CF, Arnold SE, et al. Education modifies the relation of AD pathology to level of cognitive function in older persons. Neurology. 2003;60(12):1909–15.
27. Roe CM, Xiong C, Miller JP, Morris JC. Education and Alzheimer disease without dementia: support for the cognitive reserve hypothesis. Neurology. 2007;68(3):223–8.
28. Valenzuela MJ. Brain reserve and the prevention of dementia. Curr Opin Psychiatry. 2008;21(3):296–302.
29. Piras F, Cherubini A, Caltagirone C, Spalletta G. Education mediates microstructural changes in bilateral hippocampus. Hum Brain Mapp. 2011; 32(2):282–9.
30. Kesler SR, Adams HF, Blasey CM, Bigler ED. Premorbid intellectual functioning, education, and brain size in traumatic brain injury: an investigation of the cognitive reserve hypothesis. Appl Neuropsychol. 2003;10:153–62.
31. Willerman L, Schultz R, Rutledge JN, Bigler ED. In vivo brain size and intelligence. Intelligence. 1991;15:223–8.
32. Brown J, Cooper-Kuhn CM, Kemperman G, van Praag H, Winkler J, Gage FH. Enriched environment and physical activity stimulate hippocampal but not olfactory bulb neurogenesis. Eur J Neurosci. 2003;17:2042–6.
33. van Praag H, Shubert T, Zhao C, Gage FH. Exercise enhances learning and hippocampal neurogenesis in aged mice. J Neurosci. 2005;25:8680–5.
34. Lazarov O, Robinson J, Tang YP, Hairston IS, Korade-Mirnics Z, Lee VM, et al. Environmental enrichment reduces Abeta levels and amyloid deposition in transgenic mice. Cell. 2005;120(5):701–13.
35. Manly JJ, Touradji P, Tang MX, Stern Y. Literacy and memory decline among ethnically diverse elders. J Clin Exp Neuropsychol. 2003;25(5):680–90.
36. Boyle PA, Wilson RS, Schneider JA, Bienias JL, Bennett DA. Processing resources reduce the effect of Alzheimer pathology on other cognitive systems. Neurology. 2008;70(17):1534–42.
37. Stern Y. Cognitive reserve and Alzheimer disease. Alzheimer Dis Assoc Disord. 2006;20(3 Suppl 2): S69–74.
38. Stern Y, Habeck C, Moeller J, Scarmeas N, Anderson KE, Hilton HJ, et al. Brain networks associated with cognitive reserve in healthy young and old adults. Cereb Cortex. 2005;15(4):394–402.
39. Siedlecki KL, Stern Y, Reuben A, Sacco RL, Elkind MS, Wright CB. Construct validity of cognitive reserve in a multiethnic cohort: the Northern Manhattan Study. J Int Neuropsychol Soc. 2009;15(4):558–69.
40. Benedict RH, Morrow SA, Weinstock Guttman B, Cookfair D, Schretlen DJ. Cognitive reserve moderates decline in information processing speed in multiple sclerosis patients. J Int Neuropsychol Soc. 2010;16(5):829–35.
41. Sumowski JF, Chiaravalloti N, Wylie G, Deluca J. Cognitive reserve moderates the negative effect of brain atrophy on cognitive efficiency in multiple sclerosis. J Int Neuropsychol Soc. 2009;15(4): 606–12.
42. Sumowski JF, Wylie GR, Deluca J, Chiaravalloti N. Intellectual enrichment is linked to cerebral efficiency in multiple sclerosis: functional magnetic resonance imaging evidence for cognitive reserve. Brain. 2010;133(Pt 2):362–74.
43. Sumowski JF, Wylie GR, Gonnella A, Chiaravalloti N, Deluca J. Premorbid cognitive leisure independently contributes to cognitive reserve in multiple sclerosis. Neurology. 2010;75(16):1428–31.
44. Smith A. Symbol digit modalities test manual. Los Angeles, CA: Western Psychological Services; 1982.
45. Cutter GR, Baier ML, Rudick RA, Cookfair DL, Fischer JS, Petkau J, et al. Development of a multiple sclerosis functional composite as a clinical trial outcome measure. Brain. 1999;122(Pt 5):871–82.

46. Richards M, Sacker A. Lifetime antecedents of cognitive reserve. J Clin Exp Neuropsychol. 2003;25(5): 614–24.
47. Valenzuela MJ, Sachdev P. Assessment of complex mental activity across the lifespan: Development of the lifetime of experiences questionnaire (LEQ). Psychol Med. 2007;37(7):1015--25.
48. Hall CB, Lipton RB, Sliwinski M, Katz MJ, Derby CA, Verghese J. Cognitive activities delay onset of memory decline in persons who develop dementia. Neurology. 2009;73(5):356–61.
49. Holdnack JA. Wechsler test of adult reading (WTAR) manual. San Antonio, TX: The Psychological Corporation; 2001.
50. Nelson HE. Nelson adult reading test manual. London: The National Hospital for Nervous Disease; 1982.
51. Wechsler D. WAIS-IV administration and scoring manual. San Antonio, TX: Pearson; 2008.
52. Crawford JR, Parker DM, Stewart LE, Besson JAO, De Lacey G. Prediction of WAIS IQ with the national adult reading test: cross-validation and extension. Br J Psychol. 1989;27:181–2.
53. Hart S, Smith CM, Swash M. Assessing intellectual deterioration. Br J Clin Psychol. 1986;25:119–24.
54. Nelson HE, O'Connell A. Dementia: the estimation of premorbid intelligence levels using the New Adult Reading Test. Cortex. 1978;14(2):234–44.
55. O'Carroll RE, Gilleard CJ. Estimation of premorbid intelligence in dementia. Br J Clin Psychol. 1986; 25:157–8.
56. Sharpe K, O'Carroll RE. Estimating premorbid intellectual level in dementia using the National Adult Reading Test: a Canadian study. Br J Clin Psychol. 1991;30:381–4.
57. Jones RN, Manly J, Glymour MM, Rentz DM, Jefferson AL, Stern Y. Conceptual and measurement challenges in research on cognitive reserve. J Int Neuropsychol Soc. 2011;17:1–9.
58. Satz P, Cole MA, Hardy DJ, Rassovsky Y. Brain and cognitive reserve: mediator(s) and construct validity, a critique. J Clin Exp Neuropsychol. 2011;33(1):121–30.
59. Reed BR, Mungas D, Farias ST, Harvey D, Beckett L, Widamen K, et al. Measuring cognitive reserve based on the decomposition of episodic memory variance. Brain. 2010;133(Pt 8):2196--209.
60. Stern Y, Zarahn E, Habeck C, Holtzer R, Rakitin BC, Kumar A, et al. A common neural network for cognitive reserve in verbal and object working memory in young but not old. Cereb Cortex. 2008;18(4):959–67.
61. Del Ser T, Gonzalez-Montalvo JI, Martinez-Espinosa S, Delgado-Villapalos C, Bermejo F. Estimation of premorbid intelligence in Spanish people with the Word Accentuation Test and its application to the diagnosis of dementia. Brain Cogn. 1997;33(3):343–56.
62. Mackinnon A, Mulligan R. The estimation of premorbid intelligence levels in French speakers. Encéphale. 2005;31(1 Pt 1):31–43.
63. Matsuoka K, Uno M, Kasai K, Koyama K, Kim Y. Estimation of premorbid IQ in individuals with Alzheimer's disease using Japanese ideographic script (Kanji) compound words: Japanese version of National Adult Reading Test. Psychiatry Clin Neurosci. 2006;60(3):332–9.
64. Rolstad S, Nordlund A, Gustavsson MH, Eckerstrom C, Klang O, Hansen S, et al. The Swedish National Adult Reading Test (NART-SWE): a test of premorbid IQ. Scand J Psychol. 2008;49(6):577–82.
65. Rentz DM, Huh TJ, Sardinha LM, Moran EK, Becker JA, Daffner KR, et al. Intelligence quotient-adjusted memory impairment is associated with abnormal single photon emission computed tomography perfusion. J Int Neuropsychol Soc. 2007;13(5):821–31.
66. Garibotto V, Borroni B, Kalbe E, Herholz K, Salmon E, Holtoff V, et al. Education and occupation as proxies for reserve in aMCI converters and AD: FDG-PET evidence. Neurology. 2008;71(17):1342–9.
67. Kemppainen NM, Aalto S, Karrasch M, Nagren K, Savisto N, Oikonen V, et al. Cognitive reserve hypothesis: Pittsburgh Compound B and fluorodeoxyglucose positron emission tomography in relation to education in mild Alzheimer's disease. Ann Neurol. 2008;63(1):112–8.
68. Smith CD, Chebrolu H, Wekstein DR, Schmitt FA, Jicha GA, Cooper G, et al. Brain structural alterations before mild cognitive impairment. Neurology. 2007;68(16):1268–73.
69. Smith CD, Andersen AH, Kryscio RJ, Schmitt FA, Kindy MS, Blonder LX, et al. Altered brain activation in cognitively intact individuals at high risk for Alzheimer's disease. Neurology. 1999;53(7):1391–6.
70. Sperling RA, Dickerson BC, Pihlajamaki M, Vannini P, LaViolette PS, Vitolo OV, et al. Functional alterations in memory networks in early Alzheimer's disease. Neuromolecular Med. 2010;12(1):27–43.
71. Asllani I, Habeck C, Scarmeas N, Borogovac A, Brown TR, Stern Y. Multivariate and univariate analysis of continuous arterial spin labeling perfusion MRI in Alzheimer's disease. J Cereb Blood Flow Metab. 2008;28(4):725–36.
72. Friese U, Meindl T, Herpertz SC, Reiser MF, Hampel H, Teipel SJ. Diagnostic utility of novel MRI-based biomarkers for Alzheimer's disease: diffusion tensor imaging and deformation-based morphometry. J Alzheimers Dis. 2010;20(2):477–90.
73. Hall CB, Derby C, LeValley A, Katz MJ, Verghese J, Lipton RB. Education delays accelerated decline on a memory test in persons who develop dementia. Neurology. 2007;69(17):1657–64.
74. Scarmeas N, Albert SM, Manly JJ, Stern Y. Education and rates of cognitive decline in incident Alzheimer's disease. J Neurol Neurosurg Psychiatry. 2006;77(3):308–16.
75. Stern Y, Albert S, Tang MX, Tsai WY. Rate of memory decline in AD is related to education and occupation: cognitive reserve? Neurology. 1999; 53:1942–57.

Considerations for the Neuropsychological Evaluation of Older Ethnic Minority Populations

3

Monica Rivera Mindt, Alyssa Arentoft, Kelly Coulehan, and Desiree Byrd

Abstract

The US population is rapidly becoming both older and more culturally diverse [1]. These changes in the demographic profile of the US highlight the need for clinical neuropsychologists to be equipped to competently evaluate the growing population of older individuals from culturally diverse backgrounds. However, there is a relative dearth of empirically based, practical resources specifically targeted toward serving such individuals. The aim of this chapter is to identify some of the most salient challenges in the evaluation of culturally diverse ethnic minority older adults and provide some guidelines to help face these challenges. We will examine sociocultural issues germane to older ethnic minority patients referred for neuropsychological evaluation and discuss relevant assessment considerations. Although the focus of this chapter is on ethnic minority older adults, this discussion may also be germane to other nontraditional, older populations including those from rural and low socioeconomic backgrounds.

Keywords

Racial/ethnic minorities • Dementia • Neuropsychological evaluation • Assessment • Diversity • Cultural competence • Neurocognitive impairment

M.R. Mindt, Ph.D. (✉)
Department of Psychology, Fordham University, 113 West 60th Street, LL 808F, New York, NY 10023, USA

Departments of Pathology and Psychiatry, The Mount Sinai School of Medicine, One Gustave Levy Place MHBB 1134, New York, NY 10029, USA
e-mail: riveramindt@fordham.edu

A. Arentoft, M.A. • K. Coulehan, M.A.
Department of Psychology, Fordham University, 113 West 60th Street, LL 808F, New York, NY 10023, USA
e-mail: alyssa.arentoft@gmail.com; kcoulehan@gmail.com

D. Byrd, Ph.D.
Departments of Pathology and Psychiatry, The Mount Sinai School of Medicine, One Gustave Levy Place MHBB 1134, New York, NY 10029, USA
e-mail: desiree.byrd@mssm.edu

L.D. Ravdin and H.L. Katzen (eds.), *Handbook on the Neuropsychology of Aging and Dementia*, Clinical Handbooks in Neuropsychology, DOI 10.1007/978-1-4614-3106-0_3,

The US population is rapidly becoming both older and more culturally diverse [1]. Currently, there are over 38 million people in the USA over 65 years old, comprising over 10% of the US population [2]. In 2030, there will be approximately 72 million individuals over 65 years, comprising about 20% of the US population [3]. Among older adults, ethnic minority populations, particularly Latinos and African Americans, are growing much faster than the non-Hispanic white population [4]. In 2050, ethnic minority individuals will represent approximately 42% of the older adult (65 and older) population in the USA. These changes in the demographic profile of the US highlight the need for clinical neuropsychologists to be equipped to competently evaluate the growing population of older individuals from culturally diverse backgrounds. However, there is a relative dearth of empirically based, practical resources specifically targeted toward serving such individuals.

Sociocultural Framework

Working from a biopsychosociocultural theoretical framework [5], the sociocultural level of analysis includes consideration of how social, socioeconomic, institutional, and cultural (i.e., the shared attitudes, values, goals, and practices that characterize a group from one generation to the next) [6–8] factors modulate an individual's or a group's behaviors. Sociocultural issues are critical for understanding neuropsychological test performance and neurobehavioral functioning [9–14]. In particular, it is important to consider sociocultural issues as they relate to health disparities, cognitive aging, and neurologic disease among ethnic minority older adults.

Health Disparities

A health disparity refers to a significant discrepancy in the overall disease incidence, prevalence, morbidity, mortality, or survival rates in a specific population as compared to the general population. This is mutable and disproportionately affects vulnerable populations [15, 16]. In the USA, many ethnic minority populations are disproportionately impacted by higher rates of poverty and limited access to, or use of, healthcare services, which contribute to greater vulnerability for particular medical disorders and worse disease burden [17–19]. Of particular interest to neuropsychologists, several ethnic minority groups (particularly African Americans, Hispanics/Latinos, and American Indians/Alaska Natives) are disproportionately affected by medical conditions (e.g., hypertension, HIV/AIDS, Hepatitis, diabetes, etc.) that may increase their need for neuropsychological services compared with the general population [20].

Culture and Cognitive Aging

Dementia

Evidence suggests that rates of diagnosed dementia differ between ethnic minority and non-Hispanic white older adults, with the former receiving higher rates of dementia diagnoses. Prevalence estimates suggest that African American, Latinos, and Asian American elders have higher rates of vascular dementia compared to non-Hispanic white elders [21–24], and African American and Latino elders have higher rates of Alzheimer's disease compared to non-Hispanic whites [25]. Evidence also suggests that Latinos have an earlier onset of Alzheimer's symptoms compared to their non-Hispanic white counterparts [26]. In contrast, some research has shown that African Americans have lower rates of Parkinsonian dementia and Latinos have lower rates of Alzheimer's disease compared to non-Hispanic whites [21, 27]. Preliminary research suggests that rates of dementias (i.e., Alzheimer's and vascular dementia) among Asian Americans are similar to non-Hispanic whites [28, 29], although this has not been thoroughly investigated, particularly with representative samples of Asian American populations (e.g., Chinese, Japanese, Vietnamese, Hmong, Korean, Native Hawaiian). Although the current literature is somewhat equivocal, there is a growing body of evidence that suggests that African American and Latino populations are at greater risk for both vascular and Alzheimer's-related dementias than non-Hispanic whites, with Asian Americans also at greater risk for vascular dementia.

The mechanisms that contribute to the differing rates of dementia between ethnic groups remain poorly understood. Ethnic minority individuals are at greater risk of developing cardiovascular disease, particularly individuals of low socioeconomic status (SES) [30, 31]. Ethnic minority individuals also have higher rates of hypertension, diabetes, heart disease [32], cancer, obesity, and HIV/AIDS [33]. Many of these conditions are risk factors for illnesses with neuropsychological sequelae, such as dementia. For instance, evidence indicates that the presence of vascular risk factors (e.g., diabetes and hypertension) among persons diagnosed with Alzheimer's dementia is associated with worse neuropsychological test performance at the time of diagnosis compared to those without such risk factors [34]. However, higher rates of diagnosed dementia among these ethnic groups may also be significantly affected by the lower diagnostic accuracy of many of the neuropsychological measures utilized to diagnose ethnically diverse individuals [35, 36].

Risk for Misdiagnosis

Multicultural research has demonstrated that neuropsychological performance among neurologically healthy younger and older adults significantly differs between ethnic minority and non-Hispanic white groups, even after statistically adjusting for other demographic factors (e.g., age, education, and gender) [37–44]. Further, the poor specificity of many neuropsychological tests often results in misdiagnosis of neurocognitive disorders among African Americans and Latinos [38, 45–56]. Although utilizing normative data that correct for race/ethnicity (in addition to age, education, and gender) substantially reduce the risk for misdiagnosis [39], such norms do not address the source of these performance differences.

Emerging literature points to the significant impact of numerous sociocultural factors on test performance among ethnic minority individuals, including quality of education [57–59], acculturation [37, 60–62], language (including bilingualism) [59, 63–66], and stereotype threat [67]. There is also potential test bias related to the lack of support for the cultural equivalence and construct validity of several measures with ethnic minority populations [13, 68, 69]. Thus, it is important for clinical neuropsychologists to be aware of these research findings to more accurately diagnose and serve ethnic minority patients.

In addition, disproportionate rates of disease and disease burden (health disparities), potentially increased risk for dementia due to related health disparities, and risk for misdiagnosis due, at least in part, to poor construct validity and limited appropriate normative data together set the stage for a unique set of assessment challenges for working with ethnic minority older adults. In the following section, these challenges, and suggestions for addressing them, are considered at each point in the evaluation process.

Considerations for Neuropsychological Evaluation with Ethnic Minority Older Adults

Ethical Issues and Competence

The American Psychological Association's (APA) *Ethical Principles of Psychologists and Code of Conduct* [70] provides some guidance on the ethical standards necessary to conduct a culturally competent neuropsychological evaluation. For example, Ethical Standard 2.01 [71] explains that "cultural expertise or competence at the individual level is essential for the clinician who is working with cross-cultural populations." But how does a clinician actually ascertain whether or not s/he is competent to evaluate an ethnic minority older adult?

Rivera Mindt et al. [13] proposed a cultural competence in neuropsychology (CCN) model [71–74] that assists neuropsychologists in examining their cultural competence by evaluating their own cultural awareness and knowledge of the ethnically diverse populations they would like to serve. If a neuropsychologist determines that they s/he does not currently have the requisite competence to evaluate a particular ethnic minority patient, s/he may be able to cultivate that competence through the acquisition of specific, culturally appropriate assessment, intervention, and communication skills necessary to effectively work with individuals from specific ethnic minority groups [13]. For instance, supplemental training can be acquired through continuing education courses or workshops focused on working with culturally diverse populations (such as those offered through APA Division 40, the National Academy of Neuropsychology, the American Academy of Clinical Neuropsychology, or the Hispanic Neuropsychological Society) [75], readings, and consultation [13]. In addition, neuropsychologists are also responsible for carefully considering the cultural competence of their psychometrists or graduate students, if used in the assessment process.

In terms of day-to-day practice, prior to the evaluation of an ethnic minority older patient, some relevant demographic information about the patient should first be collected (i.e., patient's age, years of education, race/ethnicity, birthplace, and language use and history) preliminarily to determine if one is competent to evaluate the older client. The issue of linguistic competence is particularly important for planning the evaluation. Although detailed discussion of linguistic competence is beyond the scope of the current chapter, useful guidance on determining one's own linguistic competence to examine non-English or bilingual patients is available elsewhere [5, 76–78]. To further inform this decision, the neuropsychologist may also consider explicitly asking about a patient's linguistic preference.

In cases in which a neuropsychologist is unsure of her or his cultural competence to examine a particular ethnic minority patient, consultation with colleagues who are familiar with multicultural neuropsychology is recommended. Extensive resources for such consultation are available elsewhere [13]. If a neuropsychologist determines that he or she does not have the requisite competence (either due to language or other concerns), it is recommended that the patient be referred to a more appropriate clinician. If such a referral is not feasible (due to geographic location or other barriers), then the neuropsychologist should consider how best to evaluate the patient, through use of a well-trained interpreter (which is less than ideal, but sometimes necessary) or in consultation with a neuropsychologist who does have the necessary cultural competence to ethically provide supervision. More thorough discussion of ethical obligations and competency issues related to neuropsychological evaluation with ethnic minority individuals is provided elsewhere and the interested reader is encouraged to review the available literature [13, 70, 71, 78–81].

The Physical Space

Once the decision has been made to evaluate an ethnic minority older patient, neuropsychologists are encouraged to consider each aspect of the evaluation through a "sociocultural lens." For instance, what is the potential impact of a neuropsychologist's physical space (i.e., the office or hospital environment) on their ethnic minority older patients? Expanding on Rivera Mindt et al.'s [13] original recommendations, neuropsychologists are encouraged to consider the following:

1. *First impressions*. Does your practice (or facility) contain images of diverse people (i.e., age, gender, race/ethnicity, etc.) via brochures, websites, or flyers, anti-discrimination statements, diversity intentions, or related services? Is your practice accessible and convenient for patients with physical or transport limitations (i.e., parking and close to public transport)?
2. *Waiting area*. Is your waiting area a welcoming place for ethnic or linguistic minorities (i.e., written signs, symbols, magazines, art, decorations, greetings, staff)?

Clinical Interview and History

The clinical interview and history taking portion of a neuropsychological evaluation is critical for the purposes of establishing rapport, ensuring accurate diagnosis, and developing appropriate follow-up recommendations. However, sociocultural issues can significantly impact this process.

Pre-interview

Working from the CCN model, it is recommended that neuropsychologists have some empirically based knowledge of the culture of origin of their older ethnic minority patients prior to beginning the clinical interview, if possible. The literature in multicultural counseling and community psychology may be particularly useful in this regard and may help identify any culturally accepted social norms that may come into play during the interview or latter portions of the evaluation.

Establishing and Maintaining Rapport

Prior to test administration, sufficient time should be dedicated to rapport building. Research indicates that level of formality, authority, eye contact, and personal space can all have an impact on establishing and maintaining rapport among persons of different ethnic groups [75, 82, 83]. These issues, along with cultural attitudes about the age and gender of the neuropsychologist or psychometrist, may be especially salient points for consideration among older ethnic minority patients who may be less acculturated to majority culture (i.e., mainstream US culture). For instance, in terms of verbal and nonverbal communication, consider how to initially approach the patient. The communication of respect may be particularly important with older patients. For instance, it may be best to have the patient introduce herself/himself to determine whether or not they wish to be called by their first or last name. Do not assume that the patient is comfortable with the use of their first name unless s/he specifies, as this may be interpreted as disrespectful or overly familiar [75].

It is also important to be aware of and sensitive to specific cultural or religious guidelines that may affect the interaction with a particular older ethnic minority patient. For example, it may be inappropriate for some women to attend their appointment without a male family member being present. Some Orthodox Jewish individuals do not shake hands with members of the opposite sex [84]. Some individuals from American Indian, Native Alaskan, or Asian/Asian American backgrounds, particularly older individuals, may view direct eye contact as a sign of disrespect [85]. Therefore, neuropsychologists should be aware of sociocultural norms that may pertain to their patient in order to interact appropriately and ensure that the patient is comfortable with the testing process. If a cultural accommodation requires any deviation from standardized testing procedure, it should be noted in the report.

Interviewing Considerations

In terms of the "nuts and bolts" of interview and history taking, neuropsychologists are encouraged to consider whether the content of their interview is culturally appropriate for the various ethnic minority patients they encounter [85, 86]. During the interview, information is typically gathered that relates to the referral question, current symptoms and complaints, and the patient's developmental, medical, psychiatric, and psychosocial history. In collecting this information, neuropsychologists are again encouraged to approach this task through a "sociocultural lens," and explicitly consider how sociocultural issues might impact an individual at each level of analysis.

In terms of current symptoms and complaints, knowledge of culturally based idioms of distress is particularly important as symptom reporting can vary greatly across individuals of different ethnic backgrounds and acculturation levels. For example, some literature suggests that Asian and Latino individuals are more likely to report somatic rather than depressive symptoms [87, 88]. From a development perspective, assess whether the person grew up with stable housing and adequate nutrition. From a medical perspective, might there be any comorbid medical conditions that disproportionately impact a certain ethnic population? In terms of past psychiatric history, it may be useful to know about the different base rates of psychiatric disorders, as well as disparities in access and utilization of psychological and psychiatric services, across different ethnic minority populations. These issues could significantly inform both current diagnosis and follow-up treatment recommendations.

With regard to psychosocial history, issues related to quality of education (QoE) are particularly important with ethnic minority elders. Caution should be exercised with older patients educated in other countries (particularly non-Western or less-industrialized countries, as this may affect familiarity with Western construct-laden measures), as well as disadvantaged areas in the USA. In both of these cases, using years of education to determine expected performance level may overestimate the individual's expected performance on Westernized neuropsychological tests. Therefore performance on the Wide Range Achievement Test (WRAT) reading subtest or the Wechsler Test of Adult Reading (WTAR) should be examined. Both estimate reading level, and are often used as proxies for quality of education [57]. When total years and quality of education vary significantly, this should be noted as a limitation and considered when examining performance on neuropsychological tests that are normatively corrected for education. In such instances, it will be important to ensure that the reading materials used during testing are written at an appropriate educational level so that the patient can reasonably be expected to understand them. Further, when large discrepancies between education and reading level (i.e., QoE) exist, utilizing Dotson et al 's. [89] battery and literacy-based norms may be a useful option for patients who are up to age 64, African American, and of predominantly low SES background. Moreover, gathering information regarding SES is important considering that there is some evidence indicating SES affects neuropsychological performance, although this has not been thoroughly investigated [11, 14].

Finally, it is strongly recommended that information related to sociocultural history is collected when working with ethnic minority elders. While the following is not an exhaustive list, below are some suggestions to consider when taking the sociocultural history. For an exceptional review of sociocultural considerations for working with Latino patients, see Llorente [81].

1. *Race and ethnicity.* It is important to ask patients to self-identify their race and ethnicity, rather than solely relying on physical appearance. Sometimes, these questions may be challenging for patients. Listing out racial/ethnic categories provided through the US Census can serve as a useful starting point. Further explanation of these categories may be needed, but at least this provides a common nomenclature.
2. *Country of origin and region.* Western or non-Western? Was the region rural, urban, or suburban? Safety and access to resources in the community? Issues related to acculturation are also important and discussed later in this chapter.
3. *Current US region of origin/neighborhood.* Rural, urban, or suburban? Safety and access to resources in the community?
4. *Immigration history (if applicable).* This would include years in the USA and years educated in the USA, as well as any relevant sociopolitical issues related to immigration.
5. *Linguistic background.* For linguistic minorities, questions about language of origin, how often a patient uses English versus the language of origin (and in which contexts), their ease with the respective languages, and preference for testing are all potentially useful areas of inquiry. Comprehensive discussion about this issue is beyond the scope of this chapter. For more information, readers are referred elsewhere [5, 76, 81, 90].
6. *Quality of education.* Tests of reading level (such as WTAR and WRAT-4) are helpful to disentangle quality of education issues. Further, questions regarding patient's type of school and classroom experience, as well as geographic region are helpful in this regard.
7. *Social support.* This may include questions about both biological and nonbiological family, church-related and spiritual resources, and other potential, nontraditional resources (e.g., community organizations).
8. *Current and childhood SES and nutrition.* This may include questions about having enough to eat and financial resources at present and during childhood.
9. *Access and utilization of health and mental-health services.* Beyond health insurance, this may include questions about healthcare access and perceived quality, attitudes about traditional and nontraditional health and mental-health services and providers, and health literacy.

Informants

When obtaining collateral information on older patients, it is important to gather reports from a reliable source (e.g., a cognitively intact caregiver, child, or spouse), as older adults may not be reliable historians if they are experiencing memory or executive dysfunction. Among patients with mild cognitive impairment (MCI), some research shows that African American informants may be more likely to under-report the patient's symptoms or functioning, while non-Hispanic white informants may be more likely to over-report [91]. However, anecdotally, one investigator reported that in his clinical experience with Mexican American patients with dementia, many of his patients' children were hesitant to report their parent's cognitive or functional decline, despite having observed such declines [92]. He noted that the children were only willing to report these observations after lengthy interview when rapport had been well established, and many apologized to their parent prior to reporting their observations. This example demonstrates the powerful potential impact of culture on the interview process, and clinicians should consider that reporting deficits may be uncomfortable or culturally inappropriate for many informants and patients [93]. Therefore, rapport building and culturally sensitive but thorough interviewing is imperative.

Testing Considerations

Socioculturally, many ethnic minority elders may be less familiar with assessment procedures than elders from majority culture [94, 95]. They may also have misperceptions about or be wary of the assessment process, so it is important that the neuropsychologist clarify the purpose of the evaluation and make sure that instructions are understood. For example, it may be useful to explain test format or when speeded performance is being assessed, as these constructs may be unfamiliar or carry different valence to certain ethnic minority older patients [95, 96]. Thus, it is critical to clearly explain the purpose of the neuropsychological evaluation to the individual—making sure to avoid using jargon, and to explain aspects of the testing that may be unfamiliar or are particularly important for the patient to understand. In addition, as noted earlier, if there is any deviation from standardized testing procedure, it should be noted in the report and considered in the final interpretation of the data.

Neuropsychological Test and Normative Data Selection

According to APA Ethical Standard 9.02b [70], "psychologists use assessment instruments whose validity and reliability have been established for use with members of the population tested." Therefore, neuropsychologists have an ethical responsibility to use appropriate and non-biased assessment instruments whenever they are available. However, relatively few neuropsychological tests have been specifically standardized and validated with culturally diverse samples. Therefore, it is often unclear how performance may vary with cultural background and whether or not the intended construct is appropriately assessed [68]. Whenever possible, neuropsychologists should use tests that have been normed and validated with individuals from the same cultural background as the patient being evaluated.

Screening Instruments

In terms of screening instruments, there are some cross-cultural assessments for dementia available, including the Rowland Universal Dementia Assessment Scale (RUDAS) [97]. Moreover, in screening general cognitive abilities, Wolfe [98] suggested that the Cognitive Abilities Screening Instrument (CASI) [99] be used in place of the Mini-Mental Status Exam (MMSE), since it has been culturally validated in Japan, China, and the USA, or the Cross-Cultural Cognitive Examination (CCCE) [100], which was developed in Guam and may be particularly useful for individuals with low literacy. Additional brief screening instruments, which have been used for detecting possible dementia among ethnically diverse older adults, include both a measure for patients (i.e., the Taussig Cross-Cultural

Memory Test), [101] and informants (i.e., the Informant Questionnaire on Cognitive Decline in the Elderly, also known as IQCODE) [102].

English Language Tests and Normative Data

A key aspect of determining which neuropsychological tests to administer often lies in the availability and appropriateness of the relevant normative data. Demographically corrected normative data that can be used with English-speaking ethnic minority elders are available for some neuropsychological batteries and tests. Heaton et al. [103] provide excellent normative data (corrected for age, education, gender, and race/ethnicity) on the expanded Halstead-Reitan battery for non-Hispanic white and African American adults up to age 85. The WAIS-IV and WMS-IV provide normative data (corrected for age, education, gender, and race/ethnicity) for non-Hispanic white, African American, and Latino adults up to age 90 [104]. As mentioned earlier, Dotson et al. [89] provide literacy-based normative data (corrected for age, gender, and WRAT-3 Reading Total Score) for African American adults up to age 64, for the following tests: California Verbal Learning Test, Benton Visual Retention Test (5th ed.), COWAT Animal Fluency, Card Rotation Test, Brief Test of Attention, Digit Span, Trail Making Test, and Identical Pictures. A particular weakness in the literature is the paucity of normative data available for English-speaking Asian-American/Pacific Islander and Latino elders. One notable exception is Kempler et al.'s [105] normative data (corrected for age, education, and race/ethnicity) for verbal fluency measures, which provide norms for non-Hispanic white, African American, Latino, and Asian American adults up to age 99.

Non-English Language Tests and Normative Data

For linguistic minorities, it is important to note that use of nonverbal measures does not mitigate the impact of linguistic and cultural differences on neuropsychological measures. These tests contain verbal instructions and may still involve verbally mediated approaches. Even when this is not the case, nonverbal measures are still culturally laden and interpretation may be limited if they have not been validated with culturally diverse samples. For example, research has shown that healthy Spanish-speaking elders performed significantly worse on several visuospatial and visuoconstructional tasks compared to their non-Hispanic white peers [40]. Therefore, the use of well-validated, empirically supported, and linguistically appropriate neuropsychological tests or batteries for linguistic minority individuals is essential.

Although this overview is certainly not exhaustive, herein we provide resources that we believe would be useful for those working with older ethnic minority individuals. In the case of Spanish-speaking older adults, there are a number of available batteries that may be appropriate for this population, including La Batería Neuropsicológica en Español [76], the NEUROPSI [106], the Batería-III Woodcock-Muñoz [107], Woodcock-Muñoz Language Survey-Revised [108], the Neuropsychological Screening Battery for Latinos (NeSBHIS) [109], and the Spanish and English Neuropsychological Assessment Scales (SENAS) [110].

In addition, the Canadian Study of Health and Aging (CSHA) neuropsychological test battery provides English and French versions of their tests, along with normative data [111]. What is notable about both the SENAS and the CSHA batteries is that they utilized statistical modeling methods to test the cultural equivalence (i.e., invariant structures) of their respective batteries in their dual respective languages. Both Mungas et al. [110] and Tuokko et al. [111] provide empirical support for the cross-linguistic construct validity of their respective neuropsychological batteries utilizing state-of-the-art statistical modeling. (e.g., item response theory (IRT) techniques to reduce test bias and covariance structure analysis [112] in the case of the SENAS battery and a relatively straightforward multi-group confirmatory factor analysis (CFA) framework in the case of the CSHA battery.) These approaches represent promising methodologies for examining the construct validity (via measurement invariance) of other neuropsychological instruments across a variety of ethnic and linguistic groups [69, 110, 111, 113].

For Mandarin-speaking older adults, Hsieh and Tori [114] provide normative data on cross-cultural neuropsychological tests across the life span (up to age 81). For Korean-speaking older adults, there is a Korean version of the California Verbal Learning Test (K-CVLT) [115] available, which provides norms correcting for ages 20–79.

While the resources available for examining ethnic minority elders have significantly improved over the course of the past 20 years, several important limitations merit discussion. First, only two neuropsychological batteries (of which we are aware) provide rigorous empirical support for their cultural equivalence and construct validity (the SENAS and the CHSA). Providing such support is important not only in the case of tests or batteries utilized in different languages but also for tests and batteries utilized across different ethnic groups [68]. The absence of this research remains a significant weakness in the discipline. Second, no comprehensive batteries or norms exist for adequately characterized English-speaking Latinos; Spanish-speakers who are *not* from Spain, Mexico, or of Mexican-American origin; Asian Americans (including Native Hawaiians, Pacific Islanders, and South Asians); American Indians or Alaska Natives; persons from Middle-Eastern backgrounds; and bilinguals. For a more comprehensive discussion of these issues, see Rivera Mindt et al. [13]. Third and perhaps most importantly, use of race/ethnicity-based norms do not explain performance differences between groups and may inadvertently leave unexplained racial/ethnic differences in neuropsychological test performance open to harmful misinterpretation [13, 116, 117].

Sociocultural Testing Issues

Culture and Acculturation

As noted above, neuropsychologists should inquire about patient-specific cultural background (e.g., is the patient/patient's family from the Dominican Republic, Puerto Rico, Cuba, etc.). They should also ascertain the individual's degree of acculturation to majority US culture. For instance, when assessing a Latino patient, one should determine their birthplace and the birthplace of the parents. This will help guide the selection of appropriate tests, norms, and interpreters (if needed). For example, in the case of Spanish language tests, the neuropsychologist should consider the country where the test was developed, particularly in regard to language and dialect—a test developed in Puerto Rico may contain colloquialisms unfamiliar to a patient from Mexico [118]. Further discussion of the issue can be found elsewhere [13, 59, 81, 109].

For Latino patients, formal assessments of level of acculturation are available and should be completed. As described in a recent position paper from the National Academy of Neuropsychology [78], the following measures can be used to assess acculturation: Acculturation Rating Scale for Mexican Americans-II [119], the Bidimensional Acculturation Scale for Hispanics [120], and Short Acculturation Scale for Hispanics [121]. The abbreviated multidimensional acculturation scale (AMAS) is also a well-validated tool, which assesses both Latino and US American identity and acculturation [122]. Unlike other acculturation instruments, which largely used Mexican-American or Puerto Rican standardization samples, the AMAS utilized a heterogeneous Latino sample that included individuals of Central and South American, Caribbean, and Mexican origins. For other ethnic groups, where standardized measures of acculturation are not available, language use (English versus language of origin) and years in the USA have been shown to serve as proxies of acculturation [61, 123, 124].

The practical application of acculturation information to the interpretation of neuropsychological test data is limited by the lack of formalized algorithms or normative data that incorporate acculturation level. However, research indicates that lower levels of acculturation to majority culture are associated with worse neuropsychological test performance, particularly in the areas of abstraction/executive functioning, attention, working memory, language, visuoconstruction, learning, and memory [37, 60–62, 92, 125–127]. Therefore, neuropsychologists should consider the *potential* contribution of acculturation level when impaired scores are present in these areas among ethnic minority older patients with low acculturation levels.

Bilingual Older Adults

When evaluating a bilingual older patient, test selection also involves several specific considerations. Factors that should be considered include (1) which language is the individual's first or native language, or did they learn both languages simultaneously? If they did not, at what age was the second language acquired? (2) Which language is currently their primary language? What is their degree of bilingualism (e.g., balanced bilingual, English-dominant bilingual, Spanish-dominant bilingual, etc.)? It may also be important to consider how many years of formal education the individual completed in their primary language. Rivera Mindt et al. [5] should be consulted for further discussion of these issues. Briefly, individuals should be tested in their most competent (e.g., strongest or primary) language whenever possible and appropriate. Ideally, language competency should be determined on the basis of both objective language measurement and subjective report, although it is also important to note that older individuals are more likely to underestimate their language fluency [5, 66]. Some objective measures for assessing Spanish–English language dominance include the Woodcock-Muñoz Language Survey-Revised and examination of the difference in performance between the English and Spanish versions of verbal fluency or naming measures [5]. Care should be taken to select tests that have been standardized and normed with the population and language of interest, whenever possible.

Awareness of the bilingualism literature can further aid in interpreting the neuropsychological test performance of bilingual ethnic minority elders, especially given the lack of normative data for this population. Research has generally shown a robust bilingual disadvantage in terms of performance on verbal measures when compared with monolinguals (who can be viewed as *hyperproficient* in their language) [66]. Specifically, bilinguals may perform worse in expressive vocabulary [128], receptive vocabulary (including response latency times) [129], and verbal fluency (particularly semantic) [130, 131]. In contrast, there are subtle bilingual advantages on measures of attention/executive functioning, particularly cognitive control, and these advantages may confer some neuroprotection in the face of normal cognitive aging and Alzheimer's disease [64, 132]. These disadvantages and advantages should be considered when interpreting test data of bilingual older adults, and should be explicitly discussed in reports. For a thorough review of the neuropsychological implications of bilingualism, see Rivera Mindt et al. [5].

Qualitative Information

For some ethnic minority patients for whom a standard evaluation may not be appropriate because of language or other cultural limitations, a process approach may be useful [133, 134] in estimating level of neuropsychological abilities. This provides qualitative information by examining the types of errors the patient makes, their approach to the tests, and their response to testing limits. For example, one may allow a patient to continue past the standard time limit on a test, such as *Block Design*. Although points would not be awarded for a response given after the specified amount of time, this would allow the examiner to assess whether or not the patient's difficulty is due to time constraints.

Post-evaluation Considerations

Upon completion of the neuropsychological evaluation, which has been conducted in a culturally competent manner, using the best available tests, the results must be examined and interpreted. There are several factors that must be considered, including which norms to apply to tests and caveats that limit test interpretation.

Neuropsychologists should consider their use of race/ethnicity-based norms depending on the situation and the referral question. For example, as Brickman et al. [80] point out, "comparing test scores from a highly educated African American man from New York City to an African American normative data set collected in the rural South might not be appropriate." Additionally, one should consider whether the goal of the referral question is to determine how well the individual is likely to be functioning in their environment, or whether the goal is to determine whether decline is suspected relative to peers. In the first instance, race–ethnicity-based norms would likely be inappropriate, while in the second instance, they may be more appropriate [135].

Next, neuropsychologists must incorporate and synthesize the sociocultural information collected during the clinical interview, history, and throughout the evaluation into the test interpretation and case conceptualization. This can be accomplished utilizing an empirically based, hypothesis testing approach grounded in the quantitative and qualitative data gathered during the evaluation. How does this converging evidence point to a particular conclusion and how does this fit (or does not) with the existing empirical literature? Equally important, it is recommended that neuropsychologists explicitly discuss in the report how the sociocultural data from the evaluation and the empirical literature factored into the test interpretation, case conceptualization, diagnosis, and recommendations.

Careful consideration should also be taken to avoid over-interpreting low performance that may be attributed, at least in part, to sociocultural factors. For example, if a test has been shown to have cultural biases, but is administered because a more appropriate alternative does not exist, the neuropsychologist should be sure to include this information in the report and to limit any conclusions drawn from these scores. For bilingual patients, Ardila et al. [136] recommend explicitly noting in the report the language the patient was tested in, formal documentation of the patient's degree of bilingualism, and whether or not an interpreter was used. In terms of differential diagnosis and the recommendations for ethnic minority older adults, it is also especially important to consider the possible influence of other factors (i.e., comorbid medical or psychiatric conditions, SES, access to care, etc.). In bringing together all of the information, including the sociocultural information, it is hoped that neuropsychologists will be better able to improve diagnostic accuracy and develop more relevant, culturally tailored recommendations for their ethnic minority older patients.

Finally, in terms of providing feedback, attention to the same sociocultural norms and communication issues (clear, jargon-free language) also apply to this "final" aspect of the neuropsychological evaluation (see section "Establishing and Maintaining Rapport"). The critical goals of the feedback session are (1) that the patient, or her/his family member, or caregiver understand the pertinent test findings and follow-up recommendations; (2) that the neuropsychologist confirms that these recommendations are appropriate and feasible for the patient; and (3) that the neuropsychologist maintains a stance of respect, flexibility, creativity, and advocacy to modify the recommendations if needed and to help advocate on behalf of the patient, if necessary, to ensure appropriate follow-up. For a more thorough discussion regarding the provision of feedback, the reader is referred elsewhere [137, 138].

Final Thoughts

Given the paucity of empirically based and practical resources that are specifically targeted toward serving ethnic minority older adults in neuropsychology, this chapter reviewed sociocultural issues germane to this population and discussed considerations for the culturally competent evaluation of older ethnic minority adults. Overall, a number of factors must be considered to provide a competent neuropsychological evaluation with ethnic minority individuals, and neuropsychologists are reminded to maintain a "sociocultural lens" throughout each step of the evaluation.

Specifically, neuropsychologists must first consider whether or not they have the appropriate training and experience to conduct a competent evaluation with a given ethnic minority elder. Neuropsychologists should consider the influence that cultural factors may play in patient self-report, informant report, and expression of symptoms. The neuropsychologist should be culturally sensitive during the evaluation, including in the selection of appropriate tests and norms, and in the manner in which they interact with the patient and her/his family members or caregivers from the clinical interview until the feedback session. While the focus of this chapter has been ethnic minority older adults, much of this information may also be relevant for nontraditional, older populations including those from rural or low socioeconomic backgrounds.

Clinical Pearls

- Remember to maintain a "sociocultural lens" and to be mindful of potential sociocultural norms throughout the evaluation, from the clinical interview to the feedback session.
- In working with informants of ethnic minority elders, be cognizant that there may be hesitance to report the cognitive or functional decline of a loved one, despite having observed such declines. Such reticence may be reduced through taking the time to establish solid rapport.
- Utilize the best available neuropsychological instruments and norms and acknowledge the potential limitations in the interpretation section of your neuropsychological report.
- Consult literature regularly for recent developments in measures and norms.
- Carefully evaluate the psychometric appropriateness of tests under consideration, particularly if the patient is bilingual.
- Consider the purpose of the evaluation (diagnostic or descriptive) and whether race/ethnicity corrected norms are indicated.
- Gather as much sociocultural information as possible (i.e., acculturation, quality of education, linguistic background, etc.) to best contextualize the neuropsychological findings.
- For non-English speaking elders or those from ethnic groups for which the neuropsychologist does not feel competent to examine, refer to a neuropsychologist who has expertise with the population or consult with such a neuropsychologist when referring out is not feasible.
- Use an interpreter when outside referral is not feasible. Only use professional interpreters (not children of patients, hospital staff, or other nonprofessionals) [5].
- Consider psychometric characteristics to determine how "low" scores should be interpreted to avoid misdiagnosis and mismanagement of neurocognitive disorders.
- Suggest longitudinal assessments to better disentangle the impact of sociocultural factors versus neurodegenerative processes.
- Explicitly state the normative data sets used within the report, if different from the manual, and discuss any limitations to the interpretability of the data based on these norms.
- Be careful not to erroneously attribute problems to cultural or linguistic issues.
- Consider the whole person, including their sociocultural context, in the development and communication of recommendations.
- Become actively involved in advancing your own cultural competence, as well as that of our field (see Rivera Mindt et al. [13] for resources).

Acknowledgements The authors wish to thank Ms. Franchesca Arias, MA for her assistance with this manuscript. Supported by grant K23MH079718 (to MRM) from the National Institutes of Health.

References

1. Heron MP, Hoyert DL, Xu J, Scott C, Tejada-Vera B. Deaths: preliminary data for 2006. Natl Vital Stat Rep. 2008;56(16):1–50.
2. US Census Bureau News. (2010, May 20). Aging population: aging boomers will increase dependency ratio, census bureau projects. Retrieved from http://www.census.gov/newsroom/releases/archives/aging_population/cb10-72.html.
3. US Census Bureau News. (2008, Aug. 14). Press releases: an older and more diverse nation by midcentury. http://www.census.gov/Press. http://www.census.gov/newsroom/releases/archives/population/cb08-123.html.
4. Robnett RH, Chop WC. Gerontology for the health care professional. Sudbury: Jones & Bartlett; 2010.
5. Rivera Mindt M, Arentoft A, Kubo Germano K, D'Aquila E, Scheiner D, Pizzirusso M, Sandoval TC, Gollan T. Neuropsychological, cognitive, and theoretical considerations for the evaluation of bilingual individuals. Neuropsychol Rev. 2008;18(3):255–68.
6. Bentacourt H, Lopez ER. The study of culture, ethnicity, and race in American psychology. Am Psychol. 1993;48:629–37.
7. Okazaki S, Sue S. Methodological issues in assessment research with ethnic minorities. Psychol Assess. 1995;7(3):367–75.

8. Phinney JS. When we talk about American ethnic groups, what do we mean? Am Psychol. 1996;51: 918–27.
9. Ardila A. Cultural values underlying psychometric cognitive testing. Neuropsychol Rev. 2005;15(4): 185–95. doi:10.1007/s11065-005-9180-y.
10. Byrd D, Miller S, Reilly J, Weber S, Wall ST, Heaton R. Early environmental factors, ethnicity, and adult cognitive test performance. Clin Neuropsychol. 2006;20:243–60.
11. Dotson VM, Kitner-Triolo M, Evans MK, Zonderman AB. Effects of race and socioeconomic status on the relative influence of education and literacy on cognitive functioning. J Int Neuropsychol Soc. 2009;15:580–9.
12. Manly JJ. Critical issues in cultural neuropsychology: profit from diversity. Neuropsychol Rev. 2008;18:179–83.
13. Rivera Mindt M, Byrd D, Saez P, Manly J. Increasing culturally competent neuropsychological services for ethnic minority populations: a call to action. Clin Neuropsychol. 2010;24:429–53.
14. Schwartz BS, Glass TA, Bolla KI, Stewart WF, Glass G, Rasmussen M, Bressler J, Shi W, Bandeen-Roche K. Disparities in cognitive functioning by race/ethnicity in the Baltimore Memory Study. Environ Health Perspect. 2004;112(3):314–20.
15. Minority Health and Health Disparities Research and Education Act of 2000. Public Law 106-525, S. 1880, 2000. p. 2498.
16. Richardson LD, Babcock Irvin C, Tamayo-Sarver JH. Racial and ethnic disparities in the clinical practice of emergency medicine. Acad Emerg Med. 2003;10:1184–8. doi:10.1197/S1069-6563(03)00487-1.
17. Cargill VA, Stone VE. HIV/AIDS: a minority health issue. Med Clin N Am. 2005;89:895–912.
18. Fiscella K, Franks P, Gold MR, Clancy CM. Inequality in quality: addressing socioeconomic, racial, and ethnic disparities in health care. J Am Med Assoc. 2000;283:2579–84.
19. US Census Bureau. Press release CB07-FF, Facts for features: (2007, July 16). Hispanic Heritage Month: Sep 15–Oct 15. www.census.gov/newsroom/releases/pdf/cb07-ff14.pdf.
20. Centers for Disease Control. (2007, June 6). About minority health. http://www.cdc.gov/omhd/AMH/AMH.htm.
21. Fitten LJ, Ortiz F, Ponton M. Frequency of Alzheimer's disease and other dementias in a community outreach sample of Hispanics. J Am Geriatr Soc. 2001;10:1301–8.
22. von Strauss E, Fratiglioni L, Viitanen M, Forsell Y, Winblad B. Morbidity and comorbidity in relation to functional status: a community-based study of the oldest old (90+ years). J Am Geriatr Soc. 2000; 48(11):1462–9.
23. Husaini BA, Sherkat DE, Moonis M, Levine R, Holzer C, Cain VA. Racial differences in the diagnosis of dementia and in its effects on the use and costs of health care services. Psychiatr Serv. 2003;54(1): 92–6.
24. Kuller LH, Lopez OL, Jagust WJ, Becker JT, DeKosky ST, Lyketsos C, Kawas C, Breitner JC, Fitzpatrick A, Dulberg C. Determinants of vascular dementia in the Cardiovascular Health Cognition Study. Neurology. 2005;64(9):1548–52.
25. Livney MG, Clark CM, Karlawish JH, Cartmell S, Negrón M, Nuñez J, Xie SX, Entenza-Cabrera F, Vega IE, Arnold SE. Ethnoracial differences in the clinical characteristics of alzheimer's disease at initial presentation at an urban alzheimer's disease center. Am J Geriatr Psychiatry. 2011;19(5):430–9.
26. Clark CM, DeCarli C, Mungas D, Chui HI, Higdon R, Nuñez J, Fernandez H, Negrón M, Manly J, Ferris S, Perez A, Torres M, Ewbank D, Glosser G, van Belle G. Arch Neurol. 2005;62(5):774–8.
27. Froehlich TE, Bogardus ST, Inouye SK. Dementia and race: are there differences between African Americans and Caucasians? J Am Geriatr Soc. 2001; 49:477–84.
28. Flaskerud JH. Dementia, ethnicity, and culture. Issues Ment Health Nurs. 2009;30(8):522–3.
29. Chiu HEK, Zhang M. Dementia Research in China. Int J Geriatr Psychiatry. 2000;15:947–53.
30. National Institutes of Health. (2010, Oct.). Fact Sheet—Health Disparities. http://report.nih.gov/NIHfactsheets/ViewFactSheet.aspx?csid=124.
31. Dodani S. Excess coronary artery disease risk in South Asian immigrants: can dysfunctional high-density lipoprotein explain increased risk? J Vasc Health Risk Manag. 2008;4:953–61.
32. Gallant MP, Spitze G, Groove JG. Chronic illness delf-care and the family lives of older adults: a synthetic review across four ethnic groups. J Cross Cult Gerontol. 2010;25(1):21–43.
33. Office of Minority Health, US Department of Health and Human Services. (2007, Dec. 7). Minority health disparities at a glance. http://minorityhealth.hhs.gov/templates/content.aspx?ID=2139.
34. Reitz C, Patel B, Tang M, Manly J, Mayeux R, Luchsinger JA. J Neurol Sci. 2007;257(1–2):194–201.
35. Rilling LM, Lucas JA, Ivnik RJ, Smith GE, Willis FB, Ferman TJ, Petersen RC, Graff-Radford NR. Mayo's older African American normative studies: norms for the mattis dementia rating scale. Clin Neuropsychol. 2005;19(2):229–42.
36. Evans JD, Miller SW, Byrd DA, Heaton RK. Cross-cultural applications of the Halstead-Reitan batteries. In: Fletcher-Janzen E, Strickland TL, Reynolds CR, editors. Handbook of cross-cultural neuropsychology. New York: Springer; 2000. p. 287–303.
37. Arnold BR, Montgomery GT, Castaneda I, Longoria R. Acculturation and performance of Hispanics on selected Halstead-Reitan neuropsychological tests. Assessment. 1994;1:239–48.
38. Gladsjo JA, Evans JD, Schuman CC, Peavy GM, Miller SW, Heaton RK. Norms for letter and category fluency: demographic corrections for age, education, and ethnicity. Assessment. 1999;6:147–78.

39. Heaton RK, Taylor M, Manly J. Demographic effects and demographically corrected norms with the WAIS-III and WMS-III. In: Tulsky DS, Saklofske DH, Chelune GJ, Heaton RK, Ivnik RJ, Bornstein R, Prifitera A, Ledbetter M, editors. Clinical interpretation of the WAIS-III and WMS-III. San Diego: Academic; 2003. p. 181–210.
40. Jacobs DM, Sano M, Albert S, Schofield P, Dooneief G, Stern Y. Cross-cultural neuropsychological assessment: a comparison of randomly selected, demographically matched cohorts of English- and Spanish-speaking older adults. J Clin Exp Neuropsychol. 1997;19:331–9.
41. Longobardi P, Cummings J, Anderson-Hanley C. Multicultural perspectives on the neuropsychological and neuropsychiatric assessment and treatment of the elderly. In: Fletcher-Janzen E, Strickland TL, Reynolds CR, editors. Handbook of cross-cultural neuropsychology. New York: Springer; 2000. p. 123–42.
42. Lowenstein DA, Duara R, Arguelles T, Arguelles S. Use of the fuld object-memory evaluation in the detection of mild dementia among Spanish- and English-speaking groups. Am J Geriatr Psychiatry. 1995;3:300–7.
43. Manly JJ, Jacobs DM, Sano M, Bell K, Merchant CA, Small SA, Stern Y. Neurocognitive test performance among non-demented elderly African Americans and Whites. Neurology. 1998;50:1238–45.
44. Stricks L, Pittman J, Jacobs D, Sano M, Stern Y. Normative data for a brief neuropsychological battery administered to English- and Spanish-speaking community-dwelling elders. J Int Neuropsychol Soc. 1998;4:311–8.
45. Adams RL, Boake C, Crain C. Bias in a neuropsychological test classification related to education, age, and ethnicity. J Consult Clin Psychol. 1982;50:143–5. doi:10.1037/0022-006X.50.1.143.
46. Diehr MC, Cherner M, Wolfson TJ, Miller SW, Grant I, Heaton RK. The 50 and 100-item short forms of the Paced Auditory Serial Addition Task (PASAT): demographically corrected norms and comparisons with the full PASAT in normal and clinical samples. J Clin Exp Neuropsychol. 2003; 25:571–85.
47. Taylor MJ, Heaton RK. Sensitivity and specificity of WAIS-III/WMS-III demographically corrected factor scores in neuropsychological assessment. J Int Neuropsychol Soc. 2001;7:867–74.
48. Klusman LE, Moulton JM, Hornbostel LK, Picano JJ, Beattie MT. Neuropsychological abnormalities in asymptomatic HIV seropositive military personnel. J Neuropsychiatry Clin Neurosci. 1992;3:422–8.
49. Manly JJ, Jacobs DM, Sano M, Bell K, Merchant CA, Small SA, et al. Cross-cultural comparison of neuropsychological test performance and diagnosis of dementia. Neurology. 1998;50:91.
50. Norman MA, Evans JD, Miller WS, Heaton RK. Demographically corrected norms for the california verbal learning test. J Clin Exp Neuropsychol. 2000;22:80–94.
51. Bohnstedt M, Fox PJ, Kohatsu ND. Correlates of mini-mental status examination scores among elderly demented patients: the influence of race-ethnicity. J Clin Epidemiol. 1994;47:1381–7.
52. Gurland BJ, Wilder DE, Cross P, Teresi J, Barrett VW. Screening scales for dementia: toward reconciliation of conflicting cross-cultural findings. Int J Geriatr Psychiatry. 1992;7:105–13.
53. Mungas D, Marshall SC, Weldon M, Haan M, Reed BR. Age and education correction of mini-mental state examination for English and Spanish-speaking elderly. Neurology. 1996;46:700–6.
54. Patton D, Duff K, Schoenberg M, Mold J, Scott J, Adams R. Performance of cognitively normal African Americans on the RBANS in community dwelling older adults. Clin Neuropsychol. 2003;17:515–30.
55. Welsh KA, Fillenbaum G, Wilkinson W, Heyman A, Mohs RC, Stern Y, Harrell L, Edland SD, Beekly D. Neuropsychological test performance in African-American and white patients with Alzheimer's disease. Neurology. 1995;45:2207–11.
56. Whitfield KE, Weidner G, Clark R, Anderson NB. Sociodemographic diversity and behavioral medicine. J Consult Clin Psychol. 2002;70(3):463–81.
57. Manly JJ, Jacobs DM, Touradji P, Small SA, Stern Y. Reading level attenuates differences in neuropsychological test performance between African American and white elders. J Int Neuropsychol Soc. 2002;8:341–8.
58. Manly JJ, Touradji P, Tang MX, Stern Y. Literacy and memory decline among ethnically diverse elders. J Clin Exp Neuropsychol. 2003;25:680–90.
59. Rivera Mindt M, Byrd D, Ryan E, Robbins R, Monzones J, Arentoft A, Kubo Germano K, Henninger D, Morgello S, for the Manhattan HIV Brain Bank. Characterization and sociocultural predictors of neuropsychological test performance in HIV+ Hispanic individuals. Cultur Divers Ethnic Minor Psychol. 2008;14(4):315–25.
60. Manly JJ, Jacobs DM, Sano M, Bell K, Merchant CA, Small SA, Stern Y. African American acculturation and neuropsychological test performance among nondemented community elders. J Int Neuropsychol Soc. 1998;4:77.
61. Harris JG, Tulsky DS, Schultheis MT. Assessment of the non-native English speaker: assimilating history and research findings to guide clinical practice. In: Tulsky DS, Saklofske DH, Chelune GJ, Heaton RK, Ivnik RJ, Bornstein R, Prifitera A, Ledbetter M, editors. Clinical interpretation of the WAIS-III and WMS-III. San Diego: Academic; 2003. p. 343–87.
62. Kennepohl K, Douglas S, Nabors N, Hanks R. African American acculturation and neuropsychological test performance following traumatic brain injury. J Int Neuropsychol Soc. 2004;10:566–77.
63. Bialystok E, Craik FIM. Bilingualism and naming: implications for cognitive assessment. J Int Neuropsychol Soc. 2007;13:209–11.
64. Bialystok E, Craik FIM, Freedman M. Bilingualism as a protection against the onset of symptoms of dementia. Neuropsychologia. 2007;45:459–64.

65. Bialystok E, Craik FIM, Ruocco AC. Dual-modality monitoring in a classification task: the effects of bilingualism and ageing. Q J Exp Psychol. 2006;26: 1968–83.
66. Gollan T, Montoya R, Cera C, Sandoval T. More use almost always means a smaller frequency effect: aging, bilingualism, and the weaker links hypothesis. J Mem Lang. 2008;58:787–814.
67. Steele CM, Aronson J. Stereotype threat and the intellectual test performance of African Americans. J Pers Soc Psychol. 1995;69:797–811.
68. Helms JE. Why is there no study of cultural equivalence in standardized cognitive ability testing? Am Psychol. 1992;47:1083–101.
69. Teresi JA, Holmes D, Ramírez M. Performance of cognitive tests among different racial/ethnic and education groups: findings of differential item functioning and possible item bias. J Ment Health Aging. 2001;7(1):79–89.
70. American Psychological Association. Ethical principles of psychologists and code of conduct. Am Psychol. 2002;57:1060–73.
71. American Psychological Association. Guidelines for multicultural education, training, research, practice, and organizational change for psychologists. Am Psychol. 2003;58:377–402.
72. Sue DW. Multidimensional facets of cultural competence. Counsel Psychol. 2001;29:790–821.
73. Sue DW, Arredondo P, McDavis RJ. Multicultural competencies/standards: a pressing need. J Counsel Dev. 1992;70:477–86.
74. Sue DW, Carter RT, Casas JM, Fouad NA, Ivey AE, Jensen M, LaFromboise T, Manese JE, Ponterotto JG, Vasquez-Nuttall E. Multicultural counseling competencies: individual and organizational development. Thousand Oaks: Sage; 1998.
75. Wong TM, Strickland TL, Fletcher-Janzen E, Ardila A, Reynolds CR. Theoretical and practical issues in the neuropsychological assessment and treatment of culturally dissimilar patients. In: Fletcher-Janzen E, Strickland TL, Reynolds CR, editors. The handbook of cross cultural neuropsychology. New York: Kluwer-Plenum; 2000. p. 3–18.
76. Artiola i Fortuny L, Mullaney HA. Assessing patients whose language you do not know: can the absurd be ethical? Clin Neuropsychol. 1998;12:113–26.
77. Artiola i Fortuny L, Garolera M, Hermosillo Romo D, Feldman E, Fernandez Barillas H, Keefe R, et al. Research with Spanish-speaking populations in the United States: lost in translation a commentary and a plea. J Clin Exp Neuropsychol. 2005; 27:555–64.
78. Judd T, Capetillo D, Carrión-Baralt J, Mármol LM, San Miguel-Montes L, Navarrete MG, Silver CH. Professional considerations for improving the neuropsychological evaluation of hispanics: A National Academy of Neuropsychology education paper. Arch Clin Neuropsychol. 2009;24(2):127–35.
79. American Psychological Association. Guidelines for providers of psychological services to ethnic, linguistic, and culturally diverse populations. Am Psychol. 1993;48:45–8.
80. Brickman AM, Cabo R, Manly JJ. Ethical issues in cross-cultural neuropsychology. Appl Neuropsychol. 2006;13(2):91–100.
81. Llorente AM. Principles of neuropsychological assessment with Hispanics: theoretical foundations and clinical practice. New York: Springer; 2007.
82. Shiraev E, Levy DA. Cross-cultural psychology: critical thinking and contemporary applications. 4th ed. Boston: Allyn & Bacon; 2010.
83. Sue DW, Sue D. Counseling the culturally different: theory and practice. New York: Wiley; 1990.
84. Schnall E. Multicultural counseling and the Orthodox Jew. J Counsel Dev. 2006;84:276–82.
85. Jackson Y. Encyclopedia of multicultural psychology. Thousand Oaks: Sage; 2006.
86. Weiss M. Explanatory model interview catalogue (EMIC): framework for comparative study of illness. Transcult Psychiatry. 1997;34:235–63.
87. Lewis-Fernandez R, Das AK, Alfonso C, Weissman MM, Olfson M. Depression in US Hispanics: diagnostic and management considerations in family practice. J Am Board Fam Pract. 2005;18:282–96.
88. Gotlib IH, Hammen CL. Handbook of depression. New York: Guilford; 2002.
89. Dotson VM, Kitner-Triolo M, Evans MK, Zonderman AB. Literacy-based normative data for low socioeconomic status African American. Clin Neuropsychol. 2008;22:989–1017.
90. Pontón M. Research and assessment issues with Hispanic populations. In: Pontón M, León-Carrión J, editors. Neuropsychology and the Hispanic patient: a clinical handbook. Mahwah: Erlbaum; 2001. p. 39–58.
91. Potter GG, Plassman BL, Burke JR, Kabeto MU, Langa KM, Llewellyn DJ, Rogers MA, Steffens DC. Cognitive performance and informant reports in the diagnosis of cognitive impairment and dementia in African Americans and whites. Alzheimers Dement. 2009;5(6):445–53.
92. O'Bryant S. Exploring the relationship between culture and cognition. J Clin Exp Neuropsychol. 2008;30(8):967–70.
93. Millet PE, Sullivan BF, Schwebel AI, Myers LJ. Black Americans' and White Americans' views of the etiology and treatment of mental health problems. Community Ment Health J. 1996;32:235–42.
94. Poreh A. Neuropsychological and psychological issues associated with cross-cultural and minority assessment. In: Ferraro RF, editor. Minority and cross-cultural aspects of neuropsychological assessment. Studies on neuropsychology, development, and cognition. Bristol: Swets & Zeitlinger; 2002. p. 329–43.
95. Echemendia RJ, Julian L. Neuropsychological assessment of Latino children. In: Ferraro FR, editor. Minority and cross-cultural aspects of neuropsychological assessment. Lisse: Swets & Zeitlinger; 2002. p. 182–203.
96. Perez-Arce P. The influence of culture on cognition. Arch Clin Neuropsychol. 1999;14(7):581–92.

97. Storey JE, Rowand JTJ, Conforti DA, Dickson HG. The rowland universal dementia assessment scale (RUDAS): a multicultural cognitive assessment scale. Int Psychogeriatr. 2004;16:13–31.
98. Wolfe N. Cross-cultural neuropsychology of aging and dementia: an update. In: Ferraro FR, editor. Minority and cross-cultural aspects of neuropsychological assessment. Bristol: Swets & Zeitlinger; 2002. p. 285–97.
99. Teng LE, Hasegawa K, Homma A, Imai Y, Larson E, Graves A, Sugimoto K, Yamaguchi T, Sasaki H, Chiu D, White LR. The cognitive abilities screening instrument (CASI): a practical test for cross-cultural epidemiological studies of dementia. Int J Psychogeriatr. 1994;6:45–58.
100. Glosser G, Wolfe N, Albert ML, Lavine L, Steele JC, Calne DB, Schoenberg BS. Cross-cultural cognitive examination: validation of a dementia screening instrument for neuroepidemiological research. J Am Geriatr Soc. 1993;41(9):931–9.
101. Taussig IM, Dick M, Teng E, Kempler D. The taussig cross-cultural memory test. Los Angeles: Available from Andrus Gerontology Center, University of Southern California; 1993.
102. Fuh J, Teng E, Lin K, Larson E, Wang S, Liu C, Chou P, Kuo BI, Liu H. The informant questionnaire on cognitive decline in the elderly (IQCODE) as a screening tool for dementia for a predominantly illiterate Chinese population. Neurology. 1995; 45(1):92–6.
103. Heaton RK, Miller SW, Taylor MJ, Grant I. Revised comprehensive norms for an expanded Halstead-Reitan Battery: demographically adjusted neuropsychological norms for African American and Caucasian adults. Odessa: Psychological Assessment Resources, Inc.; 2004.
104. Weiss LG, Saklofske DH, Coalson D, Raiford SE. WAIS-IV clinical use and interpretation scientist-practitioner perspectives. London: Academic; 2010.
105. Kempler D, Teng EL, Dick M, Taussig IM, Davis DS. The effects of age, education, and ethnicity on verbal fluency. J Int Neuropsychol Soc. 1998;4:531–8.
106. Ostrosky-Solís F, Gomez-Perez M, Matute E, Rosselli M, Ardila A, Pineda D. Neuropsi attention and memory: a neuropsychological test battery in Spanish with norms by age and education level. Appl Neuropsychol. 2007;14:156–70.
107. Muñoz-Sandoval AF, Woodcock RW, McGrew KS, Mather N. Batería III Woodcock-Muñoz. Itasca: Riverside Publishing; 2005.
108. Woodcock RW, Munoz-Sandoval AF, Ruef ML, Alvarado CG. Woodcock-munoz language survey-revised. Itasca: Riverside Publishing; 2005.
109. Pontón MO, Satz P, Herrera L, Ortiz F, Urrutia CP, Young R, D'Elia LF, Furst CJ, Namerow N. Normative data stratified by age and education for the neuropsychological screening battery for latinos (NeSBHIS): initial report. J Int Neuropsychol Soc. 1996;2:96–104.
110. Mungas D, Reed BR, Haan MN, Gonzalez H. Spanish and English neuropsychological assessment scales: relationship to demographics, language, cognition, and independent functioning. Neuropsychology. 2005;19:466–75.
111. Tuokko H, Chou P, Bowden S, Simard M, Ska B, Crossley M. Partial measurement equivalence of French and English versions of the canadian study of health and aging neuropsychology battery. J Int Neuropsychol Soc. 2009;15:416–25.
112. Mungas D, Reed BR, Crane PK, Haan MN, González H. Spanish and English neuropsychological assessment scales (SENAS): further development and psychometric characteristics. Psychol Assess. 2004;16: 347–59.
113. Bowden SC, Cook MJ, Bardenhagen FJ, Shores EA, Carstairs JR. Measurement invariance of core cognitive abilities in heterogeneous neurological and community samples. Intelligence. 2004;33:363–89.
114. Hsieh J, Tori C. Normative data on cross-cultural neuropsychological tests obtained from Mandarin-speaking adults across the life span. Arch Clin Neuropsychol. 2007;22:283–307.
115. Kang YW, Kim JK. Korean-California verbal learning test (K-CVLT):a normative study. Kor J Clin Psychol. 1997;16:379–96.
116. Manly JJ, Schupf N, Tang MX, Stern Y. Cognitive decline and literacy among ethnically diverse elders. J Geriatr Psychiatry Neurol. 2005;18(4):213–7.
117. Nell V. Cross-cultural neuropsychological assessment: theory and practice. Mahwah: Erlbaum; 2000.
118. Taussig M, Pontón MO. Issues in neuropsychological assessment of hispanic older adults: cultural and linguistic factors. In: Yeo G, Gallagher-Thompson D, editors. Ethnicity and the dementias. San Francisco: Taylor & Francis; 1996. p. 47–58.
119. Cuellar I, Arnold B, Maldonado R. Acculturation rating scale for Mexican Americans-II: a revision of the original ARSMA scale. Hispanic J Behav Sci. 1995;17:275–304.
120. Marin G, Gamba RJ. A new measurement of acculturation for Hispanics: the bidimensional acculturation scale for hispanics (BAS). Hispanic J Behav Sci. 1996;18:297–316.
121. Marin G, Sabogal F, Marin BV, Otero-Sabogal R, Perez-Stable EJ. Development of a short acculturation scale for Hispanics. Hispanic J Behav Sci. 1987;9:183–205.
122. Zea MC, Asner-Self KK, Birman D, Buki LP. The abbreviated multidimensional acculturation scale: empirical validation with two Latino/Latina samples. Cultur Divers Ethnic Minor Psychol. 2003;9(2): 107–26.
123. Berry J. Conceptual approaches to acculturation. In: Chun KM, Organista PB, Marin G, editors. Acculturation: advances in theory, measurement, and applied research. Washington: American Psychological Association; 2003. p. 83–93.

124. Choi J, Madhavappallil T. Predictive factors of acculturation attitudes and social support among Asian immigrants in the USA. Int J Soc Welfare. 2009;18:76–84.
125. Boone K, Victor T, Wen J, Razani J, Ponton M. The association between neuropsychological scores and ethnicity, language, and acculturation variables in a large patient population. Arch Clin Neuropsychol. 2007;22(3):355–65.
126. Razani J, Burciaga J, Madore M, Wong J. Effects of acculturation on tests of attention and information processing in an ethnically diverse group. Arch Clin Neuropsychol. 2007;22:333–41.
127. Coffey DM, Marmol L, Schock L, Adams W. The effects of acculturation on the wisconsin card sorting test by Mexican Americans. Arch Clin Neuropsychol. 2005;20(6):795–803.
128. Nicoladis E, Giovanni S. The role of a child's productive vocabulary in the language choice of a bilingual family. First Lang. 2000;20:3–28.
129. Martin-Rhee M, Bialystok E. The development of two types of inhibitory control in monolingual and bilingual children. Biling Lang Cognit. 2008; 11(1):81–93.
130. Gollan TH, Montoya RI, Werner G. Semantic and letter fluency in Spanish–English bilinguals. Neuropsychology. 2002;16:562–76.
131. Rosselli M, Ardila A, Araujo K, Weekes VA, Caracciolo V, Padilla M, Ostrosky-Solis F. Verbal fluency and repetition skills in healthy older Spanish–English bilinguals. Appl Neuropsychol. 2000;7:17–24.
132. Bialystok E, Klein R, Craik FIM, Viswanathan M. Bilingualism, aging, and cognitive control: evidence from the simon task. Psychol Aging. 2004;19:290–303.
133. Milberg WP, Hebben N, Kaplan E. The boston process approach to neuropsychological assessment. In: Grant I, Adams K, editors. Neuropsychological assessment of neuropsychiatric disorders. 2nd ed. New York: Oxford University Press; 1996. p. 58–80.
134. White R, Rose F. The boston process approach: a brief history and current practice. In: Goldstein G, Incagnoli TM, editors. Contemporary approaches to neuropsychological assessment: critical issues in neuropsychology. New York: Plenum; 1997. p. 171–211.
135. Manly JJ, Echemendia R. Race-specific norms: using the model of hypertension to understand issues of race, culture, and education in neuropsychology. Arch Clin Neuropsychol. 2007;22(3):319–25.
136. Ardila A, Rodriguez-Menendez G, Rosselli M. Current issues in neuropsychological assessment with Hispanics/Latinos. In: Ferraro FR, editor. Minority and cross-cultural aspects of neuropsychological assessment. Lisse: Swets & Zeitlinger; 2002. p. 161–79.
137. Gass C, Brown M. Neuropsychological test feedback to patients with brain dysfunction. Psychol Assess. 1992;4(3):272–7.
138. Post and Armstrong (in preparation). Feedback that sticks: the art of effectively communicating neuropsychological assessment results. New York, NY: Oxford University.

The Assessment of Change: Serial Assessments in Dementia Evaluations

4

Gordon J. Chelune and Kevin Duff

Abstract

The focus of the clinical neuropsychologist in everyday practice is on neurocognitive *change*. Because the diagnosis of dementia as well as mild cognitive impairment requires evidence of cognitive decline over time, the assessment of meaningful neurocognitive *change* is especially relevant in the evaluation of older adults. We briefly discuss the clinical use of norm-referenced tests used in traditional single-point assessments and then focus on the use of serial assessments to objectively monitor and assess cognitive changes over time, discussing the unique advantages and challenges of serial assessments. An overview and distillation of reliable change methods are presented and applied to a case example, demonstrating how these methods can be used as effective tools to inform the clinical evaluation of the individual patient. In the end, we hope to leave the reader with an appreciation that *change* is a unique variable with its own inherent statistical properties and clinical meaning.

Keywords

Predicting reliable change • Practice effects • Dementia and cognitive decline • Serial assessment

The Assessment of Change: Serial Assessments in Dementia Evaluations

As a multidisciplinary area of scientific inquiry, *neuropsychology* is often defined as the study of brain–behavior relationships. However, as an area of psychological practice, *clinical neuropsychology* has been described as the application of neuropsychological principles of brain–behavior

G.J. Chelune, Ph.D., ABPP(CN) • K. Duff, Ph.D., ABPP(CN) (✉)
Department of Neurology, Center for Alzheimer's Care, Imaging and Research, University of Utah School of Medicine, 650 Komas Drive, Ste. 106a, Salt Lake City, UT 84108, USA
e-mail: gordon.chelune@hsc.utah.edu; kevin.duff@hsc.utah.edu

L.D. Ravdin and H.L. Katzen (eds.), *Handbook on the Neuropsychology of Aging and Dementia*, Clinical Handbooks in Neuropsychology, DOI 10.1007/978-1-4614-3106-0_4,

relationships to the assessment, diagnosis, and rehabilitation of *changes* in human behavior that arise across the lifespan from known or suspected illnesses or injuries affecting the brain [1]. To this definition, we can also add the assessment of cognitive changes associated with medical interventions (e.g., open heart surgery, epilepsy surgery) and treatments (e.g., deep brain stimulation, pharmacologic treatments). Whether the focus is on changes in cognition induced by abnormal medical conditions or those in response to treatments and interventions, the focus of the clinical neuropsychologist in everyday practice is on *change*.

The assessment of meaningful neurocognitive change is particularly relevant for the evaluation of older adults suspected of having underlying neurodegenerative disorders. Because the diagnosis of dementia as well as mild cognitive impairment (MCI) requires evidence of cognitive decline over time [2], it is critical to distinguish between age-related decrements in cognition (e.g., memory, processing speed, executive functions) believed to be part of "normal" aging [3–5] and those early clinical changes that are pathological and disease-related (e.g., neurodegenerative disorders, cerebrovascular disease, stroke, diabetes, etc.). Traditional single-point evaluations are limited in this context as they only capture a picture of the patient's current abilities at a single point in time. Unless the patient's performances deviate markedly from an *inferred* premorbid baseline, it is difficult for the practitioner to know whether these point estimates of a patient's abilities are meaningfully different from expectation [6]. To overcome the limitations of single-point assessments, clinicians increasingly are turning to serial assessments to determine whether patients' *observed* trajectories of change over time significantly deviate from those seen in normal aging [7, 8]. Unlike single-point assessments where the clinician must infer a premorbid baseline, the patient's initial scores serve as their *observed* baseline. Armed with an appropriate conceptual framework and some simple tools, serial assessments provide the informed practitioner a powerful means for assessing diagnostically meaningful change.

In this chapter, we will briefly discuss the clinical use of norm-referenced neuropsychological tests, contrasting two underlying approaches to interpreting these norms in traditional single-point assessments. With this as a backdrop, we will then turn our attention to the use of serial assessments to objectively monitor and assess cognitive changes over time, discussing the unique advantages and challenges of serial assessments. An overview and distillation of reliable change methods will be presented and applied to a case example, demonstrating how these methods can be used as effective tools to inform the clinical evaluation of the individual patient. In the end, we hope to leave the reader with an appreciation that *change* is a unique variable with its own inherent statistical properties and clinical meaning.

Norms and How We Use Them in Single-Point Assessments

In clinical practice, when we see a patient for the first time, we use norm-referenced tests so that we can compare the performances of the individual patient to an external reference group. The norms simply describe the distribution of scores on a given test obtained by a reference group, which can be a sample from the general population, a well-screened group of healthy community-living individuals (i.e., robust norms), or a patient group with a specific condition of interest. To infer meaning from our patient's scores, we can take two very distinct approaches to answer different clinical questions [6]. The first approach is *descriptive*, that is, *where* does my patient's score fall with respect to the reference population along a standardized metric (e.g., standard scores, *z*-scores, percentile ranks)? We often apply descriptive labels such as "above average" or "below average" for ranges of scores in relation to the mean of the sample, and using standardized measures of the distribution of scores, we can assign percentile ranks that tell us how common or uncommon the specific score is *within* the reference population.

While the descriptive approach is useful in identifying where our patient's scores fall within a reference population, it does not address whether our patient's scores are impaired or not. To do this, we must take a *diagnostic* approach where we ask the question "does my patient's score *deviate* from premorbid expectations (i.e., where I expect the score to have been in the absence of an intervening illness or injury), and if so, by how much?" The reference standard is now the individual's premorbid status, *not* the mean of the reference population. In the absence of having baseline information, the clinician must infer this and often relies on demographic information [9] and performance on crystallized ability measures such as oral reading derived from normative reference groups (e.g., the Test of Premorbid Functioning [10]). Deviations from this *individual comparison standard* can also be placed on a standardized metric (e.g., *T*-scores, *z*-scores), and percentile ranks assigned to the deviations *if* we know the characteristics of the *distribution of the deviation scores* between the premorbid estimate and observed performance on a given test. Note that the focus is on the distribution of the deviation scores, *not* the distribution of either the premorbid estimates or the observed scores on a given test.

While the diagnostic approach allows us to quantify whether an individual's current performance deviates from estimates of his or her demographically predicted premorbid ability level, we are still constrained to describing the deviation in terms of base rates—how common or uncommon the deviation is for our patient relative to premorbid expectations. To be diagnostically useful, the clinician must further establish validity evidence, through a review of the test manual, his or her personal case records, or perhaps through an evidence-based review of the literature [11], that discrepancies of a certain magnitude are statistically more frequent in populations that have a specific condition of interest, such as amnesic MCI, than would be expected at this level of discrepancy in a normal population.

To illustrate the points above, let us consider the example of super clinician, Dr. Bob, who works in a memory disorders clinic and uses the test MegaMemory to evaluate memory complaints. Knowing that a patient's memory score on MegaMemory is one standard deviation below the estimated premorbid level informs Dr. Bob that the base rate of deviations of this magnitude occurs in only 16% of cases where there is an absence of an intervening illness or injury. However, after carefully reading the chapter on validity in the test manual for MegaMemory, Dr. Bob finds that the publisher conducted a case-controlled study using MegaMemory that compared equal numbers of patients with amnesic MCI and normal controls, a prevalence rate similar to what Dr. Bob sees in his clinic. The manual reports that individual deviations of one standard deviation or more from estimated premorbid levels occurred in 64% of cases with amnesic MCI compared to only 16% of controls. Performing a Bayesian analysis of the base rates between the two groups [11] yielded an odds ratio of 9.3 and a likelihood ratio of 4.0. Based on this empirical evidence, Dr. Bob now feels he can interpret a deviation score of one standard deviation or more on MegaMemory as not only relatively uncommon among healthy older adults but also as being "impaired" since deviations of this magnitude are four times more likely to occur in patients with amnesic MCI than in healthy controls, and among patients with amnesic MCI, deviations of this magnitude are nine times more likely to occur than deviations of lesser magnitude.

Using Serial Assessments to Identify Meaningful Change

Although neuropsychological tests are generally designed to assess the current state or capacity of an individual, repeated assessments are increasingly common in neuropsychological practice and outcomes research [12, 13]. This has become especially true in geriatric settings where the determination of meaningful changes in cognition over time is essential for both the diagnosis of dementia and for planning therapeutic provisions and long-term care for patients and caregivers [6, 14]. Serial observations and longitudinal comparisons are classic tools in science, and their use in clinical practice requires clinicians to understand test–retest change scores as unique cognitive variables with their own statistical and clinical properties that are different from the test measures from which they were derived [15].

Like single-point diagnostic assessments discussed above, serial assessments share (a) a focus on *change* between two points in time (albeit one observed and the other inferred); (b) estimates of change based on *individual comparison standards* rather than population standards; (c) a focus on the psychometric properties of the discrepancy or change scores rather than on the test scores themselves (i.e., the properties of the distribution of change scores); (d) use of base-rate information to determine whether a change or discrepancy score is common or uncommon; and (e) *impairment* inferred on the basis of validity studies that demonstrate that large and relatively rare change scores are statistically more common in patient groups with a known condition of interest than would be expected among the reference population.

Although serial assessments share much in common with single-point assessments, they also pose unique interpretative challenges because two or more sets of scores are involved. Under ideal test–retest conditions, a patient's retest performance should be the same as that observed at baseline, and any change or deviation from baseline would be clinically relevant. However, in the absence of perfect test stability and reliability, the clinician must deal with the residuals of these statistical properties, namely bias and error.

Bias. Bias represents a systematic change in performance. The most important source of systematic bias in clinical practice is the variable of interest, that is, the effect of disease progression over time, the impact of a surgical or pharmacological intervention, or the effect of rehabilitation. However, second only to the variable of interest, the most common source of bias in serial cognitive assessment is a positive *practice effect* in which performance is enhanced by previous test exposure, although negative biases can also occur such as those seen in aging [16]. Other forms of systematic bias on retest performance are education, gender, baseline level of performance, and retest interval [17–19]. Where large, positive practice effects are expected, the absence of change may actually reflect a decrement in performance. To make accurate diagnoses, the clinician must separate the effects of the variable of interest from other sources of bias.

Error. In addition to systematic biases, tests themselves are imperfect tools and can introduce an element of random error. For our purposes here, we will only consider two sources of error affecting serial assessment, both of which are inversely related to the test's reliability. The first is *measurement error* or the fidelity of the test, and it refers to the theoretical distribution of random variations in observed test scores around an individual's true score, which is characterized by the *standard error of measurement* (*SEM*). Because the *SEM* is inversely related to a test's reliability, tests with low reliability (<0.70) have large *SEMs* surrounding a person's true score at both baseline and on retest, and large test–retest differences can occur simply as random fluctuations in measurement. Conversely, small test–retest changes can be reliable and clinically meaningful for tests with high reliability (>0.90). Test–retest reliabilities of 0.70 or greater are often considered to be the minimum acceptable standard for psychological tests in outcome studies [20], and practitioners should be wary when interpreting cognitive change scores on tests that have lower reliabilities.

The second source of error affecting change scores is *regression to the mean*, which refers to the susceptibility of retest scores to regress toward the mean of the scores at baseline. The more a score deviates from the population mean at baseline, the more likely it will regress back toward the mean on retest. How much a score regresses depends on the reliability of the test. Again, scores on tests with high reliability show less susceptibility to regression to the mean than those on tests with lower reliability. The bottom line for clinicians when planning to perform serial assessments and faced with two tests purported to assess the same cognitive construct—choose the one with the better reliability!

Alternate forms. Alternate forms are often touted as an effective means for avoiding or minimizing practice effects due to test familiarity. Carefully constructed alternative forms may attenuate the effects of content-specific practice for some measures [21]. However, research demonstrates that alternate forms used in serial assessments still show significant practice effects [22]. While alternate forms may dampen practice effects due to content familiarity, they do not control for procedural learning and other factors that contribute to the overall practice effect. More importantly, rote use of alternate forms in serial assessment ignores other factors that impact interpretation of test–retest change scores, namely reliability and error [15].

Reliable Change in Serial Assessments with Older Adults

It should be clear that the interpretation of test–retest change scores is not a straightforward matter, and making accurate diagnostic judgments about whether an older adult has shown significant deterioration (or improvement) in cognitive status over a retest interval requires us to consider the role of bias and error in our measurements. Bias and error are problems only to the degree that they are unknowns and not taken into account when interpreting change scores. In this section, we will discuss *reliable change methods*, a family of related statistical procedures that attempt to take into account the impact of differential practice effects and other systematic biases, measurement error, and regression to the mean on the interpretation of change scores. We do not intend to do a comprehensive or in-depth review of these procedures, and the interested reader is directed to other sources for more complete coverage [13, 15, 18, 19, 23, 24]. Rather, we wish to distill the essential features of reliable change methods and demonstrate how these tools can be used diagnostically to evaluate meaningful cognitive change in older adults.

Reliable Change: A Statistical Approach to Meaningful Change

To understand the concept of reliable change, we need to distinguish between what is statistically significant at a group level and what is clinically meaningful at the individual level. Repeated measures tests of statistical significance tell us whether the mean difference between two groups of a given magnitude is a reliable difference that would not be expected to occur by chance at some predefined probability level (e.g., $p<0.05$). However, the base rates of such differences at the level of the individual may actually occur with some regularity even when no real behavioral difference. For this reason, Matarazzo and Herman have urged clinicians to routinely consider base-rate data in their clinical interpretation of test–retest evaluations [25].

Reliable Change: The Basic Model

Reliable change methods all fundamentally strive to evaluate the base rates of difference scores in a population and to determine whether the difference between scores for an individual is statistically rare and cannot be accounted for by various sources of bias (e.g., practice) or error (e.g., measurement error and regression to the mean). Like a ruler or yardstick that measures *change* from point A to point B along a standard metric (inches/yards), the basic form for any reliable change method is a ratio: reliable change (RC) = (*change score*)/(*standard error*), *where the standard error describes the dispersion of change scores that would be expected if no actual change had occurred* [26]. This is simply the distribution of test–retest scores one would see in a reference population. RC is typically expressed as a standardized *z*-score under the unit curve that has a mean of 0 and a standard deviation of 1.0. The base rate of a given RC value being equal to the percentile associated with the *z*-score, for example, a *z*-score or RC of −1.64, falls at the bottom fifth percentile. The various reliable change methods reported in the literature primarily vary along two dimensions: whether the *change score* in the numerator is a simple-difference or a predicted-difference score and whether the *standard error* in the denominator represents a measure of dispersion (observed or estimated) around the mean of difference scores or around a regression line.

Simple versus predicted-difference change scores. For the *change score* component of the RC ratio, when we do follow-up evaluations on a patient, we generally look at the retest scores and compare them with the baseline score (retest − baseline) to see if the difference is positive or negative.

This is the simple-difference approach. When no difference is expected over the retest interval (perfect stability), the simple-difference change score reflects the patient's individual deviation from a population mean difference score of 0 or no expected change. However, as we have noted earlier, there are many sources of bias affecting retest scores, with practice often exerting a strong positive bias. As a result, the actual population mean of the test–retest *change scores* is positive and has led to the development of a practice-adjusted simple-difference approach [27]. For example, the mean retest performance on the Wechsler Memory Scale-III (WMS-III) Immediate Memory Index is 13.4 points higher than at baseline when readministered several weeks later [28]. If our 68-year-old male patient that we are following for suspected dementia has a baseline score of 97 and a retest score of 100, has he actually shown an improvement of 3 points when the average retest *change score* is 13.4 or a decrement of −10.4 points (13.4 − 3 = −10.4) from expected change? To adjust for expected practice effects, Chelune and colleagues have suggested centering the *change score* component of the RC deviations around the mean of the expected practice effect and calculating the *change score* discrepancy from this mean [27].

The second approach to calculating the *change score* component of the RC ratio is the predicted-difference method. This is a regression-based approach that uses a patient's baseline performance to predict what his/or her retest score is expected to be at retest, with the regression equation being one derived from an appropriate reference sample. The discrepancy between the patient's actual observed retest score and the predicted retest score ($Y - Y'$) constitutes the *change score* discrepancy. Entering the baseline score as a predictor of the retest score into the regression equation allows practice effects to be modeled as a function of baseline performance (rather than as a constant) while also accounting for regression to the mean [29], two aspects not accounted for by the simple-difference approach. As in any regression approach, the equation can be univariate, using only the baseline score as the sole predictor, or multivariate, using additional information from other potential sources of bias as predictors, such as age, education, gender, and retest interval. In the example above of the 68-year-old male patient suspected of dementia, a regression-based equation using baseline WMS-III Immediate Memory Index scores and age was computed for the WMS-III test–retest standardization sample [15]. Given a baseline score of 97 for a 68-year-old normal individual, the predicted retest score would be 108.8. Our patient's predicted *change score* deviation is −8.8 points (observed retest score of 100 minus the predicted test score of 108.8). The reader will note that the −8.8-point predicted *change score* discrepancy is smaller than the −10.4-point simple-difference *change score*. The reason for this is that the regression-based predicted *change score* modeled not only practice effects (a positive bias) but also age (a negative bias), which dampened the expected practice effect, resulting in a smaller (although perhaps more accurate) expected retest score.

Measures of dispersion for the simple-difference method. Once the individual's *change score* discrepancy has been computed, we have a measure of *change* but do not know whether the change is large or small without having a standard metric to evaluate the dispersion of *change scores* that would occur in the absence of real change (i.e., changes simply due to error). This is reflected in the denominator of the RC ratio, and the choice of the measure of dispersion has been the subject of much debate and refinement in the reliable change literature [13, 15, 19, 23, 24, 30]. The simplest version of the *standard error* component of the RC ratio is simply the *standard deviation* of the observed *change score* discrepancies. In our dementia case example with the WMS-III, the mean test–retest *change score* obtained from the WAIS-III/WMS-III Technical Manual is 13.4 [28]. However, like many test manuals and normative studies that report the means and standard deviations of the test and retest scores, the *standard deviation* of difference (change) scores was not reported. With permission from the test publisher, Chelune calculated the actual *standard deviation* of *change scores* for the WMS-III Immediate Memory Index from the retest sample and found it to be 10.2 [15]. With this measure of dispersion, we can calculate the RC magnitude of our patient's change score by dividing the observed practice-adjusted simple-difference score (−10.4) by the standard deviation of differences (10.2) and obtain an RC *z*-score of −1.02. A *z*-score of this magnitude would be expected to occur in only about 15% of cases when no real change has occurred. Is this sufficiently rare to classify our patient's *change score* as meaningful? Most studies of reliable change invoke a 90% RC confidence interval (*z*-score ± 1.64), in which only 5% of cases would be above or below this level of change. For our patient's change score to reach this level of decline, he would have needed a retest score between 93 and 94. It is worth emphasizing that a seemingly minor decrement in performance (e.g., 3–4 standard score points in this case), a change that many clinicians might call "within the range of the test's variability," actually reflects a reliable change when corrected for expected practice effects and measurement error.

In the absence of having the actual *standard deviation* of difference scores, it is possible to estimate it in one of several ways. Jacobsen and Truax initially introduced the Reliable Change Index (RCI) as a means for calculating RC with only knowledge of the simple-difference *change score* and the *standard error of the difference* scores (S_{diff}), a measure of dispersion derived from *SEM* for the test at baseline [31]. Chelune and colleagues later adapted the RCI by adjusting for the mean practice effect [27]. In a further refinement, Iverson suggested a modified RCI that used the *SEM* at both baseline and at retest to calculate the S_{diff} [32]. Comparison of the two versions of the S_{diff} suggests that Iverson's method produces a closer estimate of the actual dispersion of *change scores* than that of Jacobsen and Truax. In the case of our WMS-III Immediate Memory example, the Iverson method produces a S_{diff} of 9.9 compared to 8.8 for the Jacobson and Truax method, where the actual *standard deviation* of differences was 10.2. A final common estimate of the observed dispersion of *change scores* is the *standard error of prediction*, which represents the standard error of a retest score predicted from a baseline score in a regression equation where the test-reliability coefficient is the standardized beta coefficient [15]. In our WMS-III example, the *standard error of prediction* for the Immediate Memory Index is 10.1, very close to the observed standard deviation of actual change scores, namely 10.2.

Standardized regression-based (*SRB*) *approach.* As noted in our discussion of the simple versus predicted methods of calculating the *change score* discrepancy in the RC ratio, the predicted-difference method generates predicted retest scores (Y') for individuals based on their specific baseline performances (X) using linear regression and then subtracts this from their observed retest scores (Y) to obtain their personal *change score* discrepancy ($Y - Y'$). Additional sources of potential bias (e.g., age, education, gender) can be added to the regression equation in a multivariate manner [29]. As noted earlier, this approach allows practice effects to be modeled as a function of individual baseline performance as well as accounting for regression to the mean. This might be particularly important as these two variables interact (e.g., the practice effects may be attenuated by regression to the mean for someone with a high baseline score, whereas practice effects are enhanced by regression to the mean for an individual with a low initial baseline score). However, unlike the simple-difference approach where the standard error term in the denominator of the RC ratio reflects the dispersion of change scores around the mean of the *change scores*, the predicted-difference approach typically uses the *standard error of the estimate* (*SEE*) for the regression equation in the denominator of the RC ratio to reflect the dispersion of scores around the regression line. In our case example with the WMS-III Immediate Memory Index [15], the regression equation for predicting retest scores was given as:

$$Y' = (\text{Baseline score} * 1.00) + (\text{Age} * -0.097) + 18.45, \text{ with an SEE of } 10.24$$

The first part of this equation gives us an individual's predicted retest score that can be used to calculate the *change-score* discrepancy component of the RC ratio, whereas the *SEE* gives us the standard error term for the denominator. The reader will note that the *SEE* for the regression line is the same as the observed *standard deviation* of the simple-difference *change scores*.

While several authors have noted that the various RC methods produce relatively similar results [19, 26], the SRB RC-approach has generally become the preferred method for individual prediction, provided that the clinician has access to prediction equations derived from reference samples appropriate to their patients. While there is a growing body of such SRB equations for a variety of tests commonly used with older adults [8, 9, 14, 17, 33, 34], and some tests such as the fourth edition of the Wechsler Adult Intelligence and Memory Scales are incorporating RC algorithms into their scoring software [10], there is still a paucity of published longitudinal SRB data. Fortunately, as will be seen in the next section, John Crawford and Paul Garthwaite have developed a simple but powerful tool for building regression equations from summary data that can be applied to the individual case [35].

Regression models of reliable change derived from summary data. As noted by Crawford and Garthwaite [35], not all neuropsychologists are aware that it is possible to construct regression equations for predicting an individual's retest performance from their baseline performance simply using sample summary data, for which there is a potential wealth of clinically useful information available in test manuals and the published literature. To build univariate regression equations from summary data alone, one only needs the means and standard deviations for test and retest scores, the size of the sample, and the test–retest reliability coefficient (or alternately the t-value from a pair-samples t test). In their 2007 paper, Crawford and Garthwaite delineate the statistical steps necessary to build such regression equations, as well as the further steps needed to compute the associated statistics for drawing inferences concerning the individual case. Recognizing that the computations involved are tedious and prone to error, Crawford and Garthwaite also developed a compiled calculator that is available for download at no cost from the following web address:

Table 4.1 Output from Crawford and Garthwaite's [35] calculator to build regression equations from sample summary data for a hypothetical patient with test–retest scores of 97 and 100 on the Wechsler Memory Scale-III Immediate Memory Index

Inputs
Mean for predictor variable (X) in sample used to build the equation = 100.2
Standard deviation for predictor variable (X) in sample = 15.9
Mean for the criterion variable (Y) in sample = 113.7
Standard deviation for the criterion variable (Y) in sample = 19.2
Correlation between predictor and criterion variable = 0.85
Sample size = 297
Individual's score on the predictor (X) variable = 97
Individual's obtained score on Y = 100
Outputs
Regression equation built from the summary data: $Y = 10.8532 + (1.0264 * X)$
Standard error of estimate for regression equation = 10.1314
Analysis of the individual case
Individual's predicted score from regression equation = 110.4155
Discrepancy (obtained minus predicted) between individual's obtained and predicted scores = −10.4155
Standardized discrepancy between individual's obtained and predicted scores = −1.0262
Significance test (t) on the standardized discrepancy between individual's obtained and predicted scores: One-tailed probability = 0.1528
Estimated percentage of population obtaining a discrepancy more extreme than individual = 15.280799%

http://www.abdn.ac.uk/~psy086/dept/regbuild.htm.

To use this calculator, one only need input the sample summary data and the patient-specific test–retest scores. Using the summary data from Chelune [15], Table 4.1 illustrates the output generated for our hypothetical 68-year-old patient whose baseline Immediate Memory Index was 97 at baseline and 100 on retest. The output is remarkably similar to that presented in previous sections for our patient example using various RC methods. Generally, the various approaches would predict our patient to have a retest score of 109–110 given his baseline score of 97. His observed retest score of 100 is 9–10 points below expectations (RC z-score deviation of about −1.0), which would likely occur in only about 15% of a sample for which there were no significant intervening events affecting cognition.

Although the Crawford and Garthwaite's regression calculator presented here is univariate [35], it has recently been expanded to handle multiple predictors, and this executable calculator is also available for download online at: http://www.abdn.ac.uk/~psy086/dept/RegBuild_MR.htm [36].

Advanced concepts and models of reliable change. The various RC methods we have described so far only consider measuring change as a discrete event across two points in time. However, there are many clinical situations where individuals are assessed serially across multiple time points, and change may be better described in terms of *trajectories of change* and intra-individual *rates of cognitive decline*. Early attempts to assess reliable change across multiple time points either averaged reliability coefficients and measures of dispersion between the various time points to arrive at composite indices of RC [37] or computed separate RC indices between each pair of time points [34]. Recently, more innovative approaches have been employed to model *change* as a trajectory or slope across multiple time points.

It is beyond the scope of this chapter to do more than alert the reader to some of these innovative approaches and to provide exemplars. Some investigators are using regression models that attempt to predict an individual's performance at time point_{2+n} by entering into regression formula not only baseline performance but the practice effects between previous time points. For example, Duff and associates [8] developed multivariate SRB equations for several neuropsychological tests widely used with older adults that used baseline performance, demographic variables, and short-term practice effects (baseline to 1 week) in predicting retest scores 1 year later. Attix and colleagues [38] developed SRB normative neuropsychological trajectories for a variety of test measures administered five times at 6-month intervals by entering in successive performances at each time point as predictors of subsequent performance at the next time point. Other investigators have focused on developing regression models that compare an individual's slope of performance across multiple time points to that of a control sample [39, 40]. Still others are using variations of longitudinal linear mixed models to estimate age-adjusted mean slopes and confidence intervals of change to identify individuals whose performances begin to deviate from expectation [7, 41]. Growth mixture modeling has also been applied to longitudinal data sets to identify subgroups of individuals who show different cognitive trajectories over time [42–45]. Clearly, we are on the verge of seeing a new generation of RC methods to assess reliable change in patients' performances over time.

A Case Example: Application of Reliable Change Methods in Clinical Practice

The accumulation of pathophysiological changes characteristic of Alzheimer's disease (AD) is believed to develop years, if not decades, before the clinical expression of frank memory loss and general cognitive decline [46]. To maximize the efficacy of emerging disease-modifying therapies and to support continued functional independence, early detection of Alzheimer's disease (AD) and other neurodegenerative disorders is paramount [42, 47]. Descriptive clinical states such as *cognitive impairment but not dementia* (CIND) and MCI have been introduced to describe abnormal cognitive states that place individuals at increased risk for progressing to AD [48]. However, these clinical states describe individuals who are already symptomatic. One does not wake up one day with dementia or MCI. Rather, cognitive decline, like neurodegenerative disease, is a dynamic process that evolves over time. Hence, serial neuropsychological evaluations have come to play an important role in documenting cognitive decline in geriatric settings.

Let us consider a case example of a 63-year-old, right-handed man with a Ph.D. Our patient is a successful professor of sociology at a major university and a married father of three children.

His past medical history is significant for depression and some cardiac issues, both currently well controlled. He has been stable on his medications for many years, and they are not thought be an issue with respect to cognition. Our patient has noticed insidious and progressive memory difficulties for about 2 years and presents to our Cognitive Disorders Clinic for evaluation. His neurologist obtains a Mini Mental State Exam score of 30/30 but on further bedside testing notes some subtle memory difficulties. The neurologist decides to refer the patient to us for comprehensive neuropsychological evaluation. We perform our evaluation and find that the patient has a relatively circumscribed pattern of memory deficit within the context of otherwise normal findings (see Baseline Scores in Table 4.2). Our impression is that this patient has amnesic MCI. We know from the research literature that patients with MCI have an increased risk of showing further decline and developing a frank dementia. However, we also know that some of these individuals revert back to "normal" when seen in follow-up [49, 50]. We share these observations with our referring neurologist and recommend that the patient be referred for a follow-up evaluation in 1 year to assess whether there has been any evidence of significant interval change in his neurocognitive status. Seeing the wisdom in our recommendations, the neurologist agrees and orders repeat testing in a year.

The patient returns 12 months later, and we repeat his evaluation. As we can see from the test–retest data summarized in Table 4.2, some of our patient's scores have gotten worse and some have gotten better. To understand which of these changes are reliable and meaningful given the different psychometric properties of the tests in our battery and to place them on a common metric, we turned to RC methods. For our purposes here, we computed reliable change information using the predicted-difference method. Using the test–retest data presented in the manuals for the tests or from longitudinal research studies with samples of healthy older adults, we entered the sample summary data into Crawford and Garthwaite's regression calculator [35] along with our patient's baseline and retest scores. In the right-hand columns of Table 4.2, we present the patient's predicted retest scores given his baseline performances, the observed–predicted discrepancy ($Y - Y'$), and the associated z-scores and population percentiles associated with the predicted-difference discrepancies. From these data, we can see that the patient's memory has continued to significantly deteriorate. We also note that his global mental status on the Mattis Dementia Rating Scale [51] and on the WAIS-III Verbal Comprehension Index [28] show signs of notable deterioration. At this point, we can confidently say that the patient's current test results reflect some further deterioration in his capacity to learn and remember new information as well as some increased difficulties with verbal intellectual abilities. While he is still likely to meet the criteria for MCI rather than dementia, his increased difficulties with verbal skills are worrisome for a neurodegenerative disorder such as Alzheimer's disease.

Future Directions: Change as a Neurocognitive Biomarker

As noted earlier, practice effects are defined as improvements in test scores due to repeated exposure to the testing materials. Traditionally, practice effects have been viewed as error variance that need to be controlled, managed, or otherwise accounted for in our interpretation of change. However, practice effects, like cognitive change in general, seems to be a unique variable that can potentially provide clinically useful information about diagnosis, prognosis, and treatment recommendations for our patients. Over the past several years, we have been prospectively examining practice effects as a neurocognitive biomarker in the development of dementia in older adults.

In an initial study examining practice effects in community-dwelling seniors with MCI, we observed two subgroups: those that benefited from practice across 1 week and those that did not [52]. Those that showed significant gains after repeat testing could no longer be classified as MCI, as they now appeared intact. These MCI participants might reflect "accidental" MCI [49, 50].

Table 4.2 Clinical case example of test–retest scores and reliable change (RC) information based on data in bold using Crawford and Garthwaite's [35] approach to derive RC regression equation from sample summary data

Test	Baseline scores			Follow-up scores			Reliable change (RC) information			
	Raw	Standard score	*T*-score	Raw	Standard score	*T*-score	Predicted retest score	Discrepancy ($Y-Y'$)	RC *z*-score	Population percentile
Global mental status										
Mini mental state exam[a]	**29**			**28**			28.57	−0.58	−0.33	37
Mattis Dementia Rating Scale: Total[b]	**140**	11		**133**	8		135.5	−6.36	−1.48	7
Wechsler tests										
Test of premorbid functioning[c]		**125**			**118**		124.25	−6.25	−1.13	13
WAIS-III Adult Intelligence Scale[d]										
General ability index	82	126	58	77	119	43				
Verbal comprehension	46	**131**	61	40	**118**	49	130.43	−12.43	−3.07	<1
Perceptual organization	36	**111**	47	37	**114**	50	115.11	−1.11	−0.19	43
Processing speed	19	**96**	41	20	**99**	43	100.14	−1.14	−0.17	43
Memory measures										
WMS-III memory[e]										
Logical memory-immediate	30	**8**	35	20	**4**	21	9.88	−5.88	−3.14	<1
Logical memory-delayed	14	**8**	37	4	**3**	18	10.61	−7.61	−3.87	<1
Digit span[d]	20	**13**	53	21	**13**	53	13.26	−0.26	−0.20	42
Hopkins Verbal Learning Test[f]										
Total trials 1–3	**22**		37	**17**		28	23.36	−6.36	−1.35	9
Delay	**0**		<20	**0**		<20	2.61	−2.61	−0.95	17
Brief Visuospatial Memory Test[f]										
Trials 1–3	**12**		31	**2**		<20	13.46	−11.46	−2.21	<1
Delay	**0**		<20	**0**		<20	2.25	−2.25	−1.01	16
Language										
Boston Naming Test[g]	**58**	13		**58**	13		57.72	0.28	0.12	55
Controlled Oral Word Association[f]	**46**	13		**49**	13		45.32	3.68	0.41	66
Visuospatial functions										
Judgment of line orientation[h]	**30**	16		**28**	14		23.48	4.52	0.83	79
KBNA complex figure and clock drawing total[i]	54	**12**		55	**14**		10.98	3.02	1.21	88
Executive functions										
Trail-making A time[f]	**38**	8		**33**	10		39.39	−6.93	0.44	67
Trail-making B time[f]	**63**	11		**97**	8		70.89	26.12	−0.51	30
KBNA practical problem and conceptual shifting total[i]	29	**13**		29	**13**		11.53	1.47	0.58	70

Notes: Sources of normative data used in developing RC prediction equations
[a][34]
[b][51]
[c][10]
[d][28]; Table 3.8
[e][28]; Table 3.11
[f][8]
[g][57]
[h][58]
[i][59]

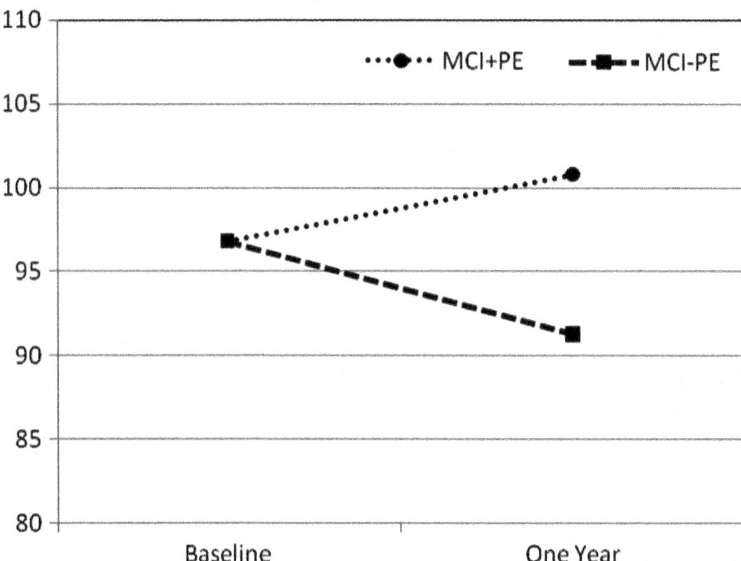

Fig. 4.1 Cognitive change across 1 year in patients with differential practice effects. Note MCI + PE = individuals with mild cognitive impairment who showed large practice effects across 1 week; MCI − PE = individuals with mild cognitive impairment who showed minimal practice effects across 1 week; *y*-axis = age-corrected standard score ($M = 100$, SD = 15) on total scale score of the Repeatable Battery for the Assessment of Neuropsychological Status

Conversely, the MCI participants that did not benefit from practice retained their original diagnostic classification, and these participants more likely demonstrate the concept of MCI. In this way, short-term practice effects provide diagnostic information that was not available with baseline data. Others also have found practice effects to be diagnostically useful in MCI [53].

Prognostically, the presence of practice effects suggests a better outcome, whereas the absence of practice effects suggests a poorer outcome. In two independent samples of individuals with MCI, we have observed that practice effects predict future cognition, above and beyond baseline cognition [8, 54]. As seen in the Fig. 4.1, when we followed our two MCI subgroups across 1 year, those that benefitted from practice across 1 week tended to remain cognitively stable across 1 year and those that did not show the expected practice effects across 1 week tended to decline across 1 year [55].

Lastly, we have examined the utility of practice effects in predicting treatment response. In a small sample of community-dwelling and cognitively intact older adults, within-session practice effects predicted response to a memory training course: those that showed practice effects displayed larger gains related to the cognitive intervention than those that did not show robust practice effects [56]. Although these findings need to be replicated, practice effects appear to contribute to a clinician's decision about diagnosis, prognosis, and treatment response, especially in older adults with memory difficulties.

Conclusions

The assessment of cognitive change lies at the very heart of clinical neuropsychology. Understanding change and how we assess it with our various test measures is complex and challenging, yet given an appropriate conceptual framework and some simple statistical tools, it is something that neuropsychologists can do uniquely well. Test–retest practice effects are not simply statistical artifacts and something to be suppressed but rather something to be understood. Especially among older adults, the capacity to learn and benefit from exposures to new experiences to potentially guide future behavior has adaptive value and may be a biological marker of neural integrity that has diagnostic significance.

Clinical Pearls

- Test–retest change scores are unique variables with their own statistical and clinical properties that are different from the test measures from which they were derived.
- Where large positive practice effects are expected, the absence of change may actually reflect a decrement in performance.
- When planning to perform serial assessments and faced with two tests purported to assess the same cognitive construct, choose the one with the better reliability.
- Use of alternate forms in serial assessment may attenuate, but not eliminate, practice effects and do not address other factors that affect the interpretation of change scores, namely bias and error.
- Test–retest reliabilities of 0.70 or greater are often considered to be the minimum acceptable standard for psychological tests in outcome studies, and practitioners should be wary when interpreting cognitive change scores on tests that have lower reliabilities.
- The basic form for any reliable change method is a ratio: reliable change (RC) = *(change score)/(standard error), where the standard error describes the dispersion of change scores that would be expected if no actual change had occurred.*
- The various reliable change methods reported in the literature primarily vary along two dimensions: (a) whether the *change score* in the numerator is a simple-difference or a predicted-difference score and (b) whether the *standard error* in the denominator represents a measure of dispersion (observed or estimated) around the mean of difference scores or around a regression line.
- Not all neuropsychologists are aware that it is possible to construct regression equations for predicting an individual's retest performance from his/her baseline performance by simply using sample summary data, for which there is a potential wealth of clinically useful information available in test manuals and the published literature.
- For computing regression equations using sample summary data for individual cases, see Crawford and Garthwaite's univariate online calculator and enter your patient specific test–retest scores: http://www.abdn.ac.uk/~psy086/dept/regbuild.htm. For multivariate data, see the website at: http://www.abdn.ac.uk/~psy086/dept/RegBuild_MR.htm.
- Although traditionally viewed as a source of bias, practice effects may provide valuable information about a patient's diagnosis, prognosis, and treatment response, especially for older adults with memory difficulties.

References

1. Barth JT, Pliskin N, Axelrod B, et al. Introduction to the NAN 2001 definition of a clinical neuropsychologist. NAN Policy and Planning Committee. Arch Clin Neuropsychol. 2003;18:551–5.
2. Winblad B, Palmer K, Kivipelto M, et al. Mild cognitive impairment—beyond controversies, towards a consensus: report of the International Working Group on Mild Cognitive Impairment. J Intern Med. 2004; 256:240–6.
3. Salthouse TA. Does the meaning of neurocognitive change change with age? Neuropsychology. 2010;24: 273–8.
4. Howieson D, Holm LA, Kaye JA, Oken BS, Howieson J. Neurologic function in the optimally healthy oldest old: neuropsychological evaluation. Neurology. 1993;43:1882–6.
5. Cullum CM, Butters N, Troster AI, Salmon DP. Normal aging and forgetting rates on the Wechsler Memory Scale—Revised. Arch Clin Neuropsychol. 1990;5:23–30.
6. Busch RM, Chelune GJ, Suchy Y. Using norms in the neuropsychological assessment of the elderly. In: Attix DK, Welsh-Bohmer KA, editors. Geriatric neuropsychology: assessment and intervention. New York: Guilford; 2006. p. 133–57.
7. Howieson D, Carlson NE, Moore MM, et al. Trajectory of mild cognitive impairment onset. J Int Neuropsychol Soc. 2008;14:192–8.
8. Duff K, Beglinger LJ, Moser DJ, Paulsen JS, Schultz SK, Arndt S. Predicting cognitive change in older adults: the relative contribution of practice effects. Arch Clin Neuropsychol. 2010;25:81–8.
9. Duff K. Predicting premorbid memory functioning in older adults. Appl Neuropsychol. 2010;17:278–82.

10. Pearson. Advanced clinical solutions for WAIS-IV and WMS-IV clinical and interpretative manual. San Antonio, TX: Pearson; 2009.
11. Chelune GJ. Evidence-based research and practice in clinical neuropsychology. Clin Neuropsychol. 2010; 24:454–67.
12. Heilbronner RL, Sweet JJ, Attix DK, Krull KR, Henry GK, Hart RP. Official position of the American Academy of Clinical Neuropsychology on serial neuropsychological assessments: the utility and challenges of repeat test administrations in clinical and forensic contexts. Clin Neuropsychol. 2010;24:1267–78.
13. Hinton-Bayre AD. Deriving reliable change statistics from test-retest normative data: comparison of models and mathematical expressions. Arch Clin Neuropsychol. 2010;25:244–56.
14. Stein J, Luppa M, Brahler E, Konig HH, Riedel-Heller SG. The assessment of changes in cognitive functioning: reliable change indices for neuropsychological instruments in the elderly—a systematic review. Dement Geriatr Cogn Disord. 2010;29:275–86.
15. Chelune GJ. Assessing reliable neuropsychological change. In: Franklin R, editor. Prediction in forensic and neuropsychology: new approaches to psychometrically sound assessment. Mahwah, NJ: Erlbaum; 2003.
16. Salthouse TA. Influence of age on practice effects in longitudinal neurocognitive change. Neuropsychology. 2010;24:563–72.
17. Duff K, Schoenberg MR, Patton D, et al. Regression-based formulas for predicting change in RBANS subtests with older adults. Arch Clin Neuropsychol. 2005;20:281–90.
18. Lineweaver TT, Chelune GJ. Use of the WAIS-III and WMS-III in the context of serial assessments: interpreting reliable and meaningful change. In: Tulsky DS, Saklofske DH, Chelune GJ, et al., editors. Clinical interpretation of the WAIS-III and WMS-III. New York: Academic; 2003. p. 303–37.
19. Temkin NR, Heaton RK, Grant I, Dikmen SS. Detecting significant change in neuropsychological test performance: a comparison of four models. J Int Neuropsychol Soc. 1999;5:357–69.
20. Slick DJ. Psychometrics in neuropsychological assessment. In: Strauss E, Sherman EMS, Spreen O, editors. A compendium of neuropsychological tests. New York, NY: Oxford University Press; 2006. p. 1–43.
21. Benedict RHB, Zgaljardic DJ. Practice effects during repeated administrations of memory tests with and without alternate forms. J Clin Exp Neuropsychol. 1998;20:339–52.
22. Beglinger LJ, Gaydos B, Tangphao-Daniels O, et al. Practice effects and the use of alternate forms in serial neuropsychological testing. Arch Clin Neuropsychol. 2005;20:517–29.
23. Collie A, Darby DG, Falleti MG, Silbert BS, Maruff P. Determining the extent of cognitive change after coronary surgery: a review of statistical procedures. Ann Thorac Surg. 2002;73:2005–11.
24. Crawford JR. Quantitative aspects of neuropsychological assessment. In: Goldstein LH, McNeil JE, editors. Clinical neuropsychology: a practical guide to assessment and management for clinicians. 2nd ed. Chichester: Wiley; 2011.
25. Matarazzo JD, Herman DO. Base rate data for the WAIS-R: test-retest stability and VIQ-PIQ differences. J Clin Neuropsychol. 1984;6:351–66.
26. Hinton-Bayre AD. Methodology is more important than statistics when determining reliable change. J Int Neuropsychol Soc. 2005;11:788–9.
27. Chelune GJ, Naugle RI, Luders H, Sedlak J, Awad IA. Individual change after epilepsy surgery: practice effects and base-rate information. Neuropsychology. 1993;7:41–52.
28. The Psychological Corporation. Updated WAIS-III WMS-III technical manual. San Antonio, TX: The Psychological Corporation; 1997.
29. McSweeny AJ, Naugle RI, Chelune GJ, Luders H. "T-scores for change": an illustration of a regression approach to depicting change in clinical neuropsychology. Clin Neuropsychol. 1993;7:300–12.
30. Maassen GH. Principles of defining reliable change indices. J Clin Exp Neuropsychol. 2000;22:622–32.
31. Jacobson NS, Truax P. Clinical significance: a statistical approach to defining meaningful change in psychotherapy research. J Consult Clin Psychol. 1991; 59:12–9.
32. Iverson GL. Interpreting change on the WAIS-III/WMS-III in clinical samples. Arch Clin Neuropsychol. 2001;16:183–91.
33. Knight RG, McMahon J, Skeaff CM, Green TJ. Reliable Change Index scores for persons over the age of 65 tested on alternate forms of the Rey AVLT. Arch Clin Neuropsychol. 2007;22:513–8.
34. Tombaugh TN. Test-retest reliable coefficients and 5-year change scores for the MMSE and 3MS. Arch Clin Neuropsychol. 2005;20:485–503.
35. Crawford JR, Garthwaite PH. Using regression equations built from summery data in the neuropsychological assessment of the individual case. Neuropsychology. 2007;21:611–20.
36. Crawford JR, Garthwaite PH, Denham AK, Chelune GJ. Using regression equations built from summary data in the psychological assessment of the individual case: Extension to multiple regression. Psychol Assessment. 2012; in press.
37. Ivnik RJ, Smith GE, Lucas JA, et al. Testing normal older people three or four times at 1- to 2-year intervals: defining normal variance. Neuropsychology. 1999;13:121–7.
38. Attix DK, Story TJ, Chelune GJ, et al. The prediction of change: normative neuropsychological trajectories. Clin Neuropsychol. 2009;23:21–38.
39. Chelune GJ, Ivnik R, Smith G. Application of reliable change methods for identifying abnormal rates of cognitive decline in dementia. Alzheimers Dement. 2006;2(S1):374.
40. Crawford JR, Garthwaite PH. Statistical methods for single-case studies in neuropsychology: comparing the slope of a patient's regression line with those of a control sample. Cortex. 2004;40:533–48.

41. Darby DG, Pietrzak RH, Fredrickson J, Woodward M, Moore L, Fredrickson A, Sach J, Maruff P. Intra-individual cognitive decline using a brief computerized cognitive screening test. Alzheimers Dement. 2012; 8(2):95–104.
42. Albert M, Blacker D, Moss MB, Tanzi R, McArdle JJ. Longitudinal change in cognitive performance among individuals with mild cognitive impairment. Neuropsychology. 2007;21:158–69.
43. Stern Y, Liu X, Albert M, et al. Application of a growth curve approach to modeling the progression of Alzheimer's disease. J Gerontol A Biol Sci Med Sci. 1996;51:M179–84.
44. Small BJ, Backman L. Longitudinal trajectories of cognitive change in preclinical Alzheimer's disease: a growth mixture modeling analysis. Cortex. 2007;43: 826–34.
45. Hayden KM, Reed BR, Manly JJ, et al. Cognitive decline in the elderly: an analysis of population heterogeneity. Age Aging. 2011;40(6):684–9.
46. Morris JC, Storandt M, Miller JP, et al. Mild cognitive impairment represents early-stage Alzheimer disease. Arch Neurol. 2001;58:397–405.
47. Amieva H, Le Goff M, Millet X, et al. Prodromal Alzheimer's disease: successive emergence of the clinical symptoms. Ann Neurol. 2008;64:492–8.
48. Petersen RC, Smith GE, Waring SC, Ivnik RJ, Kokmen E, Tangelos EG. Aging, memory, and mild cognitive impairment. Int Psychogeriatr. 1997;9 Suppl 1:65–9.
49. Brooks BL, Iverson GL, White T. Substantial risk of "Accidental MCI" in healthy older adults: base rates of low memory scores in neuropsychological assessment. J Int Neuropsychol Soc. 2007;13: 490–500.
50. de Rotrou J, Wenisch E, Chausson C, Dray F, Faucounau V, Rigaud AS. Accidental MCI in healthy subjects: a prospective longitudinal study. Eur J Neurol. 2005;12:879–85.
51. Pedraza O, Smith GE, Ivnik RJ, et al. Reliable change on the Dementia Rating Scale. J Int Neuropsychol Soc. 2007;13:716–20.
52. Duff K, Beglinger LJ, Van Der Heiden S, et al. Short-term practice effects in amnestic mild cognitive impairment: implications for diagnosis and treatment. Int Psychogeriatr. 2008;20:986–99.
53. Darby D, Maruff P, Collie A, McStephen M. Mild cognitive impairment can be detected by multiple assessments in a single day. Neurology. 2002;59:1042–6.
54. Duff K, Beglinger LJ, Schultz SK, et al. Practice effects in the prediction of long-term cognitive outcome in three patient samples: a novel prognostic index. Arch Clin Neuropsychol. 2007;22:15–24.
55. Duff K, Lyketsos CG, Beglinger LJ, et al. Practice effects predict cognitive outcome in amnestic mild cognitive impairment. Am J Geriatr Psychiatry. 2011; 19(11):932–9.
56. Duff K, Beglinger LJ, Moser DJ, Schultz SK, Paulsen JS. Practice effects and outcome of cognitive training: preliminary evidence from a memory training course. Am J Geriatr Psychiatry. 2010;18:91.
57. Zec RF, Markwell SJ, Burkett NR, Larsen DL. A longitudinal study of confrontation naming in the "normal" elderly. J Int Neuropsychol Soc. 2005; 11:716–26.
58. Montse A, Pere V, Carme J, Francesc V, Eduardo T. Visuospatial deficits in Parkinson's disease assessed by judgment of line orientation test: error analyses and practice effects. J Clin Exp Neuropsychol. 2001; 23:592–8.
59. Leach L, Kaplan E, Rewilak D, Richards B. Kaplan KBNA baycrest neurocognitive assessment: manual. San Antonio, TX: The Psychological Corporation; 2000.

After the Diagnosis of Dementia: Considerations in Disease Management

5

Steven Hoover and Mary Sano

Abstract

Once diagnosed with Alzheimer's disease or related disorders, patients and caregivers must integrate treatment and management plans. While there are no cures for these disorders, there are opportunities to optimize function and quality of life. There are pharmacological treatments available for dementia as well as for the behavioral and psychiatric symptoms that often accompany these diagnoses. Persistence can insure that drug treatments provide optimal benefit. Also nonpharmacological interventions including environmental modifications can be helpful, particularly for the behavioral problems. Supervision to insure adequate medical care, maximize independence and social interaction, and preserve patient dignity will require ongoing review of the patient's changing condition. A comprehensive approach to management will also consider legal and financial needs, support for the caregiver, and the possibility of research participation. Clinicians can introduce the possibility of research for the hope it offers to their patients and to the generations to come.

Keywords

Dementia treatment • Disease management • Caregiving • Experimental therapeutics

S. Hoover, Ph.D.
Department of Psychiatry, Mount Sinai School of Medicine, New York, NY, USA

M. Sano, Ph.D. (✉)
Department of Psychiatry, Mount Sinai School of Medicine, New York, NY, USA

James J Peters Veterans Administration Medical Center, 130 W. Kingsbridge Rd, Code 150 Rm 1F01, Bronx, NY 10468, USA
e-mail: mary.sano@mssm.edu

Introduction

When an individual begins to notice a decline in his/her memory and cognitive functioning, the instinctual reaction is often one of denial and fear. People often rationalize these changes as simply being a part of normal aging, feeling as if the concerns of friends and family are excessive and unnecessary. The additional stigma of being

L.D. Ravdin and H.L. Katzen (eds.), *Handbook on the Neuropsychology of Aging and Dementia*, Clinical Handbooks in Neuropsychology, DOI 10.1007/978-1-4614-3106-0_5,

formally diagnosed with dementia creates a challenge to coping strategies for both patients and their families. For decades, both the general public as well as the medical community held the misconception that individuals with cognitive deficits or dementia, even in the initial stages of the disease, lacked insight into their disease and were unable to grasp the implications and future repercussions of their diagnoses. However, recent research provides increasing evidence that even those with dementia, including Alzheimer's disease, retain a level of awareness into their own health and prognosis [1]. In addition, the progression of dementia can be quite variable [2]. Particularly during the early stages of the disease, those with dementia are often acutely aware of not only the relative impact of the disease on their own functioning but also of the responses and reactions of others to their diagnosis. This reaction is exacerbated by the misconceptions about the disorder promulgated by popular culture, such as comparisons of those with dementia to the "walking dead" [3]. These factors create a very vulnerable population with unique needs and special considerations.

When dealing with a patient who has been recently diagnosed with dementia, it is crucial to acknowledge that this is a disease and there are approved treatments and recommendations for medical management. It is also important to facilitate an understanding of what it means to be diagnosed with dementia, its course, and prognosis. This chapter will describe some of the hurdles that lie ahead for patients and families, and provide information to help manage these hurdles. It is important not only to educate those coping with a diagnosis of dementia but also to instill perspective and ensure quality of life for both patients and their families. This chapter aims to discuss frequently encountered questions, special considerations, and resources available to this population. It also discusses the importance of identifying and treating comorbid behavioral conditions and nonpharmacological approaches to treatment of both the patient and their family/caregivers. The identification and use of community resources and social services by patients and their families will also be discussed. The opportunities available to patients to participate in dementia research and clinical trials are described and the crucial role these studies play in ensuring continued advancement in understanding both the disease and its treatment.

Treating Dementia

Although there are approved treatments for the cognitive symptoms of dementia, the effectiveness is modest (see Table 5.1), with cholinesterase inhibition being the most established approach to treatment. This approach blocks the action of the enzyme acetylcholinesterase (AChe), an enzyme that breaks down the neurotransmitter acetylcholine in the synapse. The inhibitors permit the transmitter to sustain activation of the postsynaptic neuron, allowing the synapse to remain active longer. This class of agents has been used for the treatment of Alzheimer's disease since 1993, when tacrine was first approved. Tacrine, the first drug in this class, is not commonly used today as it is short acting, requiring treatment four times a day and routine assessment of liver enzymes. The second agent to be approved in this class, donepezil, has proven easier to use with once-a-day dosing. Donepezil is indicated for the treatment of Alzheimer's disease and has been demonstrated to be effective in patients with mild, moderate, and severe disease. Donepezil is approved for mild to moderate (5 or 10 mg) as well as severe disease (10 and 23 mg). Other drugs in this class include galantamine, which is available in a sustained release at a dose of 16–24 mg per day, and in a generic form. Rivastigmine, another agent in the same class, is available both as an oral agent and as a transdermal preparation and has been approved for the treatment of mild to moderate dementia, including Parkinson's dementia, at a dose of 6–12 mg per day, given as twice-a-day dosing. The side effect profile of these agents includes nausea and vomiting in 10–30% of the cases, which may be reduced with exposure. Although cholinesterase inhibitors have been studied in many types of dementia, approval is limited to Alzheimer's disease and Parkinson's disease. There is anecdotal

Table 5.1 Pharmacological treatments of dementia

Drug	Drug class	Indication	Target dose	Most common side effects
Tacrine[a]	Reversible acetylcholinesterase inhibitor	Mild to moderate dementia	40–160 mg/day (10–40 mg, four times daily)	Transaminase elevations requiring LFT monitoring Nausea and/or vomiting, diarrhea, dyspepsia, and anorexia (dose dependent)
			4 weeks titration	Myalgia, anorexia, and ataxia
Donepezil	Reversible acetylcholinesterase inhibitor	Mild to moderate AD	5 and 10 mg daily 1 week titration	Nausea, diarrhea, vomiting, insomnia, muscle cramp, fatigue, anorexia
		Severe AD	10 mg 23 mg	Nausea, diarrhea, vomiting, anorexia
Galantamine	Reversible acetylcholinesterase inhibitor	Mild to moderate AD	16–24 mg/day (8–12 mg twice daily) OR 16–24 ER daily 4–8 weeks titration	Nausea, vomiting, diarrhea, weight decrease, anorexia, dizziness, headache, depression
Rivastigmine	Reversible acetylcholinesterase inhibitor	Mild to moderate AD Dementia of Parkinson's disease	6–12 mg/day (3–6 mg twice daily) 2–6 week titration[b]	Nausea, vomiting, anorexia, diarrhea, dyspepsia, dizziness, headache
Memantine	NMDA antagonist	Moderate to severe AD	20 mg (10 mg twice daily) 3 weeks titration	Dizziness, headache, constipation, confusion

AD Alzheimer's disease, *ER* extended release formulation
[a]Tacrine, the first drug to be approved for the treatment of AD, is rarely used because of the burden of QID administration and the need for routine assessment for liver enzyme elevations
[b]Available as liquid and patch

evidence that cholinesterase inhibitors may be ineffective or cause clinical worsening in frontal temporal dementia [4]. Although not approved for treatment of mild cognitive impairment (MCI), several trials have demonstrated the benefit of cholinesterase inhibitors on cognitive, functional, and global clinical outcomes.

Memantine is another agent approved for the treatment of moderate to severe AD. It is an orally active NMDA receptor antagonist. The recommended starting dose is 5 mg once daily, and the recommended target dose is 20 mg per day. Despite several trials, to date there is no evidence that this drug has an effect in mild disease. There is evidence that the combination of memantine and donepezil is more effective than donepezil alone in the moderate to severe dementia population [5], which has been the basis of usage of memantine in combination with cholinesterase inhibitors. While the benefits from this agent have been labeled as minimal, it is robust with most trials demonstrating statistically significant benefits on measures of cognition and of clinical global change in subjects with AD [6].

Vitamins, Supplements, and Medical Foods

Many vitamin and neutraceutical regimens have been examined in studies to determine benefit in subjects with AD. For example, a multicenter randomized trial of vitamin E in moderately severe AD subjects demonstrated an effect in clinical outcomes, including delayed time until nursing home placement [7]. However, no benefit was identified in studies in milder individuals with MCI in either cognition or clinical outcomes [8]. Lowering of homocysteine through regimens of folate, vitamin B6 and B12, has also been studied with no evidence of benefit in patients with mild to moderate AD [9]. Further, there was some indication of increased depressive symptomatology in those receiving the vitamin regimen [9]. Omega-3 fatty acids have also been proposed as treatments for cognitive loss and dementia. A trial of DHA demonstrated no benefit in clinical or cognitive outcomes in AD, even among those who had relatively low levels of omega-3 in their diet [10]. Effects in malnourished elderly populations have not been studied, but these are infrequently seen in US aging cohorts.

Medical foods, a relatively new category regulated by the FDA as part of the Orphan Drug Act in 1988, are defined as products intended for the specific dietary management of a disease or condition that has distinctive nutritional requirements, established by medical evaluation. In contrast to FDA-approved drugs, no premarket review process exists for medical foods. Instead, they are regulated after they have become available to consumers. Axona, an example of a medical food that became available in 2009, claims to target the nutritional needs of people with AD. Specifically, it has been proposed that AD hinders the brain's ability to break down glucose, and Axona provides an alternative source of glucose that the brain can use for energy. Axona has been shown to improve cognition in AD [11], and a review of available data indicates relative safety [12]. Another medical food, Souvenaid, which is not currently marketed, is now in clinical trials. A single trial reported in 2010 describes small positive effects on memory testing but not on other traditional measures of cognition, function, and quality of life [13]. In general, there is little evidence of benefit to recommend medical foods for the treatment of AD; however, there appears to be little identified risk with their use.

Nonpharmacological Interventions for Cognitive Symptoms

Nonpharmacological interventions have been proposed for the range of symptoms in AD and other dementias. In a recent review that included both randomized and nonrandomized studies, Hulme et al. [14] identified 33 studies of nonpharmacological interventions, 10 of which addressed cognitive symptoms (described in Table 5.2). Of these, eight also examined functional and behavioral outcomes. The single most common nonpharmacologic approach described in the literature is cognitive stimulation/cognitive training. While individual studies report moderate effects on a number of different cognitive domains, no single domain was consistently improved. There is great diversity in the type of training proposed in these studies, making it difficult to prescribe any single approach. Counseling was found to have no beneficial effect on cognition or any other symptom. Two research groups studied transcutaneous electrical nerve stimulation (TENS) and found some cognitive benefit of very brief duration but no lasting benefit.

In general, the critical elements of nonpharmacological interventions are not well described, study designs are weakened by poor or absent control groups, and effects are poorly characterized. Most importantly, there is little information on how these interventions might be translated for broad use, including limited discussion on required training of individuals who deliver the intervention, and no information on the cost or required resources needed to disseminate the intervention in the community.

Importance of a Comprehensive Physical and Psychological Exam

When a patient receives a diagnosis of dementia, it is crucial to continue to address the presence of comorbid medical and psychiatric disorders. The presence of comorbid disorders may exacerbate a patient's symptoms and create additional burden that can challenge the patient's quality of life. In addition, the presence of these symptoms can have a significant influence on family members as well. These comorbid disorders can also increase the use of health-care resources and ultimately, the outcomes of care [15,16]. Many medical and psychiatric comorbidities can be treated with

Table 5.2 Nonpharmacological treatments for the cognitive symptoms of dementia (Adapted from Ref. [14])

	Description	Effectiveness	Weaknesses
Cognitive stimulation therapy/ cognitive training	Focus on information processing rather than rehearsal of factual knowledge	May work for improving memory, cognitive functioning, neuropsychiatric symptoms, behavior, depression, quality of life, learning, and activities of daily living	Less effective in more advance stages of dementia
Light therapy	Improving the patient's exposure and timing to natural and artificial light sources	May work when used to improve behavioral and psychological symptoms (sleep, behavior, mood, agitation) and cognition	–
Music therapy	Exposing patients to music	Effective in reducing behavioral and psychological symptoms, including agitation, aggression, wandering, restlessness, irritability, social and emotional difficulties, and improving nutritional intake	Effect of therapy did not persist over time
Physical activity	Promoting physical activity such as dance, support, drama, etc.	Effective for behavioral and psychological symptoms and functional ability. Moderate intensive exercise may reduce wandering and improve the quality of sleep	–
Reality orientation	Reality orientation aims to decrease confusion and dysfunctional behavior patterns in people with dementia by orientating patients to time, place, and person	May work to improve cognitive ability, depression, and apathy	Inflexible and may be confrontational in its administration
Reminiscence therapy	Involves discussion of past experiences. Photographs, familiar objects, or sensory items are used to prompt recall	May work to improve cognition, mood, and general behavior	–
Snoezelen/multisensory stimulation	Consists of visual, auditory, tactile, and olfactory stimulation offered to people in a specially designed room or environment. Used to increase the opportunity for communication and improved quality of experience	May improve disruptive behavior, mood, depression, aggression, apathy, cognition, social/emotional behaviors, wandering, and neuropsychiatric symptoms. May reduce apathy in the latter stages of dementia	Many improvements reported were not statistically significant. Overall beneficial effects were not sustained
Transcutaneous electrical nerve stimulation (TENS)	The application of an electric current through electrodes attached to the skin	May produce short-term benefits (directly after treatment) in recall, face recognition, and motivation	–
Validation therapy	Focuses on the emotional content of what someone is saying rather than the factual content. The patient is validated by acknowledging the emotions being expressed	May improve affect and behavioral disturbance	–

either pharmacological or nonpharmacological interventions. Identification of these conditions is the first step, and appropriate management and follow-up care are essential.

Depression

Depression is common in the aging population and is highly associated with cognitive loss and dementia. Prevalence estimates suggest that approximately 20–25% of those with AD also experience clinical depression, with some estimates as high as 50% [17]. Depressive symptoms in dementia may be due to the perceived loss of independence and the patient's awareness of their own cognitive decline, particularly in the early stages of the disorder [16]. Depression has also been associated with increased aggression and agitation in those with dementia [18]. Caregivers report that a patient's depression is the single most distressing symptom, and high rates of depression are also observed in caregivers themselves [19].

Depression and dementia have several overlapping symptoms, and the differential diagnosis can be difficult. Special diagnostic criteria have been proposed by the National Institutes of Mental Health (NIMH) in order to differentiate depressive symptoms associated with the patient's primary cognitive decline or dementia and those due to a secondary diagnosis of depression [20]. The guidelines indicate that when diagnosing depression, symptoms that can better be explained by the patient's primary dementia diagnosis should be excluded (e.g., increased apathy). For the diagnosis of depression in the presence of dementia, it is recommended to rely more on objective evaluation of symptoms (i.e., observed tearfulness or more easily discouraged, presence of irritability, or social isolation) rather than exclusively on self-report of depressive symptoms. Depressive symptoms include changes in mood, decreased positive affect, changes in sleep or appetite, psychomotor changes, fatigue, feelings of guilt, worthlessness, or hopelessness, increased discouragement or tearfulness, or possible suicidal ideation, and treatment should focus on these specific symptoms. It is helpful for patients and their families to understand which symptoms are likely to improve as a result of treatment and which are not. For example, antidepressants are unlikely to have a noticeable impact on a patient's memory or level of cognitive functioning. However, treatment of depression can have an impact on a patient's mood and their ability to function on a daily basis.

The pharmacology of depression in the presence of dementia has some special considerations. Tricyclic antidepressants are contraindicated in dementia patients due to their anticholinergic activity, which can adversely affect cognition [21]. Selective serotonin reuptake inhibitors (SSRIs) are often used in this population; however, these medications have been associated with an increased risk of falls and to a lesser degree with the syndrome of inappropriate antidiuretic hormone secretion (SIADH) [22].

Both cognitive and behavioral therapies have shown to produce improvement in depressive symptoms in a dementia population [23]. Cognitive strategies are more successful in the earlier stages of the disorder when a patient's cognitive abilities are still conducive to this style of therapy [23]. Cognitive therapy has been successful in challenging the patient's negative thought patterns and reducing cognitive distortions [24].

When depression is reactive, focusing on increasing pleasant events and interactions and minimizing aversive events that maintain the depression can be helpful [25] and can reduce disruptive behaviors [26]. Behavioral therapies can be used at all stages of dementia severity to focus attention on simple and familiar single-step tasks that will likely lead to success and avoid demanding activities with a high probability of failure [27].

Anxiety

Anxiety may be common in the early stages of cognitive loss when a patient's insight into his/her cognitive decline is high. At any stage of dementia, anxiety has been associated with an increased irritability, aggression, and pathological crying [28], as well as repetitive or stereotypical behaviors such as pacing, chanting, or focused motor movements [29]. Anxiety can impair the patient's ability to function, including refusal to allow necessary care. These symptoms continue to increase as an individual's cognitive decline and confusion become more severe [25]. Anxiety is present in more than 20% of patients with cognitive decline or dementia [30]. Anxiety often manifests as irritability, fear, paranoia, aggression, or depression [16]. Patients can have difficulty with articulating their emotional and psychiatric symptoms, particularly in the later stages of the disorder. It is often preferable to treat a patient's symptoms without medications because the most commonly used pharmacological agents have well-established side effects. For example, benzodiazepines, which may be useful as antianxiety agents in younger individuals, can exacerbate cognitive deficits and be associated with increased falls [31], and both the typical and atypical antipsychotics can be associated with significant risks in older adults, including increased mortality [32]. Behavioral management focuses on simplifying the environment, providing a structured routine, reducing choices, and avoiding new learning. It is also useful to minimize anticipation of either positive or negative events, keeping a patient focused on the present day [27]. Anxiety may manifest as repetitive questioning to family members or caregivers, despite efforts to continually providing newer or better answers. For these patients, the answer to the question is not as important as maintaining contact with the caregiver. It is typically the patient's need for reassurance and comforting that leads to additional questioning [27], thus providing a supportive and calming environment can be effective.

Treatment with antidepressants (e.g., SSRI) has been reported with some success [22]. Cholinesterase inhibitors have been shown to reduce symptoms of anxiety in those with minimal symptoms [33], but there is little evidence that they can successfully treat more severe anxiety. In general, treatment with benzodiazepines should be avoided as they have been shown to increase the risk of falls and delirium [16,34]. If benzodiazepines are employed, it is generally preferable to use nonoxidated, short-acting benzodiazepines (e.g., lorazepam) because they are less likely to accumulate and lead to eventual toxicity [35].

Other Behavioral Disturbances

Delusions and hallucinations also occur in dementia, tend to increase as a patient's disease progresses, and have been correlated to increased agitation and aggression [36]. For some, these delusions may be an attempt to organize information in the face of poor memory. For example, commonly reported delusions such as the belief that people are stealing things (occurring in 18–43% of dementia patients), that the patient is being abandoned (3–18% of dementia patients), and that the patient's spouse is being unfaithful (1–9% of dementia patients) [37] may be a result of forgetting the antecedent observations (e.g., losing things, not recalling the details of a planned absence of a spouse). Delusional or paranoid beliefs are associated with changes in a patient's daily routine or the presence of strangers [27]. The onset of delusional beliefs may be an indication that the patient's current level of activity is too stressful. Proper treatment of anxiety can also assist in alleviating suspicion and the formation of delusions. These environmental circumstances can often be avoided if a caregiver is made aware of them.

Hallucinations occur in 12% to 15% of patients with AD and can be auditory or visual [38]. However, in some cases, these experiences may actually represent an independently treatable disorder. For example, the presence of both tactile and visual hallucinations may actually indicate a reversible drug-induced delirium (described below), and auditory hallucinations instructing the patients to harm themselves may be a symptom of clinical depression [27]. Hallucinations may also be a manifestation of a patient's specific wishes and fears, particularly the fear of abandonment [27]. This fear is often improved by keeping caregivers visible and providing a controlled environment, adequate distractions, and continued reassurance. Pharmacological treatment of these symptoms can be quite difficult. Studies have shown modest improvement of hallucinations, delusions, and the accompanying agitation in dementia patients when being treated with antipsychotic medications such as olanzapine and risperidone [16,39]. In addition, these medications have significant side effects including sedation and extrapyramidal symptoms. In one study, quetiapine was associated with worsening of cognition and no improvement in psychiatric symptomatology [16]. Both conventional and atypical antipsychotics have also been linked to increased mortality and risk of cerebrovascular events in elderly patients [40].

Aggression

Aggression in patients with dementia is the most common reason that caregivers contact their clinicians requesting assistance [41], and is a common reason for placement a residential facility [42]. Physically aggressive behaviors are estimated to be present in 25–50% of community-based dementia patients and even more frequently within a nursing home setting [43]. Some patients will experience increased agitation that is isolated to later in the day (sundowning), which is particularly common in moderate to severe dementia. This may be related to fatigue or the loss of visual cues in the environment. An early awareness of these behavioral problems may help in planning for future care but must be weighed against anticipation anxiety in family members.

Treatment of aggressive behaviors requires identifying the underlying reason for the agitation. Some behavioral interventions for aggressive behaviors have shown promise. When aggression occurs as a consequence of a patient's anxiety or delusional beliefs, then the contributing symptoms should be addressed as described above. Reassuring patients and providing them with a controlled environment can alleviate their fears and suspicions. Marginal success has been noted in studies involving physical exercise, distraction-based interventions, and increased caregiver training [44]; however, additional research is necessary in order to determine their broad efficacy.

Delirium

Delirium is a sudden change in mental status characterized by severe confusion that is attributed to a discrete physical or mental illness that is usually temporary and reversible [45]. Within an elderly population, the most common causes of delirium are electrolyte disturbance (often from dehydration), infection, and postsurgical recovery. The presence of a dementia diagnosis increases a patient's susceptibility to developing a delirium [46], and this risk continues to increase as the dementia becomes more severe [47]. Prevalence estimates of delirium within a dementia population range from 22% to 89% in community and hospital studies [16], increasing the risk of developing delirium roughly twofold over elderly individuals without dementia [48]. Benzodiazepines increase the duration of a delirium, and as a result should primarily be used when the delirium is related to withdrawal from alcohol, a benzodiazepine, or another cross-tolerant sedative hypnotic [34]. After a delirium is successfully treated, the underlying cognitive and emotional symptoms of primary MCI or dementia will remain.

Considerations for Specific Non-Alzheimer Dementias

Vascular dementia is the most common dementia after AD. Memory impairment may be secondary while executive and attention deficits are typically more prominent, particularly early in the disease course. Vascular dementia is associated with increased depression and anxiety [49] and disrupted sleep–wake cycles [50]. It is important to consider that vascular dementia and AD may co-occur, and the expectation would be a combined symptom constellation.

Another relatively common neurodegenerative disorder is Lewy body dementia (LBD), which is estimated to affect 1.3 million people in the United States. It is characterized by cognitive impairment, parkinsonian motor symptoms, fluctuating mental status, and visual hallucinations [51]. Rapid eye movement (REM) sleep disorders [52] and an increased sensitivity to neuroleptics [53] have also been associated with LBD.

Frontotemporal dementia (FTD) represents 10–20% of all dementias and is characterized by changes in behavior, personality, and language or motor skills, but memory may be relatively intact. The most disturbing symptoms in FTD are inappropriate and disinhibited behaviors in social and work settings, including impulsivity, compulsivity, and verbal outbursts. Patients may have difficulty organizing activities, and self-care may be impaired resulting in increasing dependence. The average age of onset is 60, although earlier and later onset have been observed. Treatments with cholinesterase inhibitors are not effective and may actually have deleterious effects [54,55].

Utilizing Support Groups, Social Services, and Planning for the Future

Patients and their families may benefit from education and psychosocial services to provide support and assistance with coping as they confront a dementia diagnosis [56]. Services are most useful when tailored to consider the patient's specific level of functioning, support structure, and cultural background. Education and services can also address legal issues and financial planning. Early attention to these issues can take advantage of a patient's ability to participate in their own decision making and treatment planning [57]. While the availability of resources and services may vary in different locations, the current chapter attempts to discuss the types of options available and where to begin looking for appropriate groups and services.

Patient Support Groups

An effective approach for providing support and coping strategies for patients, particularly in the initial stages of the disease, is to connect with others experiencing the same emotions. The group setting can provide evidence that one is not alone and provide comfort in shared experiences. In response to this need, the Alzheimer's Association (www.alz.org) has instituted programs to help bring these patients together and provide both education and support. These groups allow patients to share their experiences and concerns, learn more about the disease, reduce feelings of isolation, and assist with coping and long-term planning [58]. These groups are often flexible in structure to accommodate an individual patient's availability, level of function, specific concerns, and inclusion of caregivers.

Patients may be resistant to the idea of attending support groups due to reluctance to accept their diagnosis or fear of having their stereotypes of the disease confirmed; however, several studies have explored the efficacy of these early-stage support groups and have consistently shown them to be beneficial. Patients enrolled in these programs report an increased sense of camaraderie, affirmation, improved confidence, education, and a decrease in their perceived helplessness and frustration [58–61]. Caregivers also reported increased awareness and acceptance, and stated that they helped to initiate difficult discussions about planning for the future (e.g., future medical, legal, and financial planning) and improved caregiver education regarding available community resources [58,61]. Those with the greatest level of distress at enrollment demonstrate the most significant improvement in quality of life by attending these groups [58].

Support Groups for Caregivers

Caregiving by family and friends can prove both satisfying and challenging. For informal caregivers, challenges include a shift in a relationship confronted by the patient's loss of independence and the caregiver's new responsibility, which requires time and energy, and can take a psychological toll. This toll can result from the loss of companionship of the patient, the weight of the responsibility, and the uncertainty regarding the course of the illness. High rates of depression and increased medical problems are observed in caregivers [19]. Caregiver support groups provide an opportunity to exchange information and benefit from the experience and knowledge of those in a similar situation [62]. Within these groups, caregivers are offered the opportunity to discuss their stressors and problems, and receive emotional support [63]. Support groups have been shown to provide a positive effect on a caregiver's knowledge, increase a caregiver's well being and reduce the sense of burden [64]. Mittelman et al. [65] demonstrated that structured caregiver support groups had direct effects on patients including delay in nursing home placement by nearly 1 year. National organizations such as the National Association of Area Agencies on Aging (www.n4a.org) can provide information on resources for programs, training, and support.

Support groups are underutilized, and estimates of participation range from 5% to 14% of caregivers [62]. It is important to make caregivers aware of the options that are available to help them cope with these stressors and to help them understand that attending caregiver support groups is not an indication of "failure" by the caregiver.

Social Services and Patient Care

Service needs in aging and dementia may include care for patients as well as support for caregivers; these needs will change over time and require reassessment during the course of the disease. At each stage of the disease, service goals include maximizing independence in a safe environment for the patient and supporting the social, psychological, and physical needs of the caregiver. A case manager can be useful in assisting with identifying these services. Typically trained in social work, their tasks are to assess needs, including the needs of the caregiver, and establish care planning and implementation. This may include an assessment of current resources and financial constraints, evaluation of coexisting medical needs of the patient, and establishing the capacity of the informal caregiving provided by family and friends. The assessment may identify a need for patients and family members to acknowledge their limitations and accept help. Case management can be particularly helpful for families who oversee care from a distance and when the process begins as early as possible so that continuity of care can be achieved.

Online resources are also available for managing care needs. For example, the Alzheimer's Association provides a CareFinder service at www.alz.org/carefinder. While web-based resources can be helpful and easy to access, it is important to understand their sponsorship, purpose, and mission. Those sponsored by patient advocacy groups such as Alzheimer's Association or by governmental entities such as the National Institute on Aging usually vet information through credible sources and disclose financial conflict. While providing easy-to-use information, commercial sites are likely to have product sales as a goal, and caution should be used.

During the initial stages of dementia, the need to modify the environment may be minimal and the patient may remain very active in the decision-making process. If informal caregiving is available, insuring that the caregiver is supported and stable may be all that is required. Supplemental services at this early stage may include identifying support groups, community day programs, or respite care. Additional support in the home may include help with housekeeping and companion services. Assistance from a home health aide may also be useful if medical problems interfere with independence. Home health aides can also provide assistance managing medications and appointments, and facilitate travel. As the dementia progresses, patients will require more assistance including additional medical help such as a visiting nurse or other professional, constant supervision, or even hospice for comfort care at end stages of the disease. For the majority of patients, at home services such as visiting nurses and home health aides are sufficient throughout the progression of the disease. In addition, insurance providers and Medicare typically supply coverage for respite services designed to lighten the burden of the caregiver such as homemaking, housekeeping, and companionship services.

For some, circumstances necessitate consideration of residential placement. Patients may not have family members who are available or in adequate health to assist with patient care, or the patient's cognitive decline or behavioral symptoms may require greater resources than are available in a home setting. Residential facilities can provide different levels of care in these circumstances, and one should consider the level of care that is most appropriate for each individual patient at each stage of their illness. Assisted living facilities may provide a transition between living independently and residing in a nursing home. These facilities typically provide a combination of housing and meals, as well as supportive and health-care services. Skilled nursing facilities provide continued medical supervision and have services designed specifically to address advanced care issues such as patient nutrition and medical care.

Medical–Legal Considerations

When cognitive loss and dementia are present, making plans to assist in future care decisions is advisable. It is useful to review existing advanced care directives or health-care proxy, and if they do not exist, it is advisable to put them in place. It is important to note that as long as a patient maintains his/her ability to competently make decisions on his/her own behalf, these opinions will take precedence over family or caregiver wishes, even if a health-care proxy or power of attorney has been appointed. Below we review important options and considerations for advance care initiatives.

Health-Care Proxy, Advance Care Directives, and Legal Planning

One of the key decisions to be made is who will be responsible for making health-care decisions if the patient loses the ability to make his/her own decisions. The diagnosis of dementia is not synonymous with incompetence, but as the dementia progresses, the likelihood of losing the ability to make decisions is high. It is therefore advisable for a patient to appoint a health-care proxy while they are still able. By appointing a health-care proxy, patients are assigning a person (typically a family member) to act on their behalf with regard to medical and end-of-life decisions. A patient may choose to document specific wishes regarding future medical care and decisions, either by advance care directives or a living will. These decisions can record a patient's wishes regarding issues such as the use of artificial life support, feeding tube placement, and comfort measures. By providing families and caregivers with specific instructions regarding what actions should be taken in different health-care scenarios, the patient ensures that their wishes will be followed. In the absence of these advance directives, a patient's health-care proxy will make decisions regarding their care. When assigning a proxy, patients also have the option of providing the person with varying degrees of authority. A proxy can be granted total control of medical decisions or can be given authority over only certain ones. When a patient decides to grant a proxy with only limited authority, consideration should be given to other types of scenarios in order to ensure that appropriate accommodations are made.

If a proxy has not been appointed or if a proxy's authority does not address the issue at hand, then health-care decisions are made by either the patient's family or the doctors involved in their care. Using substituted judgment, doctors and family members try to make the decision that the patient would have made if they were able to make decisions. Given the difficulty of these decisions, as well as the moral considerations involved, it is generally preferable to rely on advance care directives and appointed health-care proxies whenever possible.

A power of attorney assigns a person with the ability to speak (and sign documents) on a patient's behalf with regard to legal and financial matters. However, the power of attorney does not provide an individual with the authority to override a patient's wishes. Patients maintain the power to also make their own legal decisions, as long as they maintain the capacity to do so. In addition, unless a power of attorney is irrevocable, patients have the authority to change and withdraw the appointment as they see fit (again, assuming the patient is still deemed to have the capacity to make this decision). Powers of attorney may also be "durable," which allows this appointment to be maintained even after a patient is no longer able to make decisions for himself/

herself. The power of attorney will also make decisions regarding a patient's finances and assets.

Legal Capacity and Guardianship

In order to appoint representatives (i.e., health-care proxy or power of attorney) or make legal decisions, a patient must maintain the capacity to do so. Legal capacity is generally defined as an individual's ability to understand and appreciate the consequences of one's actions and to make rational and informed decisions. The diagnosis of cognitive loss or dementia is not synonymous with lack of capacity, and judgments of capacity may actually differ for each type of decision. When patients maintain capacity to participate in their own legal planning, the wishes of others are subordinate. However, as a dementia progresses, a patient can become increasingly impaired and confused, and may even demonstrate paranoia directed toward those trying to assist them.

In order to determine an individual's capacity to sign legal documents during the initial stages of a dementia, family members are often able to simply speak to the patient to ensure that they adequately understand and can rearticulate the implications of the documents they are signing. In other cases in which uncertainty regarding a patient's capacity persists, additional assistance can often be obtained by speaking to a lawyer or by referring the patient to a psychologist to assess his/her mental status and cognitive limitations. For cases in which a patient is deemed to lack capacity to make decisions on his/her own behalf, the court may appoint a guardian (typically a family member) to speak for the patient. A court-appointed guardian (also referred to as a conservator) can be responsible for making financial and health-care decisions for the patient.

Finding a Lawyer

While health-care proxy, advanced care directives, responsibility and power of attorney can all be executed without an attorney, it may be preferable to seek legal advice to avoid undesired consequences of these actions. Elder law focuses on estate planning and administration, disability, long-term care issues, and issues of guardianship including fiduciary. Elder law attorneys in a specific area can be obtained from the local chapter of the Alzheimer's Association (www.alz.org). Free legal advice is also available in some areas. Available resources can be found at the local Eldercare Locator (www.eldercare.gov).

Dementia Research: Current State, Future Trends, and Opportunities to Participate

There are many stakeholders in the efforts to find a treatment for AD, and themes of research include both better diagnostics to provide early detection and distinctions among types of dementias as well as initiatives to understand the underlying pathological mechanisms of the disease in order to identify new treatments. Neuritic plaques composed of amyloid and neurofibrillary tangles composed of the protein tau, the hallmark pathology of the disease, have been the primary target for drug discovery with the hope that modifying the aggregation of these proteins into pathological structures will modify the course of the disease. The breadth of research initiatives is wide, and there are three broad areas that have received significant attention and support from the National Institute on Aging (NIA): diagnostics, interventions, and genetics.

Research on Diagnostics

Early detection of AD may provide the ability to intervene more effectively. To this end, many studies of the transition from health to cognitive impairment and dementia are under way. One of the most prominent findings is that memory deficits predict the progression to AD, and from this work the criteria for recognition of MCI were developed. Work continues, defining other cognitive and biological markers that predict the disease. A large effort in this area is the Alzheimer Disease Neuroimaging Initiative (ADNI) [66]. This public–private partnership has been working to identify biomarkers that predict disease in the mildly symptomatic and nonsymptomatic individual.

Specific biomarkers that are being studied are quantitative MRI, PET images, and cerebrospinal fluid (CSF) and blood biomarkers. The imaging techniques measure the size of specific brain structures (MRI) and the energy used by specific brain areas (PET). Additional imaging studies use ligands that label proteins in the brain to identify the presence of amyloid and tau. Other studies are measuring amyloid and tau in the CSF to find early evidence of AD-like changes. These studies have been enrolling research participants with and without dementia to determine which biomarkers differentiate the groups and to track change over time. Today, these studies continue with the hope of recruiting very mildly impaired individuals, who may only demonstrate biomarker evidence of disease without accompanying impairment [67]. The hope is that finding a marker to detect those at risk will help to target a population most likely to benefit from early intervention. More information is available about ADNI at their Web site (www.adni-info.org).

Studies have suggested that these biomarkers are as important as the clinical presentation of the patient, and recent guidelines for the diagnosis of Alzheimer's disease have been reevaluated to focus on cognitive change, regardless of type, and the presence of an amyloid biomarker. Additionally, research guidelines have been proposed which include the concept of "prodromal" Alzheimer's disease, a research diagnosis that requires a positive biomarker with no evidence of clinical impairment [68].

Research on Interventions

Current treatments for Alzheimer's disease are referred to as "symptomatic" in that they produce a benefit on the cognitive, functional, and behavioral symptoms associated with the disease. Today, experimental therapeutics focus on treatments that modify the disease course. This may include slowing or stopping the disease progression or preventing the onset of the clinical symptoms of the disease. Some approaches to therapy focus on modifying biomarkers of the disease in the hope that it will change its clinical course, and many clinical trials have examined agents that would reduce amyloid in the brain. Areas that remain active today are gamma secretase inhibition and immunization (both active and passive). Blocking the gamma secretase enzyme appears to reduce the accumulation of amyloid into plaques. However, to date, this mechanism has not proven effective in modifying clinical outcomes in AD. Immunization therapeutics, both active and passive, are also being developed. Animal data support the notion that antibodies against amyloid beta (Aβ) can lead to clearance of cerebral Aβ deposits, and human trials have further demonstrated this clearance [69]. However, clinical improvement has not always accompanied the clearance, leading researchers to believe that effectiveness requires administration at much earlier stages of the disease, such as the "prodromal" stage proposed in new diagnostic criteria. Another mechanism under study is neural regeneration, and the NIA along with Ceregene pharmaceuticals has sponsored one such trial of nerve growth factor, which is stereotaxically implanted in the brain. Other regenerative agents are also in development. Drug development in Alzheimer's disease is very active with more than 96 studies actively recruiting, as reported on the clinicaltrials.gov Web site.

Genetics

Three genes associated with the development of rare early-onset forms of familial AD have been known for many years: mutations in the amyloid precursor protein (APP) gene found on chromosome 21, the presenilin 1 gene on chromosome 14, and the presenilin 2 gene on chromosome 1. The most common form of the disease, late-onset (typically defined as over the age of 60) AD, is a complex disorder, and it is likely that many genes may play a role in disease development. Until recently, however, only one gene variant, apolipoprotein E-ε4 (APOE-ε4), has been confirmed as a significant risk factor gene for late-onset Alzheimer's disease. In the past several years, however, researchers have confirmed additional gene variants of complement receptor 1 (CR1), clusterin (CLU), and the phosphatidylinositol-binding clathrin assembly protein (PICALM) as possible risk factors for late-onset Alzheimer's. The newest genome-wide association scan (GWAS) confirms that a fifth gene variant, Myc box-dependent-interacting protein 1 (BIN 1), also affects the development of late-onset AD. Several other genetic variants were identified at EPHA 1, MS4A, CD2AP, and CD33; these genes may implicate pathways involved in inflammation, movement of proteins within cells, and lipid transport as being important in the disease process. These studies utilized DNA samples from more than 56,000 study participants and are made possible through the Alzheimer's Disease Genetics Consortium (ADGC), a collaborative body established and funded by the NIA [70].

Identification of new genes may provide major clues as to the cause of AD. Genetic variants may influence risk of disease, the age of onset of symptoms, rate of progression, the amount of amyloid plaques or neurofibrillary tangles, concentrations of amyloid beta and tau in CSF, and responses to environmental factors such as medications. In addition, genetic studies can also provide new insights critical for drug discovery. The identification of new genes associated with AD is a very important preliminary step toward identifying biological pathways leading to disease. These pathways help to identify new targets for therapeutic strategies to treat and prevent the disease.

Participation in Research

There are many reasons why an individual may be motivated to participate in research. First, many individuals appreciate the opportunity for additional standardized follow-up. Often, experimental instruments and techniques are used to assess novel aspects of disease or health, and tracking that performance can provide support and insight for research participants. Research participation can also provide early access to new techniques and treatments. While there is no guarantee of a positive outcome, the requirement for safety in research demands close observation to ensure that untoward results are identified early and modifications to procedures, treatments, and study designs are made quickly. This attention can add confidence to participating in studies that might expose an individual to unnecessary or ineffective procedures. In the case of positive results, participants get the earliest exposure. In many studies, even those initially assigned to the placebo group are given the opportunity to receive the active intervention, even before the agent is fully available for marketing or before a diagnostic is fully approved.

The nature of participation in research in dementia and cognitive impairment often requires participation of a study partner, usually a friend or family member. Because they play an important role, support for family and friends is often provided in research. This can take the form of activities to maximize retention such as support groups or informational material that is often provided by study staff who are experts in the particular aspect of dementia care and management. It can also occur informally through exposure to others participating in research who offer peer support and shared experiences.

The most common and sustaining reason for research participation is altruism. The ability to make contributions that benefit others with the disease remains the highest motivator. This is an important factor in research recruitment. Longstanding characteristics of generosity in an individual are often unchanged in the presence of illness, and in the face of mortality, they may even be enhanced. Offering research participation is acknowledging the patient as an important contributor to knowledge of his/her disease and to the welfare of others.

Critical Information About Research Participation

While many practitioners acknowledge the benefit of research participation for their patients, it is not always clear how to go about identifying and evaluating studies or preparing patients for the rejection they may feel if not eligible for a given study. Additionally, many commercial entities can solicit participation with little oversight. However, there are several resources that are well established that can be helpful to patients, families, and friends. For example, because of both regulatory and publication guidance, most clinical trials as well as many other clinical studies are posted on www.Clinicaltrials.gov. Clinicaltrials.gov offers up-to-date information for locating federally and privately supported research studies that use human volunteers to answer specific health questions. The Web site was developed by the US National Institutes of Health (NIH), through its National Library of Medicine (NLM), and in collaboration with the Food and Drug Administration (FDA), as a result of the FDA Modernization Act (Public Law Number 105-1 15, 1997). The registry describes studies conducted in all 50 States and in 174 countries. The website receives over 50 million page views per month and 65,000 visitors daily. This registry has an easy-to-use search engine, and as of this writing, is posting over 900 studies in AD with more than 200 currently recruiting. The study postings describe basic entry criteria for given studies along with location and contact information. The website requires annual updating of information and posting of study results. Another opportunity for those with AD is the Alzheimer's Association TrialMatch,™ a clearing house designed to help people with AD, caregivers, families, and clinicians locate clinical trials based on specific criteria such as diagnosis, stage of disease, and location. More than 100 research studies pertaining to AD and related dementias are underway and recruiting volunteers through this service, and Alzheimer's Association TrialMatch lets you search these trials quickly and easily. It also narrows results to those trials where there is a reasonable chance to be accepted for enrollment. Individuals may register by providing information about a potential participant, and with the registrant's permission, an Alzheimer's Association Contact Center specialist will provide unbiased trial result options and trial site contact information. Specialists will not recommend any particular trial but will identify trials that match specific eligibility criteria.

Finally, the National Center for Research Resources, part of the NIH, sponsors ResearchMatch through the Clinical and Translational Science Awards (CTSA) program. ResearchMatch has a simple goal—to bring together two groups of people who are looking for one another: (1) people who are trying to find research studies and (2) researchers who are looking for people to participate in their studies. It is a secure registry that has been developed by major academic institutions across the country in order to develop a nationwide effort to enrich participation in research. This effort is not disease specific and offers opportunities to both patients and healthy individuals.

Research participation may not be for all individuals, and both the investigator and the participant have opportunities to evaluate the specific match of the potential subject and the project. From the investigator perspective, a study must be designed to answer a specific question. Selection criteria therefore focus on identifying subjects who can help answer specific questions. Inclusion criteria might define the severity of the disease or the age of a participant or exposure to other treatments. Other criteria may be used to ensure safety, requiring exclusion of some individuals based on the presence of comorbid conditions or concurrent medications that could increase risks if exposed to a new treatment or test. Some criteria may be based on ensuring that the effectiveness can be measured. For example, studies involving cognitive evaluation may exclude subjects with significant hearing or visual loss that might potentially interfere with testing.

From a participant's point of view, it is critical to work with a trusted group. The research group may be identified by a physician or vetted through one of the Web sites described in this chapter. It is also important to evaluate how much participation is right for the participant. A study may require frequent visits. Some procedures may be particularly noxious. The participant needs to weigh these against the benefit of making a contribution. An important aspect for participants to keep in mind is that participation is voluntary and one can always change his/her mind if circumstances change. In the end, it is the faithful participation in clinical research that will identify the treatments of tomorrow.

Clinical Pearls

- Pharmacological treatments available for Alzheimer's disease require careful titration to find the best dose; modest effects have been observed at all stages of the disease.
- Nonpharmacological interventions can be particularly helpful for behavioral problems associated with dementia. Environmental modifications can improve safety and extend functional independence.
- Behavioral and psychiatric symptoms are common and should be treated using both pharmacological and nonpharmacological means.
- Acute medical problems can potentially exacerbate cognitive and behavioral symptoms; routine health maintenance should be an integrated part of dementia care.
- Identifying the etiology of the dementing disorder is critical for planning and management, as subtypes have differential presenting symptoms and rates of disease progression.
- Support groups and resources are available and can improve the quality of life of both patients and their caregivers.
- Care needs in dementia will change with the progression of the disease. Matching the level of care with the patient's disease severity will contribute to maximizing independence. Case management can be helpful in identifying and accessing care needs.
- The cognitive decline associated with dementia has both legal and financial implications, and patients and their families should explore of assigning health-care proxy, power of attorney, and making advance care directives.
- There are many opportunities for those with dementia and cognitive loss to participate in clinical research and clinical trials. Clinicians can introduce the possibility of research participation for the hope it offers to their patients and to the generations to come.

Table 5.3 Additional internet resources

Information available	Web site
For information, resources, and support groups specifically pertaining to Alzheimer's disease	www.alz.org
For recent news and events specifically pertaining to Alzheimer's disease	www.nia.nih.gov/Alzheimers
For information, resources, and support groups specifically pertaining to Lewy body dementia	www.lbda.org
For information, resources, and support groups specifically pertaining to frontotemporal dementia	www.theaftd.org
For a directory of local programs and resources	www.eldercare.gov
For additional programs, training, and support	www.n4a.org
For information regarding legal and financial advice	www.caringinfo.org
For a list of clinical trials currently enrolling	www.clinicaltrials.gov

Resources

The websites listed in Table 5.3 are excellent resources for information, programs, support groups, and other resources (Table 5.3).

Acknowledgments This work was supported in part by the Alzheimer Disease Research Center at Mount Sinai funded by the following NIA grant: AG 005138

References

1. Burgener SC, Berger B. Measuring perceived stigma in persons with progressive neurological disease: Alzheimer's dementia and Parkinson's disease. Dementia. 2008;7:31–53.
2. Kraemer HC, Tinklenberg J, Yesavage JA. 'How far' vs 'how fast' in Alzheimer disease: the question revisited. Arch Neurol. 1994;51:275–9.
3. Behuniak SM. The living dead? The construction of people with Alzheimer's disease as zombies. Ageing Soc. 2011;31:70–92.

4. Kaye ED, Petrovic-Poljak A, Verhoeff NPLG, Freedman M. Frontotemporal dementia and pharmacologic interventions. J Neuropsychiatry Clin Neurosci. 2010;22:19–29.
5. Tariot PN, Farlow MR, Grossberg GT, Graham SM, McDonald S, Gergel I, Memantine Study Group. Memantine treatment in patients with moderate to severe Alzheimer disease already receiving donepezil: a randomized controlled trial. JAMA. 2004;291(3):317–24.
6. Riordan KC, Hoffman Snyder CR, Wellik KE, Caselli RJ, Wingerchuk DM, Demaerschalk BM. Effectiveness of adding memantine to an Alzheimer dementia treatment regimen which already includes stable donepezil therapy: a critically appraised topic. Neurologist. 2011;17:121–3.
7. Sano M, Ernesto C, Thomas RG, Klauber MR, Schafer K, Grundman M, et al. A controlled trial of selegiline, alpha-tocopherol, or both as treatment for Alzheimer's disease. The Alzheimer's Disease Cooperative Study. N Engl J Med. 1997;336:1216–22.
8. Petersen RC, Thomas RG, Grundman M, Bennett D, Doody R, Ferris S, et al. Vitamin E and donepezil for the treatment of mild cognitive impairment. N Engl J Med. 2005;352:2379–88.
9. Aisen PS, Schneider LS, Sano M, Diaz-Arrastia R, van Dyck CH, Weiner MF, et al. High-dose B vitamin supplementation and cognitive decline in Alzheimer disease: a randomized controlled trial. J Am Med Assoc. 2008;300:1774–83.
10. Quinn JF, Raman R, Thomas RG, Yurko-Mauro K, Nelson EB, Van Dyck C, et al. Docosahexaenoic acid supplementation and cognitive decline in Alzheimer disease: a randomized trial. J Am Med Assoc. 2010;304:1903–11.
11. Henderson ST, Vogel JL, Barr LJ, Garvin F, Jones JJ, Costantini LC. Study of the ketogenic agent AC-1202 in mild to moderate Alzheimer's disease: a randomized, double-blind, placebo-controlled, multicenter trial. Nutr Metab (Lond). 2009;10:31.
12. Roman MW. Axona (Accera, Inc): a new medical food therapy for persons with Alzheimer's disease. Issues Ment Health Nurs. 2010;31:435–6.
13. Scheltens P, Kamphuis PJ, Verhey FR, Olde Rikkert MG, Wurtman RJ, Wilkinson D, et al. Efficacy of a medical food in mild Alzheimer's disease: a randomized, controlled trial. Alzheimers Dement. 2010;6:1–10.
14. Hulme C, Wright J, Crocker T, Oluboyede Y, House A. Non-pharmacological approaches for dementia that informal carers might try or access: a systematic review. Int J Geriatr Psychiatry. 2009;25:756–63.
15. Desai AK, Grossberg GT. Diagnosis and treatment of Alzheimer's disease. Neurologic disorders update: current thinking and practices. Neurology. 2005;64:34–9.
16. Swanson KA, Carnahan RM. Dementia and comorbidities: an overview of diagnosis and management. J Pharm Pract. 2007;20(4):296–317.
17. Martin BK, Frangakis CE, Rosenberg PB, Mintzer JE, Katz IR, Porsteinsson AP, et al. Design of depression in Alzheimer's disease study-2. Am J Geriatr Psychiatry. 2006;14:920–30.
18. Lyketsos CG, Steele C, Galik E, Rosenblatt A, Steinberg M, Warren A, et al. Physical aggression in dementia patients and its relationship to depression. Am J Psychiatry. 1999;156:66–71.
19. Teri L. Behavior and caregiver burden: behavioral problems in patients with Alzheimer disease and its association with caregiver distress. Alzheimer Dis Assoc Disord. 1997;11:35–8.
20. Olin JT, Katz IS, Meyer BS, Schneider LS, Lebowitz BD. Provisional diagnostic criteria for depression of Alzheimer's disease: rationale and background. Am J Geriatr Psychiatry. 2002;10:129–41.
21. Breitbart W, Marotta R, Platt MM, Weisman H, Derevenco M, Grau C, et al. A double-blind trial of haloperidol, chlorpromazine, and lorazepam in the treatment of delirium in hospitalized AIDS patients. Am J Psychiatry. 1996;153:234–7.
22. Herrmann N. Use of SSRIs in the elderly: obvious benefits but unappreciated risks. Can J Clin Pharmacol. 2000;7:91–5.
23. Teri L, Gallagher-Thompson D. Cognitive-behavioral interventions for treatment of depression in Alzheimer's patients. Gerontologist. 1991;31:413–6.
24. Teri L, Gibbons LE, McCurry SM, Logsdon RG, Buchner DM, Barlow WE, et al. Exercise plus behavioral management in patients with Alzheimer disease: a randomized controlled trial. J Am Med Assoc. 2003;290:2015–22.
25. Zec RF, Burkett NR. Non-pharmacological and pharmacological treatment of the cognitive and behavioral symptoms of Alzheimer disease. NeuroRehabilitation. 2008;23:425–38.
26. Teri L, Logsdon RG. Identifying pleasant activities for Alzheimer's disease patients: the pleasant events schedule-AD. Gerontologist. 1991;31:124–7.
27. Weiner MF, Teri L. Psychological and behavioral management. In: Weiner MF, Lipton AM, editors. The dementias: diagnosis, treatment and research. Washington, D.C.: American Psychiatric Publishing, Inc; 2003. p. 181–218.
28. Chemerinski E, Petracca G, Manes F, Leiguarda R, Starkstein SE. Prevalence and correlates of anxiety in Alzheimer's disease. Depress Anxiety. 1998;7:166–70.
29. Luxenberg JS. Clinical issues in the behavioural and psychological symptoms of dementia. Int J Geriatr Psychiatry. 2000;15:5–8.
30. Lyketsos CG, Lopez O, Jones B, Fitzpatrick AL, Breitner J, DeKosky S. Prevalence of neuropsychiatric symptoms in dementia and cognitive impairment: results from the Cardiovascular Health Study. J Am Med Assoc. 2002;288:1475–83.
31. Madhusoodanan S, Bogunovic OJ. Safety of benzodiazepines in the geriatric population. Expert Opin Drug Saf. 2004;3:485–93.
32. Ballard C, Creese B, Corbett A, Aarsland D. Atypical antipsychotics for the treatment of behavioral and

psychological symptoms in dementia, with a particular focus on longer term outcomes and mortality. Expert Opin Drug Saf. 2011;10:35–43.
33. Cummings JL. Cholinesterase inhibitors: a new class of psychotropic compounds. Am J Psychiatry. 2000;157: 4–15.
34. Gleason OC. Delirium. Am Fam Physician. 2003; 67:1027–34.
35. Fick DM, Cooper JW, Wade WE, Waller JL, Maclean R, Beers MH. Updating the Beers criteria for potentially inappropriate medication use in older adults: results of a U.S. panel of experts. Arch Intern Med. 2003;163:2716–24.
36. Gilley DW, Wilson RS, Beckett LA, Evans DA. Psychotic symptoms and physically aggressive behavior in Alzheimer's disease. J Am Geriatr Soc. 1997;45: 1074–9.
37. Tariot PN, Blazina L. The psychopathology of dementia. In: Morris JC, editor. Handbook of dementing illnesses, neurological disease and therapy. New York: Marcel Dekker, Inc; 1994. p. 461–76.
38. Whitehouse PJ, Patterson MB, Strauss ME, Geldmacher DS, Mack JL, Gilmore GC, et al. Hallucinations. Int Psychogeriatr. 1996;8:387–92.
39. Schneider LS, Pierre N, Tariot PN, Dagerman KS, Davis SM, Hsiao JK, et al. Effectiveness of atypical antipsychotics in patients with Alzheimer's disease. N Engl J Med. 2006;355:1525–38.
40. Sink KM, Holden KF, Yaffe K. Pharmacological treatment of neuropsychiatric symptoms of dementia. J Am Med Assoc. 2005;293:596–608.
41. Nagaratnam N, Lewis-Jones M, Scott D, Palazzi L. Behavioral and psychiatric manifestations in dementia patients in a community: caregiver burden and outcome. Alzheimer Dis Assoc Disord. 1998;12: 330–4.
42. Cohen-Mansfield J, Mintzer JE. Time for change: the role of nonpharmacological interventions in treating behavior problems in nursing home residents with dementia. Alzheimer Dis Assoc Disord. 2005;19: 37–40.
43. Mann AH, Graham N, Ashby D. Psychiatric illness in residential homes for the elderly: a survey in one London borough. Age Aging. 1984;13(5):257–65.
44. Buchanan JA, Christenson AM, Ostrom C, Hofman N. Non-pharmacological interventions for aggression in persons with dementia: a review of the literature. Behav Analyst Today. 2007;8:413–25.
45. Inouye SK. Delirium and other mental status problems in the older patient (Chapter 26). In: Goldman L, Ausiello D, editors. Cecil medicine. 23rd ed. Philadelphia, PA: Saunders Elsevier; 2007.
46. Francis J. Delusions, delirium, and cognitive impairment: the challenge of clinical heterogeneity. Journal of the American Geriatric Society. 1992;40:844–9.
47. Fick DM, Agostini JV, Inouye SK. Delirium superimposed on dementia: A systematic review. Journal of the American Geriatric Society. 2002;50:1723–32.
48. Flaherty JH. The evaluation and management of delirium among older persons. Med Clin North Am. 2011;95:555–77.
49. Sultzer DL, Levin HS, Mahler ME, High WM, Cummings JL. A comparison of psychiatric symptoms in vascular dementia and Alzheimer's disease. Am J Psychiatry. 1993;156:1806–12.
50. Aharon-Peretz J, Masiah A, Pillar T, Epstein R, Tzischinsky OP, Lavie P. Sleep-wake cycles in multi-infarct dementia and dementia of the Alzheimer's type. Neurology. 1991;41:1616–9.
51. Ala TA, Yang KH, Sung JH, Frey II WH. Hallucinations and signs of parkinsonism help distinguish patients with dementia and cortical Lewy bodies from patients with Alzheimer's disease at presentation a clinico-pathological study. J Neurol Neurosurg Psychiatry. 1997;62:16–21.
52. Boeve BF, Silber MH, Ferman TJ, Kokmen E, Smith GE, Ivnik RJ, et al. REM sleep behavior disorder and degenerative dementia—an association likely reflecting Lewy body disease. Neurology. 1998;51:363–70.
53. McKeith I, Fairbairn A, Perry R, Thompson P, Perry E. Neuroleptic sensitivity in patients with senile dementia of Lewy body type. Br Med J. 1992;305:673–8.
54. Lindau M, Almkvist O, Johansson SE, Wahlund LO. Cognitive and behavioral differentiation of frontal lobe degeneration of the non-Alzheimer's type and Alzheimer's disease. Dement Geriatr Cogn Disord. 1997;9:205–13.
55. Mendez MF, Perryman KM, Miller BL, Cummings JL. Behavioral differences between frontotemporal dementia and Alzheimer's disease: a comparison on the BEHAVE-AD rating scale. Int Psychogeriatr. 1998;10:155–62.
56. Whitehouse P, Frisoni G, Post S. Breaking the diagnosis of dementia. Lancet Neurol. 2004;3:124–8.
57. Gauthier S. Advances in the pharmacotherapy of Alzheimer's disease. Can Med Assoc J. 2002;166: 616–23.
58. Logsdon RG, Pike KC, McCurry SM, Hunter P, Maher J, Snyder L, et al. Early-stage memory loss support groups: outcomes from a randomized controlled clinical trial. J Gerontol B Psychol Sci Soc Sci. 2010;65:691–7.
59. Goldsilver PM, Gruneir MRB. Early stage dementia group: an innovative model of support for individuals in the early stages of dementia. Am J Alzheimers Dis Other Demen. 2001;16:109–14.
60. Logsdon RG, McCurry SM, Teri L. Timelimited support groups for individuals with early stage dementia and their care partners: preliminary outcomes from a controlled clinical trial. Clin Gerontol. 2006;30:5–19.
61. Zarit SH, Femia EE, Watson J, Rice-Oeschger L, Kakos B. Memory club: a group intervention for people with early-stage dementia and their care partners. Gerontologist. 2004;44:262–9.
62. Gräßel E, Trilling A, Donath C, Luttenberger K. Support groups for dementia caregivers—predictors for utilisation and expected quality from a family caregiver's point of view: a questionnaire survey PART I. BMC Health Serv Res. 2010;10:219–26.
63. Kurz A, Hallauer J, Jansen S, Diehl J. Efficacy of caregiver support groups for dementia. Der Nervenarzt. 2005;76:261–9.

64. Thompson C, Spilsbury K. WITHDRAWN: Support for carers of people with Alzheimer's type dementia. Cochrane Database Syst Rev. 2007:CD000454.
65. Mittelman MS, Ferris SH, Shulman E, Steinberg G, Levin B. A family intervention to delay nursing home placement of patients with Alzheimer disease: a randomized controlled trial. J Am Med Assoc. 1996;276:1725–31.
66. Weiner MW, Aisen PS, Jack Jr CR, Jagust WJ, Trojanowski JQ, Shaw L, et al. The Alzheimer's disease neuroimaging initiative: progress report and future plans. Alzheimers Dement. 2010;6:202–11.
67. Aisen PS, Petersen RC, Donohue MC, Gamst A, Raman R, Thomas RG, et al. Clinical core of the Alzheimer's disease neuroimaging initiative: progress and plans. Alzheimers Dementia. 2010;6:239–46.
68. Jack Jr CR, Albert MS, Knopman DS, McKhann GM, Sperling RA, Carrillo MC, et al. Introduction to the recommendations from the National Institute on Aging-Alzheimer's Association workgroups on diagnostic guidelines for Alzheimer's disease. Alzheimers Dementia. 2011;7:257–62.
69. Pul R, Dodel R, Stangel M. Antibody-based therapy in Alzheimer's disease. Expert Opin Biol Ther. 2011;11:343–57.
70. National Institutes of Health. Studies find possible new genetic risk factors for Alzheimer's disease [Press Release]. http://www.nia.nih.gov/newsroom/2011/04/studies-find-possible-new-genetic-risk-factors-alzheimers-disease (2011).

Sleep and Aging

6

Matthew R. Ebben

Abstract

The purpose of this chapter is to discuss changes in sleep quality and architecture that occur as one ages. Normal age related changes in sleep architecture will be discussed first, followed by sleep and circadian rhythm disorders that increase in prevalence as we age. Finally, a short section at the end of this chapter discusses neurological disorders more frequently seen in older adults, and their impact on sleep.

Keywords

Insomnia • Geriatric • Sleep architecture • Circadian rhythms • Treatment • REM behavior disorder • Apnea

There is a general perception that degradation of sleep quality is a normal part of aging. In fact, practitioners who see geriatric patients on a regular basis often hear complaints of sleep difficulties in their patients. As we age, a number of age-related health problems are associated with difficulty sleeping. It is often difficult to differentiate sleep problems secondary to underlying health problems or medication effects from primary sleep disorders. This chapter will review the changes that occur in sleep quality as one ages and will address sleep disorders often seen in the older adults. The data discussed within this chapter is almost exclusively based on defining age chronologically. Some have argued that subjective or physiological age and time from death are more accurate ways of defining age; however, chronological age is the most consistent definition for aging. Therefore, it is the one used within this chapter.

Changes in Sleep Architecture as We Age

A number of studies have been conducted to look at changes in sleep architecture over the life span. One of the most consistent age-related changes in sleep architecture is a decline in delta or slow-wave sleep (SWS). SWS is defined electrographically by low-frequency (0.5–2 Hz), high-amplitude (>75 μV) waveforms [1] and is primarily confined to the first half of the sleep

M.R. Ebben, Ph.D. (✉)
Department of Neurology and Neuroscience, Center for Sleep Medicine, New York Presbyterian Hospital, Weill Cornell Medical College, 425 East 61st Street, New York, NY 10065, USA
e-mail: mae2001@med.cornell.edu

L.D. Ravdin and H.L. Katzen (eds.), *Handbook on the Neuropsychology of Aging and Dementia*, Clinical Handbooks in Neuropsychology, DOI 10.1007/978-1-4614-3106-0_6,

period (as long as the person is not rebounding from a period of sleep deprivation). Behaviorally, SWS is distinct from other stages of sleep because of a higher arousal threshold. The decrease in SWS over the life span was originally described in the 1970s and has been confirmed by several studies since that time [2–6]. A recent comprehensive meta-analysis of 65 studies concluded that SWS declines at a rate of approximately 2% per decade of adult life, and plateaus at approximately 60 years of age [7]. There appears to be a gender difference, with men showing a dramatic decrease in SWS. However, in women, delta sleep is preserved across the life span [8]. Generally, the EEG frequency of SWS is maintained in older adults, whereas the amplitude of the waveform decreases [2]. It is thought that this decrease in amplitude of SWS is a result of atrophy of brain tissue over time.

As the name implies, rapid eye movement (REM) sleep is defined by REMs, mixed frequency, low-voltage EEG (similar to the waking state), and muscle atonia [1]. REM sleep at one time was also called paradoxical sleep because it is electrographically similar to waking. The majority of REM sleep is typically present in the second half of the night. However, as we age, there tends to be a shift in REM sleep to earlier in the night, resulting in a slightly decreased latency to REM sleep [7, 9]. Also, a decrease of approximately 0.6% per decade in percentage of REM sleep [7, 8] has been reported [10], but this trend toward decreased REM percentage has not been found in all studies [9].

Stage 1 sleep (now called N1 sleep) is a light, transitional stage of sleep between waking and stage 2 (N2) or REM sleep. It is defined by mixed frequency, low-voltage brain waves with slow rolling eye movements [1]. When awakened from N1 sleep, individuals often report that they were unaware that they were sleeping, which underlines the transitional nature of N1 sleep. An increased level of N1 sleep is often seen as a marker for fragmentation of the sleep architecture. Compared to the young, there is a mild to moderate increase in N1 sleep in the older adults, suggesting there is increased sleep fragmentation [7]. It is thought that the increase in N1 sleep may be, in part, due to the reduction in both REM sleep and SWS. However, like SWS sleep, the level of N1 sleep seems to be better preserved in woman than in men [8].

Table 6.1 Changes in sleep variables with aging

Sleep variable	Change in % (or min)
N1	↑
N2	–
SWS	↓
REM	↓
SE	↓
WASO (min)	↑

KEY: N1= stage 1 sleep, N2 = stage 2 sleep, SWS = slow-wave sleep, REM = rapid eye movement sleep, SE = sleep efficiency, and WASO = wake after sleep onset. All variables are listed as a percentage of total sleep time, except WASO, which is in minutes, and SE, which is the total sleep time/time in bed

Stage 2 sleep (N2) is defined by an EEG signal that contains both K-complexes (negative to positive spikes with a duration of ≥0.5 s) and sleep spindles (periods of relatively fast, synchronous EEG activity that looks like a spindle of yarn and is generated by the thalamus). These two electrographic patterns are superimposed on a background of theta (4–7 Hz) activity [1]. N2 sleep makes up the majority of the sleep period throughout the life span. Although the relative percentage of N2 sleep changes very little over time, the landscape of this sleep stage undergoes significant changes. Sleep spindles and K-complexes become less numerous, and the frequency of the spindles become slower as we age (Table 6.1) [11].

Insomnia in Older Adults

Insomnia is one of the most prevalent health concerns worldwide. Current estimates indicate that 6–15% of the population suffers from insomnia [12]. According to the International Classification of Sleep Disorders [13], insomnia is defined as a complaint of difficulty initiating or maintaining sleep, waking up too early, or experiencing sleep that is consistently not refreshing. The sleeping difficulty should also be accompanied by daytime impairment, such as difficulty concentrating, memory difficulties, fatigue, stomach problems,

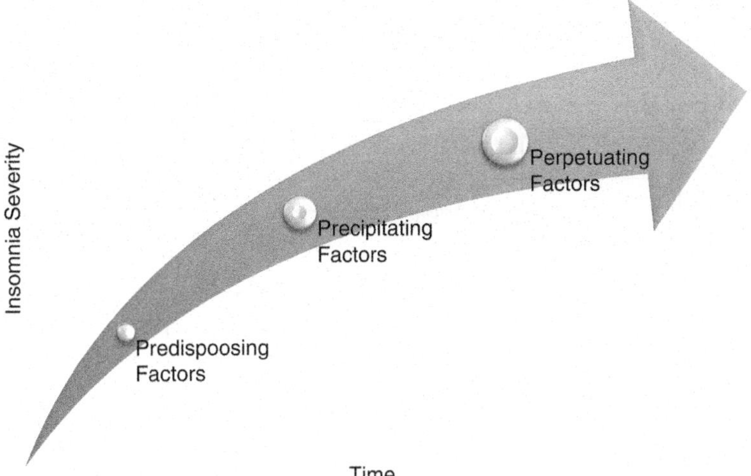

Fig. 6.1 The role of the 3Ps in the increase of insomnia severity over time. An illustration of the progression of insomnia over time. The severity of insomnia is an additive effect of each of the three factors (predisposing, precipitating, and perpetuating) described in the 3-P model. The relative importance of these factors changes over time

irritability, or reduced motivation. Studies investigating the impact of chronic insomnia demonstrated reduced quality of life, higher absenteeism, impaired job performance, and higher health-care utilization [14, 15].

In older adults, the prevalence of insomnia appears to be even higher than in the general population. In the mid-1990s, a large-scale epidemiological study was conducted that included nearly 7,000 individuals aged 65 and older. Over half of those surveyed complained of frequent difficulty sleeping [16]. Nearly a quarter of participants reported symptoms consistent with insomnia. Surprisingly, less than 20% reported little or no complaint of difficulty sleeping. When sleep quality in older compared to young adults was objectively investigated, there was a decrease in total sleep time and an increase in wake time after sleep onset [7]. However, when mood and health problems were controlled for, the prevalence of insomnia was dramatically lower at 7%. Once health or mood problems dissipate, symptoms of insomnia are also likely to disappear [17]. This suggests that insomnia is commonly a symptom of concomitant health or mood problems, and not vice versa.

To better understand how insomnia progresses over time, it is helpful to discuss this condition within the framework of the 3-P model (see Fig. 6.1). The 3Ps in this model stand for predisposing, precipitating, and perpetuating factors of insomnia. *Predisposing characteristics* are genetic or underlying personality traits such as basal level of anxiety or hyperarousal. Individuals with high levels of anxiety or hyperarousal, for example, are at increased risk of developing insomnia regardless of age [18]. These factors are considered to be relatively stable over the life span and should not be dramatically increased with age. *Precipitating events* are events that stimulate the onset of insomnia. Baseline level of predisposing factors will determine the magnitude of a precipitating event necessary to cause the onset of insomnia. Precipitating events include factors such as health and emotional problems, or death of friends or family members. Factors such as these can induce periods of difficulty sleeping [19]. As we age, we are more likely to be exposed to precipitating factors; therefore, the likelihood of developing acute insomnia increases. A *perpetuating event* is an event that causes the insomnia to continue even after the precipitating event has passed. Perpetuating activities commonly include maladaptive behaviors, such as prolonged time in bed, eating, using a computer or watching television in bed, and drinking alcohol in an effort to help

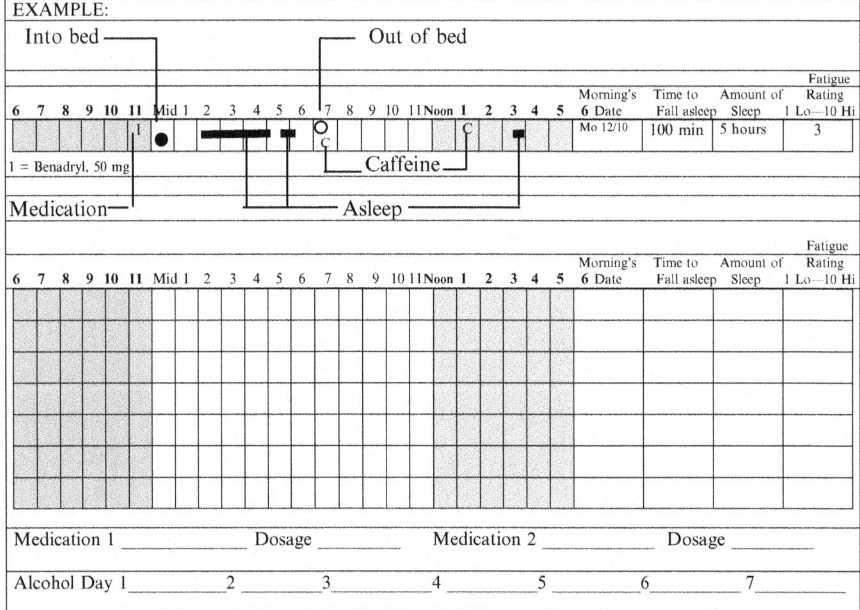

Fig. 6.2 A version of the City College of New York sleep log. Patients are instructed to complete this log upon awakening in the morning. The *black dot* indicates the time the patient got into bed, and the *black lines* represent periods of sleep. The *black circle* shows time out of bed. The number prior to the *black dot* indicates when medications were taken (if any were taken before bedtime). Medications taken at other times of the day are listed below the chart. *C* indicates time of caffeine consumption. Daily alcohol consumption for each day is listed below medications [22]

promote sleep. Acute insomnia becomes chronic due to these perpetuating habits, practices, and worrying. Older adults may be at greater risk for engaging in some perpetuating activities like spending too much time in bed because they are often retired and have more flexible schedules.

Treatment Approaches

The first line of treatment considered for insomnia for the majority of Americans is typically pharmacotherapy [20]. Many of the benzodiazepines prescribed for insomnia increase risk for falls. This is particularly problematic for older adults because they are already at a heightened risk for falls. In addition, treating insomnia with medication is typically not as durable as non-pharmacological treatments, such as cognitive behavioral therapy for insomnia (CBT-I) [21].

CBT-I is a general term that describes a host of treatments that have been shown empirically to improved quality of sleep. These commonly included sleep restriction therapy, stimulus control, cognitive therapy, and relaxation techniques. Sleep hygiene education is also commonly part of CBT-I treatment; however, it has not been shown to improve sleep quality when used in isolation of other techniques. Each of these treatments will be briefly discussed below; for a more comprehensive review, please refer to Ebben and Spielman [22].

Sleep restriction therapy was originally developed by Spielman et al. [23]. It involves drastically reducing a patient's time in bed in order to help consolidate sleep. Typically, sleep logs are completed for a period of 2–4 weeks (see Fig. 6.2). Based on the time in bed and the total sleep time documented on the sleep log, a new sleep/wake schedule is calculated. This new schedule only provides enough time (or less) in bed to achieve the patient's current sleep time. Once the patient begins the new schedule, they typically accumulate a sleep debt, which presumably helps them consolidate their sleep. Once sleep is consolidated into this relatively short period of time, total sleep time is slowly extended to satisfy the patient's sleep need. Although this technique can be difficult for the patient to execute at first, if performed correctly, sleep restriction therapy can greatly improve sleep quality and daytime functioning.

Stimulus control therapy focuses on the role of conditioned wakefulness in maintaining insomnia. Often when individuals spend sleepless nights lying in bed, they condition themselves to expect wakefulness in their bedroom environment. Once this occurs, commonly the individual will begin to spend more time in bed hoping it will increase the likelihood that they will sleep more; however, frequently the opposite occurs. When this conditioning pattern has developed, it is not uncommon for the patient to report improved sleep away from home. Emphasizing this notion of conditioned insomnia is the fact that even during laboratory polysomnograms, which involve numerous pieces of bothersome apparatus, individuals with conditioned wakefulness can achieve improved sleep quality. Therefore, the goal of stimulus control therapy is to separate sleep from wakefulness activities. This is done by encouraging the patient to reserve the bedtime for only sleep and sexual activity. Activities such as watching TV or listening to the radio in bed, for example, should be eliminated.

The practice of *cognitive therapy* to treat insomnia differs little from its practice in treating other types of psychopathology. Often patients with insomnia develop erroneous associations between their difficulty sleeping and other problems they are experiencing. For example, some may begin to worry that without high-quality sleep, they will completely lose their ability to function during the day. However, most individuals with insomnia have maintained somewhat normal daytime schedules, even after several nights of poor quality sleep. The goal of the cognitive therapist is to replace the patient's catastrophic thinking with more realistic thoughts. This process often takes longer than behavioral techniques because many thought patterns are more effectively approached indirectly (at least at first). Gaining permission from the patient to restructure their thought process requires a bond between the patient and therapist, which takes time to develop.

Relaxation techniques are treatments that focus on tension in the muscles. Progressive muscle relaxation (PMR) is the most common relaxation technique used for insomnia; however, EMG biofeedback is also occasionally used. PMR is typically used at bedtime and involves having the individual progressively tense then relax muscles throughout the body starting with the head or toes. In general, this technique has been shown to improve quality of sleep [24]. Interestingly, some data show that if this technique is used in insomniacs without muscle tension, it can worsen their sleep [25].

Circadian Rhythms in Aging

The term circadian is derived from the Latin roots circa (meaning "about") and diem ("day"). A circadian rhythm is a rhythm that is approximately 24 h or 1 day long. The pacemaker, or master clock of mammalian circadian rhythms, is located in the suprachiasmatic nucleus above the optic chiasm [26]. Circadian rhythms are generally set or reset by daytime light exposure, which naturally entrains the rhythm of the clock to a 24-h day. The human endogenous circadian rhythm (in the absence of light) in young and middle-age adults is typically longer than 24 h. Therefore, in controlled conditions that exclude light, an individual tends to fall asleep and wake-up a bit later each day.

Studies in aged animals have shown a flattening and desynchronization of circadian rhythms, which can be restored by transplanting suprachiasmatic tissue from younger animals [27]. In humans, a reduction in period length and amplitude of circadian rhythms is seen in older adults compared to the young [28]. Clinically, it is not uncommon to hear complaints from older adults regarding falling asleep too early and waking up too early. This condition is referred to as advanced sleep phase syndrome (ASPS). It is easy to confuse this type of complaint with insomnia; however, it is important to differentiate circadian rhythm disorders from insomnia because the treatments for each disorder are different.

Differentiating ASPS from insomnia is done through a careful examination of the patient's sleep/wake pattern. For example, if a patient reports a long history (usually since childhood or adolescence) of difficulty both falling asleep at night and waking up in the morning, there is a very good chance they suffer from delayed sleep phase syndrome (DSPS). It is quite common for insomniacs to report difficulty falling asleep. However, it is much less common for insomnia sufferers to report difficulty waking up in the morning. This condition is frequently seen in teenagers and young adults, although it can also be present in older individuals. In other cases, the patient may report a history of falling asleep or getting sleepy early in the evening and then waking up too early, unable to fall back to sleep. These individuals may be suffering from ASPS. This disorder has an estimated prevalence of approximately 1% overall but is more frequently seen in the older adults, with an estimated prevalence of 7% in this age group [29]. It is not uncommon to hear patients with ASPS report bedtimes of 6 pm with wake times of 2 am. In addition to physiological changes in period length of circadian rhythms such as core body temperature and melatonin that occur with age, behavioral patterns such as a less social activities in the evening and less light exposure in general may lead to the development ASPS.

In both DSPS and ASPS, if the individual has an adequate opportunity to sleep at their preferred time, total sleep time is generally within normal limits and daytime sleepiness is usually not reported. However, particularly in cases of DSPS, daytime social activities can limit the person's ability to sleep into the late morning or early afternoon on a regular basis; as a result, they often report daytime sleepiness. Patients with ASPS are often bothered by the boredom of waking at a time when other friends and family members are still sleeping. In addition, the early bedtime limits their ability to take part social activities in the evening. DSPS and ASPS are some of the most common circadian rhythm disorders in both young and older adults; however, numerous other circadian sleep disorders exist.

Generally, circadian rhythm disorders are treated with a combination of bright light, melatonin, and/or a customized sleep/wake schedule, not the typical cognitive-behavioral treatments reviewed previously in this chapter. A detailed review of the various treatment options for these disorders is beyond the scope of this chapter; for a thorough review on this topic, please refer to Zee [30].

Sleep-Disordered Breathing (Sleep Apnea)

Apnea is a Latin term that means "without breath." Sleep-disordered breathing (SDB) is a general name that includes two primary breathing disorders that occur during sleep. These two disorders are called obstructive sleep apnea (OSA) and central sleep apnea (CSA). OSA consists of a decrease or cessation in airflow secondary to a collapse in the upper airway. Another type of respiratory event included in the diagnosis of OSA is called hypopnea. This is a reduction in airflow accompanied by a decrease in blood oxygen saturation [1]. CSA, as the name implies, refers to cessation of airflow secondary to lack of signaling to breathe from the higher brain areas or "central centers."

It is normal to have some respiratory events during sleep; however, having too many is problematic. The diagnosis of sleep apnea is determined by a sleep study or polysomnogram during which sleep stages and respiratory events are monitored. Apneas and hypopneas are typically grouped into one index called the apnea-hypopnea index or AHI, which is the total number of apneas and hypopneas divided by the total hours of sleep. The typical range of AHI severity is as follows: 5–15 mild, 15–30 moderate, and ≥30 is severe [31]. The decrease in oxygen saturation associated with the respiratory events also factors into the severity of SDB. Typically, respiratory events result in brief arousals from sleep, which can cause daytime sleepiness. In fact, the majority of adults with SDB complain of excessive daytime sleepiness [32].

OSA is a serious health problem and puts patients at greater risk for hypertension, congestive heart failure, cardiac arrhythmia and ischemia, and cerebrovascular disease [33].

The prevalence of SDB in American adults is 4% for males and 2% for females [34], and the prevalence of moderate to severe apnea increases dramatically with age. The Sleep Health Heart Study found a prevalence of SDB of 20% in adults over the age of 60 [35].

Treatment for SDB most commonly involves the use of continuous positive airway pressure (CPAP). CPAP is basically a medical quality air compressor that blows air into the patient's airway causing a pneumatic splint. Once the appropriate CPAP pressure is determined, the patient begins using the CPAP machine nightly during sleep. Use of CPAP typically causes a reduction in clinical symptoms of OSA such as snoring and excessive daytime sleepiness. It is also thought to reduce the risk of the other disorders associated with sleep apnea mentioned above.

REM Behavior Disorder

REM behavior disorder (RBD) is a condition that is defined by increased motor activity during REM sleep. Dream mentation is thought to occur more frequently during periods of REM sleep. During REM, voluntary muscles are inhibited through the inhibition of spinal motor neurons [36], thereby preventing movement during dreaming episodes. However, in individuals with RBD, the inhibition of these muscles is absent or incomplete. This disinhibition presumably allows the person to act out their dreams. This may involve violent actions such as kicking, punching, or screaming (the type of movement that occurs, most likely, depends on the dream content). RBD is more common in older males with an estimated prevalence of approximately 0.5% in older adults [13]. In most cases, RBD develops after the age of 50.

There is growing evidence of the association between RBD and synucleinopathies such as Parkinson's disease, Lewy body disease, and multiple systems atrophy (MSA). In fact, one study found that 69% of patients with MSA also had RBD [37]. Another study found that 33% of patients with Parkinson's disease that underwent sleep studies were also found to have RBD. It appears that RBD can also be a prodrome of synucleinopathies. Estimates suggest there is a mean interval of approximately 10 years from the development of RBD to the diagnosis of a synucleinopathy [38]; however, RBD has been shown to precede the onset of clinical symptoms in Parkinson's disease by as long as five decades [38]. In one small study ($n=29$), 38% of men originally diagnosed with idiopathic RBD developed Parkinson's disease later in life [39]. Withdrawal from alcohol or sedative medication, as well as the use of tricyclic antidepressants, has also been associated with the development of RBD [40].

Treatment for RBD generally involves the nightly use of a low dose of clonazepam, which has been found effective in eliminating or reducing RBD symptoms in 90% of cases [41]. However, once the medication is discontinued, the symptoms of RBD return. Other benzodiazepines are also occasionally used if the patient cannot tolerate the side effects of clonazepam.

Common Neurologic Disorders That Affect Sleep

Alzheimer's disease (AD) is a progressive neurodegenerative disorder that is often associated with behavioral problems, particularly as the disease progresses. A common behavioral problem referred to as sundowning represents agitation and wandering that is often exacerbated after sundown. EEG findings in AD are typically an exacerbation of the progression normally seen in elderly patients. This includes a decrease in REM sleep and SWS, increased sleep fragmentation, and a flatting of phasic events such as K-complexes and sleep spindles normally seen in N2 sleep (reviewed in Petit et al. [42]).

Parkinson's disease (PD) is a neuromuscular disorder that causes tremors, rigidity, stiffness, bradykinesia, and coordination problems. In addition to the higher incidence of RBD described above, a significant percentage of PD patients complain of sleep problems. In a study of 149 PD patients with age-matched controls, 42% were found to have sleep difficulty compared to only

12% in the control group [43]. The most common sleep problems reported were insomnia, nightmares, and excessive daytime sleepiness (EDS). It has been hypothesized that sleepiness in PD patients is partially related to the use of dopamine agonists. This theory was recently refuted by the Canadian Movement Disorders Group who found EDS was common in PD patients.

In summary, there are a host of reasons for changes in our sleep as we age. These include significant changes in sleep architecture, as well as an increased frequency of a number of sleep disorders, some of which can be attributed to underlying health or mood disorders. Age-related behavioral changes, such as a lack of a defined daily schedule (i.e., work schedule), also contribute to sleep disorders such as insomnia or circadian rhythm disorders. Disorders that result from behavioral changes can frequently be treated successfully with behavior modification and do not necessarily need pharmacological intervention. A list of practitioners trained in the use of cognitive-behavioral treatments for sleep disorders can be found on the website of the American Academy of Sleep Medicine. In situations where the sleep disorder is secondary to another condition, treatment of the primary disorder is recommended first before sleep symptoms are the target of intervention.

Clinical Pearls

- Deterioration of sleep quality is not necessarily a normal part of aging and is most often associated with physical or psychological maladies.
- Changes in sleep architecture as we age often include a decrease in SWS and a shift of REM sleep earlier in the night.
- Use of hypnotic medication for the treatment of insomnia is often not recommended in older adults because of the increased risk of falls.
- The first line of treatment for insomnia in the elderly should be cognitive behavioral therapy for insomnia (CBT-I).
- Older persons appear to be at greater risk for certain circadian rhythm disorders such as ASPS, which can and should be differentiated from insomnia because the treatments are different.
- REM behavior disorder (RBD) is a disorder that is most common in older adult men and may be a prodrome for synucleinopathies.
- RBD can be effectively controlled in 90% of patients with the use of low-dose clonazepam.

References

1. AASM. The AASM Manual for the Scoring of Sleep and Associated Events: Rules, Terminology and Technical Specifications. Darien: American Academy of Sleep Medicine; 2007.
2. Feinberg I. Functional implications of changes in sleep physiology with age. In: Gershon S, Terry RD, editors. Neurobiology of aging. New York: Raven; 1976. p. 23–41.
3. Olivier-Martin R, Cendron H, Vallery-Masson J. [Sleep in elderly subjects. Description, analysis of various data obtained in a rural population]. Ann Med Psychol. 1975;1:77–90.
4. Feinberg I, March JD, Fein G, Aminoff MJ. Log amplitude is a linear function of log frequency in NREM sleep eeg of young and elderly normal subjects. Electroencephalogr Clin Neurophysiol. 1984;58: 158–60.
5. Ehlers CL, Kupfer DJ. Effects of age on delta and REM sleep parameters. Electroencephalogr Clin Neurophysiol. 1989;72:118–25.
6. Lauer CJ, Riemann D, Wiegand M, Berger M. From early to late adulthood. Changes in EEG sleep of depressed patients and healthy volunteers. Biol Psychiatry. 1991;29:979–93.
7. Ohayon MM, Carskadon MA, Guilleminault C, Vitiello MV. Meta-analysis of quantitative sleep parameters from childhood to old age in healthy individuals: developing normative sleep values across the human lifespan. Sleep. 2004;27:1255–73.
8. Redline S, et al. The effects of age, sex, ethnicity, and sleep-disordered breathing on sleep architecture. Arch Intern Med. 2004;164:406–18.
9. Dijk DJ, Duffy JF, Riel E, Shanahan TL, Czeisler CA. Ageing and the circadian and homeostatic regulation of human sleep during forced desynchrony of rest, melatonin and temperature rhythms. J Physiol. 1999;516(Pt 2):611–27.
10. Floyd JA, Janisse JJ, Jenuwine ES, Ager JW. Changes in REM-sleep percentage over the adult lifespan. Sleep. 2007;30:829–36.
11. Wauquier A. Aging and changes in phasic events during sleep. Physiol Behav. 1993;54:803–6.
12. Ohayon MM. Prevalence and comorbidity of sleep disorders in general population. Rev Prat. 2007;57: 1521–8.

13. Medicine, A.A.o.S. The international classification of sleep disorders. Diagnostic and coding manual. Westchester: American Academy of Sleep Medicine; 2005.
14. Kuppermann M, et al. Sleep problems and their correlates in a working population. J Gen Intern Med. 1995;10:25–32.
15. Simon GE, VonKorff M. Prevalence, burden, and treatment of insomnia in primary care. Am J Psychiatry. 1997;154:1417–23.
16. Foley DJ, et al. Sleep complaints among elderly persons: an epidemiologic study of three communities. Sleep. 1995;18:425–32.
17. Foley DJ, Monjan A, Simonsick EM, Wallace RB, Blazer DG. Incidence and remission of insomnia among elderly adults: an epidemiologic study of 6,800 persons over 3 years. Sleep. 1999;22 Suppl 2:S366–72.
18. Drake C, Richardson G, Roehrs T, Scofield H, Roth T. Vulnerability to stress-related sleep disturbance and hyperarousal. Sleep. 2004;27:285–91.
19. Bastien CH, Vallieres A, Morin CM. Precipitating factors of insomnia. Behav Sleep Med. 2004;2:50–62.
20. Walsh J, Schweitzer P. Ten-year trends in the pharmacologic treatment of insomnia. Sleep Med Rev. 1999;22:371–5.
21. Edinger JD, Wohlgemuth WK, Radtke RA, Marsh GR, Quillian RE. Cognitive behavioral therapy for treatment of chronic primary insomnia: a randomized controlled trial. JAMA. 2001;285:1856–64.
22. Ebben MR, Spielman AJ. Non-pharmacological treatments for insomnia. J Behav Med. 2009;32:244–54.
23. Spielman AJ, Caruso LS, Glovinsky PB. A behavioral perspective on insomnia treatment. Psychiatr Clin North Am. 1987;10:541–53.
24. Nicassio PM, Boylan MB, McCabe TG. Progressive relaxation. EMG biofeedback and biofeedback placebo in the treatment of sleep-onset insomnia. Br J Med Psychol. 1982;55:159–66.
25. Hauri PJ, Percy L, Hellekson C, Hartmann E, Russ D. The treatment of psychophysiologic insomnia with biofeedback: a replication study. Biofeedback Self Regul. 1982;7:223–35.
26. Moore RY, Eichler VB. Loss of a circadian adrenal corticosterone rhythm following suprachiasmatic lesions in the rat. Brain Res. 1972;42:201–6.
27. Gibson EM, Williams 3rd WP, Kriegsfeld LJ. Aging in the circadian system: considerations for health, disease prevention and longevity. Exp Gerontol. 2009;44:51–6.
28. Weitzman ED, Moline ML, Czeisler CA, Zimmerman JC. Chronobiology of aging: temperature, sleep-wake rhythms and entrainment. Neurobiol Aging. 1982;3:299–309.
29. Ando K, Kripke DF, Ancoli-Israel S. Delayed and advanced sleep phase symptoms. Isr J Psychiatr Relat Sci. 2002;39:11–8.
30. Zee P. Circadian rhythm sleep disorders. Prim Psychiatr. 2006;13:58–67.
31. The Report of an American Academy of Sleep Medicine Task Force. Sleep-related breathing disorders in adults: recommendations for syndrome definition and measurement techniques in clinical research. Sleep. 1999;22:667–89.
32. Partinen M, Guilleminault C. Daytime sleepiness and vascular morbidity at seven-year follow-up in obstructive sleep apnea patients. Chest. 1990;97:27–32.
33. Shamsuzzaman AS, Gersh BJ, Somers VK. Obstructive sleep apnea: implications for cardiac and vascular disease. JAMA. 2003;290:1906–14.
34. Young T, et al. The occurrence of sleep-disordered breathing among middle-aged adults. N Engl J Med. 1993;328:1230–5.
35. Gozal D. Morbidity of obstructive sleep apnea in children: facts and theory. Sleep Breath. 2001;5:35–42.
36. Pompeiano O. The control of posture and movements during REM sleep: neurophysiological and neurochemical mechanisms. Acta Astronaut. 1975;2:225–39.
37. Plazzi G, et al. REM sleep behavior disorders in multiple system atrophy. Neurology. 1997;48:1094–7.
38. Claassen DO, et al. REM sleep behavior disorder preceding other aspects of synucleinopathies by up to half a century. Neurology. 2010;75:494–9.
39. Schenck CH, Bundlie SR, Mahowald MW. Delayed emergence of a parkinsonian disorder in 38% of 29 older men initially diagnosed with idiopathic rapid eye movement sleep behaviour disorder. Neurology. 1996;46:388–93.
40. Ancoli-Israel S, Ayalon L, Salzman C. Sleep in the elderly: normal variations and common sleep disorders. Harv Rev Psychiatry. 2008;16:279–86.
41. Mahowald MW, Bundlie SR, Hurwitz TD, Schenck CH. Sleep violence–forensic science implications: polygraphic and video documentation. J Forensic Sci. 1990;35:413–32.
42. Petit D, Gagnon JF, Fantini ML, Ferini-Strambi L, Montplaisir J. Sleep and quantitative EEG in neurodegenerative disorders. J Psychosom Res. 2004;56:487–96.
43. Kumar S, Bhatia M, Behari M. Sleep disorders in Parkinson's disease. Mov Disord. 2002;17:775–81.
44. Hobson DE, et al. Excessive daytime sleepiness and sudden-onset sleep in Parkinson disease: a survey by the Canadian Movement Disorders Group. JAMA. 2002;287:455–63.

Medications and Cognition in Older Adults

7

Gregg L. Caporaso

Abstract

The elderly patient is particularly susceptible to negative effects on cognition that can arise from certain medications. This may occur whether or not pre-existing cognitive impairment is present. Medications whose primary target is the central nervous system (e.g., antidepressants, antipsychotics, sedative-hypnotics) or those which are targeted at other primary systems (e.g., cardiovascular drugs, urinary anti-spasmodics) should be considered as contributing factors in the patient with confusion or memory decline. Steps that can be taken to reduce this risk include: coordination of medical care among the patient's clinicians to avoid polypharmacy, judicious selection of appropriate medications, use of the lowest effective drug dose, and substitution of non-pharmacologic therapies whenever possible. This chapter addresses potential complications of medication use in older adults with cognitive decline.

Keywords

Cognition • Elderly • Medications • Tricyclic antidepressants • Antipsychotics • Neuroleptics • Anticholinergics • Benzodiazepines • Opiates

Practicing clinicians cannot escape the irony that elderly patients are more predisposed to medication side effects (e.g., due to reduced renal clearance) and to cognitive disorders (e.g., Alzheimer's disease) and that this same population is prescribed more medications, some of which may impair cognition. It is therefore incumbent upon the clinician to recognize when cognitive problems might be due to medications or combinations of medications, which medications are the most common offending agents, and how to treat these individuals optimally, by either substituting safer drugs or using non-pharmacological therapies. In addition to adverse motor effects such as impaired fine motor coordination and imbalance, many medications prescribed to elderly patients can produce adverse

*Craig D, Passmore AP, Fullerton KJ, Beringer TR, Gilmore DH, Crawford VL, McCaffrey PM, Montgomery A. Factors influencing prescription of CNS medications in different elderly populations. Pharmacoepidemiol Drug Saf. 2003;12(5):383–7.

G.L. Caporaso, M.D., Ph.D. (✉)
Division of Neurology, Westchester Health Associates, Yorktown Heights, NY 10598, USA

L.D. Ravdin and H.L. Katzen (eds.), *Handbook on the Neuropsychology of Aging and Dementia*, Clinical Handbooks in Neuropsychology, DOI 10.1007/978-1-4614-3106-0_7,

cognitive effects that impact attention, memory, and executive functions. The scope of this potential problem is immense, with upward of one-third of older adults taking psychotropic medications like antidepressants, anxiolytics, antipsychotics, and sedative–hypnotics. Many more elderly patients are prescribed medications for non-neuropsychiatric conditions that can also negatively affect cognition (e.g., antihistamines).

Clinical Assessment

History is always key in diagnosing the potential cause of cognitive decline. For example, progressive cognitive decline of insidious onset is typical for Alzheimer's disease whereas forgetfulness after new treatment for hypertension might be due to beta-blocker use. It should be kept in mind that the addition of a new medication may unmask an underlying incipient cognitive disturbance such as neurodegenerative dementia or borderline cognitive function related to prior cerebrovascular disease. Indeed, preexisting dementia puts patients at 2–3 times the risk for developing delirium [1]. In obtaining a cognitive history, reports from a spouse, adult child, or caregiver are essential since cognitive impairment or behavioral changes may not be apparent to the patient. In this regard, a correlation between the addition of a new medication or change in dose of an existing medication can be important in identifying an offending agent.

Laboratory assessment should be directed at potential effects of medications on metabolism (e.g., hypokalemia related to diuretics, decreased serum albumin with resultant higher circulating drug levels), serum levels of some medications (e.g., antiepileptic toxicity), or supervening medical conditions that can affect drug clearance or potentiate drug effects (e.g., complete blood counts and urinalysis to diagnose urinary tract infection). One must keep in mind that most elderly patients have reduced muscle mass and therefore lower serum creatinine values, so that a value within the normal laboratory range may actually represent impaired renal clearance in these individuals [2]. Consequently, most medications should be started at reduced doses in the elderly population, with upward titration proceeding slowly and cautiously.

Medications that Can Affect Cognition

Though many medications have the potential for affecting cognition, there are several classes of medications that are the most common offenders (Table 7.1). Rather than an exhaustive review of any potential problem drugs, this section will discuss those medications that the clinician is most likely to encounter in a typical hospital or office practice. In addition, toxic effects associated with drug overdose will not be discussed so that the focus will be on cognitive and behavioral problems that arise during normal prescribing practice. Cognition-enhancing drugs such as those used to treat Alzheimer's disease (e.g., donepezil, memantine) will be covered elsewhere in this volume. One convenient way to approach these various medications is by dividing them into neuropsychiatric drugs (i.e., drugs that are designed to act on the nervous system) and systemic drugs (i.e., drugs that primarily target tissues outside the nervous system).

Neuropsychiatric Drugs

Antidepressants

Depression can produce cognitive impairment (e.g., attentional deficits that can resemble memory loss, so-called pseudodementia) or worsen cognition in patients with underlying cognitive impairment. Treatment of depression in patients with or without cognitive impairment may therefore have benefits on cognitive functioning in this group [3]. However, positive effects on cognition in the elderly can depend on the choice of antidepressant [4], and certain antidepressants have the potential to worsen cognition.

Tricyclic Antidepressants

As a group, tricyclic antidepressants (TCAs, e.g., amitriptyline, nortriptyline, imipramine, clomipramine, desipramine, doxepin) are effective

Table 7.1 Medications that can affect cognition (see text for discussion)

Medical condition	Drugs that might impair cognition	Safer drug alternatives	Non-pharmacological alternatives
Depression	Tricyclic antidepressants (e.g., amitriptyline, nortriptyline, imipramine, desipramine, clomipramine, doxepin)	SSRIs (e.g., fluoxetine, paroxetine, sertraline, citalopram, escitalopram) SNRIs (e.g., venlafaxine, duloxetine)	Counseling Psychotherapy Group therapy Cognitive-behavioral therapy
Psychosis, agitation	High-potency antipsychotics (e.g., chlorpromazine, haloperidol)	Atypical antipsychotics (e.g., risperidone, olanzapine, quetiapine)	Structured environment Regular daily routines Trained caregiver
Insomnia	Benzodiazepines (e.g., alprazolam, triazolam, temazepam, diazepam, lorazepam) Diphenhydramine	Z-drugs (e.g., zolpidem, zaleplon, eszopiclone) Chloral hydrate Melatonin	Proper sleep hygiene (i.e., no late-day caffeine, no napping, regular exercise, fixed bedtime/awakening time)
Parkinson's disease	Anticholinergics (e.g., trihexyphenidyl)	L-dopa Dopamine agonists (e.g., pramipexole, ropinirole) MAO-B inhibitors (e.g., selegiline, rasagiline) COMT inhibitors (e.g., tolcapone, entacapone)	–
Epilepsy	Phenobarbital Primidone Topiramate	Carbamazepine Valproate Levetiracetam	–
Pain	Opiates (e.g., morphine, codeine, oxycodone, hydrocodone)	Acetaminophen NSAIDs Tramadol Topical agents	Biofeedback Physical therapy Acupuncture Chiropractic therapy
Motion sickness, vertigo	Scopolamine	Meclizine[a] Dimenhydrinate[a]	Vestibular exercises
Hypertension	Beta-blockers (e.g., propranolol, metoprolol)	Diuretics (e.g., hydrochlorothiazide) ACE inhibitors (e.g., captopril, lisinopril, ramipril) Angiotensin receptor antagonists (e.g., losartan)	Exercise Weight reduction
Urinary urge incontinence	Oxybutynin	M3 selective agents (e.g., tolterodine, trospium, solifenacin, darifenacin)	Scheduled toileting Fluid restriction Caffeine avoidance

ACE angiotensin-converting enzyme, *COMT* catechol-*O*-methyl-transferase, *M3* muscarinic receptor, *MAO-B* monoamine oxygenase-B, *SNRI* serotonin–norepinephrine receptor uptake inhibitor, *SSRI* selective serotonin receptor uptake inhibitor

[a]There are abundant data for scopalamine's amnesic effects but less so for these other two agents listed

antidepressants but have anticholinergic effects that can worsen memory functioning in the elderly. Given the cholinergic deficits seen in age-related illnesses such as Alzheimer's disease, Parkinson's disease, and dementia with Lewy bodies, it is not surprising that the elderly population may be especially sensitive to the negative cognitive effects of this class of medications [5]. Approximately 5–7% of geriatric inpatients who received a TCA may develop delirium [6, 7]. In a mouse model of memory and learning, the TCAs amitriptyline and imipramine worsened memory and potentiated the effects of the anticholinergic agent scopolamine, whereas the selective serotonin agent fluoxetine had no effect on memory and could reverse scopolamine's negative effects [8]. TCAs have been demonstrated to have negative effects in the elderly on measures of verbal memory [9–12]. However, low-dose imipramine (25 mg/day) was shown not to worsen memory in patients with Alzheimer's disease with or without depression [13]. In a large population-based study ($N = 1,488$ patients), TCA use was not associated in the short- or long-term with cognitive deficits or memory impairment [14].

Selective Serotonin- and Serotonin/Norepinephrine-Reuptake Inhibitors

Selective serotonin-reuptake inhibitors (SSRIs, e.g., fluoxetine, sertraline, paroxetine, citalopram, escitalopram) and serotonin/norepinephrine-reuptake inhibitors (SNRIs, e.g., venlafaxine, duloxetine, desvenlafaxine) are the most commonly prescribed antidepressants. Fortunately, they do not seem to be associated with the negative cognitive effects seen with TCAs [15]. Escitalopram improved cognition as well as mood in depressed elderly patients with memory impairment [16]. Though sertraline seemed to provide greater cognitive benefits than fluoxetine in elderly patients with depression [4, 17, 18], fluoxetine appears to be comparable with paroxetine [19], and fluoxetine may provide some benefits for memory in nondepressed patients with mild cognitive impairment [20]. Duloxetine and venlafaxine do not affect histaminergic or cholinergic receptors and have been shown to improve certain cognitive measures in older depressed patients [21–23]. Given their apparent safety in patients susceptible to cognitive impairment and their potential for improving cognition, SSRIs and SNRIs should be considered preferred treatments for depression in older patients. The prescribing physician, though, should be aware of the risk, albeit small, of delirium induced by serotonin agents as part of the serotonin syndrome, which also encompasses myoclonus, rigidity, hyperreflexia, tremors, and autonomic lability. The risk of this syndrome is increased when monoamine oxidase (MAO) inhibitors (and perhaps triptan migraine medications) are coadministered.

Antipsychotics

Antipsychotic drugs, or neuroleptics, are dopamine receptor antagonists used in the treatment of hallucinations or delusions that might occur in disorders such as schizophrenia or dementia. They are also used to treat affective diseases (e.g., bipolar disorder), Tourette's syndrome, and nausea. This group of medications carries the risk of extrapyramidal side effects (EPS) including parkinsonism (bradykinesia, rigidity, and tremors), dystonia, akathisia, and tardive dyskinesia. The older "conventional" or "high-potency" antipsychotics (e.g., chlorpromazine, haloperidol) are less selective in their blockade of dopamine receptor subtypes and are associated with greater risk of EPS. The newer "atypical" antipsychotics (e.g., risperidone, olanzapine, quetiapine) preferentially block serotonin 5-HT2A receptors more than dopamine D2 receptors and are believed to have a lower risk of EPS [24].

It should be noted that the use of either conventional or atypical antipsychotics in the elderly may be associated with increased mortality [25] and that the Food and Drug Administration has issued advisories that caution their use in this patient group [26]. The potential magnitude of this problem was highlighted by a recent study of the National Nursing Home Survey, which demonstrated that one quarter of nursing home residents are prescribed antipsychotics, and of these, perhaps 40% are prescribed antipsychotics inappropriately [27]. Though antipsychotics are commonly used in managing behavioral problems in the elderly, their use cannot be endorsed in most patients. Indeed, many patients with Alzheimer's disease can experience substantial benefits in neuropsychiatric symptoms, as well as cognition and daily functioning, with treatment using approved dementia agents such as donepezil [28], rivastigmine [29], or memantine [30]. Furthermore, though many of the neuroleptics have been shown to improve cognition in patients with schizophrenia (e.g., executive function), there are fewer data on their effects in nonschizophrenic elderly patients.

Conventional Antipsychotics

The older neuroleptics such as chlorpromazine exhibit anticholinergic activity, so one might predict that they would detrimentally affect cognition in older individuals and in particular patients with Alzheimer's disease. The results of studies examining antipsychotic use in elderly demented patients have been mixed, with some studies showing no effect on cognition [31–33] and others demonstrating negative effects on cognition [34–36]. One should interpret these studies with caution, however, since dementia patients with psychotic symptoms or behavioral disturbances have a worse prognosis than patients without these problems, and they tend to experience more rapid cognitive decline [37, 38].

Atypical Antipsychotics

The newer generation of antipsychotics seems to confer neuropsychiatric and sometimes cognitive benefits to elderly patients with psychosis, while being associated with fewer EPS [39]. However, the risk of EPS, as well as orthostatic hypotension and sedation, is not negligible, putting this group of patients at risk for falls and bone fractures.

Clozapine is a dibenzodiazepine with perhaps the lowest risk of EPS among neuroleptics. However, it carries a risk of agranulocytosis as high as 1% during the first several months (requiring weekly monitoring of blood counts) and roughly 0.01% after 1 year of use [40]. This agent also possesses anticholinergic activity, which can impair memory function, at least when studied in patients with schizophrenia [41]. Olanzapine has been shown to worsen cognition in patients with Alzheimer's disease, especially those with greater baseline impairment [42]. Compared with haloperidol, quetiapine had a wider range of benefits on psychiatric symptoms in patients with Alzheimer's disease and improved memory and daily functioning without producing significant EPS [43]. Quetiapine also showed neuropsychiatric benefits without cognition deterioration in an open-label pilot study of Alzheimer's patients [44]. Another small, open-label study using risperidone demonstrated improvement in psychosis, agitation, and aggression in patients with dementia without impacting cognition [45]. The Clinical Antipsychotic Trials of Intervention Effectiveness-Alzheimer's Disease study group (CATIE-AD) randomized over 400 patients with Alzheimer's disease and psychosis or agitation to antipsychotic medications (risperidone, olanzapine, or quetiapine) or placebo [46]. When this group examined time to discontinuation as a primary study endpoint, they concluded that adverse effects offset any advantages on neurobehavioral symptoms of antipsychotics compared to placebo [47]. In a subsequent analysis of antipsychotic medication versus placebo, though, the authors indicated that treatment with olanzapine or risperidone (and perhaps quetiapine) improved certain behavioral symptoms but had neither positive nor negative effects on cognition. Similar benefits on behavioral symptoms without cognitive deterioration were seen with these three agents in another smaller study of outpatients with Alzheimer's disease [48]. Aripiprazole is a new agent used in the treatment of schizophrenia, bipolar disorder, and as an adjunctive to antidepressants for major depression. Several recent placebo-controlled studies have demonstrated its efficacy in treating hallucinations and delusions in patients with Alzheimer's disease with little negative impact on cognition or safety [49–51]. However, head-to-head studies with other antipsychotics will be needed to test whether it really is safer than older agents. In summary, atypical antipsychotic agents may be useful in treating psychosis, agitation, and aggression in some patients with dementia without harming cognition, but the treatments must be individualized, and it would be prudent to start slowly with low doses to minimize the chance of adverse effects.

Sedative–Hypnotics and Anxiolytics

Insomnia occurs frequently in older patients and may have various causes, including a consequence of aging, sleep apnea, restless leg syndrome, or various parasomnias, such as periodic leg movement disorder. Overnight sleep studies that monitor brain electrical activity, movements, and breathing are sometimes required for diagnosing sleep disorders. Depression and anxiety are among the most common causes of insomnia, so accurate diagnosis and directed therapy should be attempted before treating sleeplessness with more generalized sleep aids. Dementia is often associated with inverted sleep–wake cycles that result in daytime sleepiness and nighttime restlessness or wandering.

In managing insomnia, a trial of non-pharmacological therapy should be completed before prescribing hypnotics or sedatives. This includes counseling on good "sleep hygiene." The patient should be told to avoid caffeinated beverages in the afternoon and evening, refrain from napping, get regular exercise, set regular bedtime and awakening hours, and restrict the bed at night for sleeping and not watching television or reading. Such non-pharmacological interventions are underutilized despite their effectiveness [52]. When needed, sleep aids should be used judiciously (e.g., only 1–2 nights/week when a patient really needs to catch up on sleep) and should not be taken nightly.

Although they are still commonly prescribed for the treatment of anxiety, the use of short-acting benzodiazepines (e.g., estazolam, triazolam, temazepam) as sleep aids has largely been supplanted by the development of non-benzodiazepines or "Z-drugs" (i.e., zolpidem, zaleplon, eszopiclone) that also act as $GABA_A$ agonists, but which are believed to have fewer side effects. It should be noted that the perceived safety vis-à-vis reduced daytime sleepiness of the latter group of medications might be due to the fact they have been unfairly compared to longer-acting benzodiazepines (e.g., nitrazepam) or inappropriate doses of short-acting agents such as temazepam (National Institute for Clinical Excellence, 2007 "Guidance on the use of zaleplon, zolpidem and zopiclone for the short-term management of insomnia," TA077).

Benzodiazepines are more potent in elderly patients due to target organ sensitivity, are cleared less efficiently due to reduced hepatic clearance and increased distribution volume, and can accumulate, resulting in cognitive impairment, psychomotor slowing, delirium, or sedation [2]. In the elderly, short-acting agents are preferred and high-potency benzodiazepines (e.g., alprazolam) should be avoided due to increased risk of side effects, such as abuse and withdrawal symptoms upon discontinuation [53]. Two large epidemiological studies in older French men and women demonstrated an association between benzodiazepine use and cognitive decline [54, 55], whereas a third did not [56]. Benzodiazepines can impair reaction time, attention, and memory [57]. Longer-acting agents are more likely to produce impairment [58]. Whenever the clinician makes a decision to stop benzodiazepines, they should be withdrawn gradually (i.e., dose tapered over one to several weeks) to lessen the risk of delirium associated with drug withdrawal in the elderly [59].

When treating anxiety, SSRIs or SNRIs should be considered before prescribing benzodiazepines. In addition, buspirone has been shown to be at least as effective as sertraline in treating anxiety in the elderly without significant adverse effects [60]. In healthy older subjects, buspirone did not affect reaction time, psychomotor speed, or memory [61]. Nefazodone seems to be a safe choice in treating elderly patients with anxiety and comorbid depression [62].

The so-called Z-drugs are the most commonly prescribed sleep aids in the elderly population. They are not without side effects and can produce hallucinations, delirium, and amnesia [63–65]. Most studies of these drugs have been conducted in younger individuals, with some showing cognitive impairment at commonly used doses [66] and others showing no significant effects [67–69]. Studies in the elderly have been limited. Following a single dose, zolpidem did not appear to affect attention or memory in healthy elderly individuals [70]. Weeklong administration of zolpidem also did not significantly impair psychomotor or cognitive functioning [71]. In contrast, another study demonstrated that older subjects experience memory impairment the day following dosing with zolpidem [72].

The antihistamine diphenhydramine is often prescribed as a sleep aid, especially by hospital staff or taken by patients seeking over-the-counter remedies. It possesses anticholinergic activity and can induce delirium in elderly patients and can impair attention and memory [73–75]. Chloral hydrate can be an effective sleep aid in older patients that carries little risk of delirium but may increase the free concentrations of certain other drugs (e.g., warfarin) due to displacement from plasma proteins [2]. Although trazodone is commonly prescribed as a sleep aid in elderly patients due to its perception as a "safe" drug, a comprehensive review of the evidence for trazodone in insomnia identified few trials that were mostly performed in depressed patients, possible tolerance, and side effects that included daytime sedation, dizziness, and psychomotor impairment [76]. Lastly, melatonin has been shown to improve sleep quality and possibly cognitive functioning in healthy elderly individuals [77]. It also appears to be an effective sleep aid in patients with dementia, reducing sleep latency and prolonging sleep duration, though long-term use may predispose to worsening affect [78]. In a randomized, crossover study comparing melatonin and zolpidem in healthy older individuals, a prolonged-release formulation of melatonin did not impact psychomotor functioning, memory, or driving skills, whereas zolpidem negatively affected all three measures [72].

Parkinson's Disease Medications

Multiple classes of medications are used in treating Parkinson's disease, including L-dopa, dopamine agonists (e.g., pramipexole, ropinirole), MAO-B (monoamine oxidase inhibitor, class B) and COMT (catechol *O*-methyltransferase) enzyme inhibitors (which increase the bioavailability of dopamine), and anticholinergic agents (e.g., trihexyphenidyl). It should be kept in mind that cognitive dysfunction is common in patients with Parkinson's disease, either in the form of dementia with Lewy bodies, as a later complication of idiopathic Parkinson's disease, or due to depression, which occurs in more than half of Parkinson's patients during some point in their illness. As such, these patients may be particularly susceptible to untoward cognitive effects of medications described in this chapter. However, drugs used specifically to treat Parkinson's disease might also have the potential for negatively impacting cognition.

L-dopa did not seem to impair cognition after 3 months of treatment in patients with Parkinson's disease with or without comorbid dementia [79]. The absence of negative cognitive effects of L-dopa seems to carry over into moderate or severe Parkinson's disease [80]. However, an earlier study failed to show any cognitive benefit of L-dopa in Parkinson's patients [81]. In patients with early Parkinson's disease, treatment either with L-dopa or the dopamine agonist bromocriptine improved cognition whereas anticholinergic therapy worsened it [82]. Addition of the MAO-B inhibitor selegiline to L-dopa treatment may help improve cognition in Parkinson's patients without dementia [83]. The newer MAO-B inhibitor rasagiline does not seem to be associated with any significant cognitive or behavioral worsening [84].

In a randomized study of patients with early/mild Parkinson's disease, the D2/D3 dopamine agonist pramipexole significantly impaired verbal memory, attention, and executive function compared to L-dopa [85]. The same study group, however, showed that the D1/D2 dopamine agonist pergolide was comparable to L-dopa in its effects on cognition [86]. However, both pergolide and pramipexole might improve working memory in medically naïve Parkinson's patients [87]. It should be noted that dopamine agonists such as pramipexole or ropinirole have been linked to impulse control disorders in patients with Parkinson's disease (e.g., pathological gambling, compulsive sexual behavior, binge eating), the risk being perhaps 2–3 times higher than in patients not treated with dopamine agonists [88]. In a small study of patients with advanced Parkinson's disease, treatment with tolcapone, a COMT inhibitor, resulted in improved scores for attention, verbal and visual-spatial memory, and praxis [89].

The anticholinergic agent trihexyphenidyl is useful in treating tremors in Parkinson's disease [90, 91] and may also be of use in patients with tardive dyskinesia [92]. Trihexyphenidyl was shown to worsen executive function in patients with Parkinson's, an effect that is mediated by subcortical frontal circuits [93]. This medication was also demonstrated to impair cognitive shifting and memory [94]. In a crossover study of patients with drug-induced EPS, cognitive performance was better on the Parkinson's medication amantadine than in trihexyphenidyl [95]. Lastly, an uncontrolled study of elderly patients with schizophrenia demonstrated a dose-dependent correlation between global cognitive and memory impairment and chronic use of trihexyphenidyl [96].

Anticonvulsants

Anticonvulsants or antiepileptic drugs (AEDs) are used primarily in treating seizure disorders but also play an important role in the management of mood disorders, neuropathic pain syndromes (e.g., trigeminal neuralgia), and migraine headaches. Since these drugs function to reduce neuronal irritability, such as cortical seizure foci, vis-à-vis inhibiting neuronal excitability, they have the potential for impairing cognition, as well as other brain and spinal cord functions such as balance [97]. At normal therapeutic doses, use of phenytoin, valproate, or carbamazepine did not seem to affect cognition significantly in most adult patients, though their safety in the elderly is less well established [98]. Carbamazepine seemed to produce fewer adverse effects on cognition compared to phenytoin, primidone, or phenobarbital in a large study of veterans [99], and a subsequent study in the same population showed no difference between carbamazepine and valproate [100].

In elderly patients on monotherapy for epilepsy (carbamazepine, phenytoin, or valproate), increasing the dose of their AED to a higher level within the normal dose range did not induce cognitive impairment or sedation [101]. A randomized study comparing valproate and phenytoin in elderly patients with new-onset epilepsy found no significant adverse cognitive effects and no difference between the two drugs [102]. However, a tolerability study of valproate in non-epileptic patients with Alzheimer's disease demonstrated cognitive worsening at a dose of 1,500 mg/day, though doses less than 1,000 mg/day might be safe [103]. Carbamazepine was shown to be superior to placebo in treating agitation and aggression in demented nursing home patients with no effects on cognition or functionality [104]. In a randomized, case–control study of Alzheimer's patients with seizures, levetiracetam improved attention and oral fluency and lamotrigine had a positive effect on mood, but phenobarbital caused persistent cognitive impairment [105]. Although it has not specifically been studied in the elderly, topiramate has been shown to impair cognitive speed, verbal fluency, and short-term memory in patients with epilepsy, whereas levetiracetam seems to lack cognitive side effects [106]. Other studies have demonstrated negative effects of topiramate on verbal fluency and attention in adults with migraines [107, 108].

Opiates

The geriatric population is particularly susceptible to musculoskeletal and rheumatologic illnesses associated with pain. Although studies directly addressing this issue are lacking, acetaminophen, nonsteroidal anti-inflammatory drugs (NSAIDs), tramadol, and topical agents (e.g., fentanyl patch or capsaicin lotion) are effective therapies that only rarely produce cognitive effects in elderly patients [109–112] (for some exceptions, see section on corticosteroids and NSAIDs). For more severe or intractable pain, patients may be prescribed opiates (e.g., morphine, codeine, oxycodone) or combination medications (e.g., acetaminophen–hydrocodone). Though any opiate may of course produce sedation or cognitive impairment in patients of any age, one study of primary care patients with nonmalignant pain found that problems with cognitive functioning were more likely related to psychological health and pain control than with specific opiate medications [113]. A review of postoperative pain management in elderly patients concluded that meperidine has consistently been shown to be associated with an increased risk of delirium whereas this has not been shown for other commonly used opiates (e.g., morphine, fentanyl, hydromorphone) [114]. In using opiates, it should be kept in mind that tolerance for a dose administered chronically may subsequently be too high and result in delirium, sedation, or cognitive impairment following another intervention to reduce absolute pain levels (e.g., spinal nerve block, surgery).

Anti-vertigo and Motion Sickness Agents

Anticholinergic and antihistaminergic agents are widely used to treat vertigo and motion sickness (e.g., seasickness). Dimenhydrinate and meclizine are antihistamines that are effective in relieving motion sickness and vertigo but which can produce psychometric slowing and sleepiness [115]. Although a case report noted memory loss and confusion in an elderly woman taking meclizine, there have been no studies specifically examining this drug's or dimenhydrinate's effects on cognition in older patients [116].

Scopolamine is an anticholinergic medication used to treat motion sickness and has been associated with memory impairment. In a blinded placebo-controlled study, it was shown to worsen cognition and behavior in a dose-dependent fashion in patients with Alzheimer's disease [117]. It has also been demonstrated to worsen memory in Parkinson's patients without preexisting cognitive impairment [118]. In a comparison between healthy individuals of different ages, scopolamine impaired memory and constructional praxis in old but not young subjects [119].

Systemic Drugs

Cardiovascular Drugs

Hypertension is a common risk factor for carotid atherosclerosis and cerebrovascular disease. Ischemic changes in the brain may in themselves produce cognitive impairment or dementia (e.g., "subcortical dementia," Binswanger's disease) or contribute to the pathogenesis or potentiate the effects of other dementias (e.g., Alzheimer's disease). However, overaggressive lowering of blood pressure in treating hypertension can also cause cognitive changes. Elderly patients with a long history of hypertension can develop cervical or cerebral blood vessels with poor compliance that require pressures greater than those considered normal in order to adequately perfuse the brain. Hypoperfusion may also be a consequence of atrial fibrillation, congestive heart failure, myocardial infarction, or coronary artery bypass grafting (CABG) [120]. As such, it can sometimes be difficult to gauge the extent to which either underlying cardiovascular pathology versus therapies used to treat them may be contributing to cognitive worsening. With the possible exception of beta-blockers (see below), antihypertensives are not thought to affect cognition significantly. A review of several randomized, placebo-controlled studies and a recent meta-analysis examining the effects of antihypertension medications on dementia suggested that these medications, and angiotensin-converting enzyme (ACE) inhibitors and diuretics in particular, may help prevent or slow the progression of dementia [121, 122].

Beta-Blockers

Although propranolol is also used to treat essential tremor and prevent migraine headaches, the clinician is most likely to use beta-adrenergic antagonists, or beta-blockers, in elderly patients with hypertension or cardiac disease. Beta-blockers may exert biological effects in the CNS either specifically via activity at downstream receptors of central adrenergic pathways (e.g., projections from the locus coeruleus) or nonspecifically via neuronal membrane stabilization [123]. Lipophilic beta-blockers such as propranolol and metoprolol cross the blood–brain barrier and accumulate in brain tissue compared to hydrophilic agents like atenolol [124]. These differences in lipophilicity seem to correspond to the relative risk of CNS effects. Switching from a lipophilic beta-blocker to a less lipophilic agent was associated with improved sleep, concentration, and memory, and atenolol was less likely to produce sleep disturbances than metoprolol [125]. However, a comprehensive review of beta-blockers concluded they in general have minimal or absent effects on memory function, as well as in causing sleep disturbances, nightmares, or hallucinations [126]. A large, randomized, controlled study of antihypertensives in elderly women failed to find evidence of cognitive decline after 5 years of treatment with a diuretic and atenolol [127]. Elderly patients with hypertension randomized to the angiotensin receptor antagonist losartan experienced improved memory, but those who received atenolol showed neither improved nor worse memory function [128]. Another study compared propranolol to placebo in young or middle-aged patients with hypertension and found little or no difference in performance on a battery of cognitive tests [129]. A small study in hypertensive veterans demonstrated no decline in cognitive performance with treatment using either propranolol or atenolol [130]. However, in a study of cognitively impaired elderly patients, use of beta-blockers was associated with a trend toward worsening memory [131].

Digoxin

Digoxin is a naturally occurring glycoside used to improve cardiac output in patients with congestive heart failure. Altered mental state and delirium can occur with toxic doses of digoxin [132] and have even been reported with so-called therapeutic serum concentrations [133]. However, at therapeutic dosages, digoxin may actually improve cognitive performance [134].

H2 Blockers and Proton-Pump Inhibitors

Histamine H2 receptor antagonists (e.g., cimetidine, ranitidine, famotidine, nizatidine) and proton-pump inhibitors (e.g., omeprazole, lansoprazole, esomeprazole, pantoprazole) are widely prescribed for the treatment of acid-reflux disease and peptic ulcer disease and to help reduce the gastric side effects of medications such as aspirin. Both classes of drug inhibit acid secretion from gastric parietal cells. Gastric acid is necessary for the release of vitamin B12 from ingested food, and H2 blockers may reduce B12 absorption [135, 136]. Since vitamin B12 deficiency can cause cognitive impairment, dementia, or delirium, prolonged inhibition of gastric acid secretion may increase the risk of neurobehavioral symptoms [137].

A case–control study of elderly patients demonstrated an association between chronic use (at least 12 months) of H2 blockers or proton-pump inhibitors and vitamin B12 deficiency [138]. Another study showed that prolonged use of proton-pump inhibitors, but not H2 blockers, was associated with vitamin B12 deficiency in the elderly, though the consequences of this on cognition were not examined [139]. A longitudinal study of elderly African-Americans demonstrated that H2 blocker use doubled the risk of developing cognitive impairment [140]. Thus, it might be prudent to periodically check serum B12 levels (or sensitive surrogate markers such as methylmalonic acid and homocysteine) when using H2 blockers or proton-pump inhibitors in elderly patients.

There have been numerous case reports describing mental confusion in patients taking the H2 blockers cimetidine, ranitidine, or famotidine. However, a randomized, placebo-controlled, crossover of healthy elderly individuals showed no adverse effects of cimetidine on cognition, leading the authors to conclude that earlier case reports might have been due to specific patient sensitivities to this class of medications [141]. A large cohort study, in contrast, suggested that H2 blocker use was associated with higher risk of cognitive impairment or decline in cognitive functioning [142].

Urinary Antispasmodics

Urge urinary incontinence due to an overactive or spastic bladder may be treated with medications that have the potential to produce cognitive symptoms. Simple measures such as restricting fluid intake, avoiding caffeine, or scheduling frequent visits to the toilet can reduce the need for medical treatment in some patients. Others, though, may be prescribed anticholinergic medications directed against muscarinic M3 receptors that decrease bladder detrusor muscle activity (e.g., oxybutynin, tolterodine, trospium, solifenacin, darifenacin). As with any anticholinergics, these drugs can produce dry mouth, constipation, dizziness, and drowsiness. The risk for these agents to impair cognitive functioning is related to their ability to penetrate the brain and their interaction with muscarinic M1 receptors [143]. In a study of healthy elderly volunteers, solifenacin did not seem to affect cognition, whereas oxybutynin impaired several measures of cognition [144]. After 3 weeks of treatment, healthy elderly subjects experienced significant memory impairment on oxybutynin in contrast to those on darifenacin, which showed no difference in memory compared to the placebo group [145]. Darifenacin was found to have no effects on cognition in another trial involving healthy elderly volunteers [146]. Tolterodine was demonstrated to produce reversible memory impairment in a single case report [147] but was found to have no effect on memory in a 3-week crossover study compared to oxybutynin [143].

Corticosteroids and NSAIDs

Corticosteroids and nonsteroidal anti-inflammatory drugs (NSAIDs) are used to treat various conditions associated with inflammation or pain (e.g., vasculitis, arthritis). Severe psychiatric symptoms, such as affective and psychotic conditions, may occur in upward of 5% of patients treated with corticosteroids [148]. Acute corticosteroid treatment, but not chronic treatment, seemed to induce memory impairment in patients with rheumatoid arthritis [149]. Steroid use has likewise been associated with reversible dementia [150, 151]. It should be noted that too rapid withdrawal of corticosteroid therapy can also affect the brain [152].

Though non-neurological side effects of NSAIDs are quite common (e.g., dyspepsia, renal impairment), they infrequently can cause aseptic meningitis, disorientation, hallucinations, and memory or attentional impairment, and the elderly may be at increased risk [153]. A large randomized, placebo-controlled study of patients with cardiovascular disease showed no difference in performance on multiple cognitive tasks with long-term low-dose aspirin therapy [154]. Aspirin failed to prevent cognitive decline in healthy older women participating in the Women's Health Study [155]. Neither naproxen nor celecoxib prevented cognitive decline compared to placebo in elderly non-demented subjects with a family history of Alzheimer's disease [156]. In contrast, a randomized, placebo-controlled study of patients with subjective memory impairment demonstrated improvements in executive functioning and memory, as well as increased cerebral metabolism on positron-emission tomography (PET) imaging with celecoxib treatment [157].

The effects of long-term NSAID use on reducing the risk of cognitive decline and dementia have been mixed [158], with most studies showing a possible protective effect [159–165] and others providing no evidence for such protection [166, 167] or demonstrating a potential detrimental effect [168, 169]. These diverse results likely reflect differences in patient or subject groups, types and doses of NSAIDs taken, age at first use, and length of therapy. Needless to say, a disappointment for those studying Alzheimer's disease is that no prospective clinical trial has yet shown that NSAID use prevents dementia.

Hormonal Therapy

There was initial enthusiasm that estrogen therapy might help prevent cognitive decline and dementia based on epidemiological studies of estrogen-replacement therapy in younger women. However, no benefits have been demonstrated in older, postmenopausal women [170, 171]. Indeed, the large Women's Health Initiative revealed that postmenopausal estrogen therapy was associated with significant risk of dementia (hazard ratio 1.76), as well as negative effects on selective cognitive measures such as verbal memory and lower brain volumes in the frontal lobe and hippocampus [172].

Testosterone levels in men decline with aging. Evidence suggests that this drop might contribute to parallel cognitive decline and that testosterone supplementation might prevent or be useful in treating cognitive impairment, though neither the association nor the benefits have been strongly demonstrated in large-scale, rigorous trials [173–175]. Treatment of elderly men with low serum testosterone levels but no cognitive impairment with exogenous testosterone (either alone or in combination with the 5-alpha reductase inhibitor finasteride, which blocks conversion of testosterone to dihydrotestosterone) did not impact cognition [176]. Further, a 6-month randomized, placebo-controlled trial of testosterone in older men with low normal serum testosterone levels failed to show any effects on cognition [177].

The long-term effects of antihormonal treatments for breast or prostate cancers on cognition in the elderly are uncertain [178]. Treatment with the antiestrogen drug tamoxifen in women with breast cancer may be associated with cognitive difficulties later in life [179, 180]. However, the selective estrogen receptor modulator raloxifene, which is used to treat osteoporosis and reduce the risk of breast cancer in postmenopausal women, was shown to improve verbal memory versus placebo [181]. Androgen deprivation in men with prostate cancer seems to be associated with decline in some cognitive domains [182]. In elderly men being treated with androgen blockade for prostate cancer, no decline in cognition was noted after 12 weeks of therapy, and addition of estrogen failed to improve verbal memory compared to androgen blockade alone [183].

Cholesterol-Lowering Drugs

The 3-hydroxy-3-methyl-glutaryl-coenzyme-A reductase inhibitors, or statins (e.g., lovastatin, pravastatin, simvastatin, atorvastatin, fluvastatin, rosuvastatin), are effective in lowering levels of total cholesterol and low-density lipoprotein (LDL) and have been important treatments in reducing the risk of coronary and cerebrovascular disease. Statin therapy in elderly non-demented women was associated with lower risk of cognitive impairment [184]. In the large Cardiovascular Health Study ($N=3{,}334$ patients), cognitive decline in the elderly was less in statin users, a finding that seemed to be in part independent of lowering cholesterol levels [185]. It has been proposed that statins affect other non-lipid-related pathways that could impact neurological disease and therefore cognition, but this has not yet been adequately studied [186].

Less is known about the cognitive effects of other cholesterol-lowering drugs on cognition. Treatment with gemfibrozil in elderly patients with hypertriglyceridemia and stroke risk factors improved cognitive scores and cerebral blood flow after several months compared to placebo [187]. Severe niacin deficiency can produce dementia (i.e., pellagra), and dietary niacin intake was found to be inversely related to risk of cognitive decline and Alzheimer's disease [188]. However, the effects on cognition in the elderly of high-dose niacin used to treat hypercholesterolemia (usually 500–2,000 mg/day) have not been examined.

Summary

The clinician must be vigilant in identifying medications that can cause or contribute to cognitive impairment in the elderly. In this age of polypharmacy, the potential for inappropriate or overprescribing has burgeoned, yet the increasing use of electronic medical records might help reverse this trend. Non-pharmacologic interventions (e.g., counseling, structured environment, group activities) should be considered in treating affective and behavioral disturbances, single agents should be used whenever possible, and drugs with potential anticholinergic (i.e., TCAs) or extrapyramidal (i.e., neuroleptics) side effects should be eschewed.

Clinical Pearls

- In prescribing any medications for elderly patients, follow the rule: "Start low, go slow." Elderly patients may require lower doses of a given medication than younger patients, so by starting at the lowest possible dose and titrating upward slowly, you will be more likely to identify the least amount of medication required as well as minimize any potential side effects.
- Avoid polypharmacy and keep abreast of what medications are being prescribed by other physicians. Increasing adoption of electronic medical records, patient-centered medical home (in which the multiple needs of a patient are coordinated through a primary/personal physician), and electronic prescribing are ways to help reduce the number of medications for a given patient and prevent deleterious interactions and side effects.
- When possible, select medications that may be used to treat more than one of the patient's medical conditions in order to reduce the patient's number of medications. For example, the SNRI duloxetine can be used to treat depression as well as painful diabetic neuropathy, or propranolol might be a good choice of

antihypertensive for a patient with essential tremor.

- Before prescribing sleep aids in elderly patients, especially those with cognitive impairment, try promoting healthy sleep habits, so-called good sleep hygiene. That is, instruct the patient or caregiver to set regular awakening and sleep times, avoid caffeine in the afternoon and evening, and restrict the bed for sleep and not reading or watching television. In addition, recommend that the patient avoid napping and get regular exercise.
- Every attempt should be made to manage behavioral problems in patients with dementia using non-pharmacological means. Simple measures such as a structured home environment (e.g., regular routines for meals, sleep, and social activities) can sometimes reduce the likelihood of behavioral outbursts or confrontations without having to resort to sedating medications.

References

1. Francis J. Delirium in older patients. J Am Geriatr Soc. 1992;40(8):829–38.
2. Thompson II TL, Moran MG, Nies AS. Drug therapy: Psychotropic drug use in the elderly (first of two parts). N Engl J Med. 1983;308(3):134–8.
3. Reynolds 3rd CF, Perel JM, Kupfer DJ, Zimmer B, Stack JA, Hoch CC. Open-trial response to antidepressant treatment in elderly patients with mixed depression and cognitive impairment. Psychiatry Res. 1987;21(2):111–22.
4. Doraiswamy PM, Krishnan KR, Oxman T, Jenkyn LR, Coffey DJ, Burt T, Clary CM. Does antidepressant therapy improve cognition in elderly depressed patients? J Gerontol A Biol Sci Med Sci. 2003;58(12): M1137–44.
5. Bartus RT, Dean 3rd RL, Beer B, Lippa AS. The cholinergic hypothesis of geriatric memory dysfunction. Science. 1982;217(4558):408–14.
6. Cole JO, Branconnier R, Salomon M, Dessain E. Tricyclic use in the cognitively impaired elderly. J Clin Psychiatry. 1983;44(9 Pt 2):14–9.
7. Livingston RL, Zucker DK, Isenberg K, Wetzel RD. Tricyclic antidepressants and delirium. J Clin Psychiatry. 1983;44(5):173–6.
8. Kumar S, Kulkarni SK. Influence of antidepressant drugs on learning and memory paradigms in mice. Indian J Exp Biol. 1996;34(5):431–5.
9. Hoff AL, Shukla S, Helms P, Aronson TA, Logue C, Ollo C, Cook B. The effects of nortriptyline on cognition in elderly depressed patients. J Clin Psychopharmacol. 1990;10(3):231–2.
10. Meyers BS, Mattis S, Gabriele M, Kakuma T. Effects of nortriptyline on memory self-assessment and performance in recovered elderly depressives. Psychopharmacol Bull. 1991;27(3):295–9.
11. Young RC, Mattis S, Alexopoulos GS, Meyers BS, Shindledecker RD, Dhar AK. Verbal memory and plasma drug concentrations in elderly depressives treated with nortriptyline. Psychopharmacol Bull. 1991;27(3):291–4.
12. Branconnier RJ, DeVitt DR, Cole JO, Spera KF. Amitriptyline selectively disrupts verbal recall from secondary memory of the normal aged. Neurobiol Aging. 1982;3(1):55–9.
13. Teri L, Reifler BV, Veith RC, Barnes R, White E, McLean P, Raskind M. Imipramine in the treatment of depressed Alzheimer's patients: impact on cognition. J Gerontol. 1991;46(6):P372–7.
14. Podewils LJ, Lyketsos CG. Tricyclic antidepressants and cognitive decline. Psychosomatics. 2002;43(1): 31–5.
15. Knegtering H, Eijck M, Huijsman A. Effects of antidepressants on cognitive functioning of elderly patients. A review. Drugs Aging. 1994;5(3):192–9.
16. Savaskan E, Muller SE, Bohringer A, Schulz A, Schachinger H. Antidepressive therapy with escitalopram improves mood, cognitive symptoms, and identity memory for angry faces in elderly depressed patients. Int J Neuropsychopharmacol. 2008;11(3): 381–8.
17. Finkel SI, Richter EM, Clary CM, Batzar E. Comparative efficacy of sertraline vs. fluoxetine in patients age 70 or over with major depression. Am J Geriatr Psychiatry. 1999;7(3):221–7.
18. Newhouse PA, Krishnan KR, Doraiswamy PM, Richter EM, Batzar ED, Clary CM. A double-blind comparison of sertraline and fluoxetine in depressed elderly outpatients. J Clin Psychiatry. 2000;61(8): 559–68.
19. Cassano GB, Puca F, Scapicchio PL, Trabucchi M. Paroxetine and fluoxetine effects on mood and cognitive functions in depressed nondemented elderly patients. J Clin Psychiatry. 2002;63(5):396–402.
20. Mowla A, Mosavinasab M, Pani A. Does fluoxetine have any effect on the cognition of patients with mild cognitive impairment? A double-blind, placebo-controlled, clinical trial. J Clin Psychopharmacol. 2007;27(1):67–70.
21. Bymaster FP, Dreshfield-Ahmad LJ, Threlkeld PG, Shaw JL, Thompson L, Nelson DL, Hemrick-Luecke SK, Wong DT. Comparative affinity of duloxetine and venlafaxine for serotonin and norepinephrine transporters in vitro and in vivo, human serotonin receptor subtypes, and other neuronal receptors. Neuropsychopharmacology. 2001;25(6): 871–80.
22. Trick L, Stanley N, Rigney U, Hindmarch I. A double-blind, randomized, 26-week study comparing the cognitive and psychomotor effects and efficacy of 75 mg (37.5 mg b.I.D.) venlafaxine and 75 mg (25 mg mane, 50 mg nocte) dothiepin in elderly patients with moderate major depression being

treated in general practice. J Psychopharmacol. 2004;18(2):205–14.
23. Raskin J, Wiltse CG, Siegal A, Sheikh J, Xu J, Dinkel JJ, Rotz BT, Mohs RC. Efficacy of duloxetine on cognition, depression, and pain in elderly patients with major depressive disorder: an 8-week, double-blind, placebo-controlled trial. Am J Psychiatry. 2007; 164(6):900–9.
24. Miller CH, Mohr F, Umbricht D, Woerner M, Fleischhacker WW, Lieberman JA. The prevalence of acute extrapyramidal signs and symptoms in patients treated with clozapine, risperidone, and conventional antipsychotics. J Clin Psychiatry. 1998;59(2):69–75.
25. Wang PS, Schneeweiss S, Avorn J, Fischer MA, Mogun H, Solomon DH, Brookhart MA. Risk of death in elderly users of conventional vs. atypical antipsychotic medications. N Engl J Med. 2005; 353(22):2335–41.
26. US Department of Health and Human Services. Public Health Advisory: Deaths with Antipsychotics in Elderly Patients with Behavioral Disturbances. Food and Drug Administration Web site.
27. Stevenson DG, Decker SL, Dwyer LL, Huskamp HA, Grabowski DC, Metzger ED, Mitchell SL. Antipsychotic and benzodiazepine use among nursing home residents: findings from the 2004 national nursing home survey. Am J Geriatr Psychiatry. 2010; 18(12):1078–92.
28. Cummings JL, McRae T, Zhang R. Effects of donepezil on neuropsychiatric symptoms in patients with dementia and severe behavioral disorders. Am J Geriatr Psychiatry. 2006;14(7):605–12.
29. Figiel G, Sadowsky C. A systematic review of the effectiveness of rivastigmine for the treatment of behavioral disturbances in dementia and other neurological disorders. Curr Med Res Opin. 2008;24(1):157–66.
30. Wilcock GK, Ballard CG, Cooper JA, Loft H. Memantine for agitation/aggression and psychosis in moderately severe to severe Alzheimer's disease: a pooled analysis of 3 studies. J Clin Psychiatry. 2008; 69(3):341–8.
31. Burton LC, German PS, Rovner BW, Brant LJ. Physical restraint use and cognitive decline among nursing home residents. J Am Geriatr Soc. 1992; 40(8):811–6.
32. Woerner MG, Alvir JM, Kane JM, Saltz BL, Lieberman JA. Neuroleptic treatment of elderly patients. Psychopharmacol Bull. 1995;31(2):333–7.
33. Steele C, Lucas MJ, Tune L. Haloperidol versus thioridazine in the treatment of behavioral symptoms in senile dementia of the Alzheimer's type: preliminary findings. J Clin Psychiatry. 1986;47(6):310–2.
34. Devanand DP, Sackeim HA, Brown RP, Mayeux R. A pilot study of haloperidol treatment of psychosis and behavioral disturbance in Alzheimer's disease. Arch Neurol. 1989;46(8):854–7.
35. Brown JW, Chobor A, Zinn F. Dementia testing in the elderly. J Nerv Ment Dis. 1993;181(11):695–8.
36. McShane R, Keene J, Gedling K, Fairburn C, Jacoby R, Hope T. Do neuroleptic drugs hasten cognitive decline in dementia? Prospective study with necropsy follow up. BMJ. 1997;314(7076):266–70.
37. Chui HC, Lyness SA, Sobel E, Schneider LS. Extrapyramidal signs and psychiatric symptoms predict faster cognitive decline in Alzheimer's disease. Arch Neurol. 1994;51(7):676–81.
38. Lopez OL, Wisniewski SR, Becker JT, Boller F, DeKosky ST. Psychiatric medication and abnormal behavior as predictors of progression in probable Alzheimer disease. Arch Neurol. 1999;56(10):1266–72.
39. Jeste DV, Rockwell E, Harris MJ, Lohr JB, Lacro J. Conventional vs. newer antipsychotics in elderly patients. Am J Geriatr Psychiatry. 1999;7(1):70–6.
40. Alvir JM, Lieberman JA, Safferman AZ, Schwimmer JL, Schaaf JA. Clozapine-induced agranulocytosis. Incidence and risk factors in the United States. N Engl J Med. 1993;329(3):162–7.
41. Goldberg TE, Greenberg RD, Griffin SJ, Gold JM, Kleinman JE, Pickar D, Schulz SC, Weinberger DR. The effect of clozapine on cognition and psychiatric symptoms in patients with schizophrenia. Br J Psychiatry. 1993;162:43–8.
42. Kennedy J, Deberdt W, Siegal A, Micca J, Degenhardt E, Ahl J, Meyers A, Kaiser C, Baker RW. Olanzapine does not enhance cognition in non-agitated and non-psychotic patients with mild to moderate Alzheimer's dementia. Int J Geriatr Psychiatry. 2005;20(11): 1020–7.
43. Savaskan E, Schnitzler C, Schroder C, Cajochen C, Muller-Spahn F, Wirz-Justice A. Treatment of behavioural, cognitive and circadian rest-activity cycle disturbances in Alzheimer's disease: haloperidol vs. quetiapine. Int J Neuropsychopharmacol. 2006;9(5): 507–16.
44. Scharre DW, Chang SI. Cognitive and behavioral effects of quetiapine in Alzheimer disease patients. Alzheimer Dis Assoc Disord. 2002;16(2):128–30.
45. Rainer MK, Masching AJ, Ertl MG, Kraxberger E, Haushofer M. Effect of risperidone on behavioral and psychological symptoms and cognitive function in dementia. J Clin Psychiatry. 2001;62(11):894–900.
46. Schneider LS, Tariot PN, Dagerman KS, Davis SM, Hsiao JK, Ismail MS, Lebowitz BD, Lyketsos CG, Ryan JM, Stroup TS, Sultzer DL, Weintraub D, Lieberman JA. Effectiveness of atypical antipsychotic drugs in patients with Alzheimer's disease. N Engl J Med. 2006;355(15):1525–38.
47. Sultzer DL, Davis SM, Tariot PN, Dagerman KS, Lebowitz BD, Lyketsos CG, Rosenheck RA, Hsiao JK, Lieberman JA, Schneider LS. Clinical symptom responses to atypical antipsychotic medications in Alzheimer's disease: phase 1 outcomes from the CATIE-AD effectiveness trial. Am J Psychiatry. 2008;165(7):844–54.
48. Rocca P, Marino F, Montemagni C, Perrone D, Bogetto F. Risperidone, olanzapine and quetiapine in the treatment of behavioral and psychological symptoms in patients with Alzheimer's disease: preliminary findings from a naturalistic, retrospective study. Psychiatry Clin Neurosci. 2007;61(6):622–9.

49. De Deyn P, Jeste DV, Swanink R, Kostic D, Breder C, Carson WH, Iwamoto T. Aripiprazole for the treatment of psychosis in patients with Alzheimer's disease: a randomized, placebo-controlled study. J Clin Psychopharmacol. 2005;25(5):463–7.
50. Mintzer JE, Tune LE, Breder CD, Swanink R, Marcus RN, McQuade RD, Forbes A. Aripiprazole for the treatment of psychoses in institutionalized patients with Alzheimer dementia: a multicenter, randomized, double-blind, placebo-controlled assessment of three fixed doses. Am J Geriatr Psychiatry. 2007;15(11): 918–31.
51. Streim JE, Porsteinsson AP, Breder CD, Swanink R, Marcus R, McQuade R, Carson WH. A randomized, double-blind, placebo-controlled study of aripiprazole for the treatment of psychosis in nursing home patients with Alzheimer disease. Am J Geriatr Psychiatry. 2008;16(7):537–50.
52. Bain KT. Management of chronic insomnia in elderly persons. Am J Geriatr Pharmacother. 2006;4(2): 168–92.
53. Bogunovic OJ, Greenfield SF. Practical geriatrics: use of benzodiazepines among elderly patients. Psychiatr Serv. 2004;55(3):233–5.
54. Paterniti S, Dufouil C, Alperovitch A. Long-term benzodiazepine use and cognitive decline in the elderly: the epidemiology of vascular aging study. J Clin Psychopharmacol. 2002;22(3):285–93.
55. Lagnaoui R, Begaud B, Moore N, Chaslerie A, Fourrier A, Letenneur L, Dartigues JF, Moride Y. Benzodiazepine use and risk of dementia: a nested case-control study. J Clin Epidemiol. 2002;55(3):314–8.
56. Dealberto MJ, McAvay GJ, Seeman T, Berkman L. Psychotropic drug use and cognitive decline among older men and women. Int J Geriatr Psychiatry. 1997;12(5):567–74.
57. Brooks JO, Hoblyn JC. Neurocognitive costs and benefits of psychotropic medications in older adults. J Geriatr Psychiatry Neurol. 2007;20(4):199–214.
58. Larson EB, Kukull WA, Buchner D, Reifler BV. Adverse drug reactions associated with global cognitive impairment in elderly persons. Ann Intern Med. 1987;107(2):169–73.
59. Foy A, Drinkwater V, March S, Mearrick P. Confusion after admission to hospital in elderly patients using benzodiazepines. Br Med J (Clin Res Ed). 1986;293(6554):1072.
60. Mokhber N, Azarpazhooh MR, Khajehdaluee M, Velayati A, Hopwood M. Randomized, single-blind, trial of sertraline and buspirone for treatment of elderly patients with generalized anxiety disorder. Psychiatry Clin Neurosci. 2010;64(2):128–33.
61. Hart RP, Colenda CC, Hamer RM. Effects of buspirone and alprazolam on the cognitive performance of normal elderly subjects. Am J Psychiatry. 1991; 148(1):73–7.
62. Cassidy EL, Lauderdale S, Sheikh JI. Mixed anxiety and depression in older adults: clinical characteristics and management. J Geriatr Psychiatry Neurol. 2005; 18(2):83–8.
63. Roehrs T, Merlotti L, Zorick F, Roth T. Sedative, memory, and performance effects of hypnotics. Psychopharmacology (Berl). 1994;116(2):130–4.
64. Toner LC, Tsambiras BM, Catalano G, Catalano MC, Cooper DS. Central nervous system side effects associated with zolpidem treatment. Clin Neuropharmacol. 2000;23(1):54–8.
65. Stone JR, Zorick TS, Tsuang J. Dose-related illusions and hallucinations with zaleplon. Clin Toxicol (Phila). 2008;46(4):344–5.
66. Mintzer MZ, Griffiths RR. Selective effects of zolpidem on human memory functions. J Psychopharmacol. 1999;13(1):18–31.
67. Troy SM, Lucki I, Unruh MA, Cevallos WH, Leister CA, Martin PT, Furlan PM, Mangano R. Comparison of the effects of zaleplon, zolpidem, and triazolam on memory, learning, and psychomotor performance. J Clin Psychopharmacol. 2000;20(3):328–37.
68. Verster JC, Volkerts ER, Schreuder AH, Eijken EJ, van Heuckelum JH, Veldhuijzen DS, Verbaten MN, Paty I, Darwish M, Danjou P, Patat A. Residual effects of middle-of-the-night administration of zaleplon and zolpidem on driving ability, memory functions, and psychomotor performance. J Clin Psychopharmacol. 2002;22(6):576–83.
69. Boyle J, Trick L, Johnsen S, Roach J, Rubens R. Next-day cognition, psychomotor function, and driving-related skills following nighttime administration of eszopiclone. Hum Psychopharmacol. 2008;23(5): 385–97.
70. Allain H, Bentue-Ferrer D, Tarral A, Gandon JM. Effects on postural oscillation and memory functions of a single dose of zolpidem 5 mg, zopiclone 3.75 mg and lormetazepam 1 mg in elderly healthy subjects. A randomized, cross-over, double-blind study versus placebo. Eur J Clin Pharmacol. 2003;59(3):179–88.
71. Fairweather DB, Kerr JS, Hindmarch I. The effects of acute and repeated doses of zolpidem on subjective sleep, psychomotor performance and cognitive function in elderly volunteers. Eur J Clin Pharmacol. 1992;43(6):597–601.
72. Otmani S, Demazieres A, Staner C, Jacob N, Nir T, Zisapel N, Staner L. Effects of prolonged-release melatonin, zolpidem, and their combination on psychomotor functions, memory recall, and driving skills in healthy middle aged and elderly volunteers. Hum Psychopharmacol. 2008;23(8):693–705.
73. Agostini JV, Leo-Summers LS, Inouye SK. Cognitive and other adverse effects of diphenhydramine use in hospitalized older patients. Arch Intern Med. 2001; 161(17):2091–7.
74. Basu R, Dodge H, Stoehr GP, Ganguli M. Sedative-hypnotic use of diphenhydramine in a rural, older adult, community-based cohort: effects on cognition. Am J Geriatr Psychiatry. 2003;11(2):205–13.
75. McEvoy LK, Smith ME, Fordyce M, Gevins A. Characterizing impaired functional alertness from diphenhydramine in the elderly with performance and neurophysiologic measures. Sleep. 2006;29(7): 957–66.

76. Mendelson WB. A review of the evidence for the efficacy and safety of trazodone in insomnia. J Clin Psychiatry. 2005;66(4):469–76.
77. Peck JS, LeGoff DB, Ahmed I, Goebert D. Cognitive effects of exogenous melatonin administration in elderly persons: a pilot study. Am J Geriatr Psychiatry. 2004;12(4):432–6.
78. Riemersma-van der Lek RF, Swaab DF, Twisk J, Hol EM, Hoogendijk WJ, Van Someren EJ. Effect of bright light and melatonin on cognitive and noncognitive function in elderly residents of group care facilities: a randomized controlled trial. JAMA. 2008; 299(22):2642–55.
79. Molloy SA, Rowan EN, O'Brien JT, McKeith IG, Wesnes K, Burn DJ. Effect of levodopa on cognitive function in Parkinson's disease with and without dementia and dementia with Lewy bodies. J Neurol Neurosurg Psychiatry. 2006;77(12):1323–8.
80. Morrison CE, Borod JC, Brin MF, Halbig TD, Olanow CW. Effects of levodopa on cognitive functioning in moderate-to-severe Parkinson's disease (MSPD). J Neural Transm. 2004;111(10–11):1333–41.
81. Radbill R, Rosenberg G, Schwartz A. Effects of levodopa therapy in Parkinson's disease. II. Measurement of behavioural changes. Can Med Assoc J. 1974;111(11):1218–22.
82. Cooper JA, Sagar HJ, Doherty SM, Jordan N, Tidswell P, Sullivan EV. Different effects of dopaminergic and anticholinergic therapies on cognitive and motor function in Parkinson's disease. A follow-up study of untreated patients. Brain. 1992;115(Pt 6):1701–25.
83. Portin R, Rinne UK. The effect of deprenyl (selegiline) on cognition and emotion in parkinsonian patients undergoing long-term levodopa treatment. Acta Neurol Scand Suppl. 1983;95:135–44.
84. Elmer L, Schwid S, Eberly S, Goetz C, Fahn S, Kieburtz K, Oakes D, Blindauer K, Salzman P, Oren S, Prisco UL, Stern M, Shoulson I. Rasagiline-associated motor improvement in PD occurs without worsening of cognitive and behavioral symptoms. J Neurol Sci. 2006;248(1–2):78–83.
85. Brusa L, Bassi A, Stefani A, Pierantozzi M, Peppe A, Caramia MD, Boffa L, Ruggieri S, Stanzione P. Pramipexole in comparison to l-dopa: a neuropsychological study. J Neural Transm. 2003;110(4):373–80.
86. Brusa L, Tiraboschi P, Koch G, Peppe A, Pierantozzi M, Ruggieri S, Stanzione P. Pergolide effect on cognitive functions in early-mild Parkinson's disease. J Neural Transm. 2005;112(2):231–7.
87. Costa A, Peppe A, Dell'Agnello G, Caltagirone C, Carlesimo GA. Dopamine and cognitive functioning in de novo subjects with Parkinson's disease: effects of pramipexole and pergolide on working memory. Neuropsychologia. 2009;47(5):1374–81.
88. Weintraub D, Koester J, Potenza MN, Siderowf AD, Stacy M, Voon V, Whetteckey J, Wunderlich GR, Lang AE. Impulse control disorders in Parkinson disease: a cross-sectional study of 3090 patients. Arch Neurol. 2010;67(5):589–95.
89. Gasparini M, Fabrizio E, Bonifati V, Meco G. Cognitive improvement during tolcapone treatment in Parkinson's disease. J Neural Transm. 1997; 104(8–9):887–94.
90. Hokendorf H. Combination therapy of extrapyramidal disease with trihexyphenidyl and l-dopa: an electromyographic study with specific reference to tremor. J Int Med Res. 1979;7(1):19–28.
91. Koller WC. Pharmacologic treatment of parkinsonian tremor. Arch Neurol. 1986;43(2):126–7.
92. Wirshing WC, Freidenberg DL, Cummings JL, Bartzokis G. Effects of anticholinergic agents on patients with tardive dyskinesia and concomitant drug-induced parkinsonism. J Clin Psychopharmacol. 1989;9(6):407–11.
93. Bedard MA, Pillon B, Dubois B, Duchesne N, Masson H, Agid Y. Acute and long-term administration of anticholinergics in Parkinson's disease: specific effects on the subcortico-frontal syndrome. Brain Cogn. 1999;40(2):289–313.
94. Van Spaendonck KP, Berger HJ, Horstink MW, Buytenhuijs EL, Cools AR. Impaired cognitive shifting in parkinsonian patients on anticholinergic therapy. Neuropsychologia. 1993;31(4):407–11.
95. Fayen M, Goldman MB, Moulthrop MA, Luchins DJ. Differential memory function with dopaminergic versus anticholinergic treatment of drug-induced extrapyramidal symptoms. Am J Psychiatry. 1988; 145(4):483–6.
96. Heinik J. Effects of trihexyphenidyl on MMSE and CAMCOG scores of medicated elderly patients with schizophrenia. Int Psychogeriatr. 1998;10(1):103–8.
97. Meador KJ. Cognitive side effects of medications. Neurol Clin. 1998;16(1):141–55.
98. Drane DL, Meador KJ. Epilepsy, anticonvulsant drugs and cognition. Baillieres Clin Neurol. 1996; 5(4):877–85.
99. Smith DB, Mattson RH, Cramer JA, Collins JF, Novelly RA, Craft B. Results of a nationwide veterans administration cooperative study comparing the efficacy and toxicity of carbamazepine, phenobarbital, phenytoin, and primidone. Epilepsia. 1987;28 Suppl 3:S50–8.
100. Prevey ML, Delaney RC, Cramer JA, Cattanach L, Collins JF, Mattson RH. Effect of valproate on cognitive functioning. Comparison with carbamazepine. The department of veterans affairs epilepsy cooperative study 264 group. Arch Neurol. 1996;53(10):1008–16.
101. Read CL, Stephen LJ, Stolarek IH, Paul A, Sills GJ, Brodie MJ. Cognitive effects of anticonvulsant monotherapy in elderly patients: a placebo-controlled study. Seizure. 1998;7(2):159–62.
102. Craig I, Tallis R. Impact of valproate and phenytoin on cognitive function in elderly patients: results of a single-blind randomized comparative study. Epilepsia. 1994;35(2):381–90.
103. Profenno LA, Jakimovich L, Holt CJ, Porsteinsson A, Tariot PN. A randomized, double-blind, placebo-controlled pilot trial of safety and tolerability of two doses of divalproex sodium in outpatients with

probable Alzheimer's disease. Curr Alzheimer Res. 2005;2(5):553–8.
104. Tariot PN, Erb R, Podgorski CA, Cox C, Patel S, Jakimovich L, Irvine C. Efficacy and tolerability of carbamazepine for agitation and aggression in dementia. Am J Psychiatry. 1998;155(1):54–61.
105. Cumbo E, Ligori LD. Levetiracetam, lamotrigine, and phenobarbital in patients with epileptic seizures and Alzheimer's disease. Epilepsy Behav. 2010; 17(4):461–6.
106. Gomer B, Wagner K, Frings L, Saar J, Carius A, Harle M, Steinhoff BJ, Schulze-Bonhage A. The influence of antiepileptic drugs on cognition: a comparison of levetiracetam with topiramate. Epilepsy Behav. 2007;10(3):486–94.
107. Romigi A, Cervellino A, Marciani MG, Izzi F, Massoud R, Corona M, Torelli F, Zannino S, Uasone E, Placidi F. Cognitive and psychiatric effects of topiramate monotherapy in migraine treatment: an open study. Eur J Neurol. 2008;15(2):190–5.
108. Kececi H, Atakay S. Effects of topiramate on neurophysiological and neuropsychological tests in migraine patients. J Clin Neurosci. 2009;16(12): 1588–91.
109. Menefee LA, Frank ED, Crerand C, Jalali S, Park J, Sanschagrin K, Besser M. The effects of transdermal fentanyl on driving, cognitive performance, and balance in patients with chronic nonmalignant pain conditions. Pain Med. 2004;5(1):42–9.
110. Blumstein H, Gorevic PD. Rheumatologic illnesses: treatment strategies for older adults. Geriatrics. 2005;60(6):28–35.
111. Ng KF, Yuen TS, Ng VM. A comparison of postoperative cognitive function and pain relief with fentanyl or tramadol patient-controlled analgesia. J Clin Anesth. 2006;18(3):205–10.
112. Kunig G, Datwyler S, Eschen A, Schreiter Gasser U. Unrecognised long-lasting tramadol-induced delirium in two elderly patients. A case report. Pharmacopsychiatry. 2006;39(5):194–9.
113. Brown RT, Zuelsdorff M, Fleming M. Adverse effects and cognitive function among primary care patients taking opioids for chronic nonmalignant pain. J Opioid Manag. 2006;2(3):137–46.
114. Fong HK, Sands LP, Leung JM. The role of postoperative analgesia in delirium and cognitive decline in elderly patients: a systematic review. Anesth Analg. 2006;102(4):1255–66.
115. Manning C, Scandale L, Manning EJ, Gengo FM. Central nervous system effects of meclizine and dimenhydrinate: evidence of acute tolerance to antihistamines. J Clin Pharmacol. 1992;32(11): 996–1002.
116. Molloy DW. Memory loss, confusion, and disorientation in an elderly woman taking meclizine. J Am Geriatr Soc. 1987;35(5):454–6.
117. Sunderland T, Tariot PN, Cohen RM, Weingartner H, Mueller 3rd EA, Murphy DL. Anticholinergic sensitivity in patients with dementia of the Alzheimer type and age-matched controls. A dose-response study. Arch Gen Psychiatry. 1987;44(5):418–26.
118. Dubois B, Danze F, Pillon B, Cusimano G, Lhermitte F, Agid Y. Cholinergic-dependent cognitive deficits in Parkinson's disease. Ann Neurol. 1987;22(1): 26–30.
119. Zemishlany Z, Thorne AE. Anticholinergic challenge and cognitive functions: a comparison between young and elderly normal subjects. Isr J Psychiatry Relat Sci. 1991;28(3):32–41.
120. de la Torre JC. How do heart disease and stroke become risk factors for Alzheimer's disease? Neurol Res. 2006;28(6):637–44.
121. Poon IO. Effects of antihypertensive drug treatment on the risk of dementia and cognitive impairment. Pharmacotherapy. 2008;28(3):366–75.
122. Shah K, Qureshi SU, Johnson M, Parikh N, Schulz PE, Kunik ME. Does use of antihypertensive drugs affect the incidence or progression of dementia? A systematic review. Am J Geriatr Pharmacother. 2009;7(5):250–61.
123. Koella WP. CNS-related (side-)effects of beta-blockers with special reference to mechanisms of action. Eur J Clin Pharmacol. 1985;28(Suppl):55–63.
124. Neil-Dwyer G, Bartlett J, McAinsh J, Cruickshank JM. Beta-adrenoceptor blockers and the blood-brian barrier. Br J Clin Pharmacol. 1981;11(6): 549–53.
125. Cove-Smith JR, Kirk CA. CNS-related side-effects with metoprolol and atenolol. Eur J Clin Pharmacol. 1985;28(Suppl):69–72.
126. McAinsh J, Cruickshank JM. Beta-blockers and central nervous system side effects. Pharmacol Ther. 1990;46(2):163–97.
127. Applegate WB, Pressel S, Wittes J, Luhr J, Shekelle RB, Camel GH, Greenlick MR, Hadley E, Moye L, Perry Jr HM, et al. Impact of the treatment of isolated systolic hypertension on behavioral variables. Results from the systolic hypertension in the elderly program. Arch Intern Med. 1994;154(19):2154–60.
128. Fogari R, Mugellini A, Zoppi A, Derosa G, Pasotti C, Fogari E, Preti P. Influence of losartan and atenolol on memory function in very elderly hypertensive patients. J Hum Hypertens. 2003;17(11):781–5.
129. Perez-Stable EJ, Halliday R, Gardiner PS, Baron RB, Hauck WW, Acree M, Coates TJ. The effects of propranolol on cognitive function and quality of life: a randomized trial among patients with diastolic hypertension. Am J Med. 2000;108(5):359–65.
130. Palac DM, Cornish RD, McDonald WJ, Middaugh DA, Howieson D, Bagby SP. Cognitive function in hypertensives treated with atenolol or propranolol. J Gen Intern Med. 1990;5(4):310–8.
131. Gliebus G, Lippa CF. The influence of beta-blockers on delayed memory function in people with cognitive impairment. Am J Alzheimers Dis Other Demen. 2007;22(1):57–61.
132. Portnoi VA. Digitalis delirium in elderly patients. J Clin Pharmacol. 1979;19(11–12):747–50.

133. Eisendrath SJ, Sweeney MA. Toxic neuropsychiatric effects of digoxin at therapeutic serum concentrations. Am J Psychiatry. 1987;144(4):506–7.
134. Laudisio A, Marzetti E, Pagano F, Cocchi A, Bernabei R, Zuccala G. Digoxin and cognitive performance in patients with heart failure: a cohort, pharmacoepidemiological survey. Drugs Aging. 2009;26(2):103–12.
135. Salom IL, Silvis SE, Doscherholmen A. Effect of cimetidine on the absorption of vitamin B12. Scand J Gastroenterol. 1982;17(1):129–31.
136. Force RW, Nahata MC. Effect of histamine h2-receptor antagonists on vitamin B12 absorption. Ann Pharmacother. 1992;26(10):1283–6.
137. Wolters M, Strohle A, Hahn A. Cobalamin: a critical vitamin in the elderly. Prev Med. 2004;39(6): 1256–66.
138. Valuck RJ, Ruscin JM. A case-control study on adverse effects: H2 blocker or proton pump inhibitor use and risk of vitamin B12 deficiency in older adults. J Clin Epidemiol. 2004;57(4):422–8.
139. Dharmarajan TS, Kanagala MR, Murakonda P, Lebelt AS, Norkus EP. Do acid-lowering agents affect vitamin B12 status in older adults? J Am Med Dir Assoc. 2008;9(3):162–7.
140. Boustani M, Hall KS, Lane KA, Aljadhey H, Gao S, Unverzagt F, Murray MD, Ogunniyi A, Hendrie H. The association between cognition and histamine-2 receptor antagonists in African Americans. J Am Geriatr Soc. 2007;55(8):1248–53.
141. Oslin DW, Katz IR, Sands LP, Bilker W, DiFilippo SD, D'Angelo K. Examination of the cognitive effects of cimetidine in normal elderly volunteers. Am J Geriatr Psychiatry. 1999;7(2):160–5.
142. Hanlon JT, Landerman LR, Artz MB, Gray SL, Fillenbaum GG, Schmader KE. Histamine2 receptor antagonist use and decline in cognitive function among community dwelling elderly. Pharmacoepidemiol Drug Saf. 2004;13(11):781–7.
143. Kay GG, Ebinger U. Preserving cognitive function for patients with overactive bladder: evidence for a differential effect with darifenacin. Int J Clin Pract. 2008;62(11):1792–800.
144. Wesnes KA, Edgar C, Tretter RN, Bolodeoku J. Exploratory pilot study assessing the risk of cognitive impairment or sedation in the elderly following single doses of solifenacin 10 mg. Expert Opin Drug Saf. 2009;8(6):615–26.
145. Kay G, Crook T, Rekeda L, Lima R, Ebinger U, Arguinzoniz M, Steel M. Differential effects of the antimuscarinic agents darifenacin and oxybutynin ER on memory in older subjects. Eur Urol. 2006;50(2):317–26.
146. Lipton RB, Kolodner K, Wesnes K. Assessment of cognitive function of the elderly population: effects of darifenacin. J Urol. 2005;173(2):493–8.
147. Womack KB, Heilman KM. Tolterodine and memory: dry but forgetful. Arch Neurol. 2003;60(5): 771–3.
148. Lewis DA, Smith RE. Steroid-induced psychiatric syndromes. A report of 14 cases and a review of the literature. J Affect Disord. 1983;5(4):319–32.
149. Coluccia D, Wolf OT, Kollias S, Roozendaal B, Forster A, de Quervain DJ. Glucocorticoid therapy-induced memory deficits: acute versus chronic effects. J Neurosci. 2008;28(13):3474–8.
150. Varney NR, Alexander B, MacIndoe JH. Reversible steroid dementia in patients without steroid psychosis. Am J Psychiatry. 1984;141(3):369–72.
151. Sacks O, Shulman M. Steroid dementia: an overlooked diagnosis? Neurology. 2005;64(4):707–9.
152. Gupta VP, Ehrlich GE. Organic brain syndrome in rheumatoid arthritis following corticosteroid withdrawal. Arthritis Rheum. 1976;19(6):1333–8.
153. Hoppmann RA, Peden JG, Ober SK. Central nervous system side effects of nonsteroidal anti-inflammatory drugs. Aseptic meningitis, psychosis, and cognitive dysfunction. Arch Intern Med. 1991;151(7):1309–13.
154. Price JF, Stewart MC, Deary IJ, Murray GD, Sandercock P, Butcher I, Fowkes FG. Low dose aspirin and cognitive function in middle aged to elderly adults: randomised controlled trial. BMJ. 2008; 337:a1198.
155. Kang JH, Cook N, Manson J, Buring JE, Grodstein F. Low dose aspirin and cognitive function in the women's health study cognitive cohort. BMJ. 2007;334(7601):987.
156. Martin BK, Szekely C, Brandt J, Piantadosi S, Breitner JC, Craft S, Evans D, Green R, Mullan M. Cognitive function over time in the Alzheimer's disease anti-inflammatory prevention trial (adapt): results of a randomized, controlled trial of naproxen and celecoxib. Arch Neurol. 2008;65(7):896–905.
157. Small GW, Siddarth P, Silverman DH, Ercoli LM, Miller KJ, Lavretsky H, Bookheimer SY, Huang SC, Barrio JR, Phelps ME. Cognitive and cerebral metabolic effects of celecoxib versus placebo in people with age-related memory loss: randomized controlled study. Am J Geriatr Psychiatry. 2008;16(12):999–1009.
158. Szekely CA, Zandi PP. Non-steroidal anti-inflammatory drugs and Alzheimer's disease: the epidemiological evidence. CNS Neurol Disord Drug Targets. 2010;9(2):132–9.
159. Andersen K, Launer LJ, Ott A, Hoes AW, Breteler MM, Hofman A. Do nonsteroidal anti-inflammatory drugs decrease the risk for Alzheimer's disease? The Rotterdam study. Neurology. 1995;45(8): 1441–5.
160. Rich JB, Rasmusson DX, Folstein MF, Carson KA, Kawas C, Brandt J. Nonsteroidal anti-inflammatory drugs in Alzheimer's disease. Neurology. 1995;45(1): 51–5.
161. Sturmer T, Glynn RJ, Field TS, Taylor JO, Hennekens CH. Aspirin use and cognitive function in the elderly. Am J Epidemiol. 1996;143(7):683–91.
162. Stewart WF, Kawas C, Corrada M, Metter EJ. Risk of Alzheimer's disease and duration of NSAID use. Neurology. 1997;48(3):626–32.

163. Szekely CA, Thorne JE, Zandi PP, Ek M, Messias E, Breitner JC, Goodman SN. Nonsteroidal anti-inflammatory drugs for the prevention of Alzheimer's disease: a systematic review. Neuroepidemiology. 2004;23(4):159–69.
164. Vlad SC, Miller DR, Kowall NW, Felson DT. Protective effects of NSAIDS on the development of Alzheimer disease. Neurology. 2008;70(19):1672–7.
165. Waldstein SR, Wendell CR, Seliger SL, Ferrucci L, Metter EJ, Zonderman AB. Nonsteroidal anti-inflammatory drugs, aspirin, and cognitive function in the Baltimore longitudinal study of aging. J Am Geriatr Soc. 2010;58(1):38–43.
166. Hanlon JT, Schmader KE, Landerman LR, Horner RD, Fillenbaum GG, Pieper CF, Wall Jr WE, Koronkowski MJ, Cohen HJ. Relation of prescription nonsteroidal antiinflammatory drug use to cognitive function among community-dwelling elderly. Ann Epidemiol. 1997;7(2):87–94.
167. Henderson AS, Jorm AF, Christensen H, Jacomb PA, Korten AE. Aspirin, anti-inflammatory drugs and risk of dementia. Int J Geriatr Psychiatry. 1997; 12(9):926–30.
168. Saag KG, Rubenstein LM, Chrischilles EA, Wallace RB. Nonsteroidal antiinflammatory drugs and cognitive decline in the elderly. J Rheumatol. 1995;22(11):2142–7.
169. Breitner JC, Haneuse SJ, Walker R, Dublin S, Crane PK, Gray SL, Larson EB. Risk of dementia and ad with prior exposure to NSAIDS in an elderly community-based cohort. Neurology. 2009;72(22):1899–905.
170. Lethaby A, Hogervorst E, Richards M, Yesufu A, Yaffe K Hormone replacement therapy for cognitive function in postmenopausal women. Cochrane Database Syst Rev. 2008;(1):CD003122.
171. Greendale GA, Huang MH, Wight RG, Seeman T, Luetters C, Avis NE, Johnston J, Karlamangla AS. Effects of the menopause transition and hormone use on cognitive performance in midlife women. Neurology. 2009;72(21):1850–7.
172. Coker LH, Espeland MA, Rapp SR, Legault C, Resnick SM, Hogan P, Gaussoin S, Dailey M, Shumaker SA. Postmenopausal hormone therapy and cognitive outcomes: the women's health initiative memory study (WHIMS). J Steroid Biochem Mol Biol. 2010;118(4–5):304–10.
173. Moffat SD. Effects of testosterone on cognitive and brain aging in elderly men. Ann N Y Acad Sci. 2005;1055:80–92.
174. Fuller SJ, Tan RS, Martins RN. Androgens in the etiology of Alzheimer's disease in aging men and possible therapeutic interventions. J Alzheimers Dis. 2007;12(2):129–42.
175. Warren MF, Serby MJ, Roane DM. The effects of testosterone on cognition in elderly men: a review. CNS Spectr. 2008;13(10):887–97.
176. Vaughan C, Goldstein FC, Tenover JL. Exogenous testosterone alone or with finasteride does not improve measurements of cognition in healthy older men with low serum testosterone. J Androl. 2007; 28(6):875–82.
177. Emmelot-Vonk MH, Verhaar HJ, Nakhai Pour HR, Aleman A, Lock TM, Bosch JL, Grobbee DE, van der Schouw YT. Effect of testosterone supplementation on functional mobility, cognition, and other parameters in older men: a randomized controlled trial. JAMA. 2008;299(1):39–52.
178. Mitsiades N, Correa D, Gross CP, Hurria A, Slovin SF. Cognitive effects of hormonal therapy in older adults. Semin Oncol. 2008;35(6):569–81.
179. Paganini-Hill A, Clark LJ. Preliminary assessment of cognitive function in breast cancer patients treated with tamoxifen. Breast Cancer Res Treat. 2000; 64(2):165–76.
180. Castellon SA, Ganz PA, Bower JE, Petersen L, Abraham L, Greendale GA. Neurocognitive performance in breast cancer survivors exposed to adjuvant chemotherapy and tamoxifen. J Clin Exp Neuropsychol. 2004;26(7):955–69.
181. Jacobsen DE, Samson MM, Emmelot-Vonk MH, Verhaar HJ. Raloxifene improves verbal memory in late postmenopausal women: a randomized, double-blind, placebo-controlled trial. Menopause. 2010; 17(2):309–14.
182. Nelson CJ, Lee JS, Gamboa MC, Roth AJ. Cognitive effects of hormone therapy in men with prostate cancer: a review. Cancer. 2008;113(5):1097–106.
183. Matousek RH, Sherwin BB. A randomized controlled trial of add-back estrogen or placebo on cognition in men with prostate cancer receiving an antiandrogen and a gonadotropin-releasing hormone analog. Psychoneuroendocrinology. 2010;35(2):215–25.
184. Yaffe K, Barrett-Connor E, Lin F, Grady D. Serum lipoprotein levels, statin use, and cognitive function in older women. Arch Neurol. 2002;59(3):378–84.
185. Bernick C, Katz R, Smith NL, Rapp S, Bhadelia R, Carlson M, Kuller L. Statins and cognitive function in the elderly: the cardiovascular health study. Neurology. 2005;65(9):1388–94.
186. Willey JZ, Elkind MS. 3-hydroxy-3-methylglutaryl-coenzyme a reductase inhibitors in the treatment of central nervous system diseases. Arch Neurol. 2010;67(9):1062–7.
187. Rogers RL, Meyer JS, McClintic K, Mortel KF. Reducing hypertriglyceridemia in elderly patients with cerebrovascular disease stabilizes or improves cognition and cerebral perfusion. Angiology. 1989; 40(4 Pt 1):260–9.
188. Morris MC, Evans DA, Bienias JL, Scherr PA, Tangney CC, Hebert LE, Bennett DA, Wilson RS, Aggarwal N. Dietary niacin and the risk of incident Alzheimer's disease and of cognitive decline. J Neurol Neurosurg Psychiatry. 2004;75(8):1093–9.

Assessment of Depression and Anxiety in Older Adults

8

Dimitris N. Kiosses

Abstract

Late-life depression and anxiety may contribute to detrimental consequences for patients and their families. They impair functioning, negatively affect quality of life, disrupt interpersonal relationships and increase utilization of medical services. Further, late-life depression is associated with increased morbidity, mortality and is the most common psychiatric diagnosis in attempted or completed suicides. This chapter explores diagnostic considerations and provides clinical pearls for the accurate assessment of the most common depression and anxiety disorders in older adults.

Keywords

Depression • Anxiety • Assessment • Diagnosis • Suicide • Disability

Epidemiology of Late-Life Depression

The prevalence of late-life depression increases as we move from the community to medical settings, home care, and nursing homes. Three percent of older adults in the community, 5–8% of medical outpatients, 11% of medical inpatients, approximately 12% of nursing home residents, and 14% of home-care recipients have major depression [1–3]. The percentages are even greater in milder forms of depression including dysthymia.

Despite its detrimental consequences, late-life depression is underdiagnosed and undertreated. Factors which contribute to underdiagnosis and undertreatment of geriatric depression likely include the following.

(a) Similarities of depression symptoms with those of medical illnesses.
(b) Many older depressed adults do not report depressed mood but rather lack of interest or pleasure in activities.
(c) Aging stereotypes.
(d) Primary care settings, where most of the depressed older adults are treated, are busy

D.N. Kiosses, Ph.D. (✉)
Department of Psychiatry, Weill-Cornell Institute of Geriatric Psychiatry, Weill Medical College of Cornell University, 21 Bloomingdale Road, White Plains, New York, NY 10605, USA
e-mail: dkiosses@med.cornell.edu

L.D. Ravdin and H.L. Katzen (eds.), *Handbook on the Neuropsychology of Aging and Dementia*, Clinical Handbooks in Neuropsychology, DOI 10.1007/978-1-4614-3106-0_8,

and emphasize medical rather than mental health problems [4]. In primary care, almost half of high utilizers receive no antidepressant treatment and 1/3 receive inadequate treatment [4, 5]. Even when antidepressants are prescribed, adherence rates are discouraging, ranging from 25 to 60% [5].

Suicide

Suicide is devastating for the victims' families, friends, and communities. Suicide rates increase with age, with white older men at greatest risk. Although there has been a decrease in suicide rates in older adults in recent years, rates may significantly rise again because of the aging of baby boomers, a cohort with increased suicide rates [6]. When compared with suicide attempts of young adults, attempts of older adults are more determined and use more lethal means, including the use of firearms or hanging. Psychiatric illnesses in general, but mood disorders and major depression in particular, are the most prominent risk factors for suicide. Other risk factors include poor physical health, disability, recent loss, and lack of social connectedness [7–9]. Assessment of these risk factors is important during the assessment of depression.

Epidemiology of Late-Life Anxiety

Late-life anxiety contributes to decreased sense of well-being, reduced satisfaction, and increased disability [10]. Even though reported prevalence rates of diagnosable anxiety in older adults vary greatly in the community (2–19%), the best estimate is about 10%, while this rate increases in medically ill populations [10]. Comorbid anxiety is common in late-life depression, with reports estimating its prevalence up to 65% [10] and it is associated with lower response to antidepressant medication treatment, longer time to response or remission, and shorter time to recurrence once remission is achieved [11–15].

Diagnosis of Clinical Depression and Anxiety

Diagnosis of Clinical Depression

There are different types of clinical depression highlighted in the DSM-IV [16], while some of them may be updated in the DSM-V. Major depressive disorder (MDD), dysthymic disorder, depressive disorder NOS, and adjustment disorder of depressed mood and anxiety are the most common diagnoses of clinical unipolar depression. Differential diagnosis is based on the severity and duration of symptoms as well as on the precipitants of the onset of depression. As we review the symptoms of different types of depression, it is evident that MDD is the most severe. In the following section, the most common depressive and anxiety disorders will be described and certain diagnostic considerations will be highlighted. The detailed descriptions of diagnoses follow the DSM-IV. The DSM-5 is expected to be released in May 2013.

Major Depressive Disorder

MDD is characterized by the presence of one or more major depressive episodes (MDEs) and the absence of any hypomanic or manic episode. A MDE is diagnosed when either depressed mood or loss of interest or pleasure (anhedonia) is present for at least 2 weeks, every day, most of the day [16]. In addition, the patient may experience five or more of the following symptoms: (a) depressed mood, (b) lack of interest or pleasure in activities, (c) significant weight loss or weight gain or appetite disturbances (in older adults, most commonly weight loss and decreased appetite), (d) sleep disturbances, i.e., insomnia or hypersomnia, (e) psychomotor agitation or retardation, (f) fatigue or loss of energy, (g) feelings of worthlessness or excessive or inappropriate guilt, (h) concentration difficulties or indecisiveness, and (i) recurrent thoughts of death, recurrent suicidal ideation, or a suicide attempt or a specific plan for committing suicide (DSM-IV) [16]. To diagnose an episode of major depression, clinically significant distress or impairment in social, occupational, or other important areas of functioning is required [16]. Within the diagnosis of MDD, there are different degrees of severity denoted in the last digit of the DSM-IV diagnosis [16]. Specifically, (1) refers to mild severity, (2) to moderate, (3) to severe without psychotic features, (4) to severe with psychotic features, whereas (5) and (6) refer to partial or full remission.

Psychotic Depression

Major depression with psychotic features is a severe disorder, which is characterized by delusions or hallucinations and is associated with slow recovery, poor outcomes, and increased disability and mortality [17–19]. Delusions are more frequent than hallucinations, and compared to delusions in dementia, delusions in psychotic depression are systematized and mood congruent [4]. Usual delusional themes include guilt, persecution, hypochondriasis, nihilism, and jealousy.

Dysthymia

Dysthymic disorder is a chronic depression of milder intensity than major depression. Specifically, depressed mood is present for most of the day, not every day but for most days than not, for at least 2 years and should not be absent for longer than 2 months [16]. Contrary to the diagnosis of major depression, lack of interest or pleasure is not a cardinal symptom of dysthymia. In addition to depressed mood, the patient may experience two or more of the following symptoms: (a) poor appetite or overeating (in older adults, most commonly poor appetite), (b) insomnia or hypersomnia, (c) low energy or fatigue, (d) low self-esteem, (e) poor concentration or difficulty making decisions, and (f) feelings of hopelessness [16]. Once again, clinically significant distress or impairment in social, occupational, or other important areas of functioning is required for diagnosis [16].

A close examination of the symptoms of major depression and dysthymia may explain why late-life depression is underdiagnosed. First, fatigue, loss of energy, concentration difficulties, weight loss, and sleep disturbances may be symptoms of other medical illnesses. As older adults frequently suffer from medical illnesses, it may be difficult to differentiate whether these symptoms are features of depression or other medical illnesses. Second, due to aging stereotypes, lack of interest or pleasure may be incorrectly perceived as a normal part of aging. This is a very critical issue as many depressed older adults do not exhibit or report depressed mood, but rather lack of interest or pleasure.

Adjustment Disorder with Anxiety and/or Depressed Mood

Adjustment disorder refers to the development of emotional and behavioral symptoms as a response to a stressor occurring within 3 months of the onset of the symptoms [16]. Usual stressors of adjustment disorder in older adults include poor physical health and disability, socioeconomic deprivation, and placement to a long-term care facility [4, 20]. Based on DSM-IV [16], the symptoms are clinically significant, may cause marked distress (more than expected from the exposure to that stressor) and significant impairment in social or occupational functioning. Adjustment disorder may occur with anxiety, depressed mood, or both.

Cognitive Deficits Associated with Depression

As mentioned above, late-life depression may be accompanied by cognitive difficulties. Poor concentration is a common symptom of depression. Moreover, nondemented depressed elders may present with disturbances in processing speed and executive functioning [21, 22]. To evaluate the etiology of cognitive difficulties in late-life depression, a thorough neuropsychological examination is strongly recommended.

Some older adults display symptoms of dementia that are due to depression. As soon as depression remits, their cognitive functioning may reach their premorbid functioning. This clinical picture is referred as "pseudodementia" or "reversible dementia." The causes of "pseudodementia" are not clearly understood; in some cases, depression may contribute to cognitive impairment whereas in others, cognitive deficits may be the result of a progressive subclinical dementia that is exacerbated by depression [4, 23]. Despite their return to almost normal cognitive functioning, older adults with "pseudodementia" may develop irreversible dementia at a rate of 9–25% per year (approximately 40% within 3 years) [4, 23]. Further research is needed to understand "pseudodementia" and its consequences.

Depression in Alzheimer's Disease

Some depressive symptoms may be similar to symptoms of Alzheimer's disease (AD). For example, diminished social activity and lack of interest, which are symptoms of depression, are prevalent in AD. The overlap of symptoms between depression and AD may complicate the diagnosis of depression in AD [24]. Further, research suggests that depression in AD may be different from other depressive disorders [24].

In 2002, the NIMH organized a workshop with a group of investigators of depression and AD to facilitate the development of provisional diagnostic criteria for depression of AD [24, 25]. The goals of the development of these criteria were to assist clinicians in diagnosing depression in AD and to provide a target for research on the mechanism and treatment of depression and AD [25]. The criteria required three (or more) of the following symptoms to be present during the same 2-week period and represent a change from previous functioning: at least one of the symptoms is either (1) depressed mood or (2) decreased positive affect or pleasure. The symptoms were: (a) clinically significant depressed mood, (b) decreased positive affect or pleasure, (c) social isolation or withdrawal, (d) disruption in appetite, (e) disruption in sleep, (f) psychomotor changes (agitation or retardation), (g) irritability, (h) fatigue or loss of energy, (i) feelings of worthlessness, hopelessness, or excessive or inappropriate guilt, and (j) recurrent thoughts of death, suicidal ideation, and plan or attempt [24, 25]. These criteria must be present in an individual diagnosed with Dementia of the Alzheimer's Type and the symptoms are believed to cause clinically significant distress or disruption in functioning [25].

The provisional diagnostic criteria for depression of AD mainly differ from DSM-IV criteria of MDD in the following ways: (a) the duration of cardinal symptoms (in DSM-IV, the symptoms must be there nearly every day, most of the day, while in provisional criteria, the symptoms may have shorter duration), (b) the number of symptoms required for the diagnosis (5 in DSM-IV vs. 3 in provisional criteria), and (c) description of anhedonia ("lack of pleasure in DSM-IV" vs. "decreased positive affect or pleasure in response to social contacts or activities" in provisional criteria) [24, 25].

Diagnosis of Anxiety

In a recent review of cognitive therapy of anxiety disorders, Clark and Beck highlight the following definitions of fear and anxiety: "Fear is a primitive automatic neuropsychological state of alarm involving the cognitive appraisal of imminent threat or danger to the safety and security of an individual," whereas "Anxiety is a complex cognitive, affective, physiological, and behavioral response system (i.e., threat mode) that is activated when anticipated events or circumstances are deemed to be highly aversive because they are perceived to be unpredictable, uncontrollable events that could potentially threaten the vital interests of an individual" [26]. Therefore, fear and anxiety have a protective value of helping us deal with actual threats. However, in anxiety disorders, the patient's perceived threats may not be accurate, last longer than expected, while the threshold for perceived threats is lowered and, therefore, the patient becomes hypersensitive to external stimuli. As a result, the response could be excessive compared to the severity of the perceived threat, while anxiety feels uncontrollable and significantly impairs functioning. Therefore, in the assessment of anxiety, the clinician has to evaluate the evidence for a realistic threat and the appropriateness and excessiveness of the patient's response to the perceived threat.

Generalized anxiety disorder (GAD) and phobias are the most common anxiety disorders in older adults [10, 27, 28], even though a number of older adults may experience clinically significant anxiety without any specific diagnosis [10]. The following section highlights the diagnoses of GAD, phobias, and panic disorder.

Generalized Anxiety Disorder

The critical features of GAD as described in DSM-IV [16] are (a) excessive and difficult to control anxiety or worry (apprehensive expectation), for more days than not, for at least 6 months; (b) at least three or more of the following symptoms: (1) restlessness, (2) being easily fatigued, (3) concentration difficulties, (4) irritability, (5) muscle tension, and (6) sleep disturbances [16]. Similar to other diagnoses in DSM-IV, the symptoms must be severe enough to cause clinically significant distress or impairment in social, occupational, or other important areas of functioning [16].

Specific Phobia

Specific Phobia is characterized by "marked and persistent fear that is excessive and unreasonable, cued by the presence or anticipation of a specific object or situation (e.g., flying, heights, animals, receiving an injection, seeing blood)" [16]. The patient recognizes that his or her fear is excessive and unreasonable and avoids the phobic situation, as the exposure of the stimulus "almost invariably provokes an immediate anxiety response" [16].

Panic Disorder

As described in DSM-IV, panic disorder is characterized by recurrent unexpected panic attacks; one of the attacks has been followed by at least 1 month of persistent concern about having additional attacks, worry about the implications or consequences of the attack, or a significant change in behavior related to the attacks [16]. Panic attacks are defined as "an intense period of fear or discomfort, in which four (or more) of the following symptoms developed abruptly and reached a peak within 10 min: (a) palpitations, pounding heart, or accelerated heart rate; (b) sweating, (c) trembling or shaking, (d) sensations of shortness of breath or smothering, (e) feeling of choking, (f) chest pain or discomfort, (g) nausea or abdominal stress, (h) feeling dizzy, unsteady, lightheaded, or faint, (i) derealization (feelings of unreality) or depersonalization (being detached from oneself), (j) fear of losing control or going crazy, (k) fear of dying, (l) paresthesias (numbness or tingling sensations), and (m) chills or hot flushes" [16]. Panic disorder may be diagnosed in the presence or absence of agoraphobia, which is characterized by anxiety and avoidance of places or situations in the event of having a panic attack.

Diagnostic Considerations

Rule out Other Diagnoses

The clinician needs to evaluate whether other mental disorders exist. For example, ruling out Bipolar I and II disorders is critical because the pharmacological or psychological treatment of bipolar depression differ from that of unipolar depression. Geriatric bipolar disorder is relatively rare in the community and its point prevalence rate is less than 0.5% [29]. However, 17% of older adults in psychiatric emergency rooms have bipolar disorder [29, 30]. Compared to young adults, fewer older bipolar patients have a diagnosis of substance abuse and more have a cognitive disorder diagnosis (i.e., dementia, amnesia, and cognitive disorder NOS) [28].

Bipolar I is characterized by the occurrence of manic episodes, with or without MDEs [16]. However, Bipolar I older patients usually have had one or more MDEs. Manic episode is defined as "a distinct period of abnormally and persistently elevated, expansive, or irritable mood, lasting at least 1 week (or any duration if hospitalization is necessary)" [16]. During this period, the patient experiences three or more of the following symptoms (four if mood is only irritable): (a) inflated self-esteem or grandiosity, (b) decreased need for sleep (e.g., patient feels rested after only 3 h of sleep), (c) more talkative than usual or pressured speech, (d) flights of ideas or racing thoughts, (e) distractibility, (f) psychomotor agitation or increase in goal-directed activities, and (g) excessive involvement in pleasurable activities that have a high potential for painful consequences (e.g., buying sprees, sexual indiscretions, or foolish business investments) [16]. The patient has significant impairment in occupational, interpersonal, or social functioning [16] that may require hospitalization. Because of the severity of the manic episodes, early-onset Bipolar I disorder has been usually diagnosed before an older adult presents with psychiatric problems, while late-onset Bipolar I disorder occurs only in a small minority of geriatric bipolar cases [31].

Bipolar II is characterized by the occurrence of MDEs and at least one hypomanic episode [16]. Hypomanic episode is of lesser severity and duration than a manic episode and is defined as "a distinct period of persistently elevated, expansive, or irritable mood, lasting throughout at least 4 days, that is clearly different from the usual nondepressed mood" [16]. During this period, the patient experiences three or more of the same symptoms described in the manic episode (four if mood is only irritable) [16]. According to the DSM-IV criteria, the hypomanic episode does not include psychotic features and is not severe enough to cause significant impairment in occupational, interpersonal, or social functioning, or to necessitate hospitalization [16].

Substance Abuse

Use of alcohol, drug, or prescription medication needs to be evaluated. The clinician shall evaluate the amount and frequency of alcohol consumption, the use of possible illicit drugs and prescription medication. Special attention must be placed on the possible abuse of prescription medications as some of them may be addictive (e.g., medications for the treatment of anxiety or pain).

Evaluation of Medical Conditions and Medications

Certain medical conditions and medications may cause depression. Specifically, medical conditions, including thyroid abnormalities, deficiency of vitamin B12, lymphomas, and pancreatic cancer, are often associated with depression [4]. Moreover, steroids, anti-Parkinsonian drugs, and benzodiazepines may cause depression [4]. As noted in DSM-IV, the symptoms of depression must not be "due to the direct physiological effects of a substance (e.g., a drug of abuse, a medication) or a general medical condition (e.g., hypothyroidism)." Treatment recommendations highlight that the medical condition may need to be treated first; however, there are cases that depression may not remit unless antidepressant medication treatment is prescribed [4].

Assessment of Depression and Anxiety

Accurate Diagnosis of Depression

During the first interview with the depressed older adult, the clinician must obtain the following information: present history of depression, onset of the current episode, precipitants of the current episode, past history of depression, current or past suicidal ideation, family history of depression and suicide attempts, history of antidepressant medication and psychotherapeutic treatments and outcomes, medical history, and list of psychiatric and nonpsychiatric medications.

The clinician should evaluate the onset of current and past depression episodes, explore any events that preceded these episodes, and evaluate the coping mechanisms that the patient used to deal with potential stressors. Helpful questions include: What were the precipitants of the episodes of depression? What were the most critical stressors that the patient experienced before the onset of depression? What were the coping mechanisms that the patient utilized? Which coping mechanisms were successful or unsuccessful?

As the clinician explores past and current depressive episodes, he should evaluate the patient's previous response to antidepressants or psychotherapies. The patient should also be asked to produce a list of all antidepressant medications (i.e., highest dosages, duration, and treatment response for each medication), a list of previous and current psychotherapeutic treatment (i.e., type of treatment, for example, cognitive behavioral therapy, behavioral therapy, or problem solving therapy; frequency and duration of treatment; and treatment response), and a list of any other treatments (e.g., electroconvulsive therapy). These lists may help the clinician to determine adequacy and response to antidepressant treatment. Finally, psychiatric hospitalizations, reasons for admissions, inpatient psychiatric treatments, and follow-up treatments should be discussed in detail.

Sometimes the patient's depression may not be easily recognized. Loss of interest and pleasure or depressed mood are cardinal symptoms of clinical depression. At least one of these two symptoms is required for the diagnosis of major depression. Therefore, a patient may suffer from depression even though he or she does not report depressed mood. In fact, many older adults report loss of interest or pleasure, as well as physical symptoms, in the absence of depressed mood. It is also important to recognize that depressed older adults may not necessarily use the words "depressed" or "sad," but rather "blue," "helpless," "hopeless," "apathetic," "disinterested," or "unmotivated." The clinician needs to evaluate the patient's words carefully and assess whether these words reflect clinical depression.

Assessment of Past or Present Suicide Ideation

Since hopelessness is associated with suicide ideation, the clinician should evaluate the degree of hopelessness and suicide ideation in past and current episodes of depression. Important questions include: What makes you feel hopeless? Have you recently felt (or have you ever felt) that life is not worth living? What parts of life are not worth living? What parts of life are worth living? How strong is your wish to live? Have you ever wished you were dead? Describe recent events that made you feel that life was not worth living or that you wished you were dead? Any specific event or stressor that precipitated these feelings? What went through your mind? Have you ever thought of hurting or killing yourself? If yes, have you thought about a specific plan? What kept you from doing anything to harm or kill yourself? Has there been a family history of suicide attempts?

The clinician should gather detailed information about past and recent suicide attempts. The patient may describe the sequence of events, as well as severity and duration of the suicide ideation that contributed to the suicide attempt. The goal of the clinician is to understand risky situations, to illuminate the hopeless thoughts that contributed to suicide ideation or suicide attempts, and to explore potential positive thoughts that have prevented the patient from harming or killing himself or herself. Access to firearms or to other potential lethal means (for example, lethal doses of medicaiton) must be evaluated during the interview of a patient at risk of suicide. In certain cases, to avoid risky access to firearms, the clinician may propose that firearms be removed from the patient's residence. Finally, the clinician may decide to hospitalize the patient if, after the evaluation, the clinician believes that the patient is a threat to himself or herself. In addition to suicide ideation, the clinician should also evaluate whether the patient is a threat to hurt others, or whether there is a history of violent outbursts and physical abuse.

Depression vs. Normal Fluctuation of Mood

Clinical depression is different from the normal "ups and downs" of everyday life in severity, duration, and its effect on the patient's functioning. Normal fluctuation of mood is usually not prolonged, is not as severe, and does not significantly impair functioning. Impairment in functioning is required for the diagnosis of clinical depression. Signs and symptoms of hopelessness, worthlessness, or excessive guilt are associated with clinical depression and are not typically part of normal mood fluctuations.

Complicated Grief

One of the most difficult situations in assessing depression and recommending treatment is when the sadness is associated with grief. In general, if the older adult's functioning is significantly impaired, psychotherapeutic or medication treatment is recommended. Because of the stigma attached to mental illness, the clinician needs to address the issue tactfully, recognizing that it is expected to experience sadness after the loss of a loved one. Grief stricken patients may also experience an exaggerated sense of guilt when they feel pleasure, which may reinforce the vicious cycle of depression.

Accurate Diagnosis of Anxiety Disorders: Productive Anxiety vs. Unnecessary Worrying

Patients with anxiety disorders often present for the treatment of anxiety with the expectation of complete elimination of their anxiety symptoms. The clinician should discuss the potential benefit of anxiety to help the patient recognize that the goal of treatment may not be the elimination of anxiety per se, but rather learning techniques to effectively deal with excessive and uncontrollable anxiety or worrying. Moderate levels of anxiety may also be a motivating factor and become a productive force.

The interview may illuminate areas of worrying, degree and duration of worrying, and its impact on the patient's functioning. It is important for the clinician to understand the patient's fears and explore his or her "catastrophic" predictions that are the basis for their anxiety or worrying. Finally, patients with anxiety may either avoid situations that produce anxiety (for example, a patient may avoid going out because he is concerned that he may have an anxiety attack) or focus extensively (obsess) on situations that trigger anxiety (for example, a patient is obsessively worried about his or her health).

Differentiating Obsessive Anxiety and Overvalued Ideas from Delusions

The clinician should assess whether the patient's obsessive concerns, anxiety, or overvalued ideas are reaching psychotic proportions. For example, a patient believes that she has cancer in the absence of any medical data to support her conviction. Questions that may help the clinician make the differential diagnosis include: (a) How convinced are you that you have cancer? (b) Do you feel relieved that the physicians have confirmed that there is no evidence of cancer? (c) Do you see any alternative explanation for your pain other than cancer? Nondelusional depressed patients usually recognize that their thoughts are exaggerated but they may not be able to reduce its effect [4]. In addition to astute questioning, the Delusional Assessment Scale for psychotic depression may help the clinician measure the intensity of delusional beliefs [32].

The Use of Formal Measures in the Assessment of Depression and Anxiety

Certain questionnaires may be helpful in identifying symptoms of depression and anxiety. These measures are not necessarily used to diagnose clinical depression but rather help the clinician identify symptoms of depression and assess their severity. Both clinician-administered and self-report measures may be administered. Clinician-administered rating scales include Hamilton Rating Scale for Depression, Montgomery-Asberg Depression Rating Scale [33]; both may be used for patients with mild cognitive impairment. Depression in patients with dementia may be evaluated with the Cornell Scale for Depression in Dementia [34], a measures which calculates a composite score based on reports from both the patients and their caregivers. Self-report questionnaires include the Beck Depression Inventory [35] and Geriatric Depression Scale [36]. Measures that may capture anxiety symptoms also include self-report (e.g., Beck Anxiety Inventory [37]) or clinician administered (e.g., Hamilton Scale for Anxiety [38]).

Involvement of Caregiver

The clinician should encourage the participation of an available and willing caregiver in the assessment process. The caregiver may be a spouse, partner, child, sibling, other family member, or an aide. If the patient does not think that the involvement of caregiver is necessary or helpful, the therapist may try to understand the reasons for the patient's reluctance (e.g., beliefs that this may be burdensome to the caregiver, tension between the patient and the caregiver, caregiver is not involved significantly in the patient's care, etc.). The clinician may explore whether these reasons may contribute to or affect patient's depression.

Caregiver participation in the assessment process may prove to be important and at times necessary. The caregiver may help in identifying periods of depression, illuminate the patient's behavior when he or she is depressed, and highlight patient's cognitive, physical, and functional limitations. This is particularly important in patients with cognitive impairment, as obtaining information from a collateral source is necessary when patients are not good historians, have advanced cognitive impairment or may lack insight into their difficulties.

Assessment of Disability

Depression may contribute to disability and disability may precipitate the onset of depression. Furthermore, recent research demonstrated that improving functioning and reducing disability mediated a reduction in depression [39]. Because of the reciprocal relationship of depression and disability, a careful assessment of patient's depression, disability, and everyday functioning is strongly recommended. Specifically, the clinician should evaluate the patient's physical and functional limitations and assess their performance in activities of daily living. Activities of daily living may be divided into instrumental activities of daily living (e.g., taking medication, walking a short distance, shopping for groceries, using the telephone, paying bills, doing housework and handyman work, doing laundry, preparing meals) or basic activities of daily living (e.g., bathing, eating, combing hair). The clinician may explore whether the patient was performing these activities before the onset of their depression, whether depression has affected the patient's performance in activities of daily living, or whether the patient *is able* to perform these activities with or without help. In addition to careful questioning, the clinician may administer instruments that evaluate a patient's functioning and disability such as the Philadelphia Multiphasic Assessment Instrument (MAI) [40], or the World Health Organization Disability Assessment Schedule II (WHODAS II) [41].

Clinical Pearls

- Clinical depression is different from the normal fluctuation of depressed mood in the severity of symptoms, their duration, and most importantly, the patient's impairment in his or her everyday functioning.
- Depressed older adults may exhibit lack of interest or pleasure and physical symptoms rather than depressed mood. This is one of the reasons late-life depression is underrecognized.
- The clinician should be aware that the patient may not report sadness or depression per se, but may report "discouragement," "lack of energy," "blue feeling," or "lack of motivation."
- Depressed elders may display "dementing" symptoms during their depression; sometimes, these symptoms subside when the depression remits. This phenomenon is called "pseudodementia" or "reversible dementia." Depression may also be a prodromal state of dementia.
- A thorough neuropsychological examination is recommended for depressed elders who present with cognitive difficulties.
- Treatment for complicated grief is recommended when the patient's functioning is significantly impaired.
- The clinician should thoroughly evaluate hopelessness given its strong correlation with suicide risk, past and present suicide ideation and attempts, and family history of suicide. Risky access to firearms or to other potential lethal means must be evaluated during the interview of a patient at risk of suicide.
- In the assessment of anxiety, the clinician has to evaluate the evidence for a realistic threat and the appropriateness and excessiveness of the patient's response to the perceived threat.

References

1. Katon W, Schulberg H. Epidemiology of depression in primary care. Gen Hosp Psychiatry. 1992;14(4): 237–47.
2. Bruce ML, McAvay GJ, Raue PJ, Brown EL, Meyers BS, Keohane DJ, Jagoda DR, Weber C. Major depression in elderly home health care patients. Am J Psychiatry. 2002;159(8):1367–74.
3. Katz IR. On the inseparability of mental and physical health in aged persons: lessons from depression and medical comorbidity. Am J Geriatr Psychiatry. 1996; 4:1–6.
4. Alexopoulos GS, Kelly Jr RE. Research advances in geriatric depression. World Psychiatry. 2009;8: 140–9.
5. Pampallona S, Bollini P, Tibaldi G, Kupelnick B, Munizza C. Patient adherence in the treatment of depression. Br J Psychiatry. 2002;180:104–9.
6. Conwell Y, Van Orden K, Caine E. Suicide in older adults. Psychiatr Clin North Am. 2011;34(2):451–68.
7. Rubenowitz E, Waern M, Wilhelmson K, Allebeck P. Life events and psychosocial factors in elderly suicides—a case-control study. Psychol Med. 2001;31(7): 1193–202.
8. Duberstein PR, Conwell Y, Conner KR, Eberly S, Caine ED. Suicide at 50 years of age and older: perceived physical illness, family discord and financial strain. Psychol Med. 2004;34(1):137–46.
9. Conwell Y, Duberstein PR, Hirsch JK, Conner KR, Eberly S, Caine ED. Health status and suicide in the second half of life. Int J Geriatr Psychiatry. 2009; 25(4):371–9.
10. Ayers CR, Sorrell JT, Thorp SR, Wetherell JL. Evidence-based psychological treatments for late-life anxiety. Psychol Aging. 2007;22:8–17.
11. Lenze EJ. Comorbidity of depression and anxiety in the elderly. Curr Psychiatry Rep. 2003;5:62–7.
12. Driscoll HC, Karp JF, Dew MA, et al. Getting better, getting well: understanding and managing partial and non-response to pharmacological treatment of non-psychotic major depression in old age. Drugs Aging. 2007;24:801–14.
13. Andreescu C, Lenze EJ, Dew MA, et al. Effect of comorbid anxiety on treatment response and relapse risk in late-life depression: controlled study. Br J Psychiatry. 2007;190:344–9.
14. Greenlee A, Karp JF, Dew MA, et al. Anxiety impairs depression remission in partial responders during extended treatment in late-life. Depress Anxiety. 2010;27:451–6.
15. Andreescu C, Lenze E, Mulsant B, et al. High worry severity is associated with poorer acute and maintenance efficacy of antidepressants in late-life depression. Depress Anxiety. 2009;26:266–72.
16. American Psychiatric Association. Diagnostic and statistical manual of mental disorders, fourth edition, text revision (DSM-IV-TR). Washington, DC: American Psychiatric Association; 2000.
17. Meyers BS, Klimstra SA, Gabriele M, Hamilton M, Kakuma T, Tirumalasetti F, Alexopoulos GS. Continuation treatment of delusional depression of older adults. Am J Geriatr Psychiatry. 2001;9:415–22.
18. Maj M, Pirozzi R, Magliano L, Fiorillo A, Bartoli L. Phenomenology and prognostic significance of delusions in major depressive disorder: a 10-year prospective follow-up study. J Clin Psychiatry. 2007;68(9): 1411–7.
19. Vythilingam M, Chen J, Bremner JD, Mazure CM, Maciejewski PK, Nelson JC. Psychotic depression and mortality. Am J Psychiatry. 2003;160(3):574–6.
20. Wilson KC, Chen R, Taylor S, McCracken CF, Copeland JR. Socio-economic deprivation and the prevalence and prediction of depression in older community residents. The MRC-ALPHA study. Br J Psychiatry. 1999;175:549–53.
21. Lockwood KA, Alexopoulos GS, Kakuma T, van Gorp WG. Subtypes of cognitive impairment in depressed older adults. Am J Geriatr Psychiatry. 2000;8:201–8.
22. Kindermann SS, Kalayam B, Brown GG, Burdick KE, Alexopoulos GS. Executive functions and P300 latency in elderly depressed patients and control subjects. Am J Geriatr Psychiatry. 2000;8:57–65.
23. Alexopoulos GS, Meyers BS, Young RC, Mattis S, Kakuma T. The course of geriatric depression with "reversible dementia": a controlled study. Am J Psychiatry. 1993;150:1693–9.
24. Olin JT, Katz IR, Meyers BS, Schneider LS, Lebowitz BD. Provisional diagnostic criteria for depression of Alzheimer disease: rationale and background. Am J Geriatr Psychiatry. 2002;10(2):129–41. Review. Erratum in: Am J Geriatr Psychiatry 2002 May-Jun;10(3):264.
25. Olin JT, Schneider LS, Katz IR, Meyers BS, Alexopoulos GS, Breitner JC, Bruce ML, Caine ED, Cummings JL, Devanand DP, Krishnan KR, Lyketsos CG, Lyness JM, Rabins PV, Reynolds 3rd CF, Rovner BW, Steffens DC, Tariot PN, Lebowitz BD. Provisional diagnostic criteria for depression of Alzheimer disease. Am J Geriatr Psychiatry. 2002;10(2):125–8.
26. Clark DA, Beck A. Cognitive therapy of anxiety disorders. New York: The Guilford Press; 2010.
27. Beekman AT, Bremmer MA, Deeg DH, Van Balkom AM, Snut JH, De Beurs E, et al. Anxiety disorders in later life: a report from the Longitudinal Aging Study Amsterdam. Int J Geriatr Psychiatry. 1998;13: 717–26.
28. Kessler RC, Berglund P, Demler O, Jin R, Merikangas KR, Walters EE. Lifetime prevalence and age-of-onset distributions of DSM-IV disorders in the National Comorbidity Survey Replication. Arch Gen Psychiatry. 2005;62:593–602.
29. Sajatovic M, Chen P. Geriatric bipolar disorder. Psychiatr Clin North Am. 2011;34(2):319–33.
30. Depp CA, Lindamer LA, Folsom DP, et al. Differences in clinical features and mental health service use in bipolar disorder across the lifespan. Am J Geriatr Psychiatry. 2005;13(4):290–8.

31. Sajatovic M, Blow FC, Ignacio RV, et al. New-onset bipolar disorder in later life. Am J Geriatr Psychiatry. 2005;13(4):282–9.
32. Meyers BS, English J, Gabriele M, Peasley-Miklus C, Heo M, Flint AJ, Mulsant BH, Rothschild AJ, STOP-PD Study Group. A delusion assessment scale for psychotic major depression: reliability, validity, and utility. Biol Psychiatry. 2006;60(12): 1336–42.
33. Montgomery SA, Asberg M. A new depression scale designed to be sensitive to change. Br J Psychiatry. 1979;134:382–9.
34. Alexopoulos GS, Abrams RC, Young RC, Shamoian CA. Cornell Scale for depression in dementia. Biol Psychiatry. 1988;23(3):271–84.
35. Beck AT, Steer RA, Brown GK. Manual for Beck Depression Inventory II (BDI-II). San Antonio, TX: Psychology Corporation; 1996.
36. Sheikh JI, Yesavage JA. Geriatric Depression Scale (GDS): recent evidence and development of a shorter version. In: Brink TL, editor. Clinical gerontology: a guide to assessment and intervention. New York: The Haworth Press; 1986. p. 165–73.
37. Beck AT, Steer RA. Beck anxiety inventory manual. San Antonio, TX: The Psychological Corporation Harcourt Brace & Company; 1993.
38. Hamilton M. The assessment of anxiety states by rating. Br J Med Psychol. 1959;32:50–5.
39. Alexopoulos GS, Raue PJ, Kiosses DN, Mackin RS, Kanellopoulos D, McCulloch C, Areán PA. Problem-solving therapy and supportive therapy in older adults with major depression and executive dysfunction: effect on disability. Arch Gen Psychiatry. 2011;68(1): 33–41.
40. Lawton MP, Moss M, Fulcomer M, Kleban MH. A research and service oriented multilevel assessment instrument. J Gerontol. 1982;37(1):91–9.
41. Ustun B. WHODAS-II disability assessment schedule. In: NIMH Mental Health Research Conference. 2000. Washington, DC.

Neuropsychological Assessment and Management of Older Adults with Multiple Somatic Symptoms

9

Greg J. Lamberty and Kimberly K. Bares

Abstract

Older adults frequently present with somatic concerns that need to be evaluated with a clear understanding of their history and context. While it is tempting to dismiss physical complaints as normal consequences of the aging process, such symptoms warrant the neuropsychologist's attention. This chapter reviews definitions, clinical presentations, assessment strategies, provision of feedback, consultation with colleagues, and treatment approaches that can be used with older adults. Rather than succumbing to therapeutic nihilism, neuropsychologists are encouraged to look into an increasingly broader range of intervention techniques that may benefit their older patients and assist their referral sources. Finally, a number of clinical "pearls" are offered to assist those in working with older patients that present with significant somatoform concerns.

Keywords

Neuropsychological assessment • Somatization • Somatoform symptoms • Intervention • Complementary and alternative medicine • Interview • Empirically supported treatment

Traditional Views of Somatoform Symptoms

Perhaps more than any group of individuals referred for neuropsychological assessment, older adults present with somatic concerns that need to be evaluated with a clear understanding of their history and context. Complaints about physical symptoms have traditionally been regarded as normal consequences of the aging process; one only needs to progress through the aging process to appreciate that basic fact. Symptoms such as pain, fatigue, sleep difficulty, and motor slowing are common and often related to generally lowered levels of activity, weight gain, and increased levels of neuropsychiatric symptoms. Certainly, such symptoms warrant

G.J. Lamberty, Ph.D. (✉) • K.K. Bares, Ph.D.
Minneapolis VA Health Care System,
Minneapolis, MN, USA
e-mail: gregory.lamberty@va.gov; kimberly.bares@va.gov

L.D. Ravdin and H.L. Katzen (eds.), *Handbook on the Neuropsychology of Aging and Dementia*, Clinical Handbooks in Neuropsychology, DOI 10.1007/978-1-4614-3106-0_9,

attention to rule out treatable medical conditions, but medical symptoms must be distinguished from the reporting of abnormally large numbers of pain, gastrointestinal, pseudoneurological, and sexual symptoms described in the criteria for somatization disorders [1]. While the diagnostic validity of the Diagnostic and Statistical Manual (DSM) criteria have been widely criticized [2], the clinical reality is that "normalcy" in older adults may well involve more complaints of pain and discomfort than that seen in younger adult samples [3,4].

There is great variability in the prevalence of the various DSM somatoform disorders, particularly somatization disorder, which prompted researchers to modify criteria for somatization disorder in a way that more accurately reflected the common and troubling presentations seen in many clinical settings. The reported prevalence of somatization disorder as described in the DSM-IV is very low (0.2–2%) [1], but rates of clinically significant somatoform symptomatology have been reported to be as high as 20–30% of all patients seen in some medical clinic settings [5–8]. Early epidemiologic studies on the DSM-based somatoform diagnoses did not typically examine differences in these presentations across the lifespan. Several reviews have failed to indicate greater prevalence of somatoform disorders with increasing age, though the association between somatoform symptoms and neuropsychiatric disorders (especially depression) is particularly high in older patients [9–11]. In other words, the presentation of multiple medically unexplained symptoms as a clinically relevant syndrome is not observed to be more common in older individuals, despite a general tendency to experience physical symptoms more commonly.

An important clinical challenge with older patients continues to be the ability to distinguish between symptoms that relate directly to physical disorders or disease processes and those that are related to what have become known in popular parlance as "mind–body" disorders [12]. With a greater overall tendency of older patients to report symptoms, this can be particularly challenging. Finally, the importance of understanding these dynamics is essential for working effectively with patients in the assessment context and subsequently making effective treatment recommendations [2].

This chapter will provide an overview of how somatic symptoms have been conceptualized in older adults and will provide guidance in making the important distinctions between "normal" presentations and those suggesting a somatic symptom disorder (the new term to be introduced in DSM-V). We will also discuss a range of treatment options for effectively managing patients with a high level of somatoform symptomatology, particularly considering the increased likelihood of cognitive dysfunction seen in aging populations in general.

Somatoform Disorders in DSM-V

Somatoform disorders were first introduced as an official diagnostic category in 1980 with the publication of the DSM-III [13]. Hysteria was the "neurotic" disorder that somatization replaced from the second DSM [14] and was based on the presumption that multiple physical symptoms were the product of underlying psychic conflicts. Rather than relying on underlying psychodynamic origins, the DSM-III focused on specific criteria that were thought to be descriptive of a distinct syndrome, as originally described in Briquet's famous monograph from the mid-nineteenth century [15]. This afforded many advantages for researchers of some disorders (e.g., schizophrenia, depression), while the lack of a proposed biological mechanism for somatization disorder relegated it to an apparently less compelling status where researchers were concerned. As noted above, it was clear that somatization disorder, as defined in DSM-III, was rare. Nevertheless, it was also the case that patients in many settings were presenting with medically unexplained symptoms that were problematic and resistant to treatment. As a result, more clinically relevant conceptualizations such as *abridged somatization* or *multisomatoform disorder* [16,17] evolved to account for the observation that patients with large numbers of medically unexplained symptoms comprised a substantial percentage of primary care and specialty clinic (e.g., neurology) visits. Over time, problems with the DSM-IV classification scheme for somatoform disorders have been identified, and calls for change have issued forth [18–21]. The reasons for these calls are numerous and include concerns about the "… dualistic nature of the diagnoses, problems with patients' acceptance of the diagnoses, lack of ability to exclude physical causes of some symptoms, restrictiveness of the diagnostic criteria, and general problems with reliability and validity…" ([2]; p. 14).

In DSM-V, Somatoform Disorders will be renamed Somatic Symptom Disorders, a change which is described on the American Psychiatric Association's DSM-V Development web site. The basic rationale for the change is described below:

> Because the current terminology for somatoform disorders is confusing and because somatoform disorders, psychological factors affecting medical condition, and factitious disorders all involve presentation of physical symptoms and/or concern about medical illness, the work group suggests renaming this group of disorders somatic symptom disorders. In addition, because of the implicit mind–body dualism and the unreliability of assessments of "medically unexplained symptoms," these symptoms are no longer emphasized as core features of many of these disorders. Since somatization disorder, hypochondriasis, undifferentiated somatoform disorder, and pain disorder share certain common features, namely, somatic symptoms and cognitive distortions, the work group is proposing that these disorders be grouped under a common rubric called complex somatic symptom disorder.
>
> (http://www.dsm5.org/ProposedRevisions/Pages/SomatoformDisorders.aspx. Downloaded on February 28, 2011) [22].

Complex somatic symptom disorder (CSSD) is proposed as a diagnosis that subsumes several DSM-IV diagnoses including somatization disorder, undifferentiated somatoform disorder, hypochondriasis, pain disorder associated with both psychological factors and a general medical condition, and pain disorder associated with psychological factors. Like the modified versions of somatization disorder that emerged after publication of DSM-III, CSSD requires one or more somatic symptoms that cause significant disruption or distress (Criterion A) as well as excessive thoughts, feelings, and behaviors that relate to the symptoms (Criterion B). Finally, the condition must be chronic (>6 months; Criterion C). These criteria are much less exclusive than those for somatization disorder, but the essential nature of a chronic and disabling condition related to an individual's concerns or preoccupation with physical symptoms seems to capture the essence of the presentations so frequently seen clinically.

Simple somatic symptom disorder (SSSD) is, as the name suggests, a more basic version of CSSD that requires only 1 month symptom duration and only one Criterion B symptom (i.e., thoughts, feelings, or behaviors associated with the symptom). In circumstances when a clinical problem is less severe or more acute, SSSD might be more appropriate and representative of a different presentation. A common example might involve such difficulties following a hospitalization or surgical procedure.

Generally speaking, the DSM-V conceptualization of somatic symptom disorders represents an effort to make the category and diagnoses more relevant and clinically useful. The proposed changes reflect a more pragmatic approach to mind–body problems. Rather than forcing dualistic distinctions, the SSD category represents a clinical reality in which patients often struggle to deal with pain, neuropsychiatric symptoms, and behavior patterns that interfere with more optimal functioning. How this applies to work with older patients is considered below.

Difficulties in Characterizing the Physical Complaints of Older Patients

Neuropsychologists who are less familiar with issues confronting older adults may be inclined to over- or underestimate the role of somatic symptoms in a given patient's health status. There are a number of ways to assure that information about a patient is objective, though care must be taken in all phases to make proper determinations.

In instances where records are available for review, the neuropsychologist should be able to obtain a reasonably objective sense of difficulties confronting the patient. This often presupposes that the referral source has expertise with older patients, which may or may not be the case. The number of physicians specializing in geriatrics is very small, and the offset between the number of specialists and the number of patients over the age of 65 is likely to increase in dramatic fashion over the next two decades (http://www.americangeriatrics.org/files/documents/Adv_Resouces/PayReform_fact5.pdf.) [23]. This means that older patients will probably be referred by an expanding and diverse base of practitioners, many of whom may have an incomplete sense of issues confronting the elderly. The appropriateness of dementia referrals can vary widely because of this variability in practitioners' expertise. Practically speaking, this means that record review, no matter how extensive, cannot replace the clinical interview and observation for an appreciation of an individual's appearance and behavior and how this squares with his self-report.

A thorough clinical interview is an essential part of the assessment process as well as an important source of information about somatic concerns. Many popular neuropsychology texts also discuss the importance of behavioral observations within the interview process and how they ultimately inform the conclusions and recommendations made in neuropsychological reports [24–26]. Careful observation of the older patient will afford insights into factors such as gait, mobility, pain behaviors, affect, orientation, and speed of processing. It is important to note differences between the patient's self-report of symptoms and whether such things are apparent in his behavioral presentation. Lamberty [2] noted two general patterns of behavior in somatizing patients—stoic and expressive. The outward appearance in these examples is strikingly different, despite the fact that the overall level of self-reported symptomatology in both kinds of presentations can be similar.

Many older adults employ a generalized normalizing strategy wherein they present themselves as "no worse off" than any of their colleagues or others their age. There is a certain charm and sensibility to this approach, though obviously the astute neuropsychologist should not be lulled into assumptions of normalcy simply because a patient takes a stoic approach to reporting his symptoms. Older patients who affect a more stoic presentation are often characterized by a different dynamic than the younger somatizing patient. With the older patient, medical history and general psychological adjustment is important to assess to look beyond stereotypes of "not wanting to be a burden." Some of these claims are fairly transparent, and within a brief period of time it becomes clear that either (1) the patient has multiple medical issues that account for his symptoms or (2) emotional or psychological distress is exerting some influence on the patient's experience and reporting of symptoms. It is also important to get a sense of the natural history of current symptoms, as well as a general history of health and medical problems over the years. The likelihood of a complex somatic symptom disorder is obviously much higher in an individual with a long history of engagement with the medical field.

Interviews with collateral sources are valuable, particularly in cases where cognitive difficulties might interfere with a patient's ability to provide a thorough and descriptive history. When patients minimize their symptoms, family members can provide a clearer sense of what kinds of problems are apparent to them. The same can be true in instances when the older patient is focused on physical complaints. Of course, the neuropsychologist must be mindful of the various roles played by friends and family members and how that might impact their reporting of what they observe in the patient or know about their history. As always, the forensic implications of an evaluation need to be considered in cases where guardianship or estate matters loom.

The cautions offered regarding the report of somatic symptoms are basically the same for complaints about cognitive difficulties. Recent work has drawn comparisons between somatoform syndromes and similar presentations that focus primarily on reports of cognitive dysfunction.

Cognitively oriented analogs of somatic symptom disorders have been suggested and have evocative names like "cogniform disorder" [27] and "neurocognitive hypochondriasis" [28], though these presentations are basically two sides of the same coin. Neuropsychologists encounter many patients that present with such a focus. Just as with physical concerns, it is important to appreciate age-related cognitive difficulties in older patients. Accounting for age-related cognitive complaints is a regular part of the assessment process for neuropsychologists, so the risk of misattributing cognitive difficulties should be lower than it is when attempting to determine the nature of physical complaints. In other words, neuropsychologists are better equipped to empirically assess cognitive difficulties than they are somatic concerns.

Understanding the Role of Physical Discomfort in the Examination Process

Older patients often find the neuropsychological evaluation process overwhelming and intimidating. The prospect of having one's cognitive functioning assessed can awaken fears about whether or not there are major deficits, degenerative changes in the brain, or impending major changes in the ability to live independently. In this context, aches and pains that complicate everyday life can become magnified and serve as significant obstacles to the successful completion of a neuropsychological examination. Older patients frequently present with limited mobility, arthritic pain, fatigue, and visual and hearing limitations secondary to a range of age-related changes. Most neuropsychologists are prepared for these basic obstacles and can alter the examination processes accordingly. Common adaptations include tables that accommodate wheelchairs, enlarged type protocols, magnifiers, sound amplifiers, allowing for extra time and breaks, and generally shortened testing protocols. Beyond these basic physical adaptations, neuropsychologists and psychometrists need to be prepared to work with the anxiety, reticence, and outright refusal to cooperate. As an exam wears on and failure experiences mount, there is increased likelihood that performance will decline and become less representative of actual abilities. The spectrum of how this presents is broad and includes decreased attentional focus and carelessness on one end, all the way to rejection of tasks and refusal to continue on the other. The parallels with pediatric assessment in this regard are substantial and can sometimes be navigated by a skilled evaluator. Regardless, it is difficult to know with certainty the impact that waning attention or investment in performance may have on the patient's overall performance. As with the clinical interview, careful observation of behaviors during testing is also important in interpreting performances that may be atypical for reasons that do not involve cognitive difficulties alone. Behaviors such as frequent sighing, moaning, pain behaviors, crying, and agitation are obviously notable and possibly suggestive of challenges to the validity of an assessment, no matter what they are motivated by.

The ability to thoroughly assess personality and psychopathology in a typical neuropsychological evaluation for the older adult is often perceived to be limited. Asking patients to complete lengthy personality inventories such as the MMPI-2 [29] after 2–3 h of testing is typically thought to place an unrealistic burden on a patient who might be experiencing difficulties with motor control, fatigue, and emotional exhaustion. Instead, more focused symptom measures such as the Beck Depression Inventory-II [30] or the Geriatric Depression Scale [31] are often employed to get a sense of whether there is notable neuropsychiatric symptomatology or, even more basically, distress. Scales specifically developed for use with older adults have typically limited the amount of somatic symptomatology assessed, presumably to avoid over diagnosing disorders such as depression that have a significant somatic component [31]. Nevertheless, to the extent that good measures of somatoform symptomatology are thought to be important in the diagnostic differential, consideration should be given to lengthier measures, such as the MMPI-2. Lamberty [2] noted that few instruments allow the extensive assessment of somatoform features that the MMPI-2 and its various subscales do. Specifically, elevations on scales 1 and 3 are prototypical indicators of a high level of somatoform symptomatology, as is an elevation on scale RC1 (somatic complaints) from the MMPI-2-RF [32]. In addition, the commonly used FBS validity scale [33] is often significantly elevated in individuals whose primary issues involve reporting of physical discomfort or concerns about cognitive difficulties. The use of more extensively validated measures allows clinicians a greater level of certainty with regard to the effects of such symptoms on general cognitive performance as a function of the literature examining these relationships.

Finally, many neuropsychologists struggle with the prospects of providing feedback to patients in cases where the results will be, frankly, difficult to hear. In some ways, talking about somatoform symptoms with older patients is facilitated by the reality that many are legitimately fearful of the prospects of having a dementing disorder. This sets up one of a few reasonable "good news/bad news" scenarios confronted by neuropsychologists. In the event that an older patient's difficulties upon testing are thought to be due to variable effort, or that they are actually performing within normative expectations, there should be some solace in knowing that their cognitive functioning is actually reasonably sound and not a great cause for concern. This also provides a good basis for a discussion about the issue of mind–body problems. Most patients are receptive to respectful feedback about how anxiety, stress, and depression symptoms can impact cognitive efficiency. Intellectually, most anyone can understand that "unseen" factors can influence cognitive or mental functioning and that there are many different ways that these problems might be treated. Again, older patients are often receptive to approaches that do not involve additional medications or surgical procedures. The remainder of this chapter focuses on a range of treatment options that are thought to represent some of the better options for working with older adults struggling with mind–body symptoms and issues.

Treatment Approaches with Older Adults

As theoretical conceptualizations and diagnostic criteria for somatoform disorders have evolved over time, so too have clinical treatment approaches expanded to better address the complex psychiatric and medical needs of patients with these conditions. Historically, treatment interventions consisted of intensive psychotherapy aimed at developing insight into psychic trauma thought to underlie the expression of psychological pain as physical symptoms. In such discovery, it was believed that patients would find relief from and resolution of their somatic ailments due to increased self-awareness and willingness to confront psychological issues more directly. These strategies were met with limited success, leading to a broadly held belief that individuals with somatoform conditions are, nearly by definition, incapable of insight and unlikely to benefit from psychological interventions. Somatizing patients became viewed as inconvenient and bothersome at best, or exasperating and draining of time and costly services at worst [34]. More recently, approaches in the field of health psychology have begun to bridge the mind/body gap between medical illness and psychological functioning. Additionally, much focus has been directed at reducing national health-care costs and finding empirically supported, cost-effective treatments for consumers of medical care. These factors have resulted in renewed interest in providing appropriate treatment interventions for individuals with somatoform conditions who are often heavy consumers of health-care services. Goals of treatment have appropriately shifted from symptom elimination and insight to symptom management, improving quality of life and daily functioning, and decreasing service utilization.

In this section, we will highlight important treatment considerations in providing care to older adults with somatoform disorders. Empirically supported treatment approaches will be reviewed, and suggestions will be made for other psychotherapeutic strategies that may hold promise in working with these patients more effectively. Challenges specific to treating older somatizing patients are presented, with an eye toward how those obstacles might be overcome. Finally, practical recommendations are made regarding the important consultative role neuropsychologists can play in helping medical colleagues work more effectively with these patients.

Treatment Considerations

It is helpful to acknowledge the many challenges involved in engaging somatizing patients in nonmedical treatments. Ironically, the first stumbling block may be a medical provider's hesitation to make a referral or a mental health clinician's hesitation to accept one. As noted above, there is a broad skepticism about the capacity of somatizing patients to benefit from therapy. This may stem from clinical training that stresses the importance of capacity for insight and a willingness to consider one's role in the development and maintenance of problems. Because the presence of somatoform conditions typically presumes a lack of conscious awareness of symptom production, with little or no insight into the condition, providers may conclude that there is little use in pursuing psychological treatment for these individuals. However, it may be helpful to keep in mind that there are many other patient groups where insight, in and of itself, is neither a prerequisite nor a goal of therapy. For example, patients with traumatic brain injuries with clearly decreased insight may still be beneficially referred for psychosocial intervention strategies. Likewise, individuals with deeply entrenched delusional belief systems are sometimes able to benefit from therapeutic strategies to decrease and manage their distress more effectively and increase quality of life.

We should also acknowledge that patients with medically unexplained symptoms are particularly challenging for health-care providers to work with. Countertransference reactions such as dislike, anger, and exasperation may cause medical providers to limit/discontinue contact with these patients and can interfere with thoughtful consideration of mental health referrals. Therapists may be unwilling to accept patient referrals and may discontinue interventions prematurely when patients are not cooperative or are otherwise aversive in session. Thus, providers (both referral sources and mental health clinicians) will benefit from acknowledging and attending to countertransference reactions. These reactions often mirror a patient's emotional state and can inform clinicians of the frustration, anger, and hostility that the patients feel in not getting the medical attention and relief they are seeking. Additionally, case consultation with peers and treatment teams can be used to get support and generate ideas about how to proceed in helpful ways.

Even when providers are open to referring for mental health services, many patients will vehemently protest such a referral, as they are symptom-driven and seeking medical solutions. By this logic, they assume that mental health providers who do not prescribe medications or order medical tests could not possibly help with their medical problems. If patients do follow through with a mental health referral, they may present with a clear goal of convincing clinicians of the legitimacy of their physical symptoms, with much focus on the failures of the medical system to properly diagnose and treat them. They may be keenly attuned to any language that implies that their symptoms are "all in their heads."

So, how do medical and mental health providers bridge this gap? Drawn from the field of addictions, motivational interviewing (MI) holds promise for facilitating readiness for therapeutic intervention and meaningful lifestyle change. First described in 1983, MI is a simple yet elegant counseling stance that meets patients where they are in their understanding of problems and readiness to explore options for improving their lives. The approach involves clinician-guided collaborative conversations during which patients' personal goals, values, and reasons for wanting things to be different are elicited. MI is increasingly used by primary care providers and has shown to be effective in preparing patients to commit to behavior change not only in alcohol and drug abuse but also in individuals with chronic illnesses such as heart disease, obesity, and even psychosis [35].

With a somatizing patient, a provider using MI would inquire about how somatic conditions impact an individual's life and how things would be different if physical concerns were less prominent. Frequent validation and reflection of concerns conveys understanding and acceptance. Clinicians listen actively and probe for "change talk," (e.g., comments from patients suggesting a wish to resume former activities). Patients are encouraged to explicitly state what they would like to be different in their lives, and what that suggests about their personal values and future goals. Ambivalence is common and validated genuinely. Any inquiries from patients about *how* change is possible are used as opportunities to discuss treatment options. Typically, over the course of 2–3 guided conversations in which clinicians actively listen, elicit personal values, explore ambivalence, and highlight change talk, patients may begin to feel more empowered to improve their quality of life, even if pain or other somatic concerns persist.

When providers and patients are committed to explore treatments for somatic conditions, there are a number of empirically supported and potentially promising treatment interventions that may be of benefit. We describe several below.

Cognitive–Behavioral Therapies

Cognitive–behavioral therapy (CBT) is perhaps the most studied psychotherapeutic intervention with demonstrated effectiveness for somatoform conditions. These approaches are based on the notion that irrational thoughts and perceptions strongly influence mood states and behavior, resulting in the development and maintenance of depression, anxiety, and other psychosocial problems [36]. As such, CBT interventions help patients to examine and change unhelpful cognitions, thereby influencing mood and behavior in a positive manner. In a recent review of randomized controlled treatments for patients with various somatic conditions (e.g., somatization disorder, medically unexplained symptoms, and others), 34 published studies involving 3,922 patients were examined [37] with CBT (group or individual therapy) as the primary intervention in 13 of those studies. Positive outcomes were noted in 85% of the studies (11 of 13), as defined by treatment groups faring better on at least one outcome measure relative to controls. Similar conclusions were drawn by Sumathipala [38] who examined six previous review articles spanning hundreds of patients treated with CBT for somatoform disorders. In general, significant beneficial effects were noted both for individual and group CBT in reducing physical complaints and mood disturbances while improving quality of life. CBT was also noted to be more efficacious than antidepressant treatments. Caution was raised, however, about the lack of data on long-term outcome in the majority of studies reviewed. Unfortunately, neither of these recent comprehensive reviews included meta-analytic procedures or specifically examined age cohort differences in response to CBT, illustrating the need for future studies in this regard.

Clinically, we have observed that older patients require some modifications to CBT due to age-related changes in their capacity to process and remember written material and to think flexibly when challenged to reframe their cognitions. This can usually be minimized by meeting with patients more frequently, slowing the pace of sessions, explaining concepts in more basic terms, and repeating/reviewing new information. One must also exercise caution to not invalidate patient's beliefs as "irrational," which quickly undermines trust and triggers defensive reactions. This can usually be addressed by resuming an empathic, reflective stance, and perhaps shifting the focus from changing cognitions to changing behaviors that stand in the way of their preferred lifestyles.

Physical and Complementary/Alternative Interventions

Patients with somatoform symptoms are generally disinclined to seek assistance in mental health settings [2]. Rather, they are more likely to see themselves as seeking relief from physical symptoms, suggesting greater receptiveness to physically oriented rather than psychologically oriented interventions. As such, treatment recommendations for approaches such as mindfulness-based stress reduction, yoga, and other exercise practices may be more beneficial for some patients. Contemporary mindfulness-based interventions developed out of traditional Far Eastern medicine practices that have acknowledged for centuries that the mind and body are intimately related. Mindfulness-based strategies involve focused attention to bring body and mind perceptions into greater awareness while assuming a nonjudgmental, observer stance. In doing so, individuals may be able to move toward greater acceptance of negative feelings (both physical and emotional) that detract from contentment and appreciation of the present moment [39]. An increasing body of literature is available to support the benefits of mindfulness-based approaches in managing a wide variety of medical ailments including chronic pain, cancer, fibromyalgia, migraine headache, and morbid obesity [40–42]. Success with these patient groups suggests the promise of similar benefit for somatoform patients. Strategies of mindfulness may include mindful breathing, body scan, mindful sitting, standing, and walking, and mindful listening to sounds and thoughts [39]. These techniques are particularly adaptable for older patients who may have decreased mobility and pain tolerance that interferes with more active physical interventions such as physical therapy and exercise.

In a randomized clinical trial conducted in Germany, an intervention termed "functional relaxation" was evaluated for its ability to reduce somatic complaints and emotional distress in patients with recurrent nonspecific chest pain [43]. The authors noted that although chest pain is a frequent complaint to cardiologists, no evidence of structural or other cardiac abnormality is found in 50% of cases after extensive and costly evaluation, and three-quarters of those individuals seek further medical attention. Functional relaxation used in this study involved guiding patients through a series of small muscle movements while exhaling. Patients were then asked to "trace" or observe changes in body awareness (e.g., move ankle, notice sensation in foot). The authors characterized this intervention as both behavioral and psychodynamic in its goal to re-experience and integrate bodily self-awareness. However, its description suggests reasonable membership among a group of mindfulness-based approaches. Results showed that patients in the functional relaxation intervention ($n=11$) reported significant declines on the Symptom Checklist-90 (SCL-90, [44]) Somatization, Anxiety, and Global Severity Index scales and on a cardiovascular complaints scale compared with those in the medical care-as-usual group ($n=11$), who showed no significant changes. Results suggested efficacy of this somatically oriented mindfulness technique in reducing body complaints and psychological distress. Again, the study was not specifically targeted to older adults and requires replication in larger samples, but may show promise for our older patients with frequent chest pain complaints.

Yoga comprises a number of mind/body practices including physical postures, controlled breathing, meditation, and relaxation. With regular practice, yoga is thought to improve the functional balance of various organ systems and to relieve muscular and nervous tension, leading to improved general health and sense of well-being [45]. In a recent review article on yoga and mindfulness, Salmon et al. [46] pointed out positive outcomes (reduced symptoms, improved quality of life, or emotional well-being) in randomized trials of yoga with several patient groups including diabetes, chronic back pain, irritable bowel syndrome, fibromyalgia, chronic pancreatitis, lymphoma, and in healthy older adults. Because several of the yoga postures, or *asanas*, involve kneeling, stretching, and twisting, older patients may require modifications to accommodate their physical capabilities and pain tolerance. Fortunately, yoga is easily adapted and, in fact, encourages a stance of "start where you are," allowing participants to accept their current mind/body state and to work patiently within their present limitations.

Older adults may also find benefit in regular physical exercise or perhaps the social support afforded by attending exercise classes. Peters et al. [47] conducted a randomized controlled study of aerobic exercise in a large sample ($n=228$) of patients ranging from 9 to 73 years with persistent medically unexplained symptoms. All participants were scheduled to attend 20 1-h sessions of either aerobic exercise or stretching, the control condition. Measures of health-care use and symptoms, emotional state, and perceived disability were completed before, during, and 6 months after training. Results showed that primary care consultations and prescriptions were significantly reduced in the 6 months following training for both groups, with no particular benefit of aerobic training over the stretching control group. The extent of reduction in medical care was dependent on the number of sessions attended. The authors suggested that these positive outcomes may have been resulted from group support from fellow sufferers and counseling by physiotherapists, resulting in reduced reliance on general practitioners and medications for symptom management.

Psychotropic Medications

Systematic reviews and meta-analytic studies provide good support for beneficial effects of antidepressant medications in the treatment of somatoform disorders. While no meta-analysis has been done that examines treatment benefit specifically for older patients, many samples in the available meta-analyses include older adults with medically unexplained illnesses and chronic pain issues. In one meta-analysis of 94 placebo-controlled studies, patients taking antidepressants showed more than three times greater improvement in medically unexplained symptoms compared to placebo controls [48]. Benefits were seen both for tricyclic antidepressants (76% of studies with positive outcomes) and selective serotonin reuptake inhibitors (SSRIs; 47% of studies with positive outcomes), though there were an insufficient number of studies with SSRIs in this meta-analysis to conclude that tricyclics were of greater benefit than SSRIs. In a smaller meta-analysis of 11 randomized controlled studies using antidepressants to treat somatoform pain disorder and psychogenic pain, patients treated with antidepressants showed significantly decreased pain intensity with a moderate effect size relative to patients treated with placebo [49]. Onghena and Van Houdenhove [50] also noted moderate to large effect sizes for treatment of chronic pain patients with antidepressants in a meta-analysis of 39 studies. It also has been shown that antidepressants that act on both serotonergic and noradrenergic receptors (tricyclics and SNRIs) may have more analgesic effects than other antidepressants [51].

While the impact of medication treatment with older somatizing patients has not been extensively studied, psychiatric consultation with a geriatric psychiatrist is recommended, especially when patients have multiple health conditions and medications that can complicate medication management. Typically, a “start low and go slow” dosing approach is taken, as older patients may experience (or anticipate) side effects which prompt them to quickly discontinue psychotropic medications before any benefit can be appreciated. Again, many older somatizing patients will resist a referral to psychiatry, both because of a preference for medical solutions and their greater generational perceived stigma of being seen by a mental health provider. This may be lessened by assurances that they are not being abandoned by their medical providers and will continue to be seen for follow-up care and renewals of psychotropics. A similar approach was found efficacious by Hoedeman et al. [52] who showed improved health outcomes in somatizing patients whose psychiatrists sent a consultation letter to the patient’s primary care providers about diagnosis and treatment options to be incorporated into their medical treatment plans. In an older study, Smith et al. [53] used a crossover randomized controlled design to evaluate the efficacy of psychiatric consultation in reducing medical costs of somatizing patients. After psychiatrists consulted with the patients’ primary care providers, quarterly health-care charges declined by 53% in the treatment group and were significantly lower than controls. After the control group crossed over, their quarterly medical charges declined by 49%. They concluded good benefit from psychiatric consultation to physicians in reducing costs, without affecting health status or patient satisfaction with health care.

Family Psychoeducation and Therapy

Clinicians often hear from exasperated spouses and family members of older somatizing patients, imploring clinicians to "do something" to relieve the patients' suffering or worries and, in turn, lessen caregiver burden. To date, no studies are available that speak to the efficacy of family interventions in working with patients with somatoform conditions. However, our clinical experience has suggested that couple/family interventions are sometimes just as or more effective in reducing somatic complaints, and quality of life than are individual interventions. Family counseling offers the opportunity for concerns to be aired and validated, reassurances to be provided, and coping strategies to be explored. Behavioral approaches such as pleasant-event scheduling (e.g., weekly brunch) can reduce loneliness and boredom and increase opportunities for physical activity, while distracting patients from physical discomfort and worries. Family members can be encouraged to reinforce positive healthy behaviors, while reducing inadvertent reinforcement of somatic complaints. Narrative therapy approaches such as those developed by White and Epston [54] invite participants to develop a richer narrative, or story, about an individual's life and capabilities, while naming and externalizing the problem (e.g., "the fibromyalgia") as separate from the person. Narrative therapy stresses that "the person is not the problem; the problem is the problem." Patients and family members are interviewed to focus on "exceptions" to the problem (e.g., "when did you not allow the fibromyalgia to get in your way this week?"). They are also encouraged to team up against the problem rather than each other and to develop ways to limit the problem's influence in their lives. By developing these broader narratives, patients often begin to view themselves as more than a sick person, with greater self-efficacy and hope to be able to live more contentedly. Family members, by extension, may also experience decreased caregiving stress and have renewed energy to continue to support their loved ones in helpful ways.

Primary Care Interventions

Neuropsychologists are uniquely suited to objectively assess brain dysfunction as well as psychological conditions that may influence cognitive performance and daily functioning. In providing feedback to referral sources, we also have the opportunity to serve an important consultative role regarding how to work more effectively with an older somatically focused patient. Some practical recommendations include the following:

- Determine a single "go-to" provider (e.g., PCP, nurse practitioner) with whom the patient can establish a collaborative alliance. This helps to reduce overlapping providers and opportunities for "splitting," or pitting of one provider against another regarding treatment approaches.
- Plan regularly scheduled appointments to reduce emergency calls or visits.
- Explicitly state that the goal of medical contacts is functional restoration and maintenance of health and well-being, not to find a cure for conditions or to eliminate all somatic worries.
- Proactively ask about new symptoms and current life stressors at each visit, making a point to acknowledge and validate distress, while providing reassurance that grave conditions have been ruled out.
- Limit medical testing and referrals to specialists that patients may seek for reassurance, but are not medically indicated.
- Avoid opiates, anticholinergic medications, and polypharmacy whenever possible, to reduce potential clouding of cognition.

- Initiate brief conversations about the mind–body connection, how chronic physical conditions often take a toll on mood, sleep, and quality of life.
- Monitor for depression, anxiety, and substance abuse issues, and seek psychiatric consultation/referral when indicated.
- Characterize referrals for mental health services as one of many available tools in medicine to address their complex needs. Reassure patients that they will continue to be followed for regular medical care.

Summary

Many clinical challenges exist for neuropsychologists and others providing services to older patients with somatoform symptoms. In this chapter, we have highlighted traditional and emerging schemes for describing somatic symptom disorders, as well as the difficulties inherent in identifying these problems in patients whose baseline often involves physical symptomatology related to normal aging. Physical concerns can impact the assessment process, and it is important to have strategies for dealing with behaviors and complaints that can limit the ability to conduct a complete assessment. In an era that emphasizes empirically supported treatments, it is important to consider treatments that have been proven effective, even if the evidence base with more specific groups of patients have not yet been extensively studied. Promising treatments that involve mindfulness-based approaches appear particularly well suited for somatizing patients given their emphasis on acceptance and increased awareness. Further, many complementary and alternative approaches appeal to somatizing patients because of a seeming lack of focus on psychological and emotional material. Neuropsychologists are in a unique position to evaluate, consult with, and recommend effective interventions for their older patients. Careful attention to the patient's needs and a collaborative approach can improve outcomes in these challenging patients, and this should be the goal of all neuropsychologists working with older adults.

Clinical Pearls

- Always attempt to obtain thorough clinical records regarding the patient's health concerns. Be mindful of whether or not the records come from experienced geriatric clinicians.
- Carefully observe patient behaviors that suggest difficulties with pain, mobility, affect, and general cognition. Attend to the context in which these behaviors are emitted.
- Consider information from family members and other collateral sources judiciously, but be aware of the relationship with the informant and the clinical context and how that might impact the nature of the report.
- Understand that over- and underestimating the impact of somatic symptoms results from not adhering to the first three suggestions.
- Be prepared for older patients to struggle with completing the neuropsychological evaluation process secondary to a range of physical, perceptual, and emotional challenges.
- Do not underestimate the importance of standardized assessment of somatic and emotional symptoms, even if older patients have limited stamina.
- Take advantage of the opportunity to reinforce an understanding of the complexity of mind–body relationships, while sharing encouraging news about a lack of cognitive findings in a positive way.
- Familiarize yourself with empirically supported treatments like MI and CBT, but understand that they can sometimes be impacted by cognitive limitations in older patients.
- Be aware of and open to complementary and alternative approaches like mindfulness meditation and yoga that can be preferable to psychologically oriented therapies for somatizing patients.
- Work closely with family members to reinforce a better understanding of the interrelatedness of stressors, somatic symptoms, and the range of treatments that can be used to lessen the impact of these symptoms.
- Work collaboratively with older patients' primary care providers to maximize the benefit

of your consultation, minimize the overuse of medications, improve therapeutic recommendations, and improve patients' and families' overall adjustment and quality of life.

References

1. American Psychiatric Association. Diagnostic & statistical manual of mental disorders, 4th edition, text revision. Washington, DC: American Psychiatric Association; 2000.
2. Lamberty GJ. Understanding somatization in the practice of clinical neuropsychology. New York: Oxford University Press; 2008.
3. McCarthy LH, Bigal ME, Katz M, Derby C, Lipton RB. Chronic pain and obesity in the elderly: results from the Einstein aging study. J Am Geriatr Soc. 2009;57:115–9.
4. Helme RD, Gibson SJ. The epidemiology of pain in elderly people. Clin Geriatr Med. 2001;17:417–31.
5. Barsky AJ, Orav EJ, Bates DW. Somatization increases medical utilization and costs independent of psychiatric and medical comorbidity. Arch Gen Psychiatry. 2005;62:903–10.
6. Carson AJ, Ringbauer B, Stone J, McKenzie L, Warlow C, Sharpe M. Do medically unexplained symptoms matter? A prospective cohort study of 300 new referrals to neurology outpatient clinics. J Neurol Neurosurg Psychiatry. 2000;68:207–10.
7. Escobar JI, Waitzkin H, Silver RC, Gara M, Holman A. Abridged somatization: a study in primary care. Psychosom Med. 1998;60:466–72.
8. Fink P, Hansen MS, Sondergaard L. Somatoform disorders among first-time referrals to a neurology service. Psychosomatics. 2005;46:540–8.
9. Drayer RA, Mulsant BH, Lenze EJ, Rollman BL, Dew MA, Kelleher K, Karp JF, Begley A, Schulberg HC, Reynolds CFIII. Somatic symptoms of depression in elderly patients with medical comorbidities. Int J Geriatr Psychiatry. 2005;20:973–82.
10. Lobo-Escolar A, Saz P, Marcos G, Quintanilla MÁ, Campayo A, Lobo A, ZARADEMP Workgroup. Somatic and psychiatric comorbidity in the general elderly population: results from the ZARADEMP project. J Psychosom Res. 2008;65:347–55.
11. Sheehan B, Banjeree S. Review: somatization in the elderly. Int J Geriatr Psychiatry. 1999;14:1044–9.
12. Sarno JE. The divided mind: the epidemic of mindbody disorders. New York: Harper; 2006.
13. American Psychiatric Association. Diagnostic and statistical manual of mental disorders. 3rd ed. Washington, DC: Author; 1980.
14. American Psychiatric Association. Diagnostic and statistical manual of mental disorders. 2nd ed. Washington, DC: Author; 1968.
15. Briquet P. Traite´ clinique et the´rapeutique de l'Hysterie. Paris: Bailliere; 1859.
16. Escobar JI, Burnam MA, Karno M, Forsythe A, Golding JM. Somatization in the community. Arch Gen Psychiatry. 1987;44:713–8.
17. Kroenke K, Spitzer RL, deGruy III FV, Hahn SR, Linzer M, Williams JB, et al. Multisomatoform disorder. An alternative to undifferentiated somatoform disorder for the somatizing patient in primary care. Arch Gen Psychiatry. 1997;54:352–8.
18. Engel CC. Explanatory and pragmatic perspectives regarding idiopathic physical symptoms and related syndromes. CNS Spectr. 2006;11:225–32.
19. Kirmayer LJ, Groleau D, Looper KJ, Dao MD. Explaining medically unexplained symptoms. Can J Psychiatry. 2004;49:663–72.
20. Mayou R, Kirmayer LJ, Simon G, Kroenke K, Sharpe M. Somatoform disorders: time for a new approach in DSM-V. Am J Psychiatry. 2005;162:847–55.
21. Sharpe M, Carson A. "Unexplained" somatic symptoms, functional syndromes, and somatization: do we need a paradigm shift? Ann Intern Med. 2001;134:926–30.
22. American Psychiatric Association. DSM-5 development. Somatoform disorders. 2012. http://www.dsm5.org/ProposedRevisions/Pages/SomatoformDisorders.aspx. 28 Feb 2011.
23. The Demand for Geriatric Care and the evident Shortage of Geriatrics Healthcare Providers. The American Geriatric Society, 2012. http://www.americangeriatrics.org/files/documents/Adv_Resouces/PayReform_fact5.pdf.
24. Axelrod BN. Neuropsychological report writing. In: Vanderploeg RD, editor. Clinician's guide to neuropsychological assessment. 2nd ed. Mahwah: Erlbaum; 2000. p. 245–73.
25. Lezak MD, Howieson DB, Loring DW, Hannay HJ, Fischer JS. Neuropsychological assessment. 4th ed. New York: Oxford University Press; 2004.
26. Strauss E, Sherman EMS, Spreen O. A compendium of neuropsychological tests: administration, norms, and commentary. 2nd ed. New York: Oxford University Press; 2006.
27. Delis DC, Wetter SR. Cogniform disorder and cogniform condition: proposed diagnoses for excessive cognitive symptoms. Arch Clin Neuropsychol. 2007; 22:589–604.
28. Boone KB. Fixed belief in cognitive dysfunction despite normal neuropsychological scores: neurocognitive hypochondriasis? Clin Neuropsychol. 2009;23: 1016–36.
29. Butcher JN, Dahlstrom WG, Graham JR, Tellegen AM, Kaemmer B. MMPI-2, Minnesota multiphasic personality inventory—2: manual for administration and scoring. Minneapolis: University of Minnesota Press; 1989.
30. Beck AT, Steer RA, Brown GK. Beck depression inventory. 2nd ed. San Antonio: The Psychological Corporation; 1996.
31. Yesavage JA, Brink TL, Rose TL, Lum O, Huang V, Adey MB, Leirer VO. Development and validation of a geriatric depression screening scale: a preliminary report. J Psychiatr Res. 1983;17:37–49.

32. Ben-Porath YS, Tellegen A. MMPI-2-RF (Minnesota Multiphasic Personality Inventory-2 Restructured Form): manual for administration, scoring, and interpretation. Minneapolis: University of Minnesota Press; 2008.
33. Lees-Haley PR, English LT, Glenn WJ. A Fake Bad Scale on the MMPI-2 for personal injury claimants. Psychol Rep. 1991;68:203–10.
34. Hahn SR, Kroenke K, Spitzer RL, et al. The difficult patient: prevalence, psychopathology, and functional impairment. J Gen Intern Med. 1996;11:1–8.
35. Rollnick S, Miller WR, Butler CC. Motivational interviewing in health care: helping patients change behavior. New York: The Guilford Press; 2008.
36. Greenberger D, Padesky CA. Mind over mood: change how you feel by changing the way you think. New York: The Guilford Press; 1995.
37. Kroenke K. Efficacy of treatment for somatoform disorders: a review of randomized controlled trials. Psychosom Med. 2007;69:881–8.
38. Sumathipala A. What is the evidence for the efficacy of treatments for somatoform disorders? A critical review of previous intervention studies. Psychosom Med. 2007;69(9):889–900.
39. Kabat-Zinn J. Full catastrophe living: using the wisdom of your body and mind to face stress, pain, and illness. 15th anniversary edition reissue. New York: Bantam Dell; 2009.
40. Bonadonna R. Meditation's impact on chronic illness. Holist Nurs Pract. 2003;17:309–19.
41. Carlson L, Speca M, Faris P, Patel K. One year pre-post intervention follow-up of psychological, immune, endocrine and blood pressure outcomes of mindfulness-based stress reduction (MBSR) in breast and prostate cancer outpatients. Brain Behav Immun. 2007;21:1038–49.
42. Sephton S, Salmon P, Weissbecker I, Ulmer C, Floyd A, Hoover K, Studts J. Mindfulness meditation alleviates depressive symptoms in women with fibromyalgia: results of a randomized clinical trial. Arthritis Rheum. 2007;57:77–85.
43. Lahmann C, Loew TH, Tritt K, Nickel M. Efficacy of functional relaxation and patient education in the treatment of somatoform heart disorders: a randomized, controlled clinical investigation. Psychosomatics. 2008;49:378–85.
44. Derogatis LR. The SCL-90-R. Baltimore: Clinical Psychometric Research; 1975.
45. Nayak NN, Shankar K. Yoga: a therapeutic approach. Phys Med Rehabil Clin N Am. 2004;15:783–98.
46. Salmon P, Lush E, Jablonski M, Sephton SE. Yoga and mindfulness: clinical aspects of an ancient mind/body practice. Cogn Behav Pract. 2009;16:59–72.
47. Peters S, Stanley I, Rose M, Kaney S, Salmon P. A randomized controlled trial of group aerobic exercise in primary care patients with persistent, unexplained physical symptoms. Fam Pract. 2002;19:665–74.
48. O'Malley PG, Jackson JL, Santoro J, Tomkins G, Balden E, Kroenke K. Antidepressant therapy for unexplained symptoms and symptom syndromes. J Fam Pract. 1999;48:980–90.
49. Fishbain DA, Cutler RB, Rosomoff HL, Rosomoff RS. Do antidepressants have an analgesic effect in psychogenic pain and somatoform pain disorder? A meta-analysis. Psychosom Med. 1998;60:503–9.
50. Onghena P, Van Houdenhove B. Antidepressant-induced analgesia in chronic non-malignant pain: a meta-analysis of 39 placebo-controlled studies. Pain. 1992;49:205–19.
51. Fallon BA. Pharmacotherapy of somatoform disorders. J Psychosom Res. 2004;56:455.
52. Hoedeman R, Blankenstein AH, Krol B, Koopmans PC, Groothoff JW. The contribution of high levels of somatic symptom severity to sickness absence duration, disability and discharge. J Occup Rehabil. 2010;20:264–73.
53. Smith GR, Monson RA, Ray DC. Psychiatric consultation in somatization disorder: a randomized controlled study. N Engl J Med. 1986;314:1407–13.
54. White M, Epston D. Narrative means to therapeutic ends. New York: W.W. Norton; 1990.

Driving Evaluation in Older Adults

10

Kevin J. Manning and Maria T. Schultheis

Abstract

Individuals increasingly maintain active driver status later into life. The prevalence of age-related medical conditions (e.g., dementia) negatively affects the cognitive, visual, and physical abilities deemed necessary for safe driving. Thus, clinicians are increasingly called upon to comment on an older patient's ability to remain an active driver. The current chapter aims to provide the clinician with a practical understanding of the literature on driving research that has been conducted in older drivers. We introduce concepts and challenges inherent in conducting driving research, and provide a review of the literature on the effects of healthy aging and neurological disease on driving performance. Special focus on cognition and driving is meant to help translate empirical studies into clinical applications. Finally, guidelines are provided for the clinician faced with evaluating driving capacity of an older adult.

Keywords

Older drivers • Driving evaluation • Alzheimer's disease and driving

Introduction

In today's fast-paced society, there is often an emphasis on autonomy and mobility. It is not surprising that our society is highly dependent on automobiles, and recent statistics indicate that individuals maintain active driver status and stay on the road later into life [1]. As a result, the number of drivers on the road over the age of 65 continues to progressively increase [2]. Advanced age and the prevalence of age-related medical conditions (e.g., dementia) have been shown to

K.J. Manning, M.S. (✉)
Department of Psychology, Drexel University, 3141 Chestnut Street, PSA Building, Room 218, Philadelphia, PA 19104, USA
e-mail: kevin.j.manning@gmail.com

M.T. Schultheis, Ph.D.
Department of Psychology and Department of Biomedical Engineering, Drexel University, 3141 Chestnut Street, PSA Building, Room 218, Philadelphia, PA 19104, USA
e-mail: schultheis@drexel.edu

L.D. Ravdin and H.L. Katzen (eds.), *Handbook on the Neuropsychology of Aging and Dementia*, Clinical Handbooks in Neuropsychology, DOI 10.1007/978-1-4614-3106-0_10,

negatively affect the cognitive, visual, and physical abilities deemed necessary for safe driving. As a result, clinicians are increasingly called upon to comment on an older patient's ability to remain an active driver. The clinical recommendation to cease or limit driving can have negative ramifications on everyday activities (i.e., getting to work, opportunity to engage in social activities, access to medical appointments/needs), sense of autonomy, and is even associated with poor health and depression [3, 4]. Clinicians are challenged to evaluate the safety of the older driver in society while balancing the patient's needs for mobility and quality of life.

The current chapter aims to provide the clinician with a practical understanding of the literature on driving research that has been conducted in older drivers. To accomplish this, we have sectioned the chapter into four main topics. The first section introduces some key concepts and challenges inherent in conducting driving research, and it is meant to provide a reference framework for the subsequent discussions. The second section provides a review of the literature on the effects of healthy aging on driving performance. By providing a description of common crash statistics and driving errors of older drivers free of neurological compromise, we aim to provide the clinician with an understanding of "typical" driving behaviors in older adults. This section also includes a summary of our current understanding of the relationship between cognition and driving in healthy aging. The third section focuses on the characterization of the older driver with neurological disease or compromise. Since the focus of this chapter is on clinical driving evaluations, we limit our review to Alzheimer's disease, Parkinson's disease, and mild cognitive impairment (MCI). The interested reader is urged to consult Schultheis et al. [5] for a review of additional age-related neurological disease or injury (e.g., stroke) that is known to effect driving performance. The final section includes a discussion of the clinical application of this research to clinical neuropsychology and aims to provide helpful guidelines for the clinician faced with evaluating driving capacity of an older adult.

Considerations in Driving Research

The relationship between driving performance and driving outcome can be conceptualized as an imaginary triangle or iceberg (see Fig. 10.1). Rizzo and colleagues [6] illustrate this point first raised by Heinrich et al. [7] and Maycock [8]. At the tip of the iceberg, above the "waterline," are driving errors that produce accidents. For example, running a red light is obviously dangerous and concerning to individual drivers and society at large, despite the fact that crashes are relatively rare events [9]. A greater portion of the iceberg is "below the waterline" and includes

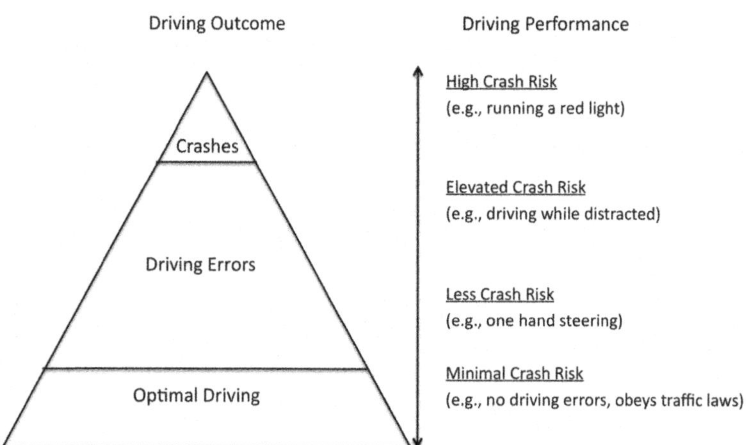

Fig. 10.1 Driving performance and driving outcome

behaviors less obvious to individual drivers and society. This portion is comprised of driving errors that increase crash risk or result in near crashes. These more frequently occurring driving errors range in crash-risk severity. For example, errors such as "texting" while driving are more related to accidents than errors related to driving with one hand on the steering wheel. Two main areas of driving research have evolved in investigating driving errors. The first aims at elucidating the relationship between specific driving errors of varying severities and crash risk or crash involvement. A second aim is to understand driver characteristics that are related to a high likelihood of committing driving errors. From a clinical application perspective, understanding how driver characteristics such as age and cognition contribute to these driving errors may aid clinicians in detecting individuals who may be at greater risk for driving difficulties.

An important consideration in driving research is the variability in how driving outcome or driving performance is defined in a laboratory. There is a lack of consistency on how this very complex behavior is quantified. Most studies have employed one of the following measures for defining driving performance: (a) behind-the-wheel examination (BTW), (b) performance on instrumented vehicles, (c) performance on driving simulators, (d) self-reported driving behaviors, (e) crash statistics, or (f) documented crash involvement (i.e., DMV reports). Despite the fact that all of these factors have been used to define "driving performance," there are significant differences across these methods (i.e., subjective vs. objective measures, real-world vs. simulated driving). A summary of the pros and cons to each of these approaches is summarized in Table 10.1. In this chapter, we have reviewed studies using any of these various methods to assess driving performance. In our own research, we have endorsed a multimethod approach, which commonly includes simultaneous measurement of more than one of these outcome measures.

It should be noted that the BTW driving evaluation is the most "clinically" useful method of evaluating driving performance. The BTW is an on-road evaluation, commonly conducted by a driving specialist (e.g., occupational therapist) in a dual-controlled vehicle, and, together with the driving specialist's off-road clinical evaluation, comprises a clinical driving evaluation. BTW evaluations can vary significantly since there are no state or federally mandated guidelines and

Table 10.1 Methods of driving assessment

Measures	Description	Driving performance pro(s)	Driving performance con(s)
Behind-the-wheel exam (BTW)	On-road test conducted by a driving specialist who observes and directs the driving of the examinee	Direct measurement of driving on the road Quantifiable measurement	Subjective rating based on clinical judgment Unable to safely measure challenging driving scenarios
Instrumented vehicle	Instrumentation (e.g., cameras, sensors) is directly linked to vehicle inputs (e.g., steering, braking)	Direct measurement of driving on the road Quantifiable measurement Objective measurement	Unable to safely measure challenging driving scenarios Expensive to implement
Virtual reality driving simulation	Mode of implementation varies from low-fidelity inexpensive computer-based to full immersion programs	Quantifiable measurement Objective measurement Allows safe presentation of challenging driving scenarios	Questionable if results from simulated driving can be translated to the real world Risk of simulation sickness
Crash statistics	Data gathered from collisions and possible contributing factors	Very strong clinical relevance	Infrequent events Usually does not account for accidents that are not reported to the authorities Data collected after the fact
Self-report	Self-report of driving history (e.g., nonreported accidents, violations, driving frequency)	Easily obtained information	Limitations of self-report include over- and underestimation of events

they are unique per setting/evaluator. In the majority of the cases, the individual being evaluated is commonly guided through identified routes while driving behaviors are observed, and a pass/fall determination is typically rendered at the end of the drive. A large percentage of individuals will successfully pass this evaluation, raising issues of sensitivity since BTW evaluations may not pick up on more subtle difficulties that could render an older diver unsafe.

There are two existing literatures of driving research—studies conducted with a clinical/medical focus and studies conducted with a transportation research focus. Arguably, these two areas of research should inform each other; however, too often this is not the case. The majority of the studies examining driving performance of the healthy older driver have been conducted by transportation researchers and are typically not published in journals that are commonly accessed by clinicians. This literature is substantial and contains important information for understanding aging and driving behaviors, regardless of the presence of neurological compromise. By contrast, the literature on driving in neurologically compromised older adults (i.e., drivers with dementia) is smaller and typically focuses on clinical contributions to driving performance (i.e., cognitive and physical changes) and the development of clinical measures for predicting driving performance.

Characterization of the Healthy Older Driver

Crash Rates of the Healthy Older Driver

A common misconception surrounding older drivers is that they have a greater likelihood of being involved in automobile crashes compared to other age groups in the general population. Empirical evidence does not support this widespread claim [10, 11]. In fact, when the crash rates of 47,500 drivers of various ages were compared after adjusting for annual miles driven, the majority of older drivers had lower crash rates than all other age groups [10]. There are two important caveats to this finding. One is that crash risk increases as driving exposure (i.e., annual miles driven) decreases. Thus, older adults who drive less than 2,000 miles annually, approximately 13% of all older drivers, have one of the largest crash rates [10]. Second, whereas older drivers are not at an *overall* increased crash risk, they are more likely to be involved in certain *types* of crashes compared to younger and middle-aged drivers. Evidence suggests that drivers aged 65 and above are significantly more likely to be involved in crashes at intersections, stop signs, while turning against oncoming traffic and changing lanes [9, 12–14]. These crashes that involve conflict with oncoming traffic or direct moving traffic flow can result in significant injuries and have been viewed as "high-risk" involvement. A closer evaluation of the specific errors provides insight into these commonly seen accidents in older adults.

Driving Errors in Healthy Older Adults

Stopping errors and errors involving the right of way elevate crash risk at intersections and stop signs. Bao and Boyle [15] compared the driving performance of 60 younger, middle-aged, and older adults at rural expressway intersections controlled by a stop sign. All participants were licensed drivers screened to ensure safe driving records. Driving performance was measured with an on-road instrumented vehicle, enabling the precise calculation of stopping profiles based on time and distance from stop signs. Overall, high crash risk was noted in older ($n=20$; age range 65–80) and younger drivers ($n=20$; age range 18–21) who were significantly more likely to run stop signs compared to middle-aged ($n=20$; age range 35–55) adults. Fully missed stop signs rarely occurred, and the majority of accidents at stop signs occur after drivers stop at least once before entering the intersection [16]. Bao and Boyle also analyzed stopping behavior and found that older drivers demonstrated a dangerous braking profile compared to middle-aged adults. Older adults braking was best characterized as sudden; they began breaking closer to the stop sign and progressed faster from the initial brake press to maximum breaking, resulting in a short stop. Described in further detail below, work using driving simulation has demonstrated that sudden stopping in older adults with Alzheimer's disease significantly increases crash risk at intersections [17].

Errors in judgment or attention are related to increased crash risk in older drivers while turning or changing lanes. Braitman et al. [18] reviewed police crash reports and photographs of accident scenes and conducted telephone interviews with at-fault drivers involved in intersection crashes. Participants were grouped according to age: drivers ages 70–79 ($n=78$), 80 and older ($n=76$), and a group of middle-aged drivers 35–54 ($n=73$). Findings confirmed that crashes that occurred when the driver failed to yield the right of way increased with age and more often occurred when the driver was turning left (i.e., against oncoming traffic). Compared to middle-aged and the oldest drivers, drivers ages 70–79 failed to evaluate the correct speed of the oncoming vehicle. That is, they saw the other vehicle, but misjudged whether there was adequate time to proceed. On the contrary, the oldest drivers reported failing to see the other vehicle involved in the accident. Likewise, failure to see another vehicle or inability to judge its oncoming speed is often cited as a reason for accidents following a lane change [19].

To summarize, older drivers are not at an overall increased crash risk compared to younger drivers. However, older drivers are more likely to commit driving errors that increase their crash risk at intersections and stop signs, and while changing lanes or turning against oncoming traffic. These errors include sudden stopping, misjudging speed and distance of other vehicles, and failure to see other vehicles on the road.

Cognition and Driving in Healthy Older Adults

Many researchers have attempted to examine the relationship between cognition and specific driving errors. Findings indicate that numerous specific cognitive abilities are significantly associated with various driving performance measures in healthy older adults free of cognitive impairment, including memory, attention, perceptual and visuospatial ability, information processing speed, and abilities falling under the broad domain of executive functioning (e.g., working memory, planning). In the following section, we provide a concise review of recent studies that investigate different aspects of driving performance in older adults free of neurological compromise. For a larger review of the literature on driving and cognition in older adults, consult Anstey et al. [20] and Mathias and Lucas [21].

Dawson et al. [22] administered a BTW exam to 111 healthy older adult drivers (age range = 65–89) and 80 middle-aged drivers (age range = 40–64). All participants were screened for neurological disorders and cognitive complaints. Rather than simply dichotomize performance on the BTW exam into "pass" or "fail," results of the exam were coded into 15 different categories of driving errors based upon the Iowa Department of Transportation's Drive Test Scoring Standards. Results clearly illustrated older adults had a propensity towards significantly more errors per drive on 7 out of the 15 categories including speed control, turning, lane changes, lane observance, parallel parking, railroad crossing, and starting the car and pulling away from the curb. Furthermore, older drivers committed significantly more high crash-risk driving errors than middle-aged drivers (such as entering an intersection during a red light). Age correlated with worse performance in the oldest group, but not in middle-aged adults. The strongest predictor of driving in the older-aged cohort was a composite measure of eight cognitive tests, including tests of visual and verbal memory, constructional praxis, visual perception, working memory, and verbal fluency. Specifically, for every one standard deviation decrease in a cognitive function composite measure in healthy older drivers, there were 3.6 more driving errors observed after adjusting for age, sex, and education.

The Salisbury Eye Evaluation and Driving Study is a longitudinal study of vision, cognition, and driving of older adults on Maryland's Eastern Shore that investigated factors associated with a frequent antecedent to crashes: lane changes [23]. There are three major strengths of this work: (1) large sample of cognitively intact licensed community-dwelling adults ($n = 981$; average Mini-Mental State Exam (MMSE) = 27.6 ± 2.2 [24]; average age 77.8 ± 5.2), (2) each participant was administered a comprehensive visual exam and five common neuropsychological tests of executive functioning, visuospatial abilities, and memory, and (3) driving performance was measured with the use of dual cameras and a driving monitoring system within each participant's vehicle for a period of 5 days. Results confirmed that older drivers often fail to check for traffic before changing lanes. Taking total lane changes into consideration, failure rates ranged from 16 to 24%, with drivers who most often changed lanes demonstrating the highest failure rate. Furthermore, findings revealed susceptibility to distraction, and higher-order visuospatial skills are important in lane-changing behavior. Worse performance on measures of visuoconstruction and auditory divided attention predicted a higher incidence of lane-changing errors after accounting for age and gender.

Freund and colleagues have used virtual reality driving simulation as an objective tool to provide older adults with clinical driving recommendations [25, 26]. Based upon driving errors measured during simulation, Freund and Colgrove [25] classified 108 older drivers (age range 61–96) as safe ($n = 35$), unsafe ($n = 47$), or restricted ($n = 26$). Safe drivers made no "hazardous errors" during simulated driving (e.g., crashes or running red lights), whereas restricted drivers committed at least one error and unsafe drivers at least two. Of several screening measures, Trail Making Test B was the only measure that significantly differed among the three groups, and a simple test of clock drawing correlated the strongest with total simulated driving errors ($r = 0.68$) and pedal confusion (i.e., confusing the gas for the brake) [26, 27]. The authors hypothesized that executive functioning may be especially relevant to driving in older adults "because executive functioning is a critical component of safe driving, and in the presence of executive dysfunction, the automatized and procedural skills learned over decades of daily living do not protect the older driver from errors" (p. 243) [26]. Although the sample consisted of community-dwelling older adults, participants had an average MMSE of 24.9 ± 4.3 and possibly met clinical criteria for MCI or dementia, limiting the generalizability of the findings. Other investigators have also provided evidence for the importance of intact executive functions in the safe driving of cognitively healthy older adults [28] as well as older adults with dementia (i.e., Alzheimer's disease and Parkinson's disease).

Driving in Older Adults with Neurological Disease

The Older Driver with Alzheimer's Disease: Crash Rates and Routine Driving Ability

Despite early work suggesting older adults with Alzheimer's disease (AD) had an increased risk of crashes compared to age-matched controls [29], more recent investigations have found no relationship between a diagnosis of dementia and crash risk [30, 31]. Although crash rates may not differ between healthy older adults and adults with AD, the groups significantly differ on driving errors committed. Dawson et al. [32] administered a BTW exam to 40 licensed drivers with mild AD (mean MMSE = 26.5 ± 2.9) and 115 older adult drivers free of cognitive impairment. Errors from the BTW were coded into 15 categories including, among others, traffic signals, stop signs, turns, lane change, speed, and parking. Considering individual error types, older adults with AD made more driving errors compared to healthy older adults in only 1 out of 15 categories: lane changes. However, when total driving errors were tallied, adults with AD made significantly more errors (42.00 ± 12.84) than healthy older adults (33.18 ± 12.22), including significantly more high crash-risk errors.

Longitudinal studies of older drivers demonstrate that a diagnosis of dementia, per se, does not universally impact the ability of individuals with Alzheimer's disease to pass a clinical driving evaluation [33, 34]. Ott et al. [34] conducted a longitudinal study of drivers with Alzheimer's disease spanning 3 years using the BTW. Greater severity of dementia determined by a Clinical Dementia Rating (CDR) [35], increased age, and lower education was associated with higher rates of BTW failure at follow-up. However, only 22% of individuals with mild Alzheimer's disease (CDR = 1.0) failed the exam at follow-up and were judged as unsafe drivers. This failure rate was even less in the group of individuals considered to have questionable dementia or severe MCI (CDR = 0.5). Therefore, despite evidence that, as a group, older drivers with AD commit more high crash-risk driving errors than healthy older adults [32], many older drivers with AD are able to safely maintain routine driving over several years when tested with the BTW [34]. As noted, the BTW, the current clinical gold standard of driving evaluations, does not allow for the administration of challenging driving scenarios [36]. The ability to older drivers with AD to adapt to novel driving situations (e.g., another vehicle suddenly swerves in front of the vehicle) is compromised compared to older adults without neurodegenerative disease.

The Older Driver with Alzheimer's Disease: Driving and Cognition

Virtual reality simulation proves a useful tool to investigate challenging driving scenarios. Rizzo et al. [17] studied 18 participants with mild to moderate AD (mean age 73) and 12 healthy older adults (mean age 70) using virtual reality driving simulation. Each participant drove an uneventful virtual route for 15 min before reaching a final intersection that triggered an illegal incursion by another vehicle. Optimal response in order to avert a crash required the driver to release the accelerator, apply the brake, and make a steering correction. Findings revealed that participants committed a safety error while driving on uneventful segments of the virtual environment. However, 6 of the 18 subjects with AD crashed as a result of intersection incursion vehicle compared to 0 control participants. Overall, cognitive performance was associated with crashes, as were individual measures of visuoconstruction, working memory, and verbal fluency.

Following up their earlier work, Uc, Rizzo, Anderson, Shi, and Dawson [31] further demonstrated the benefits of virtual reality simulation in measuring driving performance in older adults with Alzheimer's disease. They studied 61 drivers with AD (average age 73.5 ± 8.5) and 115 healthy older adults (average age 69.4 ± 6.7). All participants underwent a crash simulation; specifically, after a segment of uneventful driving, each driver suddenly encountered a lead vehicle stopped at an intersection, creating the potential for a collision with the lead vehicle or another vehicle following closely behind the driver. Contrary to their earlier findings with incursion vehicles [17], crash rates did not differ between individuals with AD (5%) and healthy older adults (3%). However, individuals with AD were more likely to engage in sudden vehicle slowing, which significantly increased the risk of being struck from behind [31]. Furthermore, sudden slowing was associated with multiple cognitive abilities, but a brief measure of executive functioning (Trail Making Part B) was associated with the greatest increase in risk of unsafe behavior. These finding suggested that with each 30-s prolongation on Trail Making Part B, the risk of abrupt slowing increased by 31%.

There has been only one meta-analytic attempt to summarize the literature on neuropsychological tests and driving performance in adults with AD [37]. In their meta-analysis, Reger et al. [37] categorized studies into three categories based on driving outcome: BTW, nonroad tests (e.g., virtual reality driving simulation), and caregiver report. Cognitive performance was grouped into six domains: mental status, attention, visuospatial abilities, memory, executive functions, and language. Results can be interpreted using Cohen's [38] classification of $r = 0.10$, 0.30, and 0.50, as small, moderate, and large effects. Overall, tests of visuospatial abilities demonstrated the strongest performance with driving outcome in adults with AD ($r = 0.29$ with BTW, $r = 0.31$ with nonroad tests, and $r = 0.19$ with caregiver report). No relationship was found between tests of executive functioning and the

BTW ($r=-0.06$), whereas a mild–moderate relationship was found between executive functioning and nonroad tests ($r=0.22$). Given findings from Uc et al. [31] and other work demonstrating the importance of executive functioning tests discriminating safe and unsafe older drivers with AD [39], results of the Reger et al. [37] meta-analysis should be interpreted with caution, and additional studies are clearly needed.

The Older Driver with Parkinson's Disease: Driving Errors and Routine Driving Ability

Compared to healthy older adults, evidence suggests that older adults with Parkinson's disease (PD) are more likely to commit driving errors involving lane changes, failing to check blind spots, reduced usage of side- and rear-view mirrors, backing out of a space, and indecisiveness at intersections [40, 41]. Uc et al. [42] compared the BTW performance of 84 older adults with PD and 182 healthy older drivers. Similar to their work with other populations [22, 31], BTW performance was classified into 15 different error categories, and total safety errors were tallied as well as serious driving errors. Individuals with PD had an average illness duration of 5.9±5.0 years, a mean Hoehn and Yahr stage of 2.2±0.59, and did not significantly differ from the healthy group on age. Drivers with PD committed more errors than healthy adults while at stop signs, turning, and maintaining lanes. Furthermore, when total errors were tallied, the PD group committed significantly more safety errors (41.6±14.6) than the cognitively healthy adults (32.9±12.3). However, the PD group did not commit more high-crash risk errors compared to healthy adults.

The majority of older adults with PD are able to pass clinical driving evaluations. Singh and colleagues [43] analyzed data on 154 PD patients referred to a clinical driving assessment service over a 15-year period. Participants had a mean duration of illness of 5.9 years, a mean Hoehn and Yahr stage of 1.9, and the average age was 67.6 years (standard deviations were not reported). As part of the driving assessment, each individual received a BTW exam rated on 17 different parameters including physical control, response to other drivers, lane discipline, roundabout management, braking, and merging. Based on these parameters, a driving specialist rated participants as "safe" or "unsafe." Out of the 154 PD patients, 50 (32.5%) were judged as unsafe to drive because of concerns over road safety.

Overall, these results suggest that individuals with PD commit more driving errors compared to age-matched peers. Error types include difficulty maintaining lane positions, turning, failing to check blind spots, reduced usage of side- and rear-view mirrors, and difficulty navigating stop signs and intersections. However, when crash risk is compared in PD subjects and healthy older adults, there are no significant differences between groups on total high crash-risk errors. Analysis of driving frequency suggests PD patients do not limit their driving compared to age-matched peers. Older adults with PD average as many miles per week and make as many trips as do healthy older adults [40]. Furthermore, the majority of PD participants are able to maintain routine driving ability when tested with the BTW, at least in early in the course of their illness.

The Older Driver with Parkinson's Disease: Driving and Cognition

Neuropsychological measures of attention, visual spatial ability, memory, and executive functioning are important in the assessment of driving performance in PD [6, 40]. Grace and colleagues [40] investigated the BTW driving performance of 21 PD subjects, 21 healthy older adults, and 20 AD subjects. PD participants had mild levels of impairment as evidenced by a mean MMSE of 28.1±1.6, a mode Hoehn and Yahr stage of 2.0, and a mean Unified Parkinson's Disease Rating Scale motor section of 28.4±7.7. Participants were classified as "safe," "marginally safe," or "unsafe" as a result of the BTW exam, and total driving errors were tallied. Results of global safety ratings are consistent with findings from Singh et al. [43] described above, where the majority of drivers with PD were characterized as "safe."

In the study by Grace et al. [40], no PD driver was characterized as "unsafe," 67% (14/21) of PD participants were characterized as "safe," and 33% (7/21) were characterized as "marginally safe." However, driving performance differences between groups were statistically significant; 100% of the healthy older adult group was characterized as "safe," and PD drivers (7.6±4.2) did commit more errors than the healthy adult group (3.7±2.7). Cognitive performances were also statistically different between groups defined by driving safety ratings. When compared to the healthy control group, PD participants characterized as "marginally safe" drivers performed significantly worse on measures of verbal learning and memory, visuospatial ability, working memory, and finger tapping. The neuropsychological performance of drivers with PD labeled as "safe" did not significantly differ from the healthy adult group. Comparisons of "safe" and "marginally safe" PD drivers confirm the importance of visuospatial abilities and working memory in discriminating the two groups. Amick et al. [44] reported that performance on Trail Making Test, Rey Complex Figure Copy Test, and the Useful Field of View Divided Attention Subtest, a measure of visual attention [45], distinguished 14 safe PD and 11 marginally safe PD drivers tested BTW.

Analysis of the neuropsychological performance of 84 PD participants revealed that visual processing speed and attention, motion perception, visuoconstruction, visual memory, and general cognition were significant predictors of total error counts on the BTW after adjusting for age and education [42]. Far visual acuity and contrast sensitivity (i.e., the ability to see objects that do not stand out from their background) were also significant predictors of total driving errors. Devos and colleagues [46] compared the clinical characteristics and cognitive performance of 29 adults with PD who "passed" a virtual reality driving simulation and 11 adults with PD who "failed" the simulation. Those adults with PD who failed the evaluation were older and had longer disease duration, worse contrast sensitivity, worse motor performance on the UPDRS, and worse performance on the Rey Complex Figure Copy Test. Disease severity did not significantly differ between groups when rated on the Hoehn and Yahr scale but was significantly different when rated with the CDR.

Review of the literature on PD and driving suggests the clinician should consider clinical and cognitive risk factors when evaluating fitness to drive in patients with PD. Important clinical factors include disease duration and severity, motor performance, visual acuity, and contrast sensitivity. Neuropsychological measures of attention, visual spatial ability, memory, and executive functioning can inform driving recommendations and identify those in need of further evaluation [44].

Characterization of the Older Driver with Mild Cognitive Impairment

The research on the driving performance of older adults with MCI is less developed that than of older adults with AD and PD. Briefly, MCI is a term that broadly defines an intermediate stage of objective cognitive decline thought to be associated with higher risk of dementia [47, 48]. Wadley et al. [49] investigated the BTW performance of 46 adults with MCI (mean age = 71.30 ± 7.79) and 59 cognitively healthy older adults (mean age = 67.07 ± 6.72) with MCI defined using Petersen criteria [50]. However, it was noted that the MCI participants performed comparably to the cognitively healthy older adults on the Dementia Rating Scale [51] with average scores (DRS) of 132.60 ± 8.49 and 137.48 ± 6.26, respectively. It is notable that 43 of the MCI participants were characterized as amnesic MCI, and the majority of these participants were described as free of cognitive impairments in domains other than memory.

Wadley and colleagues [49] recorded five BTW error types: turning, lane control, gap judgment, steering steadiness, and maintaining proper speed in MCI subjects. Driving outcome was defined using two methods: (1) as the total errors across the five error types, and (2) the driving specialist's ratings of (A) "evaluator took control of the car," (B) "unsafe," (C) "unsatisfactory," (D) "not optimal," and (E) "optimal." Results revealed that overall mean errors did not differ between adults with MCI and cognitively healthy older adults. When groups were compared on the driving specialist's ratings, a higher proportion of adults with MCI were judged as demonstrating "not optimal" performance on left turns, lane control, and an overall global rating of driving performance. These authors discuss two major implications of their findings. First, driving abilities in individuals with MCI, while "less than optimal," were not impaired. No drivers received "unsafe" or "unsatisfactory" driver ratings, nor did the evaluator ever take control of the vehicle. The authors bring this point by summarizing, "It appears that individuals with MCI are less likely than cognitively normal peers to *seamlessly* perform certain routine driving maneuvers" (p. 92, italicized added) [49]. Second, they speculate that executive functions are important cognitive abilities affected in MCI that may underlie less than optimal driving performance. This interpretation is consistent with evidence that executive functioning abilities are significantly impaired even in adults who meet criteria for pure amnesic MCI [52]. Future research is needed to further investigate the impact of executive dysfunction on driving performance and better understand changes in driving ability among individuals with MCI.

Application to Clinical Neuropsychology

Clinical neuropsychologists are often called upon to comment on the driving abilities of older adults. The recommendation to cease or continue driving entails significant responsibility, both to the patient and society. Despite the ample literature on the relationship between cognitive performance and driving, it remains challenging for clinicians to translate the statistically significant relationships between cognition and driving into clinically meaningful outcomes for older adults. Presently, there are no neuropsychological practice parameters or guidelines as to what constitutes a necessary and sufficient assessment battery for determining vehicle-driving fitness [53]. Recently, the American Academy of Neurology has updated a clinical practice parameter on patients with dementia and their families who seek advice on driving [54]. Iverson et al. [54] urge clinicians to consider risk factors for decreased driving ability (history of crashes/citations, reduced driving mileage, self-reported avoidance, aggressive personality characteristics) and to use the CDR scale and informant report as the primary methods of determining the driving risk of the older patient with dementia. We concur that consideration of risk factors and family concerns are extremely important in conducting clinical driving evaluations. However, Iverson et al. [54] fail to address the contributions of cognition and do not address how clinicians may best evaluate when cognitive performance begins to impede on driving performance. We purport that neuropsychological assessment can make a valuable contribution to clinical driving evaluations, and whenever possible, a comprehensive cognitive assessment should be included in the driver evaluation process. Presented below are recommendations for clinical neuropsychologists, and other clinicians, involved in evaluations of driving safety.

Clinical Neuropsychological Considerations on Driving

The gold standard for driving assessment remains the clinical driving evaluation, of which the BTW examination is a critical component [55]. Driving simulation, while of great potential use, remains in its infancy as a clinical tool. When specifically evaluating driving capacity, the clinical neuropsychological evaluation can serve as guide to inform whether further evaluation of driving ability is warranted. It is also important to recognize that what constitutes a sufficient clinical neuropsychological evaluation may not constitute adequate neuropsychological assessment in driving ability. Although limited, research can provide direction for the selection of neuropsychological measures to be administered. Specific cognitive domains associated with driving performance have been identified in the literature and include varying types of attention (i.e., divided attention, sustained attention), information

Table 10.2 Neuropsychological measures empirically related to crash rates or behind-the-wheel performance in older adults

Cognitive domain	Neuropsychological measure	Study sample(s)
Attention	Useful field of view [31, 45, 67–69]	AD, HC
	Cancelation task [70, 71]	HC
Processing speed	Symbol Digits Modalities Test [72, 73]	PD
	Trail Making Part A [32, 74]	AD
Executive functions	Brief Test of Attention [23, 75]	HC
	Clock drawing [76]	HC
	Mazes [39, 71]	HC, AD
	Paper folding task [67, 77]	HC
	Stroop color-word Test [78]	HC
	Tower of London test [78, 79]	HC
	Trail Making Part B [31, 69, 70, 74]	AD, HC
	Wisconsin Card Sorting Test [78, 80]	HC
Visuospatial	Judgment of Line Orientation [31, 81]	AD
	Block design [22, 82]	HC
	Complex Figure Copy [22, 31, 32]	AD, HC
	Beery–Buktenica Test of Visual Motor Integration [23, 83]	HC
	Motor-Free Visual Perception Test [68, 69, 76]	HC
Memory	Benton Visual Retention Test [31, 32, 71, 84]	HC, AD
	Complex Figure Recall [22, 31]	AD, HC
	Hopkins Verbal Learning Test [40, 85]	PD
Motor	Purdue Pegboard [73, 86]	PD

Note: References to the driving literature are in bold. *AD* Alzheimer's disease, *HC* cognitively healthy older adults, *PD* Parkinson's disease

processing speed and reaction time, working memory, visual spatial learning and memory, visual scanning, judgment, inhibition, problem-solving, and spatial perception. Table 10.2 provides examples of empirically supported neuropsychological measures associated with driving ability as defined by crash rates or BTW performance. This is not meant as a systematic review of the literature or a comment on the strength of the relationship between neuropsychological tests and driving performance. Instead, Table 10.2 is provided to guide the clinician in test selection of neuropsychological assessment of driving ability.

Case Example

Cases encountered in clinical practice are often far from "classic" and straightforward. Clinicians asked to comment on the functional performance of patients are often challenged by the relationship (or lack thereof) between objective cognitive performance and daily functioning. Furthermore, clinicians do not always have the luxury of lengthy evaluations.

Mr. Smith is a 72-year-old retired machine operator with 12 years of education, who underwent a clinical driving evaluation following complaints of his own worsening driving performance.

History of Present Illness

- Mr. Smith's family first noticed symptoms of depression and anxiety in 2001 when he was 65 years old.
- Mr. Smith's wife first noticed difficulties with his memory in 2005 when Mr. Smith was 69 years old. These difficulties were not noticeable to Mr. Smith's two children, but he was prescribed Aricept by his internist.
- Mr. Smith underwent a neurological evaluation in August 2007 following periods of increased confusion while his wife was hospitalized for a lengthy illness. The neurologist reported an MMSE of 25/30 and diagnosed "MCI, possible worsened by underlying depression."

- Medical history was significant for hypertension, hypothyroidism, hypercholesterolemia, coronary artery disease (with a stent placed in 2005), prostate cancer (surgery in 2003), and type II diabetes successfully managed with medication.
- MRI of the brain, completed in September 2007, revealed "diffuse atrophy" and a "few foci of increased T2 signal within the supratentorial white matter secondary to chronic small vessel ischemia."
- While his wife remained hospitalized, Mr. Smith lived alone and performed his own daily activities. However, he reported his driving had become more cautious, and he had struck a curb. Mr. Smith asked his neurologist to refer him for a clinical driving evaluation.

Clinical Driving Evaluation: Off-Road Assessment

- Cognitive difficulties included poor divided attention, decreased short-term memory, and impaired mental flexibility (see Table 10.3).
- Binocular visual acuity was 20/20. Depth perception, peripheral vision, and basic reaction time were judged to be within normal limits.

Clinical Driving Evaluation: On-Road Assessment

- Mr. Smith was "very nervous/cautious initially and too slow."
- With cues to "drive closer to posted speed limits," Mr. Smith's "speed improved as [he] relaxed."
- Mr. Smith required "minimal verbal reminders on multilane curved roads for lane placement."
- "Tendency to the drift to the left," but was "not unsafe" and was "aware of other vehicles in the left lane."
- He drove "55 in a 65-mph zone" but had a "good response to vehicles merging from the right."
- Mr. Smith passed his driving evaluation, and it was recommended that he only drive on local familiar roads and to familiar destinations and restrict his driving to daylight off-peak hours only.

Case Assessment

Results of Mr. Smith's clinical driving evaluation, notable for impairments on off-road cognitive measures but safe on-road driving, clearly demonstrates that cognitive impairment does not always equal driving impairment. In order to gain a comprehensive picture of the cognitive abilities of patients, multimethod assessment is important. If a decision was made for Mr. Smith to relinquish his driving privileges solely on the basis of the few off-road cognitive measures administered, it is obvious this decision would have been premature. Multiple abilities should be assessed under each cognitive domain. For example, there is empirical support for the useful field of view (UFOV) and its strong relationship to driving ability in older adults [56]. However, neither the UFOV nor any other measure alone will explain all the variance in driving performance [57, 58]. As noted, Table 10.2 provides examples of empirically supported cognitive measures.

Additional Risk Factors

There are additional risk factors for driving errors besides age and cognition. Other medical

Table 10.3 Case example: Results of Mr. Smith's off-road assessment September 2007

Measure	Raw score	Percentile	Description
Trail Making Part A	54″	10	Low average
Trail Making Part B	537″	<1st	Impaired
WAIS-R Digit Symbol	18/93	7th	Borderline
WAIS-R Picture Completion	11/20	9th	Low average
Motor-Free Visual Perceptual Test—Revised (MVPT-R)	24/36	–	Impaired*

**Note*: All normative data are based on Heaton et al. [87] or Wechsler [88] besides MVPT-R, which is based on recommendations of the American Medical Association [89]

conditions, often comorbid in older adults, can impact driving. In Mr. Smith's case, there was a complicated cardiovascular history along with diabetes, in addition to the identified cognitive problems. Age-related changes and diseases affecting vision (e.g., reduced contrast sensitivity, cataracts), respiratory diseases (e.g., sleep apnea), and musculoskeletal conditions (e.g., arthritis) are but a few.

The clinician should also carefully consider the potential impact of medications on driving performance [59, 60]. LeRoy and Morse [61], in conjunction with the National Highway Traffic Safety Administration, analyzed the medication use of 33,519 individuals involved in a traffic accident and 100,000 controls who had not crashed. Results suggested the side effects of individual medications and combinations can impair cognitive functioning and lead to unsafe driving. Mr. Smith's current medications at the time of his driving evaluation included several examples of the medication classes associated with increased likelihood of accidents:

- Clopidogrel (antiplatelet; 69% increased likelihood of accidents)
- Escitalopram (SSRI; 59% increased likelihood of accidents)
- Ranitidine (H2 blocker; 55% increased likelihood of accidents)
- Levothyroxine (thyroid hormone; 29% increased likelihood of accidents)
- Lisinopril (angiotensin-converting enzyme inhibitor; 23% increased likelihood of accidents)

The reader is referred to Looco and Staplin [62] for a comprehensive review on the impact of polypharmacy on the older driver.

Insight into cognitive impairment and awareness of functional ability is another risk factor. For example, when tested on a BTW exam and asked to gauge their performance, older adults with MCI tend to overestimate their driving ability [63]. What is remarkable in Mr. Smith's case is that *he* requested the driving evaluation. In the majority of cases, there is a reluctance to raise the issue of driving by patients and, subsequently, the burden of inquiring about changes in driving in on the treating clinician. It is also important to be aware of the fact that older drivers typically described self-limiting their driving in certain scenarios. For example, older drivers often describe not driving during heavy traffic or in poor weather conditions. However, empirical evidence does not support these claims; evidence suggests older drivers do not regulate their driving as much as they report [64]. Clinicians should therefore obtain information from collateral sources. Consultation with a knowledgeable spouse or other family member, ideally someone who drives with the patient, is a must.

Sensitive Functional Assessment

Sensitive functional assessment, in conjunction with thorough cognitive assessment, is essential to the development of evidence-based driving guidelines for older adults. The BTW exam does not typically involve challenging driving scenarios; it has been argued that the BTW exam only assesses driving performance associated with automatized procedural driving, and not driving skills dependent on higher cognitive abilities. Figure 10.2 illustrates the difficulty with using the BTW as the sole measure of driving performance. Greater emphasis on incorporating the literature from driving research into clinical practice may help

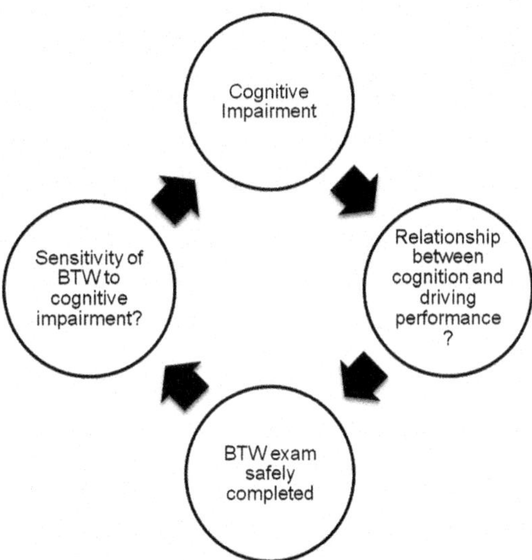

Fig. 10.2 Do clinical behind-the-wheel exams lack sensitivity to cognitive impairment?

illuminate the relationship between cognitive functioning and driving performance. For example, Uc et al. [31] investigated the effect of suddenly stopped lead vehicles on the virtual reality driving performance of older healthy adults and adults with AD. Results revealed AD patients were more likely to engage in sudden vehicle slowing, which significantly increased the risk of being struck from behind [31]. Multiple cognitive abilities were associated with sudden vehicle slowing, but time on Trail Making Part B had the strongest association with performance. In each 30-s prolongation on Trail Making Part B, the risk of abrupt slowing increased by 31%. Given his significant impairment on Trails B, it is intriguing to speculate on Mr. Smith's reaction to a vehicle suddenly stopping in front of him on the actual road. Whereas not available in the case of Mr. Smith, empirically validated driving simulation may prove a useful tool in clinical driving examinations.

Interventions and Recommendations

Potential driving cessation should be discussed as early as possible with the older patient. This is especially true for adults with a neurodegenerative illness who will eventually cease driving. In the case of progressive disorders (i.e., dementia), it is beneficial to have an ongoing dialogue about driving ability and to consider that multiple driving evaluations may be required during the course of the disease. Clinicians, especially neuropsychologists, have a responsibility to counsel and educate the patient and his or her family on the impact of relinquishing a driver's license. Inclusion of family members in this counseling process can serve to alleviate common communication strains between patients and family members about this sensitive topic. It is important to recall that one robust finding in the literature is the relationship between driving cessation and depression and loss of autonomy. Practical considerations include finding alternate transportation to doctors' appointments, work, and other activities outside the home. A useful review of interventions for older adults who have ceased driving is included in Windsor and Anstey [65].

Clinicians should also be familiar with interventions for older drivers who do not need to relinquish their driving privileges but require modification of their driving habits. These interventions include driving education (i.e., refresher course). There is moderate evidence that driving education improves behavior and awareness in older drivers [66]. Driving education may allow older drivers to successfully maintain safe driving for extended periods of time.

Neuropsychologists should be familiar with the work of driving specialists in their area who conduct clinical driving evaluations (see additional resources below for help finding a driver specialist in your area). Knowledge of the driving specialist's clinical examination will enable a frank discussion with patients as what they can expect from further evaluations. Finally, the clinician should be familiar on state laws on mandatory reporting, which vary considerably. For example, in Pennsylvania, state law requires all health-care personnel authorized to diagnose or treat disorders to report within 10 days the full name and address of any patient who has been diagnosed as having a condition that could impair his or her ability to safely operate a motor vehicle. However, not all states require mandatory medical reporting and instead temper their recommendations (e.g., Arkansas' guidelines include "We do encourage unsafe driver's to be reported to our office"). An excellent resource that includes a review of state guidelines and descriptions of driving assessment methods is the "Physician's Guide to Assessing and Counseling Older Drivers" sponsored by the National Highway Traffic Safety Administration and available free from their website (http://www.nhtsa.gov/Senior-Drivers).

Driving is a complex behavior. To date, there remains much controversy about which clinical tools or methods are the best predictors of driving capacity. One important contribution that a clinical neuropsychologist can contribute to this process is to support the evaluation of driving capacity at multiple levels. The literature provides support that using a combination of measures can provide the best data for making recommendations. As clinical neuropsychologist, the most commonly requested contribution is the identification of the cognitive impairments that may impede driving performance. As clinicians specializing in brain–behavior relationship, we should recognize the complexity of this behavior and promote the evaluation of other domains affecting driving (i.e., vision, motor, psychological, and driving history). The integration of data from these various areas is a unique contribution that neuropsychologist can provide to patients and their families.

Clinical Pearls

- *Know the law.* State laws vary in their requirements for reporting and assessing drivers. Clinicians are strongly encouraged to be familiar with their individual state requirements (additional resources listed below).
- *Ask about driving.* Clinicians should be aware that driving cessation is often a topic of conflict. Too often, older adults do not raise the issue for fear of complete loss of driving privileges. Family members are also conflicted and in many cases are unsure about how to handle/raise the discussion. Clinicians can help minimize this conflict by including questions about driving performance in their regular checkups or appointments.
- *Know what cognitive domains are most relevant.* Although there is not a specific pattern or defined group of tests that 100% predict driving performance, general domains of cognition relevant to driving are identified in the literature. Neuropsychological test selection should be based upon empirical evidence with multiple abilities assessed under the domains of attention, information processing speed, working memory, executive functions, visual-spatial abilities, visual spatial learning, and memory.
- *Be familiar with the clinical driving evaluation process.* This includes identifying referral procedures and locations offering BTW evaluations with Certified Driving Rehabilitation Specialist (CDRS) accreditation. The neuropsychological evaluation should serve as guide to inform further evaluation of driving ability and should not serve as a substitute for a comprehensive driving evaluation.
- *Be familiar with age-related medical conditions* (i.e., dementia, stroke, seizures) that affect driving. Communication with the treating physician (i.e., neurologist, cardiologist) can help educate colleagues of the need to consider driving capacity.
- *Be on the lookout for medication effects.* Given the high number of medications commonly used by older adults, clinicians should consider the effect (individual or combined) of medications on driving behavior. Medications altering cognition, alertness, increasing fatigue, drowsiness, or altering sleep patterns may warrant consideration.
- *Potential driving cessation should be discussed as early as possible.* It is often beneficial to include significant others or additional family members in this dialogue as they may provide additional insight into driving performance.
- *Familiarize yourself with transportation options.* Clinicians have a responsibility to counsel and educate the patient and his or her family on the impact of relinquishing a driver's license. Being prepared with appropriate referrals (i.e., medical transportation services) or community information (i.e., transit schedules) can help adults begin to explore/plan alternate methods of transportation.
- *Consider interventions.* Interventions can benefit individuals who do not need to relinquish their driving privileges but require modification of their driving habits. These interventions can range from structured approaches (i.e., improving field of view) to more practical recommendations, such as restricting or limiting driving.

Appendix A. Additional Resources

- National Highway Traffic Safety Administration
  - Guidelines and strategies for working with older drivers; statistics on older driver's traffic safety (http://www.nhtsa.gov/Senior-Drivers).

- Association for Driver Rehabilitation Specialists
  - Includes a directory for locating a driver specialist in your area (http://www.aded.net).
- The Handbook for the Assessment of Driving Capacity (2009). Schulthies, MT., Deluca, J. and Chute, DL. Elsevier Publishers.
- CanDrive
  - Website for driving research with older adults; includes publications and other resources (http://www.candrive.ca/).

References

1. Fildes BN. Future directions for older driver research. Traffic Inj Prev. 2008;9:387–93.
2. Dobbs BM. Aging baby boomers: a blessing or challenge for driver licensing authorities. Traffic Inj Prev. 2008;9:379–86.
3. Martolli RA, de Leon CFM, Glass TA, Williams CS, Cooney LM, Berkman LF. Consequences of driving cessation: decreased out-of-home activity levels. J Gerontol B Psychol Sci Soc Sci. 2000;55:S334–40.
4. Oxley J, Whelan M. It cannot be all about safety: the benefit of prolonged mobility. Traffic Inj Prev. 2008;9:367–78.
5. Schultheis M, DeLuca J, Chute D, editors. Handbook for the assessment of driving capacity. New York: Academic; 2009.
6. Rizzo M, Uc EY, Dawson J, Anderson S, Rodnitzky R. Driving difficulties in Parkinson's disease. Mov Disord. 2010;25 Suppl 1:S136–40.
7. Heinrich HW, Petersen D, Roos N. Industrial accident prevention. New York: McGraw-Hill; 1980.
8. Maycock G. Accident liability: the human perspective. In: Rothengatter ET, Vaya EC, editors. Traffic and transport psychology: theory and application. Oxford: Pergamon; 1997. p. 65–76.
9. McGwin Jr G, Brown D. Characteristics of traffic crashes among young, middle-aged, and older drivers. Accid Anal Prev. 1999;31:181–98.
10. Langford J, Methorst R, Hakamies-Blomqvist L. Older drivers do not have a high crash risk-a replication of low mileage bias. Accid Anal Prev. 2006;38: 574–8.
11. Hakamies-Blomqvist L, Raitanen T, O'Neill D. Driver ageing does not cause higher accident rates per km. Transport Res F Traffic Psychol Behav. 2002;5: 271–4.
12. Ryan GA, Legge M, Rosman D. Age related changes in drivers' crash risk and crash type. Accid Anal Prev. 1998;30(3):379–87.
13. Hakamies-Blomqvist LE. Fatal accidents of older drivers. Accid Anal Prev. 1993;25(1):19–27.
14. Cooper PJ. Differences in accident characteristics among elderly drivers and between elderly and middle-aged drivers. Accid Anal Prev. 1990;22(5): 499–508.
15. Bao S, Boyle L. Driver performance at two-way stop-controlled intersections on divided highways. Transport Res Rec J Transport Res Board. 2008;2069: 26–32.
16. Retting RA, Weinstein HB, Solomon MG. Analysis of motor-vehicle crashes at stop signs in four US cities. J Safety Res. 2003;34:485–9.
17. Rizzo M, McGehee DV, Dawson JD, Anderson SN. Simulated car crashes at intersections in drivers with Alzheimer disease. Alzheimer Dis Assoc Disord. 2001;15(1):10–20.
18. Braitman KA, Kirley BB, Ferguson S, Chaudhary NK. Factors leading to older drivers' intersection crashes. Traffic Inj Prev. 2007;8(3):267–74.
19. Sen B, Najm WG, Smith JD. Analysis of lane change crashes, performed by John A. Volpe National Transportation System Center, Cambridge, MA. Washington DC: Department of Transportation, Administration NHTS; 2003.
20. Anstey KJ, Wood J, Lord S, Walker JG. Cognitive, sensory and physical factors enabling driving safety in older adults. Clin Psychol Rev. 2005;25(1):45–65.
21. Mathias JL, Lucas LK. Cognitive predictors of unsafe driving in older drivers: a meta-analysis. Int Psychogeriatr. 2009;21(4):637–53.
22. Dawson JD, Uc EY, Anderson SW, Johnson AM, Rizzo M. Neuropsychological predictors of driving errors in older adults. J Am Geriatr Soc. 2010;58(6):1090–6. doi:10.1111/j.1532-5415.2010.02872.x.
23. Munro CA, Jefferys J, Gower EW, et al. Predictors of lane change errors in older drivers. J Am Geriatr Soc. 2010;58:457–64.
24. Folstein MF, Folstein SE, McHugh PR. "Mini mental state": a practical method for grading the cognitive state of patients for the clinician. J Psychiatr Res. 1975;12:189–98.
25. Freund B, Colgrove LA. Error specific restrictions for older drivers: promoting continued independence and public safety. Accid Anal Prev. 2008;40(1):97–103.
26. Freund B, Gravenstein S, Ferris R, Burke BL, Shaheen E. Drawing clocks and driving cars. J Gen Intern Med. 2005;20(3):240–4.
27. Freund B, Colgrove LA, Petrakos D, McLeod R. In my car the brake is on the right: pedal errors among older drivers. Accid Anal Prev. 2008;40(1):403–9.
28. Zook NA, Bennett TL, Lane M. Identifying at-risk older adult community-dwelling drivers through neuropsychological evaluation. Appl Neuropsychol. 2009;16:281–7.
29. Friedland RP, Koss E, Kumar A, et al. Motor vehicle crashes in dementia of the Alzheimer type. Ann Neurol. 1988;24(6):782–6.
30. Carr DB, Duchek J, Morris JC. Characteristics of motor vehicle crashes of drivers with dementia of the Alzheimer type. J Am Geriatr Soc. 2000;48(1):18–22.
31. Uc EY, Rizzo M, Anderson SW, Shi Q, Dawson JD. Unsafe rear-end collision avoidance in Alzheimer's disease. J Neurol Sci. 2006;251(1–2):35–43.

32. Dawson JD, Anderson SW, Uc EY, Dastrup E, Rizzo M. Predictors of driving safety in early Alzheimer disease. Neurology. 2009;72(6):521–7.
33. Duchek JM, Carr DB, Hunt L, et al. Longitudinal driving performance in early-stage dementia of the Alzheimer type. J Am Geriatr Soc. 2003;51(10): 1342–7.
34. Ott BR, Heindel WC, Papandonatos GD, et al. A longitudinal study of drivers with Alzheimer's disease. Neurology. 2008;70:1171–8.
35. Hughes CP, Berg L, Danziger WL, Coben LA, Martin RL. A new clinical scale for the staging of dementia. Br J Psychiatry. 1982;140:566–72.
36. Boyle L, Lee JD. Using driving simulators to assess driving safety. Accid Anal Prev. 2010;42:785–7.
37. Reger MA, Welsh RK, Watson GS, Cholerton B, Baker LD, Craft S. The relationship between neuropsychological functioning and driving ability in dementia: a meta-analysis. Neuropsychology. 2004;18(1):85–93.
38. Cohen J. A power primer. Psychol Bull. 1992;112: 155–9.
39. Ott BR, Festa EK, Amick MM, Grace J, Davis JD, Heindel WC. Computerized maze navigation and on-road performance by drivers with dementia. J Geriatr Psychiatry Neurol. 2008;21(1):18–25.
40. Grace J, Amick MM, D'Abreu A, Festa EK, Heindel WC, Ott BR. Neuropsychological deficits associated with driving performance in Parkinson's and Alzheimer's disease. J Int Neuropsychol Soc. 2005; 11(6):766–75.
41. Cordell R, Lee HC, Granger A, Vieira B, Lee AH. Driving assessment in Parkinson's disease—a novel predictor of performance? Mov Disord. 2008;23(9): 1217–22.
42. Uc EY, Rizzo M, Johnson AM, Dastrup E, Anderson SW, Dawson JD. Road safety in drivers with Parkinson disease. Neurology. 2009;73(24):2112–9.
43. Singh R, Pentland B, Hunter J, Provan F. Parkinson's disease and driving ability. J Neurol Neurosurg Psychiatry. 2007;78:363–6.
44. Amick MM, Grace J, Ott BR. Visual and cognitive predictors of driving safety in Parkinson's disease patients. Arch Clin Neuropsychol. 2007;22(8):957–67.
45. Ball K, Owsley C, Sloane ME, Roenker DL, Bruni JR. Visual attention problems as a predictor of vehicle crashes in older drivers. Invest Ophthalmol Vis Sci. 1993;34(11):3110–23.
46. Devos H, Vandenberghe W, Nieuwboer A, Tant M, Baten G, De Weerdt W. Predictors of fitness to drive in people with Parkinson disease. Neurology. 2007;69(14):1434–41.
47. Flicker C, Ferris SH, Reisberg B. Mild cognitive impairment in the elderly: predictors of dementia. Neurology. 1991;41(7):1006–9.
48. Petersen RC, Smith GE, Waring SC, Ivnik RJ, Tangalos EG, Kokmen E. Mild cognitive impairment: clinical characterization and outcome. Arch Neurol. 1999;56(3):303–8.
49. Wadley VG, Okonkwo O, Crowe M, et al. Mild cognitive impairment and everyday function: an investigation of driving performance. J Geriatr Psychiatry Neurol. 2009;22(2):87–94.
50. Petersen RC. Mild cognitive impairment as a diagnostic entity. J Intern Med. 2004;256:183–94.
51. Jurica PJ, Leitten CL, Mattis S: DRS-2: Dementia Rating Scale-2. Professional Manual. Lutz, FL, Psychological Resources, 2004.
52. Brandt J, Aretouli E, Neijstrom E, et al. Selectivity of executive function deficits in mild cognitive impairment. Neuropsychology. 2009;23(5):607–18.
53. Hopewell CA. Driving assessment issues for practicing clinicians. J Head Trauma Rehabil. 2002;17: 48–61.
54. Iverson DJ, Gronseth GS, Reger MA, Classen S, Dubinsky RM, Rizzo M. Practice parameter update: evaluation and management of driving risk in dementia. Neurology. 2010;74:1316–24.
55. Korner-Bitensky N, Bitensky J, Sofer S, Man-Son-Hing M, Gelinas I. Driving evaluation practices of clinicians working in the United States and Canada. Am J Occup Ther. 2006;60:428–34.
56. Clay OJ, Wadley VG, Edwards JD, Roth DL, Roenker DL, Ball KK. Cumulative meta-analysis of the relationship between useful field of view and driving performance in older adults: current and future implications. Optom Vis Sci. 2005;82(8):724–31.
57. Bedard M, Weaver B, Darzins P, Porter MM. Predicting driving performance in older adults: we are not there yet! Traffic Inj Prev. 2008;9(4):336–41.
58. Langford J. Usefulness of off-road screening tests to licensing authorities when assessing older driver fitness to drive. Traffic Inj Prev. 2008;9(4):328–35.
59. Lotfipour S, Vaca F. Commentary: polypharmacy and older drivers: beyond the doors of the emergency department for patient safety. Ann Emerg Med. 2007;49:535–7.
60. Ray WA, Thapa PB, Shorr RI. Medications and the older driver. Clin Geriatr Med. 1993;9(2):413–38.
61. LeRoy AA, Morse ML. Multiple medications and vehicle crashes: analysis of databases. Washington, DC: Department of Transportation, Administration NHTS; 2008.
62. Lococo KH, Staplin L. Literature review of polypharmacy and older drivers: identifying strategies to collect drug usage and driving functioning among older drivers. Washington, DC: US Department of Transportation, Administration NHTS; 2006.
63. Okonkwo O, Griffith HR, Vance DE, Marson DC, Ball K, Wadley V. Awareness of functional difficulties in mild cognitive impairment: a multidomain assessment approach. J Am Geriatr Soc. 2009;57:978–84.
64. Blanchard RA, Myers A, Porter MM. Correspondence between self-reported and objective measures of driving exposure and patterns in older drivers. Accid Anal Prev. 2010;42:523–9.
65. Windsor TD, Anstey KJ. Interventions to reduce the adverse psychosocial impact of driving cessation on older adults. Clin Interv Aging. 2006;1:205–11.
66. Kua A, Korner-Bitensky N, Desrosiers J, Man-Son-Hing M, Marshall S. Older drivers retraining: a systematic

review of evidence of effectiveness. J Safety Res. 2007;38:81–90.
67. De Raedt R, Ponjaert-Kristoffersen I. Predicting at-fault car accidents of older drivers. Accid Anal Prev. 2001;33:809–19.
68. Staplin L, Gish KW, Wagner EK. MaryPODS revisited: updated crash analysis and implications for screening program implementation. J Safety Res. 2003;34(4):389–97.
69. Ball KK, Roenker DL, Wadley VG, et al. Can high-risk older drivers be identified through performance-based measures in a department of motor vehicle setting? J Am Geriatr Soc. 2005;54:77–84.
70. Richardson ED, Martolli RA. Visual attention and driving behaviors among community-living older persons. J Gerontol A Biol Sci Med Sci. 2003;58: M832–6.
71. Whelihan WM, DiCarlo MA, Paul RH. The relationship of neuropsychological functioning to driving competence in older persons with early cognitive decline. Arch Clin Neuropsychol. 2005;20:217–28.
72. Smith A. Symbol digits modalities test. Los Angeles: Western Psychological Services; 1982.
73. Worringham CJ, Wood J, Kerr GK, Silburn PA. Predictors of driving assessment outcome in Parkinson's disease. Mov Disord. 2005;21:230–5.
74. War Department, Adjutant General's Office. Army Individual Test Battery. Manual for directions and scoring. Washington, DC: War Department, Adjutant General's Office; 1944.
75. Schretlen D, Bobholz J, Brandt J. Development and psychometric properties of the brief test of attention. Clin Neuropsychol. 1996;10:80–9.
76. Oswanski MF, Sharma OP, Raj SS, et al. Evaluation of two assessment tools in predicting driving ability of senior drivers. Am J Phys Med Rehabil. 2007;86: 190–9.
77. Salthouse TA, Mitchell DJ, Skovronek E, Babcock RL. Effects of adult age and working memory on reasoning and spatial abilities. J Exp Psychol Learn Mem Cogn. 1989;15:507–13.
78. Daigneault G, Joly P, Frigon J. Executive functions in the evaluation of accident risk of older drivers. J Clin Exp Neuropsychol. 2002;24:221–38.
79. Shallice T. Specific impairments of planning. Philos Trans R Soc Lond B Biol Sci. 1982;298:199–209.
80. Grant DA, Berg E. A behavioral analysis of degree of reinforcement and ease of shifting to new responses in a Weigl-type card-sorting problem. J Exp Psychol. 1948;38:404–11.
81. Benton AL, Varney N, Hamsher K. Visuospatial judgment: a clinical test. Arch Neurol. 1978;35: 364–7.
82. Wechsler D. Wechsler Adult Intelligence Scale. 3rd ed. San Antonio: Psychological Corporation; 1997.
83. Beery K, Buktenica N, Beery N. Beery-Buktenica Developmental Test of Visual-Motor Integration. Upper Saddle River: Pearson; 2010.
84. Benton Sivian A. Benton Visual Retention Test. 5th ed. Upper Saddle River: Pearson; 1991.
85. Brandt J, Benedict RH. Hopkins Verbal Learning Test—Revised. Professional manual. Lutz: Psychological Assessment Resources; 2001.
86. Instrument L. Grooved pegboard user instructions. Lafayette: Lafayette Instrument; 2002.
87. Heaton RK, Miller SW, Taylor MJ, Grant I. Revised comprehensive norms for an expanded halstead-reitan battery: demographically adjusted neuropsychological norms for African American and Caucasian adults. Lutz: Psychological Assessment Resources; 2004.
88. Wechsler D. Wechsler Adult Intelligence Scale. Revised edition. San Antonio: Psychological Corporation; 1981.
89. Carr DB, Schwartzberg JG, Manning L, Sempek J. Physician's guide to assessing and counseling older drivers. 2nd ed. Washington, DC: Administration NHTS; 2010.

Environmental Design for Cognitive Decline

11

Rosemary Bakker

Abstract

Cognitive decline, especially substantial changes associated with Alzheimer's disease and other dementias, significantly changes how individuals interact with their home environment. The nature and extent of these changes are highly individual and in constant flux, and are influenced by neuropathology, normal age-related changes in physical and mental functions, medications, as well as specifics in the patient's home environment. One consistent observation is that sensitivity to the environment increases sharply with the onset of dementia. As a clinician, it is important to understand the functional challenges that the typical unadapted home presents to a dementia patient, and the guiding principles for a dementia-friendly living space. Equipped with this information, clinicians can serve as a frontline resource, advising patients and their families about practical home management strategies to enhance safety, performance of daily skills, and quality of life.

Keywords

Dementia home safety • Falls • Activities of daily living • Wandering • Smart home technology • Memory aides • Alzheimer's caregiving • Agitation • Monitoring

Environmental design is an underutilized yet effective treatment option in helping patients with cognitive decline maintain function with fewer behavioral problems [1]. In this chapter, key design solutions (e.g., memory aides, interior design, and smart home technologies) will be explored that can help patients and their caregivers lead safer and more satisfactory lives. Environmental design cannot stand alone as a therapeutic modality; therefore, the importance of the psychosocial environment, with guidelines on how caregivers can best elicit cooperation and trust from their loved ones, will be addressed. Table 11.1 highlights environment-related changes in function and perception commonly associated with dementia.

R. Bakker, M.S., ASID. (✉)
Division of Geriatrics, Department of Medicine, Weill Cornell Medical College, 525 E. 68th Street, Box 39, New York, NY 10065, USA
e-mail: rob2013@med.cornell.edu

L.D. Ravdin and H.L. Katzen (eds.), *Handbook on the Neuropsychology of Aging and Dementia*, Clinical Handbooks in Neuropsychology, DOI 10.1007/978-1-4614-3106-0_11,

Table 11.1 Environment-related changes of function and perception in dementia patients

Visual/spatial	*Hearing*
Problems with visual/spatial perception if foreground and background are not color contrasted (e.g., reduced food intake can occur if food and plate are the same color)	Inability to focus due to excessive background noise
Perceptual distortion caused by highly patterned flooring, seating, or wall covering	Confusion or agitation in noisy environments
Inability to recognize their own image (e.g., in the mirror or in a bare reflective window)	Loss of ability to interpret sounds accurately; underlying hearing disorders can also predispose a person toward auditory misperceptions (e.g., sound of telephone perceived as small dog barking)
Visual misinterpretations in low lighting	
Problems with object recognition with similarly shaped objects (e.g., waste basket mistaken for toilet bowl)	
Mobility	*Memory/judgment*
Difficulty in walking caused by changes in gait and balance, especially if area carpets and door sills are present	Problems with sequential tasks
Stair climbing difficulties – lack of handrails – only one handrail, if patient has a one-side weakness due to a stroke – risers and steps in the same color	Problems with short-term memory (e.g., forgetting food cooking on stove) Inability to focus Way finding issues and getting lost, even within the home Inappropriate judgment (e.g., putting clothes in the microwave to dry)
Forgetting they cannot walk unassisted	
Forgetting to use their walker or inability to learn how to use it	
Restricted access due to narrow doorways or lack of stair alternatives during wheelchair usage in the late stages	

Caregiver Challenges

Fluctuation in Skills and Behaviors

Patient skills, behavior, and memory can fluctuate from day to day or even within a single day, making it difficult for individuals or families to know how to intervene. Robert C took his wife for testing as he could no longer cope with her changes in memory and judgment; she was regularly flooding the apartment, forgetting that the bath water was running. An accomplished cook for 50 years, she had recently roasted a frozen chicken in the oven without removing the plastic wrapping. Yet he reports, there are days when she still seems "normal."

Unusual Behaviors

Patients may engage in unusual or unsafe behaviors that are particularly challenging to cope with, like hoarding or wandering. Mistaken perceptions can occur in low-light levels and in shadowy areas, sometimes leading to calls to the police due to "strangers in the room." Low-stress thresholds are common and seemingly minor events, such as the noise of a loud television or dishwasher, can act as a trigger for an extreme reaction. It is not surprising that more than 40% of caregivers of persons with cognitive decline rate the emotional stress of caregiving as high or very high [2], and that 34% of caregivers report needing more help with keeping the person safe at home [3].

Lack of Insight

Patients with cognitive decline often have limited insight that there is anything wrong, making it difficult for the clinician or family member to openly discuss dementia or safety issues for fear of upsetting the patient. For example, the patient may not remember that he or she has been leaving the stove on or getting lost on the way home from a shopping excursion. As a clinician, you may need to broach performance of daily activities gently, noting any resistance, and get permission from the patient to speak privately with the caregiver later on, if necessary.

Cognitive Decline or Poor Design?

When a patient has impaired function, it is commonly assumed that the problem is cognitive decline rather than the interaction between the patient and the environment. Consider the following example: On a very hot summer day, the author reported to the assisted-living staff that her mother was in her room—agitated and without air conditioning; the staff replied that her Alzheimer's had progressed and she could no longer operate her air conditioner. Upon further investigation, however, the lack of function was not due to dementia. Rather, her mother simply could not read the lettering on the air conditioner's control panel because the font was too small and the contrast between the font and the background color too low. She was not able to understand the problem, but she did express her frustration over the poor design as the discussion ensued. "Why do they do that? Why do they make your brain work so hard?" Applying an On/Off label in a large black font against a white background quickly restored her function—and her well-being.

An environment that is suited for individuals with cognitive impairments does not happen spontaneously, it takes understanding and planning. Without understanding the environment's effect on a patient's behavior, many caregivers blame declining abilities on the disease and may not engage in preventive measures. In some cases, the interventions are too restrictive, not allowing for meaningful participation by the patient. For example, if a patient forgets a couple of steps in the bathing process due to problems with sequential tasks, the caregiver may take over all steps, which often causes resentment on both sides.

Finding Out What Works

Clinicians should stress to caregivers that design and behavioral strategies need to be individualized and continually reassessed; strategies that are effective for some may only work briefly or not at all in different situations. Throughout this chapter, individualized approaches to challenging situations will be highlighted, to illustrate the wide variety of responses in this population.

Ongoing Safety and Design Issues

Caregivers should keep in mind that providing for the safety of their loved ones is an *ongoing challenge as the disease progresses*. As one caregiver recently remarked, "Even when you think you have resolved a problem, you have no clue as to what is going to hit you in the face the next day." To help reduce challenging behaviors when adapting the home environment, changes should be phased in gradually whenever possible, and caregivers should be instructed to observe how the person responds and switch course when and if necessary. If the caregiver is planning on keeping their loved one at home for as long as possible, consideration should be given to increasing the home's accessibility (e.g., wider doorways, ramps, walk-in showers, etc.).

The Environment as a Therapeutic Modality

Reducing Environmental Triggers of Agitation

It is common for caregivers to report that their loved ones are easily agitated, but when the patient's behavior is explored in greater detail, there is usually a specific event preceding the agitation that acts as a trigger for that behavior. If a patient presents with a new history of agitation, ask the caregiver to think back to the activity or conversation that took place prior to the behavior. For example, if a caregiver states that their loved one becomes agitated during bathing, ask them to document exactly when the agitation begins. Was the patient uncomfortable while disrobing, fearful of getting into or out of the bathtub, anxious when the water was turned on, or when their body was washed? Caregivers can be advised to keep a journal and document the behavioral incidents. If the cause is external, whether it is precipitated by environmental factors or by caregiver interaction, the caregiver can then act to change or modify the trigger(s) and the associated agitation [4–7].

Common triggers for agitation include environmental factors and caregiver interaction, including:

- Noise
- Room temperature
- Standard bathing techniques
- Lack of stimulation
- Overstimulation
- Denial of access
- Tasks too complicated for person's current abilities
- Caregiver tone of voice
- Caregiver behavior (e.g., controlling)

Monitoring the Effects of Interventions

It is not always clear if a person can safely engage in an activity, and balancing risk and freedom is an ongoing challenge for caregivers. At some point, the caregiver may need to set certain items or areas of the household off-limits. Most standard home safety checklists recommend denying access to "safety hazards" but do not mention that sometimes the solution causes a new problem. Patient A may simply walk away if they can no longer turn the stove on (after removal of the knobs) or open a newly locked cabinet door, but patient B may become so frustrated that they attempt to remove the lock or the door or even tear the room apart. Ron G removed the knobs and installed child safety covers on the stove before he went to work so that his mother would not cook when he was not at home; this is a common home safety recommendation. Left alone all day, his mother became so agitated that she dismantled the stove and emptied the kitchen cabinets onto the floor and countertops. Ron G was overwhelmed by this severe reaction and felt he had no choice but to place her in a nursing home. This outcome may have been prevented, or at least postponed, if he had been warned of the potential for negative outcomes and had been able to monitor the situation.

Memory Aides for Earlier Stages

In the early to mid stages, depending on the extent of the cognitive loss, reminder signs with simple language, large-sized text, and personalized images, act as an "external brain," giving needed instruction for daily living. The image and text used *must* be customized for the person and large enough to capture their attention, or the intervention will not be effective [4]. Here are a few successful examples:

1. Cecilia G remembered to brush her teeth if simple instructions were placed in her direct view:
   (a) Put toothpaste on toothbrush.
   (b) Brush teeth.
2. Arlene S identified her room when a photo of herself from her earlier days was placed on the door. But for Ed T, a former corn researcher, it was a dried corn arrangement, not a personal portrait, which enabled him to recognize his apartment door.

Finding Lost Items

Losing and searching for belongings is a common and frustrating activity; organizational strategies may be helpful for those experiencing mild cognitive decline. For example, a patient may be able to learn to place their keys in one location, especially if it is visually easy to identify, as in a bright red bowl on an uncluttered foyer table. A sign (text and icon) reminding the patient to place the keys in the bowl can help reinforce the new behavior. Electronic finder devices can also reduce distressing time spent on finding objects. The patient may not be able to learn how to use the device or may misplace the device, but caregivers have successfully used locator devices for some patients with good results [5]. As one caregiver said, "I used to get so anxious when I visited my dad, as we would spend a lot of time searching for his keys and then we would both be in a bad mood. Now, when I visit, I use the locator device, which I keep on my key ring and within minutes, I find his keys. Now we spend more time on enjoyable activities."

Visual Misperceptions and Visual Dysfunction

Problems with Depth Perception

Many patients experience visual dysfunction when there is lack of contrast, causing significant problems with depth perception. Lack of contrast makes it harder or impossible to identify objects that are set against a background of similar colors. For example, a patient may walk right past a white toilet on a white wall and continue to search for the toilet, but a color-contrasted toilet seat can enhance object recognition and may help the person remain continent for a longer period of time [6]. Patterned carpeting or carpets with dark contrasting borders also be difficult for patients with visuospatial difficulties; some individuals may not perceive the floor to be level and may attempt to jump or step over patterns or borders.

Misperception and the Environment

Some individuals have difficulty differentiating objects, especially those that have similar shapes, such as a patient who mistakes the wastebasket (oval shape) for the toilet bowl (oval shape). Others may be unable to recognize themselves in a mirror or misperceive what's there. For example, he or she may see a stranger and not themselves in the mirror or think that their own reflection in a dark window at night is a stranger. And some may see frightening shapes, like a crouching person in a large houseplant in dim lighting, or animals in a swirling, patterned fabric or carpet. Others have difficulty differentiating reality from representation. They may perceive people in photographs as real and refuse to undress or even get upset if the photograph does not respond when spoken to. If a violent TV show is on, they may think the event is actually happening right in their room. The person may become so frightened that they call the police.

The following interventions can reduce or eliminate the misperceptions, depending on the cause:

- Remove wastebaskets from bathrooms.
- Remove or cover mirrors.
- Turn photographs around (or remove, if necessary).
- Close blinds or drapes early at night.
- Increase light levels.
- Control TV viewing.
- Replace patterned furnishings.

Lighting and Function

Appropriate lighting can improve overall quality of life for people with dementia, though this is often overlooked. It can reduce the environmental misperceptions that occur in low-light conditions. Appropriate lighting can also significantly improve visual function due to age-associated visual loss [7]. Mark P regularly led the congregation during prayer service, but when he began stumbling over words, everyone thought it was due to the progression of his dementia. But after a new overhead light was installed, his reading skills went back to normal.

Mobility and Falls

Patients with dementia fall two to three times more often than individuals without cognitive impairments [8]. Patients experience not only normal age-related vision and mobility changes

Table 11.2 Common dementia-related risk factors for falls

Inability to housekeep, maintain a home, or hoarding behavior can create mounds of clutter and other home hazards
Reduced attention and/or depth perception can make certain objects, like doorsills and low tables, less noticeable and are common causes for tripping
Lowered stress thresholds and becoming easily agitated; storming off or possibly striking out and losing balance
Fear of falling and, consequently, not walking much, which further increases fall risk; reduced exercises leads to weakened muscles and stiff joints
Impaired memory and judgment can cause risky behaviors, such as descending steep stairs in the dark, searching for a mother or adult child the person believes is still in his/her care
Changes in perception and balance can cause problems, such as knowing where to place one's feet going up or down stairs, walking with a shuffle, and getting one's foot caught on area rugs or doorsills, or holding onto unsteady furniture

that increase fall risk but also dementia-related challenges increase the incidence of unsafe situations. Table 11.2 lists common dementia-related risk factors for falls.

Strategies to Reduce Falls

There are a variety of environmental strategies to employ depending on the patient's fall risk factors. Below is a list of key interventions:

- Remove area carpets and doorsills, especially if patient shuffles.
- Clear clutter (crates and baskets can be used to store clutter outside of walkways if patient is upset at removal).
- Remove low tables, especially glass.
- Provide for accessibility:
  - Ramps
  - Walk-in showers
  - Bath and shower chairs
  - Use compensatory measures:
  - Highlight edges of steps for better visibility
  - Color contrast seating, bedding, and toilet seat to floor
- Monitor high fall areas with sensors or weight-sensitive chair, bed, or floor pads to alert caregiver when person attempts to transfer or use stairs independently when it is no longer safe to do so.

Challenges with Stair Climbing

At some point, the individual may have difficulty climbing stairs, especially if there are no handrails. One-sided handrails can be problematic for an individual with weakness on the side as the handrail (e.g., due to a stroke). Risers and steps that are similar in color can also pose a challenge. If the patient is unsure of their step or becomes agitated when climbing stairs, a 2-in. strip of bright tape applied along the edge of the step may help them better distinguish the tread from the riser [9]. When it is too dangerous for someone to use the stairs without supervision, the caregiver needs to limit access. A monitoring device, such as a motion sensor, should be used. A motion sensor with a remote alert can notify the caregiver, even in another room, when the patient approaches the staircase. Advance notice may give the caregiver the time they need to be at the patient's side to offer assistance. A baby monitor may or may not work, depending on the amount of noise a person makes walking across a room. Denying access to the stairs using gates or locked doors may be necessary at times, but it should be done with caution and frequent monitoring, especially when the person is accustomed to using the stairs freely. Child safety gates are specifically designed for children, not for the strength or height of an adult. Some individuals may simply turn around and walk away when faced with a child safety gate, but others may attempt to open the gate, or worse, climb over it.

Electric Stair Lifts

Sometimes people ask if a patient with dementia can use an electric stair chair lift. There is little research on this topic, but problems with fear of falling should be expected, as most patients have little or no experience with using a "chair" that automatically moves up and down the stairs. Step-by-step instructions *before starting the chair lift* could help reduce fears. It may also be a good idea for the caregiver to walk behind the person and offer support, telling their loved one that they are safe, and they will not fall.

Wandering

Wandering and getting lost are serious problems for patients with dementia, especially since it happens so unpredictably. A patient can wander off unexpectedly, even when the caregiver thinks they are safe. It is not unusual that someone with dementia may leave their home in an effort to get to a job they no longer have, or they may go searching for someone they truly believe is still in their care, such as a child who is now fully grown. They may leave home desperately searching for their "real" home because they no longer recognize where they are living. The patient may pace and constantly move about, increasing their chances of getting lost. Finally, they may become agitated and storm off; they may be bored, disturbed by too much noise, or upset by side effects from certain medications.

What makes wandering difficult is that most people are so accustomed to leaving home whenever they wish, and individuals with dementia are no exception. At some point in the disease, the patient *will* get lost if they go out alone, and we cannot predict when that moment will come. Wandering typically occurs during the middle stages of AD, when many other disease symptoms are present. However, caregivers have brought their loved ones in for testing only *after* a serious wandering episode, stating that there was no warning that there was anything to be concerned about. It can be a shocking way to learn that the dementia process has begun.

There has been little research on which wandering solutions work best in different situations and environments, so trying to find the best strategies to deal with wandering can be challenging. How well any intervention works depends on a number of factors, including the patient's temperament, the stage of the disease, their environment, and, of course, the product or strategy employed. For example, a patient may become very agitated by locked doors, refuse to carry a tracking device like a cell phone, or wear a special monitoring device on their wrist. Further, GPS and other tracking devices do not work in all environments. Since no *single* strategy will work in all situations, it is best to recommend that the caregiver try several to see which ones work best for their situation. Combining several strategies is preferred for backup safety; for example, using both an ID bracelet as well as a monitoring device that alerts the caregiver to an open door.

Pilot studies of a nighttime home wandering monitoring system, consisting of room and bed occupancy sensors, door alarms with remote alerts, and a communication panel at the caregiver's bedside showed potential for improved caregiver well-being and quality of sleep [10], reduced injuries, and unattended home exits by persons with dementia [11]. *Redirecting* an individual's attention from leaving home to a preferred activity is a powerful preventive tool. Many patients have decreased initiation but can participate if someone else can initiate the activity for them. Going outside when the weather permits can also reduce "cooped up" feelings and associated agitation. Refer to the section on wandering at *ThisCaringHome.org* for prevention strategies; there are also reviews and descriptions of electronic devices that can help find the patient if they wander and cannot find their way home.

Chair and Bed Transfers

Assisting an adult in the sit-to-stand transfer is one of the most difficult and dangerous tasks for a caregiver, putting them at risk for injury [12]. Caregivers, especially novice caregivers, often provide more physical help than is needed, not knowing how else to proceed, and physical support is usually not performed in an ergonomically correct manner [13]. Difficulties with transferring are usually due to a combination of factors, including furniture design, the individual's health, memory, and response to the caregiver (e.g., many patients do not respond favorably to a caregiver's request to get up from a chair or bed).

Chairs

For most people with adequate strength and function, it is much easier to get up from an ergonomic chair (not too low or deep, with an opening under the seat, and side arms) than from a sofa or an easy chair, because the necessary body movements are much easier on the joints and muscles. Even individuals with Parkinson's disease who are rigid and frequently lean forward can get in and out of a good chair, especially if they rock back and forth and rise on the count of three.

Motorized, lift-up chairs can be extremely helpful when the person has severely limited movement or refuses to sleep in bed, as the chair can be put in a reclining position. Caregivers should be forewarned that a lift chair is best used with a caregiver present, as the controls are typically difficult for persons with dementia to use. A fall could occur if a person attempts to climb out of a chair that is in the reclining position. Additionally, some patients become frightened when the chair starts to move without warning, so the caregiver should tell the person what is going to happen *before* they lower or raise the chair, even if they think the person will not understand.

Beds

A mattress with the appropriate degree of firmness will be comfortable for the patient to sleep on and easier to push off from when getting out of bed. For many individuals, the most suitable bed height for a comfortable transfer is 18 in. Before attempting to help a person out of bed, instruct the caregiver to give a good reason to get up. In addition, a warm, gentle voice can do wonders. The right type of bed handle can help a person get out of bed and stand, as it offers a stable surface to hold onto and push off from, it can also help with balance. To use a bed handle safely, the person still needs good upper body strength and the ability to stand and bear weight. The bed handle should attach *securely* to the bed frame.

Impact of Memory Issues on Transfers

Although it may be hard to imagine, people with dementia sometimes forget how to get out of a chair or bed, therefore providing instructions may be helpful. Gloria T had been physically helping her husband to get up from his chair and bed, but was experiencing significant back problems. The author recommended that her husband be assessed for function to see if he still had adequate ability to help with transferring. A physical therapist's assessment showed that he had adequate transfer function and taught Gloria T "coaching" techniques to replace her physical assistance. She now offers simple step-by-step instructions, including visual cueing, like tapping the edge of the seat or bed, and physical cues, like placing one hand on his lower back and one on his shoulder to gently guide him forward. The caregiver's attitude and physical approach is an important aspect of the person's willingness to get up. Approaching the patient with a positive attitude and offering an inviting reason to get up can provide needed encouragement. To reduce feelings of intimidation and "power struggles," the caregiver should be advised to be at eye level with the patient (e.g., sit next to patient or kneel down at bedside) while inviting the patient to an enjoyable activity.

Meal Preparation, Cooking, and Dining

Organizational Strategies and Cues

Although many patients may no longer be able to cook a full meal, most can participate in a limited way with the proper instruction and kitchen organization. It is hard for anyone to find items in a cluttered environment, especially, if the storage areas are not well marked. Patients in the early stages or their caregivers can be advised to group similar items together (e.g., breakfast foods items). If the patient forgets to look inside the cupboards or drawers, signs and pictures can be put up on the outside to help him locate objects behind closed doors or drawers. If this does not work, a cupboard door can be removed. The most used items can also be left on the countertop, in see-through containers, labeled in large letters to help alert the patient as to their contents. Gregg T was able to prepare his breakfast on his own, but only when his wife set out all ingredients beforehand and left simple instructions.

Cooking Challenges

Use of cooking appliances when an individual's memory is impaired is a major safety concern [14]. Devices that automatically turn off appliances left on inadvertently can proactively help to avert crises and extend a patient's ability to cook, as long as the patient still has good stove skills and judgment. For example, Jon B installed a device to turn off the stove for his wife's nighttime cup of tea. He felt she was safe cooking independently but wanted assurance that if she were to forget and leave the stove on, it would automatically shut off after a set period of time (he chose 3 min, long enough for the kettle to boil). Alternatively, cooking appliances are available that may be safer to use for a certain subgroup of patients, including electric teakettles that automatically turn off after the water boils and microwaves with easy one-button cooking.

Not everyone, however, will be able to use a new appliance or learn a new way of cooking, *no matter how minor*. Caregivers who have replaced a gas stove with an electric stove are sometimes shocked to discover that their loved one cannot learn how to use it. Smart devices and safer household appliances can be very helpful, but they do not replace caregiver oversight. Caregivers should be advised to *frequently* assess the patient's cooking skills and judgment, for example:

- Do they still know which cookware is safe to use or do they put plastic containers on lit burners or metal containers in the microwave?
- Might an electric teakettle be placed on a hot burner?
- Do they know that paper plates that are safe to use in the microwave oven are not safe in the toaster oven?

Eating and Nutritional Status

Nutritional status can be affected by a myriad of factors, including lighting, table and tableware, food choice and appearance, cueing, and tablemates (for those living in a facility). Often, eating challenges can be overcome with a bit of trial and error.

Inadequate lighting and lack of color contrast can lead to reduced nutritional intake [15].

- High contrast between the dinnerware and the tabletop is now included in design regulations for dementia specific units in some assisted-living and nursing home residences.
- Printed tablecloths decorated with fruit may cause the cloth to be picked at instead of the actual food; therefore, plain tablecloths and placemats are recommended.
- A person's food or liquid intake can be inadequate if the drinking glass or utensils cannot be easily grasped; built-up handles and appropriate-sized glasses are the key.
- Choice of food items, texture, portion, and arrangement are critical for encouraging appetite. Some individuals will refuse to eat from a plate piled high with food or if more than one food is served at one time.
- Many patients have changes in olfactory and taste perceptions; unusual flavor combinations or excessive desire for sweets are not uncommon [16]. Caregivers report that their loved one's appetites have increased when they added sauces to dishes, including salsa, honey mustard, maple syrup, or ketchup. The choice of flavors and their combination is very

individual so it is important that the caregiver experiment to see what the patient responds to most favorably.
- Verbal cueing (e.g., "place the fork in your hand") and physical cueing (placing a fork in their hand) may encourage greater independence.
- Some individuals who can no longer manipulate utensils may be able to eat independently if finger foods are offered (e.g., baked fries or fish sticks). A key to success is to serve only foods that require like utensils at a given time, otherwise confusion can occur over which food items require the use of a utensil.

Hygiene

Bathing and Agitation

Bathing a person with dementia is one of the most stressful activities for a caregiver. It can also be an emotionally demanding experience for the patient, who may be stressed by fear of running water, discomfort in a cold drafty room, embarrassment at being seen undressed, fear of falling (especially when moving in or out of the tub), or confusion due to memory problems. The person may think he or she has already bathed, or may be simply overwhelmed by the bathing process itself, no longer understanding what to do or how to do it. Dementia-friendly bathing techniques can be highly effective in reducing bathing agitation. In the video, *Bathing Without a Battle*, nursing home residents who previously yelled, hit, and cursed during a standard bath are shown relaxing and thanking the aide for their help after the aide had received specialized training [17, 18]. If a patient refuses to bathe or experiences agitation during bathing, consider referring the caregiver to techniques such as:
- Warming up the room before the bath (feeling cold can be a stressor).
- Using a specially designed bathing privacy outfit (lack of privacy can be a stressor).
- Using a handheld shower and avoiding spraying water onto the head and facial area (overly sensitive areas in many patients with dementia).
- Placing a color-contrasted towel on the bath chair for enhanced depth perception and using a color-contrasted bath mat in the tub for a full immersion (so the person can judge the depth of the tub to reduce fear of drowning).

Toileting

Some individuals become incontinent simply because they cannot find the bathroom. They may not be able to distinguish the bathroom door from the surrounding doors, or they may have completely forgotten the bathroom's location [4]. If they are in the early to mid stage, the patient may be able to find the bathroom using the following techniques:
- Placing a large sign on the door.
- Painting the door a bright color.
- Leaving the light on in the bathroom or hallway.

Another common problem is forgetting to use toilet tissue. Increased odor and infection risk are key concerns. Reminder notes and verbal prompts can be helpful for some, but do not work for everyone. Bidet toilet seats have been used as a substitute for paper in Continental Europe and Asia for many years. There are separate units or those that attach to an existing toilet, with push button controls for washing and drying, allowing the user to wash after each use. Bidet toilet seats can increase the person's cleanliness, but they are expensive, and they require a caregiver present as operating new controls and a new way to toilet would be beyond the skills of most patients with cognitive loss.

Dressing

Patients with cognitive decline commonly experience clothing and dressing problems [19]. For example, the individual may no longer be able to organize and sort clothing and, therefore, leave piles of clothing scattered about or mix dirty clothes with clean clothes. At some point, dressing may require more skills than the patient possesses. For example, they may forget the order in which to put on various clothing items, they may wear too little or too many layers of clothing, or they may refuse/forget to change clothing when needed. Often, the patient may resist help and become terribly agitated when the caregiver tries to intervene. Here are a few simple strategies that have helped other caregivers in similar situations:

- Label drawers with words or pictures of the content (e.g., blouses, pants, underpants).
- Leave out the clothes to be worn that day, in the order in which they are to be worn either on a wall hook or on the bed.
- Buy two or three of the same clothing item. When the patient is bathing, the caregiver can quickly swap the dirty set for the fresh.

Smart Devices and Monitoring Systems

In the last decade, there has been a significant increase in the availability of home monitoring products to help extend independent living for those with cognitive decline. These systems allow caregivers to monitor the activity of a family member who is living alone, so they can check in on them from a remote location and offer support as needed. Smart devices can be used "off the shelf" for specific activities or entire home systems can be installed. Monitoring can help to identify problems as they occur so that the caregiver can intervene before they become a full-blown crisis. For example, there are medication reminders that attach to a standard phone line and will send the caregiver an alert if the person does not remove pills from a medication box. There are also devices that detect extreme changes in room temperature and can send the caregiver an alert if the home is too hot or too cold. Dan G visited his mother in Wisconsin in early winter and was alarmed to discover how cold the home was. His mother had inadvertently turned off the furnace switch and was not cognizant that there was any problem. A monitoring device could have detected the drop in temperature and sent the son an alert; then the son could have called a neighbor to check in on the mother and turn the furnace back on. Fortunately, the son visited his mother before any serious problems occurred.

Home "Behavioral" Systems

These monitoring systems work by using discreet wireless sensors placed in key locations around the home, like the bedroom, kitchen, medication areas, and bathroom. The sensors keep track of the patient's normal routines and send the designated caregiver(s) alerts regarding unusual situations or departures from the norm. For example, depending on the system, the caregiver can receive alerts if the person opens the outside door at 5:00 am instead of their usual 10:00 am time, or gets out of bed at night and does not return. Pilot studies show these systems can be helpful for the right person, who can still live safely on their own, but need daily monitoring and some backup support to do so [20–22].

Conclusion

Clinicians can serve as a valuable resource to patients and their caregivers by providing them with advice and information on how to avoid excess disability through dementia-appropriate design. By understanding the environment's effect on a person's behavior, caregivers have the opportunity to create a therapeutic environment that promotes more positive outcomes, allowing them and the person they care for lead safer, more satisfied lives.

Clinical Pearls

- Caregivers should keep in mind that providing for the safety of their loved ones is an *ongoing challenge as the disease progresses.*
- Reminder signs can act as an "external" brain for those in the earlier stages helping a person function more independently. Use simple language, large-sized text, and/or photographs.
- Usually there is a *specific* event preceding agitation that acts as a trigger for that behavior (e.g., noise, cold interior temperature, water flowing onto the face during a shower.) Advise the caregiver to find the "trigger" when the person is agitated so that he or she can act to change or

modify the trigger(s) and the associated agitation.

- Before denying access to appliances, rooms, or exit and entrance doors, monitoring technologies (e.g., motion sensors, remote door alarms, automatic turn off devices) should be tried first whenever possible. If locks need to be installed (e.g., cabinets, front door) or the stove knobs removed, advise the caregiver to monitor the person's reaction, as some patients become agitated when access is denied.
- Interventions should be *frequently* reassessed since strategies may not continue to be effective as the symptoms of the disease progress or if the environment changes.
- Salient interior features and household items should be color-contrasted from their background to enhance function (e.g., increase food intake by using a strongly contrasting plate color to the food, reduce tripping on stairs by highlighting the edges of steps with 2-in. color tape).
- To reduce environmental misperception, patterns should be kept to a minimum and lighting levels should be abundant and glare free, with no dark areas in a room.

References

1. Gitlin LN, Hauck WW, Dennis MP, Winter L. Maintenance of effects of the home environmental skill-building program for family caregivers and individuals with Alzheimer's Disease and related disorders. J Gerontol A Biol Sci Med Sci. 2005;60: 368–74.
2. Alzheimer's Association Alzheimer's disease facts and figures, Alzheimer's & dementia (6). http://www.alz.org/documents_custom/report_alzfactsfigures2010.pdf. Accessed 29 Mar 2012.
3. Caregiving in the U.S. National Alliance for Caregiving and AARP. 2004. http://www.caregiving.org/data/04finalreport.pdf. Accessed 29 Mar 2012.
4. Calkins M. Design for dementia. J Healthcare Design. 1991;3:159–71.
5. Jones K. Enabling technologies for people with dementia: report of the assessment study in England. 2004. http://www.enableproject.org/download/Enable%20-%20National%20Report%20-%20UK.pdf. Accessed 29 Mar 2012.
6. Dunne TE, Neargarder SA, Cipolloni PB, Cronin-Golmb A. Visual contrast enhances food and liquid intake in advanced Alzheimer's disease. Clin Nutr. 2004;23:533–8.
7. Torrington JM, Tregenza PR. Lighting for people with dementia. Lighting Res Technol. 2007;39(1):81–97.
8. Tinetti ME, Speechley M, Ginter SF. Risk factors for falls among elderly persons living in the community. N Engl J Med. 1988;319(26):1701–7.
9. Hurley A, Gauthier M, Horvath K, Harvey R, Smith S, Trudeau S, Cipolloni PB, Hendricks A, Duffy M. Promoting safer home environments for persons with Alzheimer's disease: the home safety/injury model. J Gerontol Nurs. 2004;30:43–51.
10. Spring H, Rowe M, Kelly A. Improving caregivers' well-being by using technology to assist in managing nighttime activity in persons with dementia. Res Gerontol Nurs. 2009;2(1):39–48.
11. Rowe M, Kelly A, Horne C, Lane S, Campbell J, Lehman B, Phipps C, Keller M, Benito AP. Reducing dangerous nighttime events in persons with dementia by using a nighttime monitoring system. Alzheimers Dement. 2009;5(5):419–26.
12. Patient care ergonomics resource guide: safe patient handling and movement. Patient Safety Center of Inquiry. Tampa, FL: Veterans Health Administration and Department of Defense; 2001 (rev 8/31/05). http://www.visn8.va.gov/patientsafetycenter/resguide/ErgoGuidePtOne.pdf. Accessed 29 Mar 2012.
13. Daikoku R, Saito Y. Differences between novice and experienced caregivers in muscle activity and perceived exertion while repositioning bedridden patients. J Physiol Anthropol. 2008;27(6):333–9.
14. Safety at home. Alzheimer's Association National Office. 2005. http://www.alz.org/national/documents/brochure_homesafety.pdf. Accessed 29 Mar 2012.
15. Calkins MP, Brush JA. Designing for dining: the secret of happier mealtimes. J Dement Care. 2002;10(2):24–6.
16. Piwnica-Worms K, Omar R, Hailstone JC, Warren JD. Flavour processing in semantic dementia. Cortex. 2010;46(6):761.
17. Barrick AL, et al. Bathing without a battle: creating a better bathing experience for persons with Alzheimer's disease and related disorders (CD-ROM). Chapel Hill, NC: University of North Carolina; 2003.
18. Barrick AL, Rader J, Hoeffer B, Sloane P, Biddle S, editors. Bathing without a battle: person-directed care of individuals with dementia, Springer series on geriatric nursing. 2nd ed. New York: Springer; 2008.
19. Cohen-Mansfield J, Creedon M, Malone T, Parpura-Gill A, Dakheel-Ali M, Heasly C. Dressing of cognitively impaired nursing home residents: description and analysis. Gerontologist. 2006;46(1):89–96.
20. Kinney J, Kart C, Murdoch L, Conley C. Striving to provide safety assistance for families of elders: the SAFE house project. Dementia. 2004;3(3):351–70.
21. Topo P. Technology studies to meet the needs of people with dementia and their caregivers: a literature review. J Appl Gerontol. 2009;28:5–37.
22. Buettner L, Yu F, Burgener S. Technology innovations: evidence supporting technology-based interventions for people with early-stage Alzheimer's disease. J Gerontol Nurs. 2010;36(10):15–9.

Additional Resources

ThisCaringHome.org, a project of Weill Cornell Medical College, is multimedia web site that offers caregivers innovative ways to learn research-based strategies that reduce caregiver stress and enhance the safety and well-being of loved ones with Alzheimer's disease or other types of dementia.

Prevention of Cognitive Decline 12

Jose Gutierrez and Richard S. Isaacson

Abstract

Effective strategies to prevent cognitive decline in the context of normal aging, mild cognitive impairment, and dementia are imperative. Existing studies have provided some clues into the puzzle of prevention, yet it is rare that the evidence is unquestionable. Specific dietary changes rich in vegetables, fruits, and fish and low in carbohydrates and saturated fat are advisable, with particular emphasis in patients at risk of developing Alzheimer's disease (AD) or vascular dementia. Patients should remain active physically and mentally. Physical exercise is among the best of all potential interventions against AD. There is no evidence that hormonal supplementation can decrease the incidence of dementia. Some agents that are touted as having cognitive protective effects should only be used under physician supervision. AD patients should be considered for medical therapy unless contraindicated. Promising novel therapies include active and passive immunization against Aβ peptides and gamma secretase inhibitors to reduce Aβ production. In this chapter, we review strategies used to prevent age related cognitive decline.

Keywords

Alzheimer's disease prevention • Delay of cognitive decline • Vitamins • Fish oil • Dementia • Cholinesterase inhibitors • Curcumin • Cognitive exercises

J. Gutierrez, M.D., MPH.
Department of Neurology, Neurological Institute, Columbia University, 710 West 168th Street, 6th Floor, New York, NY 10032, USA
e-mail: jg3233@columbia.edu

R.S. Isaacson, M.D. (✉)
Department of Neurology, Clinical Research Building, University of Miami Miller School of Medicine, 1120 NW 14th Street, Suite 1339, Miami, FL 33136, USA
e-mail: risaacson@med.miami.edu

Introduction

The prevention of cognitive decline and dementia is a complex area in which multiple prior interventions have failed to show a consistent effect. The importance of studying preventive measures for cognitive decline and dementia is directly proportional to the magnitude of the dementia

L.D. Ravdin and H.L. Katzen (eds.), *Handbook on the Neuropsychology of Aging and Dementia*, Clinical Handbooks in Neuropsychology, DOI 10.1007/978-1-4614-3106-0_12,

epidemic that our society faces. Cognitive decline encompasses a continuum of changes ranging for normal aging in the mildest expression to dementia on the more severe presentation; there is subjectivity in the definition of each category. Advancing age is accompanied by the decline of cognitive abilities such as perceptual speed, reasoning, episodic memory, and working memory [1]. The early stages of pathologic cognitive decline, often referred as mild cognitive impairment (MCI) or cognitive impairment without dementia, pertain to cognitive decline "greater than expected" for age and educational level and no more than mild functional impairment in carrying activities of daily living that does not qualify for the diagnosis of dementia [2]. Dementia is defined as a progressive global deterioration of cognitive abilities in multiple domains severe enough to interfere with daily living [3]. More precise definitions are discussed elsewhere in this volume.

The challenge posed by MCI and dementia to society is not insignificant: Ten percent of persons older than 65 years and about 50% of those older than 85 years have Alzheimer's disease (AD), the most common form of adult onset dementia [4]. By 2050, the prevalence of AD in the USA is expected to triple. This increment is largely attributed to the aging of the "baby boomer generation." The risk of dementia nearly doubles with every 5 years of age. The US Medicare economic cost of caring for people with dementia in 2008 was 91 billion dollars, and it is expected to nearly double by 2015 [5]. Of no less importance is the untold economic and emotional impact on families and friends.

The prevention of cognitive decline emerges as the main way to offset the demographic transition of our aging society and the concomitant challenge that it represents. If the onset of AD can be delayed by 5 years, the expected prevalence would decrease by more than 1 million cases after 10 years and more than 4 million cases after 50 years [6]. In this chapter, we review strategies used to prevent cognitive decline at different levels. Primary prophylaxis refers to avoidance of age-associated cognitive decline. Secondary prophylaxis refers to prevention or slowing of progression from MCI to dementia. Tertiary prophylaxis refers to the treatment of dementia that encompasses either gaining of function, stabilization of the decline, or slowing of the progression. Since the most prevalent of the dementias is AD, the majority of the interventions and strategies reviewed will be related to AD and, to a lesser degree, vascular dementia.

A large body of evidence exists in the literature, and a detailed, critical analysis of each reference has been attempted when possible. We emphasized the level of evidence available in order to preserve the scientific rigor. However, methodological heterogeneity in populations studied, study designs, case definitions, and outcome evaluations has resulted in conflicting evidence that precludes a firm conclusion on many of the prevention strategies reviewed and discussed. When reading the results of observational and experimental studies, it is important to keep in mind that statistical significance is not equivalent to clinical relevance and that the opposite is also true.

An Overview of Cognitive Decline

The normal cognitive process requires complex neural networks localized in different part of the brain such as the medial temporal lobes including the hippocampus and the entorhinal cortex and the frontoparietal cortices [7] Memory, attention, executive functions, perception, language, and psychomotor functions are components of the cognitive process [8]. The dysfunction in any of these components in the context of neurodegeneration has a pathological substrate in a corresponding brain area accounting for its processing. The pathological changes vary depending on the type of dementia. Since AD is the hallmark of the neurodegenerative diseases associated with dementia and also the most studied, many clinical trials have been exclusively focused on AD.

The early pathological changes in AD involve the deposition of Aβ42 aggregates and related tau accumulation in vulnerable brain areas such as the hippocampus and the entorhinal cortex. The activity of gamma and beta secretases is thought to be an important rate-limiting step in the pathology of AD. The Aβ and tau aggregates progress to plaques and tangles that are eventually widespread in the brain. After decades of accumulation, synaptic dysfunction and neuronal loss appear to play a major role in driving the cognitive deficit [7]. Oxidative damage, excessive glutaminergic activity, energy failure, inflammation, and apoptosis seem to be significant contributors to neuronal loss and progressive cognitive dysfunction [9–13]. The degeneration of some regions is associated with neurotransmitter deficiencies that are part of neuronal circuits important for cognition (e.g., degeneration of the basal forebrain is associated with decrements in acetylcholine-mediated neuronal activity involved in memory).

Multiple genetic, clinical, and environmental risk factors have been associated with the occurrence of AD. Vascular risk factors like diabetes mellitus (DM), hypertension (HTN), dyslipidemia (Dys), and smoking are attractive targets from a public health perspective due to their high prevalence, their relative ease to treat, and the multiple other diseases associated with these factors. The contribution of each risk factor seems additive to the occurrence and severity of the disease.

The prevention of cognitive decline involves multiple strategies directed at different stages of the pathophysiological process. Examples are Aβ and tau aggregation inhibitors, antioxidants, anti-inflammatory compounds, cognitive enhancers or facilitators, neuroprotective agents, or some combination of these approaches. The failure of recent trials to prevent cognitive decline and the complexity of the cascade leading to AD suggest that pleiotropic interventions may be more likely to succeed, although no evidence so far exists to support this statement [7].

Vitamins and Minerals

B Vitamins

Vitamin B1 (thiamine) and vitamin B2 (riboflavin) exist in a variety of food sources, including enriched and whole grain cereals, organ meats, milk, and vegetables. Vitamin B6 (pyridoxine) and vitamin B12 (cobalamin) generally come from meat, poultry, seafood, and eggs as well as enriched cereals. The major source of folates is the green leafy vegetables [14]. Thiamine, riboflavin, and niacin function in major biochemical pathways in the metabolism of glucose, amino acids, and fatty acids, while the coenzymes of vitamin B12, folate, and vitamin B6 interact together in the metabolism of homocysteine, a risk factor for vascular disease and dementia [15, 16]. The exploration of these vitamins in the context of cognition is related to their antioxidant and anti-inflammatory properties along with their role in nucleotide synthesis and nerve functions [14].

An important interaction occurs between vitamin B12, folate, and pyridoxine that could mediate some effects in cognitive decline. All three vitamins are major determinants of homocysteine levels, and high levels can be deleterious due to neurotoxic and vasotoxic effects on brain vasculature and normal cognitive functioning [17–19]. Longitudinal studies have explored the interaction between folate, vitamin B6, and B12 and cognitive decline. Folate levels are associated with different degrees of cognitive decline independent of the homocysteine and vitamin B levels [19–21]. Future studies attempting to evaluate the effects of B vitamins and folate supplementation should control for homocysteine levels to further clarify this interaction. Trials of combined vitamin supplementation are challenging to interpret due to various covariates that make it difficult to isolate an effect [2, 14].

Vitamin B1 (Thiamine)

Animal models have shown that rats with low thiamine diet have impaired cognitive performance when compared with controls fed with adequate thiamine supplementation [22], and repetitive episodes of thiamine deficiency can cause worsening of cognitive performance and severe brain damage [23, 24]. Thiamine deficiency has been associated with blood–brain barrier (BBB) dysfunction and intracellular edema in animal models, revealing pathological changes that could derail the normal functioning of the brain [14].

In a non-randomized controlled trial (RCT), Meador et al. [25] found that older individuals supplemented with 3–8 g/day of oral thiamine showed statically significant improvement in the ADAS in the initial months with slowing of the cognitive decline rate during 11–13 months after the trial stopped. The small sample and open design are concerns in this trial. Mimori et al. [26] showed that higher blood levels of thiamine after supplementation with an oral form were associated with improvement in scores on the Mini-Mental State Examination (MMSE) in an open design trial. Low thiamine levels have not been consistently associated with higher prevalence of AD [14], and there is currently not enough evidence at this point to recommend thiamine supplementation for the prevention or treatment of cognitive decline [2, 3, 27].

Vitamin B2 (Riboflavin)

Godwin et al. showed that individuals at the bottom decile of riboflavin dietary intake had worse cognitive performance in some domains compared to the upper deciles [28], and Lee et al. found that MMSE scores increased as riboflavin intake increased in women but not in men [29]. However, low riboflavin serum levels have not been associated with the presence of AD. There is no RCT specifically designed to evaluate the effects of riboflavin in cognitive decline or dementia. Riboflavin supplementation is not recommended for AD prevention or treatment [2, 3, 27, 30].

Vitamin B6 (Pyridoxine)

In rodents, the supplementation of pyridoxine did not improve cognition or learning functions. When analyzing the linear dose–response relationship, low pyridoxine was associated with worse motor skills [14]. In high-dose supplementation trials in humans [14], it was shown that pyridoxine was associated with improved long-term memory, but threats to validity make conclusions based on these trials uncertain. Mizrahi et al. found an association of low pyridoxine dietary intake with AD; however, the recall bias for dietary exposure among patients with dementia limits interpretation of this data [31]. There is currently not enough evidence to support the use of pyridoxine for the prevention or treatment of cognitive decline [2, 3, 27, 32].

Vitamin B12 (Cobalamin)

In rats with nucleus basalis magnocellularis lesions (mimicking a hypocholinergic state), the supplementation of cobalamin had no effect on movements and did not improve memory [33]. In observational studies, high methylmalonic acid level, a more specific marker for vitamin B12 deficiency, was associated with a faster rate of cognitive decline, especially in APOE ε4 carries [34]. The administration of cobalamin was associated with improvement on a12-word list learning test at 15 min, and a trend was found for improvement on other cognitive measures in an RCT of cognitively impaired individuals with B12 deficiency [35, 36]. In uncontrolled trials, there is conflicting evidence on the effects of cobalamin supplementation in normal and cognitively impaired patients. In most of the studies where cobalamin supplementation was associated with cognitive improvement, the cobalamin was administered via parenteral route. Dietary intake of cobalamin has not been associated to the presence AD in cross-sectional studies [14]. The heterogeneity of the trials, cognitive outcomes, and populations studied contribute to the inconsistency of the findings. The supplementation of cobalamin for the prevention or treatment of cognitive decline is not supported at this point [2, 3, 27, 32]. However, vitamin B12 levels are part of the workup for reversible causes of dementia as well as other neurological diseases, and deficiencies should be a target of clinical intervention.

Folate

In amyloid precursor protein (APP) mutant mice model, Kruman et al. [37] showed that the amount of deposition of Aβ amyloid did not differ among folate-deficient mice vs. a control group. However, the *cornus ammonis* (CA) 3 region of the hippocampus in folate-deficient mice had at least 20% fewer neurons compared to controls, suggesting susceptibility of this region to folate deficiency independent of Aβ production or deposition. Apolipoprotein E gene (ApoE)-deficient mice, a model thought to be at increased susceptibility to oxidative damage, were fed with folate-free diet in one group and folate-supplemented diet in the other one. The folate-supplemented group showed significant decrement in the amount of oxidative by-products when challenged with iron, an oxidizing substance [14, 38]. These results suggest that the oxidative potential of ApoE deficiency could be alleviated with folate supplementation. In a diet-induced hyperhomocysteinemia rat model, the investigators evaluated the impact of folate supplementation on the homocysteine-induced endothelial dysfunction [29]. They found that the folate supplementation reduced endothelial nitric oxide synthetase activity and glucose transporter protein-1 activity, suggesting that folate supplementation could offset the oxidative potential of homocysteine at the endothelial level.

Observational studies have shown conflicting data in regards of dietary intake of folate and the presence of AD. Tucker et al. investigated the association of dietary intake and several vitamins and found that high dietary folate offered independent protection against cognitive [21], while Morris et al. showed that high folate intake from food or supplements was associated with faster cognitive decline in a cohort of aging individuals [39]. Despite these conflicting findings, most of the cross-sectional and case–control studies suggest that lower levels of serum folate or higher prevalence of folate deficiency is found in patients with AD [14].

In human studies, one RCT showed cognitive benefit of folate supplementation in demented, cognitively impaired, and normal subjects, but no clinical benefit was reported [14]. Fioravanti et al. showed that folate supplementation improved cognitive scores in aged patients with cognitive impairment and low folate levels. Of interest, initial cognitive status did not correlate with initial folate levels [40]. Bryan et al. studied women of all ages without cognitive impairment and reported that folate supplementation improved cognition in the older women. Unfortunately, the dietary intake of these women could potentially be an interaction that was not controlled for since dietary intake of folate and other vitamins were correlation with speed of processing, recall and recognition, and verbal ability [41]. Sommer et al. showed, in a very small sample, that very high doses of folate supplementation (20 mg/day) can be associated with worsening cognitive functions [42]. Recent systematic reviews and meta-analysis do not support the use of folate with or without vitamin B supplements for the prevention or treatment of cognitive decline in the short term [2, 3, 27, 32, 43]. Long-term administration of folate supplements to healthy and cognitively impaired individuals has not yet been systematically studied. Folate levels are part of the dementia workup and should be supplemented if indicated.

Vitamins C and E

The protective factors of antioxidants are the proposed mechanism of action of vitamin C for the prevention of cognitive decline. It has been observed that higher levels of ascorbic acid (vitamin C) are associated with better cognitive performance in a cohort study [44]. Vitamin E is considered a powerful antioxidant available in oily food. In adults over 65 year of age, it was shown that individuals in the upper tercile of vitamin E consumption (data obtained by a food questionnaire) had better cognitive performance than the lower tercile [45]. Wengreen et al. studied the dietary intake of vitamins C and E in individuals older than 65 followed on average for 7 years and found that the higher intake of vitamin E and C was associated with higher MMSE scores and that the low intake of these vitamins and carotene was associated with higher rate of decline in MMSE [46]. However, trials examining the combination of vitamins E and C supplementation have failed to consistently demonstrate significant improvements, and at this time, there is no evidence to support the prescription of vitamin C and vitamin E or their combination for preventing the cognitive decline [32, 47].

Chromium

Metabolic syndrome is associated with insulin resistance and secondary hyperinsulinemia. The receptor for insulin transport across the BBB becomes saturated with the flush of plasmatic insulin, thus creating a hypoinsulinimic state in the brain. Hypoinsulinemia is associated with increased rate of Aβ aggregation. Peripheral hyperinsulinemia has also been associated with worse cognitive performance among AD and non-AD patients [48].

Chromium is an essential trace mineral used in insulin receptor signaling, and it is thought to amplify the insulin action [49]. At doses of 200–1,000 mcg, it has been shown to improve insulin resistance in diabetic patients [50, 51]. Krikorian et al. [49] randomly assigned 26 patients to receive chromium supplementation vs. placebo and followed them for 12 weeks with examination on multiple cognitive tests. No effects were seen on fasting insulin or fasting glucose, but a reduced rate of intrusion errors was found in the active group. Functional magnetic resonance imaging (fMRI) data showed that individuals in the active arm had increased activation in multiple regions of the brain including the thalamus and the frontal cortex; however, areas of activation did not correspond to the improved cognitive performance. This suggests that chromium could have functions independent on its effects on metabolism that should be further explored. Chromium supplementation shows promising results but not enough to unequivocally determine an association with AD or cognitive decline [2]. Larger and better designed studies should be undertaken to strengthen the current evidence.

Polyphenolic Compounds (Flavonoids)

One of the most well-studied hypothesis underlying AD causation has been Aβ-mediated neurodegeneration. Several phenolic compounds, such as wine-related myricetin (MYR), curcumin, nordihydroguaiaretic acid (NDGA), and rosmarinic acid (RA), have been shown to possess strong anti-Aβ aggregation properties in vitro and in vivo [52]. Flavonoids are also part of the polyphenol family, phytochemicals thought to have important antioxidative, antiviral and anticarcinogenic properties [14]. They are ubiquitous in vegetables, and they provide the plant with its color that attracts pollinators and repels insect attacks [9]. They are found in high concentrations in berries, onions, dark chocolate, broccoli, apples, tea, red wine, purple grape juice, soybean, and tomatoes [53]. Below we will discuss the more conspicuous members of the phenolic family that have been studied to date.

Berries

Berries are thought to be rich in antioxidants, and their consumption is hypothesized to provide neuroprotection against the oxidative and inflammatory process associated with aging. Strawberries, blueberries, blackberries, cranberries, and raspberries are fruits with high antioxidant capacity due to the high content of anti-inflammatory anthocyanins and/or proanthocyanidins (flavonoid compounds) [14, 54, 55].

Anthocyanins can cross the BBB and block 5′-deiodinase activity and stimulate T3 transport into rat brains [56]. In blueberry-fed rats, histopathology and cognitive test results suggest a protective effect compared with controls. Blueberry extract was associated with increased precursor cells (increased neurogenesis) in the dentate gyrus in rats that also performed better on cognitive testing [57]. Strawberry extract supplementation in animal experiments has been associated with improved biochemical markers in the brain suggestive of neuroprotection; however, an association with cognitive performance has not been reported [14]. In vitro studies suggest that various berry extracts can protect the deleterious effects of Aβ-induced oxidative damage [58]. Human studies are lacking to recommend berries extracts for the prevention of cognitive decline; however, inclusion of berries in the diet has a theoretical benefit and is recommended as part of a balanced diet.

Curcumin

Hamaguchi et al. showed that RA, CUR, and MYR inhibit the aggregation of Aβ monomers to

Aβ oligomers and from oligomers to Aβ deposition [52]. Curcumin is a potent antioxidant and an effective anti-inflammatory compound. Curcumin can inhibit the formation of Aβ oligomers and fibrils, bind plaque, and reduce plaque burden [59]. In another animal model of dementia, curcumin (20 mg/kg p.o. daily for 14 days) successfully attenuated Streptozotocin STZ-induced memory deficits. Higher levels of brain AChE activity and oxidative stress were observed in STZ-treated animals, which were significantly attenuated by curcumin [60]. Other animal studies raise the possibility that curcumin may act as a metal chelator, have anti-apoptotic or immunomodulator properties, or promote neurogenesis [7].

In human studies, one of the main challenges using curcumin is its poor bioavailability [61]. In a pilot study, a small RCT evaluated the pharmacokinetics and effects of curcumin supplementation in humans [62]. The preliminary results showed promising MMSE changes without major side effects, yet the short period of follow-up and the lack of cognitive decline in the placebo group limit the interpretation of the data. The risks associated with curcumin administration are uncertain, and further studies are warranted in regard to safety and efficacy. In the trial by Baum et al. [62], gastric, neurological, and pulmonary symptoms were reported at an equal rate among patients taking placebo and those on active treatment. Four clinical trials have studied curcumin for AD treatment (two with no significant differences in cognitive function; no results yet from the other two); however, there is no clinical trial evidence for AD prevention [62, 63]. The risk:benefit ratio of curcumin supplementation should be discussed in detail with patients and caregivers.

Docosahexaenoic Acid (DHA)

DHA is a long-chain 22-carbon omega-3 polyunsaturated fatty acid with six double bonds. It is found abundantly in marine algae, fatty fish, and fish oil [7]. The main proposed mechanism of action of DHA in the context of cognitive decline is the preservation of debrin, a vital component for the adequate synaptic function. Other pleiotropic mechanisms in which DHA can affect the progression of cognitive decline are anti-inflammatory activity, neuroprotection, neurogenesis, antioxidant, metabolic enhancer, and weak amyloid aggregation inhibitor [7].

In animal models, it has been shown that depleting DHA from the system was associated with cognitive impairment, but replacing DHA prevented pathological changes similar to those seen in AD [64, 65]. A small trial of DHA in MCI and AD groups was associated with a slower rate of cognitive decline [66, 67]. A recent randomized, double-blind, placebo-controlled study with 485 subjects (aged 55 and older) called the "Memory Improvement with Docosahexaenoic Acid Study" (MIDAS) aimed at evaluating the effects of 900 mg/day of algae-based DHA in healthy older adults with age-related cognitive decline [66, 67]. The study found that DHA taken for 6 months improved memory and learning in healthy, older adults with mild memory complaints.

A combination of DHA and choline showed improvement in delayed memory after 12 weeks of follow-up compared to placebo [68]. In a recent RCT, 402 patients with AD were given DHA or placebo and followed for 18 months. The primary outcomes were changes in ADAS-cog and clinical dementia rating (CDR) obtained every 6 months until the end of the follow-up period. Secondary outcomes were MMSE and MR brain volume measurements. The active arm did not show any significant difference in the primary or secondary outcomes when compared with the placebo group in a model adjusted for covariates. However, in a subgroup analysis based on APOE genotype, subjects without an APOE ε4 allele who received DHA showed slower progression of cognitive decline as documented by the ADAS-cog and MMSE compared with APOE ε4-negative patients in the placebo group. No significant differences were observed in the CDR and the brain volumes [69]. The APOE ε4-status interaction on the effectiveness of DHA had already been documented by Whalley et al. [70] in nondemented patients in whom erythrocyte membrane DHA content was positively associated with cognitive performance.

Recent systematic reviews of RCT and observational studies published for DHA supplementation have failed to identify unequivocal evidence suggestive of a protective effect of DHA on cognitive decline [2, 27, 32], although the association of DHA with slower cognitive decline seems to be somewhat consistent across studies [3]. Taken together, these data suggest DHA supplementation may have a potential role in the prevention of cognitive decline and that its effect may be more evident in APOE ε4-negative patients. Early supplementation as well as the long-term effects of DHA warrants further investigation.

Diet

The first suggestion that diet could provide protective effects against cognitive decline and dementia came from the Mediterranean basin where lower prevalence of cognitive decline and other neurodegenerative disease was observed. Since then, multiple studies have investigated the "Mediterranean diet" as well as other dietary patterns [71]. In general, a balanced and healthy diet should provide adequate amount of vitamins, minerals, and elemental components necessary to function. As it has been discussed above, these elements could provide protection against the neurodegeneration associated with AD and cognitive decline from various perspectives including high supply of natural fish oil, vitamins, and polyphenols [5, 13].

The traditional Mediterranean diet is rich in fruits, vegetables, whole grains, olive oil, cheese and yogurt, low-to-moderate consumption of wine, and fish or seafood products. Variation might occur according to the country or region studied, but the core elements and the proportions are relatively similar [72]. Several scores and outcome scales have been created to assess adherence to the Mediterranean diet [73]. In a recent prospective cohort study, a higher Mediterranean diet score was associated with better cognition. In this same cohort, a dose–response effect of Mediterranean diet was suggested based on the progressive lower risk for developing dementia or MCI in the middle and the upper score tertile when compared with the bottom tertile (21% and 47% risk reduction, respectively) [74, 75]. Another prospective cohort showed that high adherence to Mediterranean diet was associated with better cognitive performance and episodic memory test results over time, but did not show any protective effect for the development of AD [76].

Due to methodological difficulties with the adjustment for covariates associated with a healthier diet, such as education, exercise, and less prevalent cardiovascular risk factors, the final impact of the Mediterranean diet on cognition is still debatable. Some authors have suggested that the late onset of a healthier diet might not reverse a lifelong exposure to detrimental factors. It is generally thought that the earlier the healthy diet is introduced, the better it is for cognition as well as for other cardiovascular risks that are also known to contribute to the occurrence of AD and cognitive decline [71]. Since no well-designed RCT has proven the efficacy of Mediterranean diet vs. other type of diet, the evidence available is low to systematically recommend Mediterranean diet for the prevention of cognitive decline [2]. On the other hand, it seems that the Mediterranean diet contains a healthy combination of ingredients that could potentially lead to a better health overall.

Gu et al. [77] proposed a different approach to the evaluation of diet and the risk for cognitive decline/AD. Since there was concern that a Mediterranean diet might have a low prevalence in local communities not in the Mediterranean basin, nutrients and dietary patterns were evaluated with various statistical analyses to obtain components of the diet associated with lower risk of developing AD. It was shown that a dietary pattern consisting of greater intake of salad dressing, nuts, fish, tomato, poultry, cruciferous vegetables, fruit, and dark and green leafy vegetables was associated with lower risk of AD and negatively correlated with intake of high-fat dairy, red meat, organ meat, and butter. Based on the previous results, a healthy diet rich in vegetables, fruits, grains, and fish and nut oils is recommended [1, 3, 5]. As discussed by several authors, fragmenting ingredients in the diet has failed to produce robust evidence. To date, it has been methodologically difficult to measure diet components and to determine if a particular component has more effects than the others.

Other Supplements or Diet-Related Items

Garlic

Garlic is high in antioxidants and organosulfurs. An extract preparation has been associated with decrement in blood pressure and cholesterol levels. It is speculated that garlic may have a double benefit by lowering cardiovascular risk factors and their impact on the development of AD as well as supplying important antioxidants that counteract the ongoing neurodegenerative process. It has been shown in animal models that garlic can reduce homocysteine [78]. In vitro studies demonstrated that garlic extract can inhibit Aβ and caspase enzymes that promote the deposition of amyloid [79]. Budoff et al. [80] showed that garlic can also decrease the levels of homocysteine in humans, although it is unclear if its effect was independent of that attributable to concurrent statin therapy the subjects were receiving. More studies are needed to clarify the efficacy of garlic extract as preventive measure for cognitive decline.

Ginkgo Biloba

Ginkgo biloba contains flavonoids and terpenes that have been suggested to have pleiotropic actions that can affect inflammation and oxidative processes in the human body [81]. It is approved in some European countries for the treatment of cerebrovascular insufficiency and cognitive decline, although in the USA, it is sold as a supplement [1]. Short-term supplementation has provided conflicting results, with some studies showing marginal improvement in cognition while others fail to reproduce any significant effect [13, 82]. A small RCT showed that ginkgo extract was associated with marginal improvement in the clinical dementia rating scale (CDR) when adjusting for medication adherence [83]. The clinical significance of this marginal improvement in cognitive testing in conjunction with a higher incidence of stroke and TIA in the treatment arm could have confounded the results. A recent meta-analysis [84] on nine trials using standardized formulation of ginkgo biloba in the treatment of dementia showed statistically significant improvement in cognitive scales with no significant benefit in activities of daily living performance. In the Alzheimer's dementia subgroup analysis, ginkgo biloba supplementation was associated with statistically significant changes in cognitive scales as well as in the activities of daily living performance. The high variability of study designs hampers the generalization of these results. Ideally, a well-powered, blinded RCT should be performed to provide better quality evidence to evaluate the value of ginkgo biloba supplementation in the context of cognitive decline/dementia.

Alcohol

Low-to-moderate alcohol consumption has been associated with decrease risk of dementia in some observational studies [85, 86]. It is hypothesized that alcohol exerts its benefit through the improvement of the lipid profile, although the content of flavonoids in red wine could also contribute [9, 52]. A recent meta-analysis of 23 observational studies showed that small amounts of alcohol can be protective against dementia and AD but did not impact the rate of cognitive decline or the incidence of vascular dementia [85]. The heterogeneity of the studies included in the analysis prevents a firm conclusion on the applicability of the findings. Thus, the systematic recommendation of alcohol consumption for the prevention of cognitive decline is not supported with the current state of evidence.

Caffeine

Caffeine has been used by civilization since ancient times. Its popularity has granted its status as the more popular and most consumed behaviorally acting substance around the world [87]. Caffeine is an antagonist of adenosine receptors A_1 and A_{2A}, although it can also interact with other enzymes and receptors like $GABA_A$ or 5′ nucleotidase at higher levels [88]. In animal models, antagonist of A_{2A} receptors like caffeine decreased the levels in cerebrospinal fluid and serum of Aβ peptides and counteracted its noxious effects at the neuronal levels [89, 90]. Inhibition of phosphodiesterase is thought to be a potential mechanism to convey neuroprotection [91]. The activation of A_{2A} receptors has been associated with long-term potentiation in striatal and hippocampal synapses essential for memory processing. The excessive or insufficient activation of these receptors results in aberrant synaptic functioning [91–93]. Caffeine can act as normalizer of aberrant memory performance rather than enhancing this process, especially in conditions with excessive endogenous adenosine stimulation such as fatigue and stress [91, 94].

In humans, caffeine reaches a peak in plasma 45–120 min after oral ingestion and has a half-life that ranges from 2.5 to 4.5 h [88]. Caffeine facilitates learning on tasks in which information is presented passively, but it has not proven effective for those tasks that involve intentional learning. The caffeine effect on memory tasks seems to have an inverted U shape curve, with improvement seen during mild-to-moderate complexity tasks but impaired performance for high complexity tasks [8]. Caffeine confers a boost for cognitive performance among fatigued individuals, and it might also improve cognitive functioning with chronic consumption, although its acute effect is more evident in non-usual consumers [95, 96]. Caffeine appears to have a differential effect across the age span. In older populations, the administration of caffeine is more effective for improving attention, psychomotor performance, and cognitive functioning, possibly offsetting the decline associated with age. A large part of these effects may be explained by counteracting age-related decreased arousal [97, 98].

The relationship between AD and caffeine has been more elusive to grasp. A retrospective cohort study suggested a protective effect of caffeine intake at midlife against the subsequent development of AD [99]. In prospective studies, Ritchie et al. showed a protective effect of caffeine in women consuming more than three cups of coffee per day [100], and van Gelder et al. showed that men also benefitted from caffeine intake. In his prospective cohort, it was shown that men who drank more than three coffee cups per day had slower cognitive decline when compared with those drinking less than three cups per day and non-coffee drinkers [101]. Another prospective cohort analysis showed that cognitive performance was strongly associated with caffeine intake, with no gender differences in its protective effects. However, caffeine intake was also strongly associated with age, IQ, and social class, thus education confounding effects could not be ruled out [102]. Finally, Boxtel et al. were not able to reproduce any of the above-mentioned findings and demonstrated no associations between longtime caffeine intake and cognitive performance [103]. In the context of heterogeneous studies and results, it is difficult to strongly recommend caffeine intake as an effective measure against cognitive decline; however, it seems safe to say that caffeine can provide a boost in memory performance and has been shown to be protective in some populations.

Cardiovascular Risk Profile

Although age is the single most important risk factor for the development of dementia, cardiovascular risk factors seem to be strongly associated with cognitive decline and dementia and carry the great advantage of being modifiable. Traditional risk factors like hypertension, diabetes, dyslipidemia, and smoking are believed to convey risk for vascular disease. Vascular disease is associated with cerebral hypoperfusion, oxidative stress, neurodegeneration, and cognitive decline [104]. The clinical expression of vascular disease can manifest as either mild cognitive symptoms or a full-blown dementia that may be attributable to an AD process, mixed AD/vascular pathology, or vascular disease alone [105]. There is general agreement that the pure cases of AD account for less than 20% of all the cases and that AD with various components of vascular disease are much more common than AD alone [106–108]. The amount of AD pathology necessary to produce clinical dementia seems to be less when concurring with the presence of vascular risk factors [105]. The cumulative presence of vascular disease has a biological gradient in the severity of cognitive decline moderated by covariates like age, gender, and race [109–111]. This is difficult to disentangle, as it would be unethical to perform an RCT to evaluate the effects of controlling for risk factors in some but not other subjects.

Hypertension and Hypercholesterolemia

It seems that a lifetime exposure to cardiovascular risk factors can be associated with higher odds for dementia, suggestive of a time period where exposure is more fundamental for subsequent risk. The interaction of the risk exposure and time of onset varies according to each risk factor. There is evidence that higher levels of systolic pressure in midlife are associated with higher risk of dementia later in life, but lower levels of systolic pressure later in life can also be associated with dementia [112]. The same effect has been described for cholesterol levels [113].

In primary prevention trials of cardiovascular disease, conflicting evidence exists about the effect on controlling risk factors and the incidence of dementia. While treatment of hypertension with calcium channel blockers and ACE inhibitors showed reduction in all cardiovascular outcomes and halved the risk to develop AD [114], other trials using diuretics and beta-blockers or angiotensin receptor blockers did not reproduce the findings [115, 116]. Recent meta-analyses have not found a significant effect in the treatment of hypertension with the subsequent risk of developing AD [2, 117, 118]. Trials and meta-analysis investigating the effects of cholesterol lowering medications (statins) have failed to demonstrate protective effects of statins on the subsequent risk of developing AD [2, 119–121]. It is possible that the large number of covariates to control in these trials such as concomitant risk factors, education, diet content, levels of exercise, and genetic predisposition, might partially account for the lack of clear benefit. Regardless, cardiovascular risk factors should be aggressively treated in populations with or without cognitive decline to reduce cardiovascular mortality.

Diabetes and Insulin Resistance

Several investigators have claimed that insulin resistance is a risk factor for cognitive decline [106]. Insulin facilitates cognition when given concomitantly with glucose to support metabolism. Defects in insulin signaling are associated with increased deposition of Aβ and hyperphosphorylated tau. Insulin-degrading enzyme (IDE) is a protease involved in the degradation of insulin and Aβ. In patients with hyperinsulinemia, insulin can saturate IDE and subsequently increase the AB serum levels [122]. Patients with diabetes have lower hippocampal and prefrontal volumes when compared with nondiabetic controls [123]. The progression of dementia in patients with stroke and diabetes was more prominent when compared to patients without stroke without diabetes [124]. Diagnosed and undiagnosed diabetes have been associated with lower MMSE scores in a population-based sample [125]. Although diabetes has been strongly associated with the presence of AD [126–128], less is known about its treatment and the effects on dementia incidence [125, 129]. The treatment of diabetes should be a priority in all patients for its multiple deleterious consequences.

Smoking

Initial observational studies suggested that smoking could be associated with lower risk for developing

Alzheimer's disease in carriers of APOE ε4 [130, 131]. Former smokers had a decreased risk for developing dementia with increasing numbers of pack-per-year smoked. This was suggestive of a dose–effect relationship of higher exposure to nicotine and lower incidence of dementia [130, 132]. The interaction between APOE ε4 status and smoking exposure has been a matter of debate and that remains unclear. However, it is generally accepted that smokers have higher risk of developing dementia and that there is a dose–effect gradient with higher odds for heavier smokers [133].

Additionally, smoking can accelerate atrophy and degenerative changes resulting from neuronal loss [134, 135]. In a recent meta-analysis of prospective studies, Anstey et al. showed that current smokers had an increased risk of Alzheimer's disease compared with former smokers at baseline. Current smokers also shower greater decline in cognitive abilities, but the groups were not different regarding risk of vascular dementia or other dementias. The authors concluded that elderly smokers have increased risks of dementia and cognitive decline [136]. A recent systematic review found low-quality evidence to unequivocally support the association of tobacco use and dementia, although it was categorized as a risk factor [2]. There is no question that all smokers should be encouraged to quit. In the case of patients with cognitive decline and dementia, it should be even further emphasized.

Physical Exercise

Physical exercise is thought to exert its protective effects on cognition through the improvement of cardiovascular disease, as well as decreasing amyloid throughout the brain (e.g., frontal lobes and hippocampus) [5, 137]. Additionally, exercise induces brain neurotrophic factors that are used in repair processes [5, 137]. In observational studies, it has been demonstrated that there is lower prevalence of dementia in people who exercise regularly compared with those who do not [138, 139]. Interventional studies have demonstrated that people who become physically active can improve their cognition and can slow down the rate of decline as early as 4 months after the intervention. [140, 141]. Promoting exercise should be part of a holistic strategy to promote healthy lifestyles in patients and should be advised in patients with cognitive decline or AD unless contraindicated or not practical to implement. Tailoring of the physical exercise and routines to the patient's needs and capacities is advisable.

There is uncertainty regarding secondary prophylaxis with treatment of cardiovascular risk factors. Heterogeneous definitions of MCI and varying methodologies in conversion studies confound our understanding of the impact of these risk factors on the progression of MCI to dementia. Even assuming a stable and reproducible definition of MCI, no strong association has been found with the presence of cardiovascular risk factors [142]. To date, no strategy has been successful to halt the progression of MCI to dementia [106]. As mentioned above, general recommendations to engage in a healthy life should be applied to patients with MCI.

In summary, it would be unethical to advise against treating cardiovascular risk factors in the absence of evidence toward preventing cognitive decline or dementia. The development of cerebrovascular disease is a well-known consequence of uncontrolled risk factors, and the incidence of stroke is strongly associated with cognitive problem or dementia [143–146]. It is safe to say that addressing the cardiovascular profile should be a priority in patients with cognitive dysfunction, dementia, or those at risk of developing either.

Cognitive Engagement

The term "cognitive reserve" has been applied in the literature to describe the general idea that the greater number of neurons or advance neuropsychological competence (intelligence) can protect an individual from developing clinically evident cognitive decline or dementia [147]. A more comprehensive definition of cognitive reserve involves neurocomputational flexibility where the end goal is adaption. It proposes that high brain-reserve individuals have a larger repertoire of strategies to resolve complex tasks as well as redundant neuronal networks to carry out the same activities. As such, when a particular network malfunctions, other networks can be used to conduct the same strategy, or if not possible, other strategies can be used to solve the same tasks [148]. Environmental enrichment has been associated with neurotrophic and nerve growth factors, increased synaptogenesis, and synaptic plasticity [147].

Cognitive Training

Longitudinal studies assessing the association of mental activities and the incidence of dementia have shown that engaging in highly complex mental activities is a protective factor against the development of dementia, with a dose-dependent effect observed in some studies [149, 150]. A systematic review of observational studies evaluated 22 population-based cohorts and showed that education attainment, cognitive lifestyle activities, and occupational complexity conferred protection against the subsequent development of dementia [151]. An older trial found that individuals who received cognitive training had a favorable influence on everyday coping and on memory performance [152].

The ACTIVE trial published in 2002 was a major study in this field that randomized 2,832 patients to four groups and three intervention arms: 10-session group training for memory (verbal episodic memory; $n=711$), reasoning (ability to solve problems that follow a serial pattern; $n=705$), or speed of processing (visual search and identification; $n=712$) or a no-contact control group ($n=704$). The results showed significant improvement in 87% of processing speed, 74% of reasoning, and 26% of memory-trained participants and demonstrated reliable cognitive improvement immediately after the intervention period. Booster training significantly enhanced training gains in processing speed and reasoning interventions (speed booster, 92%; no booster, 68%; reasoning booster, 72%; no booster, 49%), which were maintained at the second year of follow-up. No training effects on everyday functioning were detected in the second year of follow-up [153]. A 5-year follow-up of the same population showed that compared with the control group, cognitive-trained subjects had improved cognitive abilities specific to the abilities trained that persisted after the intervention was stopped [154].

A computer-based cognitive training RCT aimed at improving aural language processing was linked to improvement in targeted cognition and non-trained cognitive function in the active group compared to controls [155]. In individuals with MCI, unimodal memory training might not be enough [156, 157]. A small study indicated that multimodal intervention might be more effective in patients with MCI [158]. The multidomain cognitive training approach has also been tested in patient with dementia with encouraging results [156]. However, longer follow-up is needed to investigate whether effects of cognitive training are sustained. Based on previous results, it seems advisable for individuals at risk for developing dementia to engage in cognitive training programs as part of a formal multimodal therapeutic approach.

Social Engagement

It has been well documented that individuals with reduced social networks are more risk for developing cognitive decline compared with those who have more broad social interactions. Activities that exposed the individual to interact with others and create bonding are considered protective against cognitive decline [5]. A few critics have challenged the notion that this is a predictive association, suggesting that the retraction from social networks might precede the onset of cognitive symptoms during midlife and could be a sign of premature non-cognition symptoms of neurodegeneration [159]. Other difficulties in isolating social engagement effects on the risk of dementia have been the multiple covariates associated with both such as exercise and cognitive reserve. It seems reasonable to advise engagement in social activities as tolerated to promote healthy aging.

Depression

One of the reversible causes of cognitive impairment that all aged adults with cognitive complaints should be assessed for is depression. It can be difficult to isolate depression from dementia, since patients with dementia have a higher prevalence of depression than nondemented populations, and sometimes depression could be a prodromal sign of dementia [5]. A recent meta-analysis of observational studies showed that depression doubles the risk of developing dementia in later life. Findings of increased risk were robust to sensitivity analyses. Interval between diagnoses of depression and AD was positively related to increased risk of developing AD, suggesting that rather than a prodrome, depression may be a risk factor for AD [160]. Even if the overall evidence quality is low, [2] patients with cognitive complaints should be screened for depression and treated when indicated.

Pharmacological Strategies

Hormones

Hippocampal atrophy is a major pathological change in patients with MCI or AD. Shrinkage of the hippocampus can start in early adulthood and accelerate with age; losses of 0.3–2.1% per year are reported, with slower rate of progression reported in women compared with men [161, 162]. The apparent slower degeneration in women in early adulthood reverses in the postmenopausal stage, with greater odds of dementia for women when compared with men [163]. This has led to multiple studies evaluating the role of estrogens and other gonadal hormones as neuroprotectors.

Estrogens are known to influence verbal fluency, verbal memory, performance on spatial tasks, and fine motor skills [164]. Estrogens can mediate neuroprotection due to their ability to mediate the oxidative processes in the brain, besides altering the potassium conductance, apoptosis, and transcriptional factors regulation [163]. The aging process is associated with decreased memory abilities, focusing attention efficiently and in speed of information processing. However, women tend to have smaller hippocampal volumes, decrease glucose metabolism in areas concerned with cognition, and greater age-adjusted prevalence of dementia [165]. Observational studies have suggested that memory problems are frequently associated with menopause, although otherwise healthy postmenopausal women do not have significant memory problems as measured by standard psychological testing [166, 167]. Blood levels of estrogenic hormones are not consistently associated with differential cognitive performance [168]. Another explanation of the excess of AD cases in women seen in observational designs has been the longer survival of women compared to men [169].

Several clinical trials and longitudinal studies have tried to disentangle this puzzle. Researchers observing a longitudinal cohort reported that hormone replacement therapy (HTR) was associated with better performance on psychological testing [170] although another group with a different cohort failed to reproduce this claim [171]. Two recent meta-analyses found a 29–34% risk reduction for women using HRT vs. nonusers [168, 172]. The Women's Health Initiative Memory Study (WHIMS) used a sample from a large, population-based prospective cohort to enroll in an RCT to test the hypothesis that HRT with estrogen with progestin could reduce the risk of MCI or dementia. They enrolled 4,532 patients who were randomized to active and control arms and followed up during approximately 13 months. They failed to show that estrogen in combination with progesterone offers a protective effect against cognitive decline in the form of MCI or probable dementia. On the contrary, they found an elevated risk of developing either MCI or dementia in patients using the HRT that almost double the risk for those not using it [4]. This is by far the largest and best-structured RCT to test the hypothesis that hormonal supplement could provide cognitive benefits. The possibility of hormonal replacement at earlier stages of gonadal hormone withdrawal in perimenopausal women has not been explored, and some believe that larger periods of estrogen deprivation can lead to irreversible damage to some brain structures [169, 173, 174]. This remains to be settled with future RCT specifically designed to test this hypothesis. At this point, there is no scientific evidence to recommend hormonal supplementation in postmenopausal women to prevent or treat cognitive decline. Anecdotally, many experts agree that when initiated after onset of menopause-related cognitive symptoms, hormonal supplementation may be beneficial, yet there is no established scientific evidence to support this observation.

The role of dehydroepiandrosterone (DHEA) has also been explored in the context of cognitive decline. They are the most abundant circulating hormones in young adults, and they are major precursors of androgens and estrogens in the central nervous system, [175] especially in the post-menopausal stage in aged individuals where the gonadal production of sex hormones drops [176]. Some observational studies have suggested that the drop of DHEA with aging can account for some of the cognitive difficulties associated with age, partially due to the unopposed deleterious effect of cortisol on the oxidative stress balance [10, 177]. Although the supplementation with DHEA is appealing as a way to prevent cognitive decline, human results have failed to prove any significant improvement in chronic supplementation of the hormones, and a few have shown negative effects. As theorized with HRT, it is thought the timing of supplementation is important and that future trial should explore early supplementation after the drop of "youthful" levels of the hormones [178]. Other explanations for this lack of results have been the age-associated decrement in enzymatic activity necessary to convert the hormones into their active metabolites as well as individuals with advanced disease. There is no evidence at this point to recommend the supplementation of DHEA for the prevention or treatment of cognitive decline.

Piracetam and Piracetam-Like Drugs

Piracetam is a nootropic compound ("nootrope" comes from ancient Greek meaning "for or toward the mind") [179]. The mechanisms of action of these medications are related to their effects as GABA-mimetic, antioxidants, modulators of intracellular calcium, as well as facilitators of cholinergic transmission in the hippocampal area [180]. Some members of this family are known as cognitive enhancers due to the facilitation of cognitive processes.

Piracetam is the most studied compound as a cognitive enhancer. It has been used to evaluate protection against cognitive decline in various clinical settings like traumatic brain injury, cerebrovascular insufficiency, cardiac bypass cognitive deficit, and MCI with promising results [180]. Part of its efficacy can be attributed to the offset of depressive symptoms. Conflicting evidence has been produced by meta-analysis [181, 182], and no large-scale trial has been implemented so far to demonstrate the effects of this compound in patients with MCI and dementia [181, 182]. Less studied nootropic compounds are oxiracetam, aniracetam, and pramiracetam. Phase I and II trials are promising, but the level of evidence available at this point is not enough to systematically recommend piracetam or any nootropic drugs for the prevention or treatment of cognitive decline.

Acetylcholinesterase Inhibitors

Among the widespread neurodegeneration in AD and MCI, the basal forebrain is affected. This area of the brain secretes acetylcholine that is part of an important neuronal pathway including memory. It is believed that in part, the acetylcholine deficiency is responsible for memory dysfunction in AD and MCI. Acetylcholinesterase (AChE) inhibitors are drugs that block or inhibit the enzyme in charge of degrading acetylcholine, thus favoring larger amount of acetylcholine present at the synaptic level [183]. It has also been suggested that AChE itself can somehow decrease the amyloid deposition making it also a good candidate as disease-modifying drugs [184].

In the USA, four AChE inhibitors have been approved: tacrine, donepezil, galantamine, and rivastigmine, although the last three have largely supplanted tacrine, the first AChE approved [185]. Donepezil (Aricept®) is an AChE inhibitor with an *N*-benzylpiperidine and an indanone moiety that shows longer and more selective action. It is currently FDA-approved for the treatment of mild, moderate, and severe Alzheimer's dementia. It is highly selective of AChE, and it has been shown to strongly inhibit AChE as well as to increase the levels of AChE in animal and humans models [186]. Galantamine (Razadyne®) is a selective, reversible competitive AChE inhibitor that has been approved for the symptomatic treatment of Alzheimer's disease. Galantamine is a natural product belonging to the Amaryllidaceae family of alkaloids [187]. Galantamine was the first drugs of this class to have an extended release form and also the first to come off patent and go generic. Rivastigmine (Exelon®) is a pseudo-irreversible inhibitor of both AChE and butyrylcholinesterase and has been shown in a number of clinical trials to be efficacious in AD. Unlike other cholinesterase inhibitors that are only available in oral formulations, a novel transdermal rivastigmine patch has been developed and approved for the treatment of mild-to-moderate AD [188]. Several clinical trials have shown mild to modest improvement on various cognitive tests; however, more uncertainty exists in the behavioral outcome associated with these drugs.

There have been multiple reviews and meta-analysis on whether AChE inhibitors are useful. The conflicting results are mainly due to the criteria to evaluate the evidence and the trial results. Hansen et al. included 26 RCT of all AChE inhibitors and evaluated four outcomes: cognition, function, behavior, and global score. The evidence was also rated according to its methodological strengths. Only four studies had good evidence, the majority had fair qualification, and a few did not provided enough information to rate them. In cognition, function, and behavior, the pooled means for all drugs were statistically significant. In the global domain, galantamine was borderline nonsignificant. No head-to-head comparison among AChE inhibitors was significant due to poor quality of the data available for review [185]. Another meta-analysis approach investigated the effects of AChE inhibitors in AD, vascular dementia, and MCI. Donepezil and galantamine were found to offer benefit in cognition when compared to placebo in AD and vascular dementia patients, but donepezil failed to prove a significant effect in MCI patients. The authors also evaluated a summary relative risk for improvement or stabilization with input for providers and caregivers. In this analysis, the effects remained significant in all groups and for all drugs except for donepezil in vascular dementia treatment and rivastigmine for improvement/stabilization for all types of dementia [189]. Two recent systematic reviews determined that there was no significant effect of AChE inhibitors in improvement or stabilization of cognitive decline in aged adults based on moderate quality evidence [2, 3].

The administration of AChE inhibitors is recommended for patients with AD or vascular dementia upon proper medical evaluation and when there are no contraindications to their administration. The drug of choice should be individualized based on tolerability, indications, as well as practical issues like insurance status, route of administration, and familiarity of the physician with the drugs. There is no enough evidence at this point to support the use of AChE inhibitors in patients at risk for cognitive decline or with MCI; better powered studies are needed to discern this question.

Memantine

Memantine (Namenda®) is an uncompetitive *N*-methyl-D-aspartate (NMDA) receptor antagonist with moderate affinity. In general, NMDA receptor antagonists are considered good neuroprotectors due to their ability to counterweight excessive glutamate stimulation that is associated with increased intracellular calcium, mitochondrial dysfunction, and eventually apoptosis [190]. The pharmacokinetic properties of memantine make it a theoretical good drug for exitotoxicity-related pathologies.

Memantine is approved for moderate to severe dementia and can be used in combination with AChE inhibitors when indicated. The trials that lead to the approval of memantine followed the patient over no more than 28 weeks. The outcome evaluation varied among them, and the results showed improvement in some but not all cognitive domains evaluated; the behavior domain was certainly the least affected [191–193]. Subsequently, Wilcock et al. found significant improvement in agitation/aggression markers in a 6-month follow-up trial [194]. In a recent meta-analysis, memantine was not better than placebo to improve ADAS-cog scores in patients with mild-to-moderate AD; however, it did show benefit in patients with vascular dementia and better scores in a scale used to evaluate the caregiver impression of stabilization or improvement of the disease (CIBIC-plus) [189]. There is presently not enough data to evaluate if memantine can provide protective effects in patients with MCI [2, 3].

Novel Therapies

Immune Therapy

The deposition of Aβ is considered to be a major pathway in the neurodegeneration seen in AD. Researchers have used either active or passive vaccination with antibodies against Aβ to reduce deposition and/or increase clearance of Aβ in the brain [195]. Intravenous immunoglobulins (IVIG) have been used in trials to treat Alzheimer's dementia. The proposed mechanism of action includes catalization of Aβ oligomers, conformational changes of Aβ fibrils making them less prone to aggregation, and complement activation, among others [196]. In an open-label, small-sample, dose-finding study, Relkin et al. found benefit of administering IVIG on cognitive scores in patient with Alzheimer's dementia [197]. Based on these and other preliminary results, a phase III trial is currently underway to determine the efficacy of IVIG in the treatment of AD. The first vaccination attempt was stopped prematurely due to a major adverse event associated to the vaccine (6% of the patient enrolled developed meningoencephalitis). It was hypothesized that the patients developed a strong T-cell reaction that induced an autoimmune disease to the affected areas of the brain where Aβ deposits were found. Only 19% developed a serum response with positive antibodies against Aβ found in plaques and vascular amyloid but not to soluble Aβ. It was found also that respondents had slower rate of cognitive decline, and in autopsies done subsequently, it was found that respondents had less plaque deposition that non-respondents. Of interest, the presence of meningoencephalitis was independent of the antibody response [195, 198]. Based on these encouraging results, a new epitope is being investigated that would be designed to target mainly B cells aiming at avoiding or decreasing the risk of meningoencephalitis shown in the previous trial. The results from animal models have so far been promising, although no human phase I study is currently going on [199].

Bapineuzumab is a humanized monoclonal antibody use for passive transfer of antibodies against soluble Aβ. Preclinical trials have showed a nonsignificant trend for improvement in cognition when compared to placebo in patient with AD. Post hoc analysis found significant effects on cognition for APOE ε4 noncarriers compared to no effects in carriers. A phase III trial is currently underway [200].

Gamma Secretase Inhibitors

Amyloid precursor protein is cleaved by beta and gamma secretases to produce multiple-sized Aβ fibrils. Gamma secretases can produce Aβ40 and Aβ42, the first one being the most abundant and the second one the most prone to aggregation and deposition [201]. Gamma secretase inhibition could potentially reduce Aβ production and decrease the aggregation and plaque burden in AD. A phase I trial of a gamma secretase compound called LY450139 has demonstrated that it can reduce Aβ concentrations in the brain, cerebrospinal fluid, and serum [202]. A phase II trial of the same compound showed significant reduction in the serum levels of Aβ40 and Aβ42 in serum nut not in CFS. No cognitive effects were seen in either active group compared to placebo, although the follow-up was short (14 weeks). A phase III trial is currently underway to evaluate efficacy [203].

Conclusions

Effective strategies to prevent cognitive decline in the context of normal aging, mild cognitive impairment, and dementia are imperative to face the oncoming epidemic of dementia and cognitive disease in our society. Evidence-based recommendations are imperative to avoid unnecessary expenses and the creation of false expectation in patients and their families. Methodological difficulties and biases assault several good-intentioned trials. Existing studies have provided some clues into the puzzle of prevention of cognitive decline, yet it is rare that the evidence is unquestionable. The issue of studying a complex process like cognition represents challenges that researchers must be aware of. The presence of multiple factors and covariates that can bias the results presents a major hurdle in the design stage as well as in the statistical analysis, especially in small-sample studies.

When evaluating diet components, the major difficulty is in isolating the effect that a nutrient or diet component has on cognition or the evolution of dementia. The fact that isolated vitamins, minerals, and other components have failed to demonstrate a reliable association does not mean that the intake of these is not beneficial. There is a possibility that the combination of multiple components is what makes the difference. Additionally, trying to adhere to healthy lifestyle recommendations including a diet rich in essential nutrients, smoking abstinence, regular exercise, as well as adequate cardiovascular profile is by all means a goal in any patient. Challenging the brain with new information and new experiences seems to be advisable, especially in those who already have early cognitive complains. There is no evidence at this point that pharmacological agents can slow down the progression of MCI to dementia. The administration of AChE inhibitors in combination with memantine should be prescribed when applicable to demented patients to stabilize the disease and probably slow down the progression. Promising novel therapies include active and passive immunization against Aβ peptides and gamma secretase inhibitors to reduce Aβ production. Table 12.1 summarizes the literature on prevention of cognitive decline. A summary of prevention strategies for patients and their families is presented in Table 12.2.

Table 12.1 Summary of the literature on prevention of cognitive decline

Strategy studied	Presumptive mechanism of action	State of evidence in the prevention of cognitive decline/dementia
Vitamin 1 (thiamine)[a]	– Normal functioning of the brain–blood barrier – Adequate cellular functioning	– Not sufficient to recommend it
Vitamin B2 (riboflavin)[a]	– Important cofactor in energy production	– Not sufficient to recommend it
Pyridoxine (vitamin B6)[a]	– Important cofactor for neurotransmitter production – Involved in homocysteine metabolism	– Not sufficient to recommend it
Cobalamin (vitamin B12)[a]	– Important in cell reproduction and DNA synthesis – Involved in homocysteine metabolism – Cofactor is fatty acid synthesis	– Not sufficient to recommend it – Cobalamin levels are part of the initial dementia workup
Folate[a]	– Important in cell reproduction and DNA synthesis – Involved in homocysteine metabolism – Antioxidant properties	– Not sufficient to recommend it – Folate levels are part of the initial dementia workup
Vitamins C and E[a]	– Powerful antioxidants – Adequate cellular reproduction and functioning – Important for a healthy immune system	– Not sufficient to recommend it
Chromium	– Improves insulin resistance	– Not sufficient to recommend it
Berries	– Powerful antioxidants – Neuroprotectors	– Not sufficient to recommend it

(continued)

Table 12.1 (continued)

Strategy studied	Presumptive mechanism of action	State of evidence in the prevention of cognitive decline/dementia
Curcumin	– Antioxidant – Anti-inflammatory – Aβ aggregation inhibitor – Anti-apoptotic	– Not sufficient to recommend, weigh risk:benefit ratio individually
Docosahexaenoic acid (DHA)	– Neuroprotector, specially for synaptic activity – Anti-inflammatory – Antioxidant	– Probably effective – More efficacious in APOE ε4-negative patients
Mediterranean diet	– Supply of a synergistic combination of essential nutrient and vitamins for normal metabolic functioning	– Advised as part of a healthy lifestyle but not enough evidence to claim a consistent benefit in cognition
Garlic	– Antioxidant – Hypolipemic	– Not sufficient to recommend it
Ginkgo biloba	– Anti-inflammatory – Antioxidant – Improves blood circulation	– Not sufficient to recommend it
Low alcohol consumption	– Favors lipid profile – Flavonoids in some types of wines could serve as antioxidants	– Not sufficient to recommend it
Caffeine	– Increases arousal, especially in aged individuals – Neuroprotective – Cognitive normalizer (see text)	– Can provide a boost in some cognitive processes – More evidence needed to recommend it systematically
Treatment of hypertension, diabetes, and dyslipidemia	– Decreases oxidative processes in the brain – Improves cerebral circulation – Decreases incidence of stroke – Decreases incidence of vascular dementia	– Essential component of all patients with cognitive complains – The negative results of trials treating these factors have to be taken in consideration for future strategies
Smoking abstinence	– Decreases oxidative process – Decreases incidence of stroke	– Al patient should be strongly advice to quit smoking
Physical exercise	– Stimulates neurotrophic factors production – Improves oxygenation capacity – Improves lipid profile	– It should be recommended in all patients according to their capacities and needs
Social cognitive engagement	– Improves cognitive reserve – Could offset depressive symptoms and isolation	– Likely beneficial as part of a multimodal therapeutic approach
Cognitive training	– Improves cognitive reserve	– Recommended when possible as part of a multimodal therapeutic approach
Treatment of depression	– Improves overall neurological functioning – Can impaired adequate oral intake, compliance with medications, social engagement, etc.	– Recommended when indicated – Depression screening is part of the initial dementia workup
Hormonal replacement therapy	– Can prolonged the neuroprotective effects of estrogens in postmenopausal women – Improve cardiovascular profile – Neurotrophic effects in the brain	– Not recommended – More studies needed to evaluate earlier interventions
Dehydroepiandrosterone (DHEA)	– Endogenous precursor of sexual hormones – Opposes the deleterious effects of increased cortisol in the brain	– Not sufficient to recommend it
Nootropic compounds (piracetam)	– Cognitive facilitators – Antioxidants – Weak antidepressant	– Not sufficient to recommend it
Acetylcholinesterase inhibitors	– Increase cholinergic activity in the brain facilitating cognitive processes – Weak Aβ aggregation inhibitors	– Recommended for the treatment of dementia if applicable – No sufficient evidence to recommended it for the treatment or prevention of MCI

(continued)

Table 12.1 (continued)

Strategy studied	Presumptive mechanism of action	State of evidence in the prevention of cognitive decline/dementia
Memantine	– Neuroprotection by offsetting excessive glutaminergic activity	– Recommended in patient with moderate to severe dementia when feasible
Active and passive immunization against Aβ	– Inhibits aggregation and deposition of Aβ peptides in the brain – Decreases neurodegeneration associated to Aβ plaques	– Used only under research protocols
Gamma secretase inhibitors	– Decreased the production of Aβ oligomers that are prone to aggregation	– Used only under research protocols

MCI mild cognitive impairment, *Aβ* amyloid beta
[a]In the context of proven deficiencies, it should be treated accordingly

Table 12.2 Top ten strategies for Alzheimer's disease prevention

1. Increase physical activity as tolerated and as approved by your primary care physician
2. Have a healthy diet (e.g., incorporating a Mediterranean-style diet, including fruits and vegetables, lean protein (fish, chicken, turkey), low-fat items, nuts, and seeds
3. Increase socialization, including activity programs, adult education classes, and social groups
4. De-stress! Think positive and see your primary care physician for general guidance
5. Increase mental activity
6. Listen to music (especially classical) and consider music therapy programs
7. Ongoing follow-up with your primary care doctor for routine health maintenance (i.e., control vascular risk factors such as high blood pressure, cholesterol, diabetes/high sugars) to decrease rate of progression of memory decline
8. Assure adequate dietary intake of essential vitamins. Consider a multivitamin each day, folic acid 1 mg (total) each day, and vitamin D 1,000–2,000 I.U. each day
9. Curcumin (turmeric root) one tablet twice per day. Buy in a health food store
10. Fish oil capsules, slowly increasing to at least three capsules each day – must have DHA in it, the more the better

A more detailed review of treatment and prevention strategies for Alzheimer's disease can be found at www.TheADplan.com. For a resource for patients and families, see Isaacson, Richard S. Alzheimer's Treatment Alzheimer's Prevention: A Patient and Family Guide. Florida: Alzheimer's Disease Education Consultants, 2012

Clinical Pearls

- When it comes to vitamins and minerals, if deficient, treat. There is no evidence that more of something you already have is useful.
- What is good for the heart is good for the brain; paying attention to CV risk factors is important.
- There is no evidence that hormonal supplementation can decrease the incidence of dementia. If there is an indication for hormonal supplementation, the cognitive status should not be a factor in the decision-making process.
- Some agents that are touted as having cognitive protective effects should only be used under physician supervision. This is due to wide availability, lack of FDA oversight, cost, and possible contraindications/adverse effects.
- A diet rich in vegetables, fruits, nuts, and fish is advisable to everybody, with particular emphasis in patients at risk of developing cognitive decline or Alzheimer's or vascular dementia.
- Patients should remain active physically and mentally. Physical exercise is among the best of all potential interventions against Alzheimer's disease.
- Patients with diagnosis of Alzheimer's dementia should be considered for medical therapy unless contraindicated.

References

1. Brown LA, Riby LM, Reay JL. Supplementing cognitive aging: a selective review of the effects of ginkgo biloba and a number of everyday nutritional substances. Exp Aging Res. 2010;36:105–22.
2. Plassman BL, Williams Jr JW, Burke JR, Holsinger T, Benjamin S. Systematic review: factors associated with risk for and possible prevention of cognitive decline in later life. Ann Intern Med. 2010;153: 182–93.
3. Daviglus ML, et al. National Institutes of Health State-of-the-Science Conference statement: preventing alzheimer disease and cognitive decline. Ann Intern Med. 2010;153:176–81.
4. Shumaker SA, et al. Estrogen plus progestin and the incidence of dementia and mild cognitive impairment in postmenopausal women: the Women's Health Initiative Memory Study: a randomized controlled trial. JAMA. 2003;289:2651–62.
5. Middleton LE, Yaffe K. Promising strategies for the prevention of dementia. Arch Neurol. 2009;66:1210–5.
6. Brookmeyer R, Damiano A. Statistical methods for short-term projections of AIDS incidence. Stat Med. 1989;8:23–34.
7. Frautschy SA, Cole GM. Why pleiotropic interventions are needed for Alzheimer's disease. Mol Neurobiol. 2010;41:392–409.
8. Nehlig A. Is caffeine a cognitive enhancer? J Alzheimers Dis. 2010;20 Suppl 1:S85–94.
9. Prasain JK, Carlson SH, Wyss JM. Flavonoids and age-related disease: risk, benefits and critical windows. Maturitas. 2010;66:163–71.
10. Miller DB, O'Callaghan JP. Aging, stress and the hippocampus. Ageing Res Rev. 2005;4:123–40.
11. Glade MJ. Oxidative stress and cognitive longevity. Nutrition. 2010;26:595–603.
12. Akiyama H, et al. Inflammation and Alzheimer's disease. Neurobiol Aging. 2000;21:383–421.
13. Tapsell LC, et al. Health benefits of herbs and spices: the past, the present, the future. Med J Aust. 2006;185:S4–24.
14. Balk E, et al. B vitamins and berries and age-related neurodegenerative disorders. Evid Rep Technol Assess (Full Rep). 2006;164:1–161.
15. Riggs KM, Spiro 3rd A, Tucker K, Rush D. Relations of vitamin B-12, vitamin B-6, folate, and homocysteine to cognitive performance in the Normative Aging Study. Am J Clin Nutr. 1996;63:306–14.
16. Wang HX, et al. Vitamin B(12) and folate in relation to the development of Alzheimer's disease. Neurology. 2001;56:1188–94.
17. Seshadri S, et al. Plasma homocysteine as a risk factor for dementia and Alzheimer's disease. N Engl J Med. 2002;346:476–83.
18. Garcia A, Zanibbi K. Homocysteine and cognitive function in elderly people. CMAJ. 2004;171:897–904.
19. Ravaglia G, et al. Homocysteine and folate as risk factors for dementia and Alzheimer disease. Am J Clin Nutr. 2005;82:636–43.
20. Kado DM, et al. Homocysteine versus the vitamins folate, B6, and B12 as predictors of cognitive function and decline in older high-functioning adults: MacArthur Studies of Successful Aging. Am J Med. 2005;118:161–7.
21. Tucker KL, Qiao N, Scott T, Rosenberg I, Spiro 3rd A. High homocysteine and low B vitamins predict cognitive decline in aging men: the Veterans Affairs Normative Aging Study. Am J Clin Nutr. 2005;82: 627–35.
22. Terasawa M, Nakahara T, Tsukada N, Sugawara A, Itokawa Y. The relationship between thiamine deficiency and performance of a learning task in rats. Metab Brain Dis. 1999;14:137–48.
23. Jolicoeur FB, Rondeau DB, Barbeau A, Wayner MJ. Comparison of neurobehavioral effects induced by various experimental models of ataxia in the rat. Neurobehav Toxicol. 1979;1 Suppl 1:175–8.
24. Ciccia RM, Langlais PJ. An examination of the synergistic interaction of ethanol and thiamine deficiency in the development of neurological signs and long-term cognitive and memory impairments. Alcohol Clin Exp Res. 2000;24:622–34.
25. Meador K, et al. Preliminary findings of high-dose thiamine in dementia of Alzheimer's type. J Geriatr Psychiatry Neurol. 1993;6:222–9.
26. Mimori Y, Katsuoka H, Nakamura S. Thiamine therapy in Alzheimer's disease. Metab Brain Dis. 1996;11:89–94.
27. Jia X, McNeill G, Avenell A. Does taking vitamin, mineral and fatty acid supplements prevent cognitive decline? A systematic review of randomized controlled trials J Hum Nutr Diet. 2008;21:317–36.
28. Goodwin JS, Goodwin JM, Garry PJ. Association between nutritional status and cognitive functioning in a healthy elderly population. JAMA. 1983;249: 2917–21.
29. Lee H, Kim HJ, Kim JM, Chang N. Effects of dietary folic acid supplementation on cerebrovascular endothelial dysfunction in rats with induced hyperhomocysteinemia. Brain Res. 2004;996:139–47.
30. Scileppi KP, Blass JP, Baker HG. Circulating vitamins in Alzheimer's dementia as compared with other dementias. J Am Geriatr Soc. 1984;32:709–11.
31. Mizrahi EH, et al. Plasma total homocysteine levels, dietary vitamin B6 and folate intake in AD and healthy aging. J Nutr Health Aging. 2003;7:160–5.
32. Dangour AD, et al. B-vitamins and fatty acids in the prevention and treatment of Alzheimer's disease and dementia: a systematic review. J Alzheimers Dis. 2010;22:205–24.
33. Masuda Y, Kokubu T, Yamashita M, Ikeda H, Inoue S. EGG phosphatidylcholine combined with vitamin B12 improved memory impairment following lesioning of nucleus basalis in rats. Life Sci. 1998;62: 813–22.
34. Tangney CC, Tang Y, Evans DA, Morris MC. Biochemical indicators of vitamin B12 and folate insufficiency and cognitive decline. Neurology. 2009;72:361–7.
35. Kwok T, et al. Randomized trial of the effect of supplementation on the cognitive function of older

people with subnormal cobalamin levels. Int J Geriatr Psychiatry. 1998;13:611–6.
36. Hvas AM, Juul S, Lauritzen L, Nexo E, Ellegaard J. No effect of vitamin B-12 treatment on cognitive function and depression: a randomized placebo controlled study. J Affect Disord. 2004;81:269–73.
37. Kruman II, et al. Folic acid deficiency and homocysteine impair DNA repair in hippocampal neurons and sensitize them to amyloid toxicity in experimental models of Alzheimer's disease. J Neurosci. 2002;22:1752–62.
38. Mattson MP, Chan SL, Duan W. Modification of brain aging and neurodegenerative disorders by genes, diet, and behavior. Physiol Rev. 2002;82: 637–72.
39. Morris MC, et al. Dietary folate and vitamin B12 intake and cognitive decline among community-dwelling older persons. Arch Neurol. 2005;62: 641–5.
40. Fioravanti M, et al. Low folate levels in the cognitive decline of elderly patients and the efficacy of folate as a treatment for improving memory deficits. Arch Gerontol Geriatr. 1998;26:1–13.
41. Bryan J, Calvaresi E, Hughes D. Short-term folate, vitamin B-12 or vitamin B-6 supplementation slightly affects memory performance but not mood in women of various ages. J Nutr. 2002;132: 1345–56.
42. Sommer BR, Hoff AL, Costa M. Folic acid supplementation in dementia: a preliminary report. J Geriatr Psychiatry Neurol. 2003;16:156–9.
43. Wald DS, Kasturiratne A, Simmonds M. Effect of folic acid, with or without other B vitamins, on cognitive decline: meta-analysis of randomized trials. Am J Med. 2010;123:522–7. e522.
44. Perrig WJ, Perrig P, Stahelin HB. The relation between antioxidants and memory performance in the old and very old. J Am Geriatr Soc. 1997;45:718–24.
45. Morris MC, Evans DA, Bienias JL, Tangney CC, Wilson RS. Vitamin E and cognitive decline in older persons. Arch Neurol. 2002;59:1125–32.
46. Wengreen HJ, et al. Antioxidant intake and cognitive function of elderly men and women: the Cache County Study. J Nutr Health Aging. 2007;11: 230–7.
47. Dangour AD, Sibson VL, Fletcher AE. Micronutrient supplementation in later life: limited evidence for benefit. J Gerontol A Biol Sci Med Sci. 2004;59: 659–73.
48. Wallum BJ, et al. Cerebrospinal fluid insulin levels increase during intravenous insulin infusions in man. J Clin Endocrinol Metab. 1987;64:190–4.
49. Krikorian R, Eliassen JC, Boespflug EL, Nash TA, Shidler MD. Improved cognitive-cerebral function in older adults with chromium supplementation. Nutr Neurosci. 2010;13:116–22.
50. Cefalu WT, Wang ZQ, Zhang XH, Baldor LC, Russell JC. Oral chromium picolinate improves carbohydrate and lipid metabolism and enhances skeletal muscle Glut-4 translocation in obese, hyperinsulinemic (JCR-LA corpulent) rats. J Nutr. 2002;132: 1107–14.
51. Anderson RA, et al. Elevated intakes of supplemental chromium improve glucose and insulin variables in individuals with type 2 diabetes. Diabetes. 1997;46:1786–91.
52. Hamaguchi T, Ono K, Murase A, Yamada M. Phenolic compounds prevent Alzheimer's pathology through different effects on the amyloid-beta aggregation pathway. Am J Pathol. 2009;175: 2557–65.
53. Crozier A, Del Rio D, Clifford MN. Bioavailability of dietary flavonoids and phenolic compounds. Mol Aspects Med. 2010;31(6):446–67.
54. Moyer RA, Hummer KE, Finn CE, Frei B, Wrolstad RE. Anthocyanins, phenolics, and antioxidant capacity in diverse small fruits: vaccinium, rubus, and ribes. J Agric Food Chem. 2002;50:519–25.
55. Halvorsen BL, et al. A systematic screening of total antioxidants in dietary plants. J Nutr. 2002;132: 461–71.
56. Saija A, Princi P, D'Amico N, De Pasquale R, Costa G. Effect of Vaccinium myrtillus anthocyanins on triiodothyronine transport into brain in the rat. Pharmacol Res. 1990;22 Suppl 3:59–60.
57. Casadesus G, et al. Modulation of hippocampal plasticity and cognitive behavior by short-term blueberry supplementation in aged rats. Nutr Neurosci. 2004;7: 309–16.
58. Joseph JA, Fisher DR, Carey AN. Fruit extracts antagonize Abeta- or DA-induced deficits in Ca2+ flux in M1-transfected COS-7 cells. J Alzheimers Dis. 2004;6:403–11. discussion 443–409.
59. Yang F, et al. Curcumin inhibits formation of amyloid beta oligomers and fibrils, binds plaques, and reduces amyloid in vivo. J Biol Chem. 2005;280: 5892–901.
60. Rinwa P, Kaur B, Jaggi AS, Singh N. Involvement of PPAR-gamma in curcumin-mediated beneficial effects in experimental dementia. Naunyn Schmiedebergs Arch Pharmacol. 2010;381:529–39.
61. Lao CD, et al. Dose escalation of a curcuminoid formulation. BMC Complement Altern Med. 2006;6:10.
62. Baum L, et al. Six-month randomized, placebo-controlled, double-blind, pilot clinical trial of curcumin in patients with Alzheimer disease. J Clin Psychopharmacol. 2008;28:110–3.
63. Hamaguchi T, Ono K, Yamada M. REVIEW: Curcumin and Alzheimer's disease. CNS Neurosci Ther. 2010;16:285–97.
64. Oster T, Pillot T. Docosahexaenoic acid and synaptic protection in Alzheimer's disease mice. Biochim Biophys Acta. 2010;1801:791–8.
65. Greiner RS, Moriguchi T, Hutton A, Slotnick BM, Salem Jr N. Rats with low levels of brain docosahexaenoic acid show impaired performance in olfactory-based and spatial learning tasks. Lipids. 1999; 34(Suppl):S239–243.
66. Chiu CC, et al. The effects of omega-3 fatty acids monotherapy in Alzheimer's disease and mild cognitive

impairment: a preliminary randomized double-blind placebo-controlled study. Prog Neuropsychopharmacol Biol Psychiatry. 2008;32:1538–44.

67. Freund-Levi Y, et al. Omega-3 fatty acid treatment in 174 patients with mild to moderate Alzheimer disease: OmegAD study: a randomized double-blind trial. Arch Neurol. 2006;63:1402–8.
68. Scheltens P, et al. Efficacy of a medical food in mild Alzheimer's disease: A randomized, controlled trial. Alzheimers Dement. 2010;6:1–10. e11.
69. Quinn JF, et al. Docosahexaenoic acid supplementation and cognitive decline in Alzheimer disease: a randomized trial. JAMA. 2010;304:1903–11.
70. Whalley LJ, et al. n-3 Fatty acid erythrocyte membrane content, APOE varepsilon4, and cognitive variation: an observational follow-up study in late adulthood. Am J Clin Nutr. 2008;87:449–54.
71. Feart C, Samieri C, Barberger-Gateau P. Mediterranean diet and cognitive function in older adults. Curr Opin Clin Nutr Metab Care. 2010;13:14–8.
72. Willett WC, et al. Mediterranean diet pyramid: a cultural model for healthy eating. Am J Clin Nutr. 1995;61:1402S–6S.
73. Kourlaba G, Polychronopoulos E, Zampelas A, Lionis C, Panagiotakos DB. Development of a diet index for older adults and its relation to cardiovascular disease risk factors: the Elderly Dietary Index. J Am Diet Assoc. 2009;109:1022–30.
74. Scarmeas N, Stern Y, Tang MX, Mayeux R, Luchsinger JA. Mediterranean diet and risk for Alzheimer's disease. Ann Neurol. 2006;59:912–21.
75. Scarmeas N, et al. Mediterranean diet and mild cognitive impairment. Arch Neurol. 2009;66:216–25.
76. Feart C, et al. Adherence to a Mediterranean diet, cognitive decline, and risk of dementia. JAMA. 2009;302:638–48.
77. Gu Y, Nieves JW, Stern Y, Luchsinger JA, Scarmeas N. Food combination and Alzheimer disease risk: a protective diet. Arch Neurol. 2010;67:699–706.
78. Borek C. Garlic reduces dementia and heart-disease risk. J Nutr. 2006;136:810S–2S.
79. Peng Q, Buz'Zard AR, Lau BH. Neuroprotective effect of garlic compounds in amyloid-beta peptide-induced apoptosis in vitro. Med Sci Monit. 2002;8:BR328–337.
80. Budoff MJ, et al. Inhibiting progression of coronary calcification using Aged Garlic Extract in patients receiving statin therapy: a preliminary study. Prev Med. 2004;39:985–91.
81. Gold PE, Cahill L, Wenk GL. The lowdown on Ginkgo biloba. Sci Am. 2003;288:86–91.
82. Oken BS, Storzbach DM, Kaye JA. The efficacy of Ginkgo biloba on cognitive function in Alzheimer disease. Arch Neurol. 1998;55:1409–15.
83. Dodge HH, Zitzelberger T, Oken BS, Howieson D, Kaye J. A randomized placebo-controlled trial of Ginkgo biloba for the prevention of cognitive decline. Neurology. 2008;70:1809–17.
84. Weinmann S, Roll S, Schwarzbach C, Vauth C, Willich SN. Effects of Ginkgo biloba in dementia: systematic review and meta-analysis. BMC Geriatr. 2010;10:14.
85. Peters R, Peters J, Warner J, Beckett N, Bulpitt C. Alcohol, dementia and cognitive decline in the elderly: a systematic review. Age Ageing. 2008;37: 505–12.
86. Orgogozo JM, et al. Wine consumption and dementia in the elderly: a prospective community study in the Bordeaux area. Rev Neurol (Paris). 1997;153:185–92.
87. Koppelstaetter F, et al. Caffeine and cognition in functional magnetic resonance imaging. J Alzheimers Dis. 2010;20 Suppl 1:S71–84.
88. Fredholm BB, Battig K, Holmen J, Nehlig A, Zvartau EE. Actions of caffeine in the brain with special reference to factors that contribute to its widespread use. Pharmacol Rev. 1999;51:83–133.
89. Dall'Igna OP, Porciuncula LO, Souza DO, Cunha RA, Lara DR. Neuroprotection by caffeine and adenosine A2A receptor blockade of beta-amyloid neurotoxicity. Br J Pharmacol. 2003;138:1207–9.
90. Arendash GW, et al. Caffeine protects Alzheimer's mice against cognitive impairment and reduces brain beta-amyloid production. Neuroscience. 2006;142: 941–52.
91. Cunha RA, Agostinho PM. Chronic caffeine consumption prevents memory disturbance in different animal models of memory decline. J Alzheimers Dis. 2010;20 Suppl 1:S95–116.
92. Huang CC, Liang YC, Hsu KS. A role for extracellular adenosine in time-dependent reversal of long-term potentiation by low-frequency stimulation at hippocampal CA1 synapses. J Neurosci. 1999;19: 9728–38.
93. d'Alcantara P, Ledent C, Swillens S, Schiffmann SN. Inactivation of adenosine A2A receptor impairs long term potentiation in the accumbens nucleus without altering basal synaptic transmission. Neuroscience. 2001;107:455–64.
94. Lieberman HR, Tharion WJ, Shukitt-Hale B, Speckman KL, Tulley R. Effects of caffeine, sleep loss, and stress on cognitive performance and mood during U.S. Navy SEAL training. Sea-Air-Land. Psychopharmacology (Berl). 2002;164:250–61.
95. Smith AP. Caffeine, cognitive failures and health in a non-working community sample. Hum Psychopharmacol. 2009;24:29–34.
96. Rees K, Allen D, Lader M. The influences of age and caffeine on psychomotor and cognitive function. Psychopharmacology (Berl). 1999;145:181–8.
97. Jarvis MJ. Does caffeine intake enhance absolute levels of cognitive performance? Psychopharmacology (Berl). 1993;110:45–52.
98. Lorist MM, Snel J, Mulder G, Kok A. Aging, caffeine, and information processing: an event-related potential analysis. Electroencephalogr Clin Neurophysiol. 1995;96:453–67.
99. Eskelinen MH, Ngandu T, Tuomilehto J, Soininen H, Kivipelto M. Midlife coffee and tea drinking and the risk of late-life dementia: a population-based CAIDE study. J Alzheimers Dis. 2009;16:85–91.

100. Ritchie K, et al. The neuroprotective effects of caffeine: a prospective population study (the Three City Study). Neurology. 2007;69:536–45.
101. van Gelder BM, et al. Coffee consumption is inversely associated with cognitive decline in elderly European men: the FINE Study. Eur J Clin Nutr. 2007;61:226–32.
102. Corley J, et al. Caffeine consumption and cognitive function at age 70: the Lothian Birth Cohort 1936 study. Psychosom Med. 2010;72:206–14.
103. van Boxtel MP, Schmitt JA, Bosma H, Jolles J. The effects of habitual caffeine use on cognitive change: a longitudinal perspective. Pharmacol Biochem Behav. 2003;75:921–7.
104. de la Torre JC. Alzheimer disease as a vascular disorder: nosological evidence. Stroke. 2002;33: 1152–62.
105. Snowdon DA, et al. Brain infarction and the clinical expression of Alzheimer disease. The Nun Study. JAMA. 1997;277:813–7.
106. Stephan BC, Brayne C. Vascular factors and prevention of dementia. Int Rev Psychiatry. 2008;20: 344–56.
107. Kalaria RN. Comparison between Alzheimer's disease and vascular dementia: implications for treatment. Neurol Res. 2003;25:661–4.
108. Fernando MS, Ince PG. Vascular pathologies and cognition in a population-based cohort of elderly people. J Neurol Sci. 2004;226:13–7.
109. Luchsinger JA, et al. Aggregation of vascular risk factors and risk of incident Alzheimer disease. Neurology. 2005;65:545–51.
110. Dartigues JF, Fabrigoule C, Barberger-Gateau P, Orgogozo JM. Memory, aging and risk factors. Lessons from clinical trials and epidemiologic studies. Therapie. 2000;55:503–5.
111. Launer LJ. Regional differences in rates of dementia: MRC-CFAS. Lancet Neurol. 2005;4:694–5.
112. Skoog I, et al. 15-year longitudinal study of blood pressure and dementia. Lancet. 1996;347:1141–5.
113. Mielke MM, Zandi PP. Hematologic risk factors of vascular disease and their relation to dementia. Dement Geriatr Cogn Disord. 2006;21:335–52.
114. Forette F, et al. Prevention of dementia in randomised double-blind placebo-controlled Systolic Hypertension in Europe (Syst-Eur) trial. Lancet. 1998;352: 1347–51.
115. Lithell H, et al. The Study on Cognition and Prognosis in the Elderly (SCOPE): principal results of a randomized double-blind intervention trial. J Hypertens. 2003;21:875–86.
116. Curb JD, et al. Effect of diuretic-based antihypertensive treatment on cardiovascular disease risk in older diabetic patients with isolated systolic hypertension. Systolic Hypertension in the Elderly Program Cooperative Research Group. JAMA. 1996;276:1886–92.
117. McGuinness B, Todd S, Passmore P, Bullock R. The effects of blood pressure lowering on development of cognitive impairment and dementia in patients without apparent prior cerebrovascular disease. Cochrane Database Syst Rev. 2006;19:CD004034.
118. McGuinness B, Todd S, Passmore P, Bullock R. Blood pressure lowering in patients without prior cerebrovascular disease for prevention of cognitive impairment and dementia. Cochrane Database Syst Rev. 2009;2:CD004034.
119. McGuinness B, Craig D, Bullock R,. Passmore P. Statins for the prevention of dementia. Cochrane Database Syst Rev.2009;4:CD003160.
120. Zhou B, Teramukai S, Fukushima M. Prevention and treatment of dementia or Alzheimer's disease by statins: a meta-analysis. Dement Geriatr Cogn Disord. 2007;23:194–201.
121. Agostini JV, et al. Effects of statin use on muscle strength, cognition, and depressive symptoms in older adults. J Am Geriatr Soc. 2007;55:420–5.
122. Cook DG, et al. Reduced hippocampal insulin-degrading enzyme in late-onset Alzheimer's disease is associated with the apolipoprotein E-epsilon4 allele. Am J Pathol. 2003;162:313–9.
123. Bruehl H, et al. Modifiers of cognitive function and brain structure in middle-aged and elderly individuals with type 2 diabetes mellitus. Brain Res. 2009; 1280:186–94.
124. Censori B, et al. Dementia after first stroke. Stroke. 1996;27:1205–10.
125. Bourdel-Marchasson I, et al. Characteristics of undiagnosed diabetes in community-dwelling French elderly: the 3 C study. Diabetes Res Clin Pract. 2007; 76:257–64.
126. Arvanitakis Z, Wilson RS, Bienias JL, Evans DA, Bennett DA. Diabetes mellitus and risk of Alzheimer disease and decline in cognitive function. Arch Neurol. 2004;61:661–6.
127. Allen KV, Frier BM, Strachan MW. The relationship between type 2 diabetes and cognitive dysfunction: longitudinal studies and their methodological limitations. Eur J Pharmacol. 2004;490:169–75.
128. Yaffe K, et al. Diabetes, impaired fasting glucose, and development of cognitive impairment in older women. Neurology. 2004;63:658–63.
129. Areosa SA, Grimley EV. Effect of the treatment of Type II diabetes mellitus on the development of cognitive impairment and dementia. Cochrane Database Syst Rev. 2002;4:D003804.
130. Aggarwal NT, et al. The relation of cigarette smoking to incident Alzheimer's disease in a biracial urban community population. Neuroepidemiology. 2006;26:140–6.
131. Ott A, et al. Smoking and risk of dementia and Alzheimer's disease in a population-based cohort study: the Rotterdam Study. Lancet. 1998;351:1840–3.
132. Merchant C, et al. The influence of smoking on the risk of Alzheimer's disease. Neurology. 1999;52:1408–12.
133. Juan D, et al. A 2-year follow-up study of cigarette smoking and risk of dementia. Eur J Neurol. 2004; 11:277–82.
134. Meyer J, Xu G, Thornby J, Chowdhury M, Quach M. Longitudinal analysis of abnormal domains comprising mild cognitive impairment (MCI) during aging. J Neurol Sci. 2002;201:19–25.

135. Fratiglioni L, Wang HX. Smoking and Parkinson's and Alzheimer's disease: review of the epidemiological studies. Behav Brain Res. 2000;113:117–20.
136. Anstey KJ, von Sanden C, Salim A, O'Kearney R. Smoking as a risk factor for dementia and cognitive decline: a meta-analysis of prospective studies. Am J Epidemiol. 2007;166:367–78.
137. Dishman RK, et al. Neurobiology of exercise. Obesity (Silver Spring). 2006;14:345–56.
138. Rockwood K, Middleton L. Physical activity and the maintenance of cognitive function. Alzheimers Dement. 2007;3:S38–44.
139. Ravaglia G, et al. Physical activity and dementia risk in the elderly: findings from a prospective Italian study. Neurology. 2008;70:1786–94.
140. Lautenschlager NT, et al. Effect of physical activity on cognitive function in older adults at risk for Alzheimer disease: a randomized trial. JAMA. 2008;300:1027–37.
141. Angevaren M, Aufdemkampe G, Verhaar HJ, Aleman A, Vanhees L. Physical activity and enhanced fitness to improve cognitive function in older people without known cognitive impairment. Cochrane Database Syst Rev. 2008;3:CD005381.
142. Matthews FE, Stephan BC, McKeith IG, Bond J, Brayne C. Two-year progression from mild cognitive impairment to dementia: to what extent do different definitions agree? J Am Geriatr Soc. 2008;56:1424–33.
143. Kirshner HS. Vascular dementia: a review of recent evidence for prevention and treatment. Curr Neurol Neurosci Rep. 2009;9:437–42.
144. Pohjasvaara T, et al. How complex interactions of ischemic brain infarcts, white matter lesions, and atrophy relate to poststroke dementia. Arch Neurol. 2000;57:1295–300.
145. Tatemichi TK, et al. Risk of dementia after stroke in a hospitalized cohort: results of a longitudinal study. Neurology. 1994;44:1885–91.
146. Moroney JT, et al. Risk factors for incident dementia after stroke. Role of hypoxic and ischemic disorders. Stroke. 1996;27:1283–9.
147. Valenzuela MJ. Brain reserve and the prevention of dementia. Curr Opin Psychiatry. 2008;21:296–302.
148. Stern Y. What is cognitive reserve? Theory and research application of the reserve concept. J Int Neuropsychol Soc. 2002;8:448–60.
149. Verghese J, et al. Leisure activities and the risk of dementia in the elderly. N Engl J Med. 2003;348: 2508–16.
150. Fratiglioni L, Wang HX, Ericsson K, Maytan M, Winblad B. Influence of social network on occurrence of dementia: a community-based longitudinal study. Lancet. 2000;355:1315–9.
151. Valenzuela MJ, Sachdev P. Brain reserve and dementia: a systematic review. Psychol Med. 2006;36: 441–54.
152. Oswald WD, Rupprecht R, Gunzelmann T, Tritt K. The SIMA-project: effects of 1 year cognitive and psychomotor training on cognitive abilities of the elderly. Behav Brain Res. 1996;78:67–72.
153. Ball K, et al. Effects of cognitive training interventions with older adults: a randomized controlled trial. JAMA. 2002;288:2271–81.
154. Willis SL, et al. Long-term effects of cognitive training on everyday functional outcomes in older adults. JAMA. 2006;296:2805–14.
155. Mahncke HW, et al. Memory enhancement in healthy older adults using a brain plasticity-based training program: a randomized, controlled study. Proc Natl Acad Sci USA. 2006;103:12523–8.
156. Gates N, Valenzuela M. Cognitive exercise and its role in cognitive function in older adults. Curr Psychiatry Rep. 2010;12:20–7.
157. Troyer AK, Murphy KJ, Anderson ND, Moscovitch M, Craik FI. Changing everyday memory behaviour in amnestic mild cognitive impairment: a randomised controlled trial. Neuropsychol Rehabil. 2008;18:65–88.
158. Rozzini L, et al. Efficacy of cognitive rehabilitation in patients with mild cognitive impairment treated with cholinesterase inhibitors. Int J Geriatr Psychiatry. 2007;22:356–60.
159. Saczynski JS, et al. The effect of social engagement on incident dementia: the Honolulu-Asia Aging Study. Am J Epidemiol. 2006;163:433–40.
160. Ownby RL, Crocco E, Acevedo A, John V, Loewenstein D. Depression and risk for Alzheimer disease: systematic review, meta-analysis, and metaregression analysis. Arch Gen Psychiatry. 2006;63:530–8.
161. Tisserand DJ, Visser PJ, van Boxtel MP, Jolles J. The relation between global and limbic brain volumes on MRI and cognitive performance in healthy individuals across the age range. Neurobiol Aging. 2000;21: 569–76.
162. Wolf H, et al. Structural correlates of mild cognitive impairment. Neurobiol Aging. 2004;25:913–24.
163. Markou A, Duka T, Prelevic GM. Estrogens and brain function. Hormones (Athens). 2005;4:9–17.
164. Sherwin BB. Estrogenic effects on memory in women. Ann N Y Acad Sci. 1994;743:213–30. discussion 230–211.
165. Murphy DG, et al. Sex differences in human brain morphometry and metabolism: an in vivo quantitative magnetic resonance imaging and positron emission tomography study on the effect of aging. Arch Gen Psychiatry. 1996;53:585–94.
166. Caldwell BM, Watson RI. An evaluation of psychologic effects of sex hormone administration in aged women. I. Results of therapy after six months. J Gerontol. 1952;7:228–44.
167. Portin R, et al. Serum estrogen level, attention, memory and other cognitive functions in middle-aged women. Climacteric. 1999;2:115–23.
168. Yaffe K, Sawaya G, Lieberburg I, Grady D. Estrogen therapy in postmenopausal women: effects on cognitive function and dementia. JAMA. 1998;279: 688–95.
169. Barrett-Connor E, Laughlin GA. Endogenous and exogenous estrogen, cognitive function, and dementia in postmenopausal women: evidence from epidemiologic studies and clinical trials. Semin Reprod Med. 2009;27:275–82.

170. Maki PM, Zonderman AB, Resnick SM. Enhanced verbal memory in nondemented elderly women receiving hormone-replacement therapy. Am J Psychiatry. 2001;158:227–33.
171. Lokkegaard E, et al. The influence of hormone replacement therapy on the aging-related change in cognitive performance. Analysis based on a Danish cohort study. Maturitas. 2002;42:209–18.
172. LeBlanc ES, Janowsky J, Chan BK, Nelson HD. Hormone replacement therapy and cognition: systematic review and meta-analysis. JAMA. 2001;285: 1489–99.
173. Matthews K, Cauley J, Yaffe K, Zmuda JM. Estrogen replacement therapy and cognitive decline in older community women. J Am Geriatr Soc. 1999;47: 518–23.
174. Zandi PP, et al. Hormone replacement therapy and incidence of Alzheimer disease in older women: the Cache County Study. JAMA. 2002;288:2123–9.
175. Sorwell KG, Urbanski HF. Dehydroepiandrosterone and age-related cognitive decline. Age (Dordr). 2010;32:61–7.
176. Labrie F, et al. DHEA and the intracrine formation of androgens and estrogens in peripheral target tissues: its role during aging. Steroids. 1998;63: 322–8.
177. Karishma KK, Herbert J. Dehydroepiandrosterone (DHEA) stimulates neurogenesis in the hippocampus of the rat, promotes survival of newly formed neurons and prevents corticosterone-induced suppression. Eur J Neurosci. 2002;16:445–53.
178. Wolf OT, Kudielka BM, Hellhammer DH, Hellhammer J, Kirschbaum C. Opposing effects of DHEA replacement in elderly subjects on declarative memory and attention after exposure to a laboratory stressor. Psychoneuroendocrinology. 1998;23:617–29.
179. Giurgea C. The "nootropic" approach to the pharmacology of the integrative activity of the brain. Cond Reflex. 1973;8:108–15.
180. Malykh AG, Sadaie MR. Piracetam and piracetam-like drugs: from basic science to novel clinical applications to CNS disorders. Drugs. 2010;70:287–312.
181. Waegemans T, et al. Clinical efficacy of piracetam in cognitive impairment: a meta-analysis. Dement Geriatr Cogn Disord. 2002;13:217–24.
182. Flicker L, Grimley Evans J. Piracetam for dementia or cognitive impairment. Cochrane Database Syst Rev. 2000;2:CD001011.
183. Palmer AM. Cholinergic therapies for Alzheimer's disease: progress and prospects. Curr Opin Investig Drugs. 2003;4:820–5.
184. Rees TM, Brimijoin S. The role of acetylcholinesterase in the pathogenesis of Alzheimer's disease. Drugs Today (Barc). 2003;39:75–83.
185. Hansen RA, et al. Efficacy and safety of donepezil, galantamine, and rivastigmine for the treatment of Alzheimer's disease: a systematic review and meta-analysis. Clin Interv Aging. 2008;3:211–25.
186. Sugimoto H, Ogura H, Arai Y, Limura Y, Yamanishi Y. Research and development of donepezil hydrochloride, a new type of acetylcholinesterase inhibitor. Jpn J Pharmacol. 2002;89:7–20.
187. Marco L, do Carmo Carreiras M. Galanthamine, a natural product for the treatment of Alzheimer's disease. Recent Pat CNS Drug Discov. 2006;1:105–11.
188. Kurz A, Farlow M, Lefevre G. Pharmacokinetics of a novel transdermal rivastigmine patch for the treatment of Alzheimer's disease: a review. Int J Clin Pract. 2009;63:799–805.
189. Raina P, et al. Effectiveness of cholinesterase inhibitors and memantine for treating dementia: evidence review for a clinical practice guideline. Ann Intern Med. 2008;148:379–97.
190. Thomas SJ, Grossberg GT. Memantine: a review of studies into its safety and efficacy in treating Alzheimer's disease and other dementias. Clin Interv Aging. 2009;4:367–77.
191. Winblad B, Poritis N. Memantine in severe dementia: results of the 9 M-Best Study (Benefit and efficacy in severely demented patients during treatment with memantine). Int J Geriatr Psychiatry. 1999;14:135–46.
192. Reisberg B, et al. Memantine in moderate-to-severe Alzheimer's disease. N Engl J Med. 2003;348:1333–41.
193. Tariot PN, et al. Memantine treatment in patients with moderate to severe Alzheimer disease already receiving donepezil: a randomized controlled trial. JAMA. 2004;291:317–24.
194. Wilcock G, Mobius HJ, Stoffler A. A double-blind, placebo-controlled multicentre study of memantine in mild to moderate vascular dementia (MMM500). Int Clin Psychopharmacol. 2002;17:297–305.
195. Lemere CA. Developing novel immunogens for a safe and effective Alzheimer's disease vaccine. Prog Brain Res. 2009;175:83–93.
196. Dodel R, et al. Intravenous immunoglobulins as a treatment for Alzheimer's disease: rationale and current evidence. Drugs. 2010;70:513–28.
197. Relkin NR, et al. 18-Month study of intravenous immunoglobulin for treatment of mild Alzheimer disease. Neurobiol Aging. 2009;30:1728–36.
198. Schenk D. Amyloid-beta immunotherapy for Alzheimer's disease: the end of the beginning. Nat Rev Neurosci. 2002;3:824–8.
199. Fu HJ, Liu B, Frost JL, Lemere CA. Amyloid-beta immunotherapy for Alzheimer's disease. CNS Neurol Disord Drug Targets. 2010;9:197–206.
200. Salloway S, et al. A phase 2 multiple ascending dose trial of bapineuzumab in mild to moderate Alzheimer disease. Neurology. 2009;73:2061–70.
201. Portelius E, et al. A novel Abeta isoform pattern in CSF reflects gamma-secretase inhibition in Alzheimer disease. Alzheimers Res Ther. 2010;2:7.
202. Siemers ER, et al. Safety, tolerability, and effects on plasma and cerebrospinal fluid amyloid-beta after inhibition of gamma-secretase. Clin Neuropharmacol. 2007;30:317–25.
203. Fleisher AS, et al. Phase 2 safety trial targeting amyloid beta production with a gamma-secretase inhibitor in Alzheimer disease. Arch Neurol. 2008;65:1031–8.

Clinical Neuropsychology Practice and the Medicare Patient

13

Edward A. Peck III, Lucien W. Roberts III, and Joy M. O'Grady

Abstract

Neuropsychology practices continue to see increasing constraints on utilization and reimbursement by Medicare and other payors. In this chapter, the authors share insights regarding the business aspects of providing clinical neuropsychological care to Medicare patients. They discuss the internal revenue and cost drivers of today's neuropsychology practice and emphasize a proactive approach—whether in the private or institutional setting—to business planning and management. This chapter will help neuropsychologists maintain both fiscal viability and a high level of professional quality in patient care.

This chapter is divided into three sections. First, the authors delve into cost drivers and frequent inefficiencies of the practice. Next, the authors address common Medicare scenarios, sharing both examples and helpful forms. Finally, the authors share several insights on the future of neuropsychology and their recommendations for thriving amidst the changes that will come.

Keywords

Medicare • Business issues • Managed care • Office overhead costs • Practice expenses • Cost of practice • Medicare opt-out issues

In 1965, President Johnson signed H.R. 6675 to establish Medicare for the elderly in Missouri. President Truman was the first to enroll in Medicare [1].

Fast-forward a few years. The President of the United States, in his annual message to Congress, complained about the rising cost of health-care costs, the variations in access to health care, and the variation in the quality of health care across social and income groups. He recommended a

E.A. Peck III, Ph.D., ABPP-CN. (✉)
L.W. Roberts III, MHA, FACMPE
J.M. O'Grady, Ph.D.
Neuropsychological Services of Virginia, Inc,
2010 Bremo Road, Suite 127, Richmond,
VA 23226, USA
e-mail: epeckphd@aol.com; lucien.roberts@yahoo.com; jogrady9177@yahoo.com

L.D. Ravdin and H.L. Katzen (eds.), *Handbook on the Neuropsychology of Aging and Dementia*, Clinical Handbooks in Neuropsychology, DOI 10.1007/978-1-4614-3106-0_13,

more "level playing field" approach to national health-care reform that would rely on current market forces to bring change to the US health-care system. Congress voted deny the President what he wanted. A familiar story? The President was Richard Nixon, and the date of the annual speech to Congress was 1972. The concern was how much the then current federal programs contributed to "this growing investment in health" as a portion of national expenditures [2].

Fast-forward to the early 1980s. At that time there were relatively few nationally identified federal health-care sponsors besides Champus and Medicare or multistate private insurance carriers such as Blue Cross/Blue Shield (aka Anthem/aka Wellpoint). However, the mid to late 1980s saw the first sparks leading to the now recognized baby boomer explosion of aging in the US population. Suddenly, mental health services were confronted with the expansion of the Managed Care system and the resulting attempts by employers to limit the costs of medical care, while simultaneously trying to continue to offer a comprehensive insurance plan to their employees. For a much more detailed review of this period of health-care change, the reader is directed to The Managed Care Museum website [3].

Health maintenance organizations (HMOs), the predominant managed care "cost control" strategy of the 1980s, offered an all-or-nothing option: typically, only care provided by providers in a network HMOs was covered. Through much of this period and even today, mental health has been something of an afterthought for insurance payors. HMOs evolved and Preferred Provider Organizations (PPOs) were established to counter the "all-or-nothing" nature of restrictive HMO networks. These plans still had gatekeepers to access, but they also offered patients various financial and/or easier access to specified providers. In turn, these providers had to agree to work within the limitations in practice and the fees ordained by the PPO. Eventually, more costly Point of Service (POS) plans were developed to offer patients an opportunity to circumvent the more negative aspects of the gatekeeper provisions to their plans. In recent years, we have seen other efforts to control health-care costs by putting more of the responsibility for care on the patient. Plans such as health savings accounts, flexible spending accounts, high deductible health plans, and tiered-pricing formularies are all examples of this effort to control health-care costs by involving the patient in the responsibility for their care.

The federal and state governments have continued to attempt to control Medicare and Medicaid expenditures. None of these attempts at managing health-care costs have been particularly effective in tempering the rising costs of health care significantly. Nonetheless, we expect that there will continue to be a migration toward some form of managed care alternative to traditional Part B Medicare, combined with reduced payments, in Medicare. The clinical neuropsychologist cannot ignore Medicare HMOs and other limitations on Medicare, and simply hope that they will go away. Many Medicare managed care plans generally pay close to standard Medicare, but may present the patient and the provider with additional constraints (e.g., arduous preauthorization processes or fewer testing units permitted). It is incumbent upon each Medicare provider and/or professional practice group to understand the cost and hassle factor of doing business with each plan, so that they can make informed financial decisions with regard to participation in such plans.

Purpose of the Current Chapter

This chapter is designed to provide practical information concerning the business aspects of providing clinical neuropsychological care to Medicare patients under current (and projected) access and funding parameters. The specific focus is on Medicare reimbursement as it relates to practice management issues in clinical neuropsychology.

Medicare is not going away. It already comprises about 15% of the population of our nation. Medicare enrollment grew nearly 19% between 2000 and 2010, from 39.6 million enrollees to 47.1 million enrollees. The first baby boomers (those born between 1946 and 1964) became

Medicare eligible on January 1, 2011, and will contribute to an expected *doubling* of Medicare enrollment by 2030. The existing health-care infrastructure and Medicare reserves are not prepared. As a side note, Medicaid enrollment grew nearly 60% between 2000 and 2010, further stressing federal and state funding [4].

There will be increasing pressure on providers to do more with less and to cope with increasing constraints on utilization and reimbursement. In response, it is incumbent upon every neuropsychological practice to understand its internal revenue and cost drivers and to be as efficient—with time and resources—as practically possible.

Good business is good business, and many of the matters we discuss in this chapter are applicable to your entire clinical practice and not just to your Medicare patient services. At the end of the work day, the difference between the dollars which your practice collects and what your practice pays out in expenses is critical. A practice cannot thrive—much less survive—if it focuses on revenues while ignoring expenses, or vice versa. The successful neuropsychology practice must keep an eye on both revenues and expenses.

In this chapter, we emphasize a proactive response to the management of your professional practice, whether it is in a private or institutional setting. We believe that by being proactive in your business planning and management, you can avoid many patient- and insurance-related problems. This is far more reasonable than trying to resolve a situation which has already gotten out of control.

This chapter is comprised of three sections:

1. Understanding your Cost of Practice and Living Within Your Means
2. Addressing Common Medicare Scenarios: Examples and Forms
3. Medicare and Neuropsychology: A Look Forward to the Abyss or to Eden? What will our business management practices look like in the future?

The first section offers insight into the business management of your practice. We urge our readers to use this section as a building block upon which to improve the financial operation of their practices.

Understanding Your Cost of Practice and Living Within Your Means

Let us start with a basic point for the private practitioner or institutional practitioner. For the private practitioner, the point is how much your practice brings in per month is not as important as how much you actually spend per month to pay all the bills. You need to know the extent of your financial overhead in order to meet your responsibilities. For the institutional provider, the point is to understand and appreciate what your administrator is setting as your minimum RVU or cost recovery value per time unit for a specific time period (quarterly, yearly, and so forth). You need to know to understand what you (or the institution) have to spend to keep your practice open.

Our goal is to help you calculate what it actually costs your practice to operate. Knowing this cost is essential to managing your expenses and improving your operating margins. The first thing you should do is to have your accountant or office manager develop a financial spreadsheet which lists all of the expense categories paid during each month and each year. Table 13.1 is an example of a practice income statement; it lists many of the cost categories which should be included in such a spreadsheet [5].

The sum of your expenses is your total cost of practice. To make a profit, you must recoup more than this amount. Once you have calculated the total expense for your office, you can calculate "what if" scenarios relating to profit and loss. It is also helpful to look at a 3-year period when possible to trend/forecast changes. You should plan to calculate cost escalations for each of these line items, e.g., salaries and fringe benefits, as part of projecting expenses for the coming 3 years.

Once you have an annual total cost of operation, you can calculate your average total cost per hour of practice. For example, an office which is open 8 h a day, 5 days a week, has 2,080 operating hours per year, less holidays, vacations, bad weather closings, and the like. Dividing your annual total cost by your total operating hours will

Table 13.1 A sample financial report

	Sample financial report		
Revenues	Current month October	Current year to date 10 months	Prior year to date 10 months
Fees received	46484.87	350875.00	320897.50
Other income	2490.00	30115.00	18737.00
Interest earned	30.39	429.00	190.00
Total revenue	49005.26	381419.00	339824.50
Cost of practice			
Accounting	300.00	3000.00	2800.00
Advertising	50.00	500.00	425.00
Bank charges	17.81	581.79	500.00
Co. car loan	350.00	3500.00	0.00
Co. car expenses	65.00	650.00	639.00
Charity contributions	100.00	225.00	200.00
Continuing education	120.00	250.00	250.00
Dues and subscriptions	400.00	2805.00	3000.00
Employee benefits	660.00	6660.00	5000.00
Equipment—capital	0.00	2000.00	1000.00
Equipment—other	125.00	300.00	500.00
Insurance—malpractice	100.00	900.00	900.00
Insurance—Co. car	90.00	900.00	860.00
Insurance—other	140.00	1140.00	1000.00
Interest—loans	43.49	825.74	0.00
Legal fees	125.00	350.00	675.00
Licenses	100.00	450.00	450.00
Maintenance—equipment	475.00	2900.00	2500.00
Miscellaneous	50.00	2400.00	700.00
Office expense	239.00	3100.00	3000.00
Postage	135.00	1650.00	250.00
Refunds	50.50	1117.00	1750.00
Registrations—meeting	180.00	450.00	400.00
Rent—office	2000.00	20000.00	17000.00
Repairs	0.00	1000.00	800.00
Supplies—office	54.00	1334.75	1000.00
Supplies—test	125.25	375.00	350.00
Taxes—payroll	4800.00	48000.00	39000.00
Taxes—other	0.00	375.00	375.00
Telephone	210.24	2848.90	2500.00
Telephone ans. service	90.00	900.00	800.00
Travel	616.00	3300.00	1000.00
Meals and entertainment	75.00	590.00	200.00
Wages	8711.52	77810.64	74508.97
Total expenses	20597.81	193188.82	164332.97
Net income/loss	28407.45	188230.18	175491.53

Co. is company, *ans.* is answering

calculate your practice's average cost per hour of operation. Simply stated, if your practice is not bringing in at least this much per hour of operation (e.g., per week or per month), it is losing money.

It is possible to take a more detailed look at how much it costs you to provide an hour of testing or an hour of therapy. For example, you can set up a spreadsheet which incorporates cost items such as (1) technician salary and fringe benefits, (2) cost of test equipment, (3) cost of room space rent, (4) cost of front office (scheduling to billing), and (5) your salary and benefits. However, this is secondary to getting a solid handle on your overall average cost per hour of operation. Once you have a good feel for such data, you can dig deeper and look at individual financial facets of your practice.

This juncture is a good time to review your expenses at a "line item" basis. Be critical. We urge you to focus on expenses because a dollar saved is a dollar earned, whereas a dollar charged often results in receipts of less than half that.

Some axioms for consideration: A mere 30 min of overtime a day for a technician earning $20 an hour will cost your practice $3,900 per year ($20/h times 0.50 h/day times 5 days/week times 52 weeks/year times, at time-and-a-half). Add in matching tax obligations of 7.65%, and your cost exceeds $4,000 per year.

If you have a 5-year lease for 2,500 square feet at $20 per square foot, a 4% escalation clause will cost you $5,359 more than a 3% escalation clause over the term of the lease ($20/square foot times 2,500 square feet is $50,000 in rent in year 1; in year 5, you will be paying $58,493 with a 4% escalation clause or $56,275 with a 3% escalation clause).

By avoiding the overtime and higher rent escalation in these two examples, you would save more than $26,000 over 5 years. Savings equals income.

Review annual service agreements for copiers, faxes, credit card processing, and postage meters. Ask your vendors for better deals if you will renew for 24 months instead of 12 months. Talk with other medical practices to ensure that your staff wages and annual increases are not too far above or below the average range for your geographic area. Ask the practices next door and across the hall if they would like to bid out janitorial or some other service together to get a better price.

The checklist provided as Table 13.2 offers a roadmap for managing your practice better.

Clearly, Table 13.2 goes into more detail than we can discuss in the space of this chapter. However, we felt its inclusion would provide readers a good checklist of areas where the cost of your practice operations might be improved. In this regard, while it is possible for your practice to take a more detailed look at how much it costs you to provide an hour of testing or an hour of therapy is only part of getting a solid handle on your total average cost per hour of business operation.

Having gotten a grasp on your expenses, you should develop a spreadsheet that lists the actual reimbursement amount paid by each insurance carrier, for each service you provide. Table 13.3 presents such a spreadsheet, and it lists (for the purposes of this chapter) allowed payment rates for CPT codes 96118 and 90806, Medicare Region 3, and for several other (unidentified) plans. For the record, the other insurance plans are not named due to confidentiality requirements. Many insurance plans have subplans or carve outs to their plan, which may pay at different rates. This includes Medicare HMO and PPO plans. The spreadsheet that you develop should have the information organized so that each insurance plan can be viewed and compared for the CPT codes actually used in your office. Such a spreadsheet will serve several purposes, including allowing you to evaluate which insurance plans pay a better fee for a particular CPT code unit of service. Table 13.4 provides a comparison of CPT allowed payments from different insurer sources.

The following instances warrant consideration of contract termination or negotiation with the insurance company:

- If a payor pays relatively less than others or less than what it costs your practice to provide a service.
- If you and your office staff consistently spend so much time getting testing units or evaluations preapproved, or after providing the service, having to file and refile the claim for payment, that the cost of doing business with that company is not worth the payment received. Remember, this is an overhead expense. It may not be worth it to spend that time refiling the claim. It may be better that you terminate that contract.

While fee negotiation with Medicare is not possible, it is possible to negotiate with Medicare

Table 13.2 Practice operations checklist

	2011	2012	2013	2014	2015
Budgets					
Operating budget used to track performance?					
Operating budget includes prior year (PY) comparison?					
Capital budget established?					
Expenses compared to PY, budget, benchmarks?					
Retirement plans					
Service agreements (basis points) renegotiated?					
Expenses allocated to participants vs. borne by practice?					
Former employees removed if costing practice $$?					
Contributions balanced with operating cash?					
Timing/cost of plan valuations reviewed?					
Housekeeping					
Cost per square foot compared to other practices?					
Bid out or renegotiated alone or with other practices?					
Right sized frequency of service for satellite/nonclinical areas?					
Backed out square footage for space that will not be cleaned (e.g., samples closet, electrical/server closet, extra rooms)?					
Shredding					
Quarterly check of bins for nonpatient content?					
Bid out or renegotiated?					
Eliminated junk faxes?					
Checked for duplicate office notes, etc., and rooted out causes?					
Overtime/wage management					
Given wage increases only when warranted?					
Compared wages/benefits to those of other practices?					
Tracked overtime hours as a percent of worked hours?					
Reviewed schedules for smart scheduling?					
Tracked provider start time vs. scheduled start time?					
Avoided scheduling of "same sex" at end of day?					
Avoided scheduling of procedures at end of day?					
Ensured staff has exam rooms ready at start of day?					
Kept unwarranted overtime at a minimum?					
Employee retention					
Trended turnover rate vs. PY? By office/dept?					
Maintained undesired turnover at <5%?					
Engaged employees per the Gallup Q 12 Survey?					
Employees know what is expected of them?					
Employees have what they need to do their jobs?					
Employees have a chance to do their best everyday?					
Employees recognized/thanked every week?					
Employee development encouraged?					
Employee input requested and used?					
Equipment purchases and leases					
Obtained multiple bids?					
Bid out with other practices if buying common/same items?					
Asked finalists for better pricing/terms?					
Shopped for best interest rates?					

(continued)

Table 13.2 (continued)

	2011	2012	2013	2014	2015
Negotiated caps or free years on equipment maintenance?					
For operating leases, defined "fair market value" before signing?					
Locked in pricing on future purchases before signing?					
Looked for leases/loans with no personal guarantees?					
Negotiated supplies purchasing with future caps?					
Evaluated refinancing of existing leases?					
Credit card processing					
Obtained multiple bids? Compared ALL costs/rates?					
Considered Internet-based processing services?					
Considered dual purpose "swipe" readers?					
Copiers/printers/scanners/faxes					
Inventoried existing units/leases/maintenance agreements?					
Determined cost per copy of existing units?					
Bid out with other practices?					
Asked for free consolidation audits/bids from vendors?					
Reviewed ways to reduce unnecessary/duplicate copies?					
Eliminated high cost and duplicative units?					
Reviewed processes for document retention (scan vs. print)?					
Copiers/printers/scanners/faxes					
Compared current pricing discounted plans?					
Compared current pricing to other professional organization vendors?					
Solicited others in local community or same specialty to join in group purchasing?					
When purchasing the following, look at volume buying with others:					
Copiers/faxes					
Housekeeping					
Shredding					
Supplies/equipment					
Payroll/accounting					
Legal advice					
*Contract review					
Electronic medical records and practice management systems					
Employee benefits/insurance options					
Office supplies					
Kitchen/coffee service and supplies					
If you buy it, bid it…					
Revisit provider schedules					
Provider Time Off policies reviewed for impact on schedule?					
Provider Time Off policies reviewed for carryover limits?					
Provider Time Off truly and fairly tracked?					
Reviewed schedules to make sure schedulers are optimizing?					
Looked for possible scheduling inequities?					
Determine Relative Value Unit (RVU)/hour worked for each doctor/office?					

(continued)

Table 13.2 (continued)

	2011	2012	2013	2014	2015
Provider compensation agreements					
Reviewed compensation relative to collections and overhead?					
Incentives and formulas understood by providers?					
Buy-in from providers on incentives and formulas?					
At least 50% of compensation to production incentives?					
Communications					
Evaluated elimination of pagers via cell phone use?					
Considered foregoing insurance on units if pagers are retained?					
Reviewed monthly answering service invoices?					
Negotiated better rates and eliminated extraneous charges?					
Considered group bidding?					
Reviewed existing cell phone agreements?					
Considered foregoing maintenance insurance?					
Bid out agreement?					
Evaluated "family" vs. "corporate" plans?					
Looked at size of bucket of minutes vs. usage?					
Looked at cost of data messaging options?					
Completion of patient forms					
Asked patients to fill in nonclinical parts before appt.?					
Had providers/support staff fill out remainder during appt.?					
Reviewed charge(s) for form completion?					
Increased charge for time-consuming forms?					
Ensured form collection fees are collected up front?					
Patient registration forms					
Posted online or e-mailing to reduce copying/postage expenses?					
If making copies, farmed out to minimize cost per copy?					
The rent					
Negotiated cap on Common Area Maintenance increases?					
Negotiated annual rent increase limits?					
Obtained guaranteed construction timeline in writing?					
Analyzed financing options and rates?					
Locked in renewal terms, including $$$ for refurbishment?					
Included "No Trade" provisions in lease to protect against involuntary relocation?					
Asked landlord to pay for all construction, architectural, and space planning drawings?					
Refinanced existing loans?					
Insurance benefits					
Medical malpractice					
Right sized limits to state caps?					
Bid out to ensure rates are competitive?					
Secured "tail" coverage for retiring docs at no cost?					
Ensured provider employment agreements are clear on tail coverage?					
Health/dental/disability/Section 125					
Bid out to ensure rates are competitive?					
Ensured all alternatives considered have the key providers in network that your staff, your docs, and their families use?					

(continued)

Table 13.2 (continued)

	2011	2012	2013	2014	2015
Considered alternatives along a continuum of co-pays, deductibles, and drug plans?					
Offered multiple options (PPO, HMO, HAS)?					
Set practice's contribution to employee premiums as a fixed dollar amount rather than a percentage?					
Evaluated a Section 125 plan for employee premiums?					
Asked for group billing discounts for individual long term disability (LTD) policies?					
Looked to American Psychological Association (APA) and others for discounts?					
Updated asset schedules for tax and business insurance calculations?					
Deleted unused assets?					
Used good descriptions/serial numbers for new assets?					
Most costs are fixed, so…					
Evaluated adding one patient/provider/day or/half-day?					
Evaluated scheduling for efficient filling of schedules?					
Evaluated scheduling for potential creation of overtime?					
Ensured electronic remittance is in place and working?					
Looked to limit your nonrevenue-producing task producers?					
Credentialing?					
Mail review (and other distractions)?					
Patient/family phone calls?					
Exam room turnover?					
Ensured exam/testing rooms are stocked and ready?					
Shared "best kept" secrets with referrers to help them?					
Evaluated/reduced avoidable "no shows"?					
Looked at space utilization/efficiency/alternative uses?					
Subleasing?					
Shared satellite offices?					
Optimized coding and documentation?					
Most costs are fixed, so…					
Bell curve analyses vs. national norms and PY?					
Audited coding and documentation for problems/opportunities?					
Reviewed denial rates and trends by payor?					
Payor contracts					
Calculated operating expense and total expense per RVU?					
Compared payments for top 15–20 high dollar and high volume codes by payor to operating and total expense for same?					
Eliminated or renegotiated money-losing and marginal agreements?					
Actively managed "% of Medicare" contracts to ensure proper payment?					
Established base Medicare year for contracts to protect against cuts?					
Asked for annual fee schedule increases?					
Asked for relevant fee schedules (not sample fee schedule)?					
Completed a Strengths, Weaknesses/Limitations, Opportunities, and Threats (SWOT) analysis to assess negotiating strategy?					
Asked your providers and staff to complete Payor Report Cards?					
Asked for carve-outs for certain services or codes?					

(continued)

Table 13.2 (continued)

	2011	2012	2013	2014	2015
Loaded updated fee schedules in practice management system?					
Audited payments on signed contracts?					
If giving notice, considered 45+45 strategy?					
Co-pays, deductibles					
Ensured patients know what they owe before visit?					
Offered multiple payment options?					
Tracked collection of co-pays, deducts by site, by employee?					
Reminded staff what it costs to collect a co-pay after the fact?					
Ensured eligibility and deductible status are being checked previsit?					
Reminded providers that downcoding for friends only helps the payor?					
No shows					
Tracked "no show" excuses for patterns, noncompliance?					
Established "no show" fees not to anger but to deter?					
Empowered your front office to make decisions on excuse validity?					
After the fact collections					
Using Lockbox Services?					
Wasting $$ by sending pre-explanation of benefit (EOB) patient statements?					
Considering collections placement after two statements?					
After the fact collections					
Looked at service charges for second/third statements?					
Looked at service charges for statements for co-pays?					
Accounts payable					
Verifying ALL nonrecurring invoices?					
Reviewed renewing contracts for onerous "evergreen" clauses?					
Tracking and managing inventory?					
Considered online bill pay?					
Used a "rewards" credit card for paying bills where possible?					

Table 13.3 Tracking of Medicare allowed payments 2007 to 2011 for CPT codes 96118 and 90806

Year	CPT code	
	96118	90806
2007	$111.79	$87.71
2008	$106.45	$85.26
2009	$103.96	$91.77
2010	$97.01	$85.11
2011	$95.74	$87.97

managed plans offered by regional and national payors. This is particularly true when they need your specialty services due to local service supply shortages. It is better to walk away from an agreement that costs you more to provide the service than to provide the service for that plan.

This is also a time to review your commercial payor contracts and ensure you are being paid what you are due. Surprise, surprise, some payors have been known to pay less than what they have told you they will pay you! Medicare claims are generally paid accurately in terms of the number of units allowed and billed. However, you must stay current with what are the published approved/allowed payment rates.

If your current approved/allowed fee schedules have not been loaded into your practice management software system, make this a priority. This should be carried out for each insurance company and plan you bill. Updated and current fee schedules in your practice management system are the *best way* of tracking whether your

Table 13.4 Comparison of CPT allowed payments from different insurer sources

		Ins 1	Ins 2	Ins 3	Ins 4	Ins 5	Ins 6	Ins 7	Ins 8	Ins 9	Ins 10
		HMO	PPO	Medicaid	Commercial	Commercial	Medicare	Medicare	Medicaid	Commercial	Medicare
				Commercial			Region 3	Commercial 1			Commercial 2
90801	DI Int	97.85	102.88	85.00	72.00	72.00	112.98	151.55	107.63	85.00	168.00
90806	Therapy	81.37	81.35	70.00	72.00	72.00	62.61	87.97	67.49	75.00	90.00
96101	Psy test	81.37	81.45	70.00	72.00	80.00	60.87	95.74	58.65	75.00	90.00
96102	PT	81.37	81.45	70.00	72.00	45.00	48.83	69.10	37.48	75.00	49.00
96103	PT	30.90	30.90	30.00	72.00	20.00	41.35	44.00	35.19	75.00	44.00
96118	Np test	81.37	81.45	70.00	67.10	85.00	71.35	95.74	71.14	75.00	103.00
96119	NT	81.37	81.45	70.00	67.10	50.00	51.74	69.10	47.94	75.00	69.00
96120	NT	30.90	30.90	30.00	67.10	20.00	60.31	65.00	51.52	75.00	65.00

practice is being paid the correct amount per unit of each plan contract. Make sure your billing staff is cognizant of what you should be paid when they are posting payments. We cannot overemphasize this point. Your billing staff should know how much is paid per unit and when there is a deviation from the expected payment amount. They need to know that you want to know when problems in reimbursement arise.

Other spreadsheets can be prepared which calculate various ratios of actual payment versus the average length of time it takes to receive payment once your claim is submitted; number of first submissions (called "clean claims") leading to payment versus multiple submission/resubmissions of claims; and frequency of other problems leading to delay in payment and/or refusal of payment by the insurance company. Many of these spreadsheets are premade as part of commercial software billing programs.

Over time, you will determine that some insurance companies pay a lower fee per unit of service but that they actually cost less in terms of the actual cost to your practice. This is because they have a very high rate of clean claims, thereby lowering your claims processing costs. In turn, others may promise a high rate of payment but cost more to service the claim (or, as noted earlier, cost you so much more in staff and doctor time getting preauthorizations than your actual reimbursement per hour or per unit due to having to resubmit claims and so forth).

Most of the above applies to Medicare as well as other federal, private, and commercial insurance plans. With respect to Medicare, let us look at the hard reality of what is going on at the time we wrote this chapter (January to May 2011). The United States has reached its national debt limit, and Congress has only just agreed to increase the debt limit and thereby increase the debt burden in the future. This may lead to further significant spending cuts in federally funded insurance plans. Medicare and Medicaid spending accounted for 5.7% of Gross Domestic Product in fiscal year 2008 and is expected to more than double in the next 30 years [4].

The Sustainable Growth Rate, or SGR, is a major component of Medicare's current formula for determining annual updates to physician reimbursements for services. The SGR was intended to be a budgetary restraint on Medicare's total expenditures to maintain budget neutrality. Absent Congressional intervention, the SGR will dramatically cut provider reimbursement rates, while practice costs continue to rise. The SGR effectively caps total Medicare expenditures on provider services [6].

So, why should you be concerned with the SGR and Medicare payment cuts? All you want is to keep a full practice and pay your bills, and earn your salary? Well, how are you going to know if your practice is going to (a) make a profit, (b) break even, or (c) operate at a loss on Medicare services such as psychotherapy or testing if you do not know what the amount of fee reimbursement is going to be a month, 3 months, or a year from today. You HAVE to think about the basic cost of delivering your professional service to the public from a business management point of view.

Table 13.3 presents the hard reality of the decline in Medicare allowed payment (the actual amount you are paid) over the past 5 years. As you can see, the actual CPT 96118 fee in Region 3 has declined from a 2007 level of 111.79 to a 2011 level of 95.74 (14%). In contrast, the CPT 90806 fee has increased by 26 cents. Without a doubt, your overhead has continued to increase during this time period. Can you afford to see Medicare patients for these rates? Where can you make up the difference in lost revenue?

At the institutional level, the same situation regarding Medicare reimbursement is going to direct how the institution will allocate resources for patient care and professional salaries. Most of us have heard the real stories from our peers who have been told bluntly by their hospital administrator to balance their department budget (including their continued salary and other overhead) by increasing actual cash receipts (not just billable hours to indigent patients) to a level which covers salary and other expenses, or their position would be canceled.

Here is a basic example using CPT 96118. If your office cost of service is $150.00 per hour and you currently receive $150.00 per unit of

96118, then you are breaking even, with no profit or loss. Now, if the amount you receive is $95.74 for each unit of 96118 provided to a Medicare patient, that is a loss of 54.26 per unit. Thus, an 8-h service with 96118 leads to a loss of $434.08. Where will you make up this loss? Have you calculated the total number of Medicare-based CPT units of service billed by your practice in the past 12 months? Please take a minute or two and calculate this amount versus your actual overhead. Consider what an additional projected 21% SGR cut would do to your office financial picture. This is only one of the many reasons why large numbers of physicians and psychologists are considering whether they can afford to continue to provide services to Medicare patients.

How you spend your professional time is a decision based upon multiple issues. Having an accurate picture of your office's financial status and how it can be affected by seeing patients who lead to financial profit or loss for your practice is critical to your business decision making. Once you actually analyze your costs for carrying out a neuropsychological evaluation to a patient with a specific insurance plan, is continued service to patients with that plan justified from a business perspective?

Another concern that drives up office costs is the matter of patient "no shows." These are the instances in which patients do not show for their scheduled appointments. "No shows" cost your practice money since they represent unproductive "no income" time in which you still have the cost associated with running a practice. Virtually all insurance companies (Medicaid is a notable exception in most states) permit neuropsychologists and other providers to charge patients who fail to show for their appointments. While "no show" charges do not offset all the lost revenue from a "no show," they can provide an incentive to patients to keep their appointments.

As of October 1, 2007, Medicare allows the clinical neuropsychologist to charge patients a "no show" fee, provided the following conditions are met [7]:

1. The "no show" charge must be applied consistently to all patient insurance groups (Medicaid being an allowed exception) and not just to Medicare patients.
2. Patients must be informed in advance of the "no show" charge (we recommend that you inform patients at the time appointments are made, at the time appointments are confirmed, and in your patient registration material).
3. The charge must be reasonable (there is no guideline for "reasonable," though we are aware of $25–50 being common for "no show" charges per hour in our community). A simple method to find out what is the common charge in your community is to call YOUR personal physician's office and ask what they charge for a "no show." Just remember, most PCP visits are much shorter that the typically 1-h minimal unit of time you set aside for a patient.
4. "No show" charges are billed directly to patients as a "noncovered" service; they *cannot* be billed to Medicare or other insurance companies.

Medicare Participation Options

Neuropsychologists and other providers are not required to see Medicare patients. Three options exist for contracting with Medicare: (1) participating (PAR), (2) nonparticipating (NON-PAR), and (3) opting out/private contracting (OPT-OUT) [8].

As a general rule, Medicare contractors send letters to providers in mid-November of each year, informing them of the upcoming calendar year's payment rates and offering them an opportunity to change their participation status. Providers then have until December 31 of that year to make their participation decisions. Unless CMS reopens this "open enrollment period," participation is binding for the entire calendar year.

1. PAR: When a neuropsychologist agrees to "participate" in Medicare, they agree to accept Medicare's reimbursement rates as payment in full for the calendar year in question. Medicare reimburses participating providers at 100% of the approved payment rate and pays them more rapidly than nonparticipating providers. Generally speaking, 80% of the payment comes from Medicare, with the balance coming from the patient.

2. NON-PAR: If a neuropsychologist elects not to participate in Medicare, they have the option whether or not to "accept assignment." If the NON-PAR provider accepts assignment, Medicare pays claims at 95% of the participating provider amount, with 80% of that amount coming from the contractor and 20% from the patient. If the NON-PAR provider decides not to accept assignment, they must fill out a Medicare beneficiary's claim form and submit the claim directly to Medicare. Medicare then pays the patient directly, leaving the physician to bill the patient for services rendered. Physicians cannot charge Medicare patients for filing their claims, but by refusing assignment, NON-PAR providers can balance bill patients up to the "limiting charge" (federal law restricts Medicare nonparticipating providers from balance billing more than 115% of the Medicare nonparticipating reimbursement rate. This is called the "limiting charge." The potential reimbursement rate for NON-PAR providers is 115% of the Medicare NON-PAR reimbursement rate, which is 109.25% of the participating provider reimbursement rate). Of course, as a NON-PAR provider, the onus is on your practice to bill and collect from your patients. For many practices, the cost of billing Medicare on behalf of their patients, then billing the patients to collect what Medicare paid directly to them, and then attempting to collect from these patients is not worth it.
3. OPT-OUT: Neuropsychologists also may elect to opt out of the Medicare system entirely. To do so, one agrees to not participate in the Medicare program for 2 years and privately contracts with Medicare beneficiaries for services rendered. Neuropsychologists can then bill patients directly for their services at rates agreed to between the patient and neuropsychologist. To meet the legal requirements for the opt-out option, one must sign and file an affidavit in which they agree not to bill or receive payment from Medicare for at least 2 years.

The affidavit of participation status must be completed at least 30 days before the first day of the next calendar quarter; there is a 90-day window for rescinding the affidavit. The opted-out neuropsychologist and Medicare patient must sign a written contract *before* any service is rendered. The contract must clearly state that, by signing the contract, the patient (1) declines all Medicare payments for services rendered by the neuropsychologist, (2) is liable for all charges without Medicare balance billing limitations *or* assistance from Medigap or other supplemental insurance, and (3) acknowledges that the patient has the right to receive services from other medical providers.

Where a neuropsychologist opts out and is a member of a group practice or otherwise reassigns his or her rights to Medicare payment to an organization, the organization may no longer bill Medicare or be paid by Medicare for services that the neuropsychologist furnishes to Medicare beneficiaries. However, if the neuropsychologist continues to grant the organization the right to bill and be paid for the services he furnishes to patients, the organization may bill and be paid by the Medicare patient for the services that are provided under the private contract. The decision of an individual provider to opt out of Medicare does not affect the ability of the group practice or organization to bill Medicare for the services of those and practitioners who continue in a participating or nonparticipating status with Medicare.

Other Critical Medicare Issues

We would be remiss if we did not discuss two enormous claims-related issues facing practices before 2014: the transition to the 5010 claims transaction standard and the transition to ICD-10. *Both have the potential to bring cash flow from most insurance payors to an absolute standstill.*

The first deadline of January 1, 2012, is for the adoption of a new standard—the 5010 standard—for electronic claims transactions. This change *must* be done to accommodate core processes such as claims submission and remission and additional processes such as claim status inquiry, eligibility inquiry, and transaction acknowledgment.

The second deadline is the long-awaited deadline for moving from ICD-9 to ICD-10. This deadline is slated for October 1, 2013. In addition to changes neuropsychologists will have to make in recording diagnoses and procedures, the move to ICD-10 will require extensive programming and testing of practice management systems, revision of encounter and testing forms, and numerous other changes. [Note: Many neuropsychologists use DMS-IV/TR for billing. Many of the same issues will occur when the revised DSM-V is published.]

It is critical that practices be ready for these two deadlines. Failure to prepare for either could bring a practice to its operational—and financial—knees.

Moving from X12 4010A1 to 5010

HIPAA law requires the Department of Health and Human Services (HHS) to adopt standards that "covered entities" (i.e., all practices, health plans, electronic billing clearinghouses) must use when electronically conducting core administrative transactions. The current version of this standard is the Accredited Standards Committee's X12 Version 4010/4010A1. Beginning January 1, 2012, the required standard will be Version 5010, which will allow for additional functionality. The new standard holds the promise of more efficient claims transactions for your staff and, if your practice is ready, will have no impact on your clinical routine.

Moving from ICD-9 to ICD-10

From a clinical perspective, ICD-10 will require much more specificity. The number of diagnoses increases from about 13,000 to more than 68,000, while the number of procedures will go from 4,000 to 72,589. The more you understand the ICD-10 nomenclature, the better off you will be on October 1, 2013.

From a business perspective, ICD-10 matters, too…a great deal. Why? Because ICD-10 codes consist of between 3 and 7 alphanumeric characters; ICD-9 codes consist of 3–5 digital characters. This expansion from a maximum of five characters to seven characters and the change from a numeric field to an alphanumeric field will require numerous behind-the-scene changes to the "business" of neuropsychology.

The following list of questions for your practice management system vendor should guide your practice in its preparations [9].

Practice Management System Vendor Questions: 5010

- When will your product be upgraded to support the 5010 standard?
- When will we be able to run test claims using the 5010 standard? [If the date they provide you is later than October 1, 2011, push for an earlier date].
- In addition to claims submission, what transactions will we be able to test?
- What preparation is needed on our end to test the 5010 standard?
- Is the upgrade to 5010 included in my ongoing maintenance expense?
- Will your product support both the 4010A1 and the 5010 standard during a transition phase?
- Will we be permitted to migrate to the 5010 standard prior to January 1, 2012?

There are several questions you should ask of your clearinghouse and payors along these same lines:

- When will you be ready to support the 5010 standard for all of our electronic transactions?
- Will your software be upgraded to support all features of the 5010 standard?
- What changes must be made on our end to support the 5010 standard? Are additional registrations/notifications required?
- Will there be additional fees associated with this migration? This is a question for your clearinghouse.
- When can we test the 5010 standard process in total with our practice management software,

our clearinghouse, and payors all testing the same data set(s)?
- What are your plans to support both the 4010A1 and 5010 standards concurrently?

Practice Management System Vendor Questions: ICD-10

- When will your product be upgraded to support ICD-10?
- When will we be able to run test claims using ICD-10? [If the date they provide you is later than June 1, 2013, push for an earlier date. This transition is going to be a huge one for all of us.]
- What preparation is needed on our end to test ICD-10?
- Is the upgrade to ICD-10 included in my ongoing maintenance expense?
- Will our practice management (and/or electronic health record) software include a searchable ICD-10 database?
- Will your product support both ICD-9 and ICD-10 during a transition phase? Do you have projected dates for the transition phase?
- Will we be permitted to migrate to ICD-10 prior to October 1, 2013?

Questions for Clearinghouses and Payors

- When will you be ready to accept ICD-10 codes on claims?
- What changes must be made on our end to support ICD-10? Are additional registrations/notifications required?
- Will there be additional fees associated with ICD-10?
- What "claim scrubbing" edit changes will be made to your software to process ICD-10 claims? When will you be able to provide us with an explanation of how these new edits will impact operations?
- When can we test ICD-10 submissions in total with our practice management software, our clearinghouse, and payors all testing the same data set(s) using ICD-10 codes in 5010 transactions?
- What are your plans to support both ICD-9 and ICD-10 concurrently?
- Will you be ready for migration to ICD-10 prior to October 1, 2013?

Some Common Medicare Patient Request Situations: What Is the Appropriate Response?

These responses are based upon a review of the current APA ethics code as well as our years of clinical and business-related experience. Our responses should be viewed as guidelines to be considered by the reader. You may develop other responses to these situations that are also appropriate or, perhaps, even more appropriate than what is noted below. The main thrust of each response deals with (a) making a priori service delivery decisions about the contractual arrangements you set up with the patient and (b) using your understanding of how the patient's insurance approval and reimbursement system works.

Situation A. The patient who wants you to carry out a comprehensive, attorney-requested or court-ordered, forensic examination, which is to be billed in its entirety to Medicare. The purpose of this evaluation is for a forensic opinion(s) to be developed and used in a legal matter.

Response. Do not accept the referral with the proviso of billing Medicare for a forensic (administrative) service. This is not a medically necessary service. You may be in violation of several ethical rules as well as run the risk of committing fraud in terms of your contractual relationship with the insurance payor. Ask yourself the question, "Is the referral question and the resultant testing medically necessary as they relate to the making of a diagnosis or alleviating a medical or mental problem? Would the testing be necessary if there was no active litigation?"

Medicare specifically states. The services of CPs are not covered if the service is otherwise excluded from Medicare coverage even though a clinical psychologist is authorized by State law to perform them. For example, the Social Security Act (Section 1862(a)(1)(A)) excludes from coverage services that are not "reasonable and necessary for the diagnosis or treatment of an illness or injury or to improve the functioning of a malformed body member." Therefore, even though the services are authorized by State law, the services of a CP that are determined to be not reasonable and necessary are not covered [10].

Situation B. The patient has always wondered if they could have a learning disability, and now they want to be tested under Medicare for that service. They want educational testing to identify a diagnosis of a learning disability, and the patient wants you to bill the services to Medicare. They are not complaining of any other form of medical, neurological illness or injury or mental health problem that may be causally associated with such an educational condition.

Response. It is our understanding that Medicare does not cover testing for educational purposes, such as to identify a learning disability, as it does not meet the criteria for medical necessity/covered service.

Situation C. The patient asks or demands that you waive either their co-pay, their deductible, or both.

Response. Do not waive the co-pay or deductible. Not only are you providing a service well below your cost basis but you may find that you have violated the law! The Centers for Medicare & Medicaid Services (CMS) has mandated that physicians and other providers of health care MUST collect co-pays and deductibles [11].

The reasoning behind this is as follows: If you (the neuropsychologist) waive the co-pay or deductible, you are, in effect, giving the patient a discount. Therefore, if you are willing to "sell" your service to the patient at a discount, you should also give a discount to the insurer. A second (and lesser) reason for requiring co-pays and deductibles is to cause the patient to have a share in the cost of their health care, thereby reducing unnecessary consumption of covered services.

A Review of Some Sample Forms for a Private Practice in Clinical Neuropsychology

The items that follow are examples of the types of forms that we have developed to address common situations which occur in management of our practice. Please feel free to adapt them to your practice as needed. Versions of some of these forms have been presented elsewhere [5].

Please note the following caveats. Many of the forms have been reviewed by our company attorney for acceptable legal standards according to the laws of the Commonwealth of Virginia. You will need to determine whether the wording in these forms is legally valid in your jurisdiction. Also, we feel that these forms reflect an appropriate professional standard of practice according to current APA ethics standards. Please do not try to interpret these documents out of context. Our office will change these forms whenever it is deemed necessary so as to maintain acceptable legal and ethical standards. Finally, each of these forms is designed to be completed on an a priori service delivery basis. This issue is critical in many of the circumstances relevant to these forms.

(a) Referral form (Fig. 13.1): This intake form is typically completed as part of a telephone call from either the referral source or the patient/patient's family. Please note that it also prompts for secondary and tertiary insurance information. Some patients have Medicare plans that may require a preauthorization for services. You do not want to have to try to get a preauthorization while the patient is waiting at the registration window and waiting for their appointment.

(b) Registration form (Fig. 13.2): Page 1 asks for the typical information. Page 2 addresses a number of specific issues. Without going into a line by line annotation, please note several items of particular interest: first, that the time for testing includes administration, scoring, and report preparation as well as report discussion and, second, that the cost of responding to medical legal matters requires time and that fees will be charged for these services; page 3 deals with documenting the Medicare No Show policy and other general insurance matters.

(c) Waiver of insurance (Fig. 13.3): This form is a copy of the standard Medicare "Advance Notice for Medically Unnecessary Services—Waiver of Medical Necessity" form [12]. This form should be used in those situations where you have a Medicare enrollee who is requesting services which, in their specific situation, are not likely to be deemed medically

Neuropsychological Services Of Virginia
Intake Form

Referred To: _______________ Referred By: _________________________________ Date: ________________

Referral Called In By: ___________________ Phone No: _________________ Fax No: ____________________

Client Name: ____ DOB: ________________ Age: ______

Address: ______________________________________ City/State: _________________ Zip: ____________

Home Phone: ___________________ Work Phone: ____________________ Cell Phone: __________________

Preferred Phone: [Circle] Home - Work - Cell Email Address: ____

Responsible Party: ____________________________ Relationship To Patient: ____________________________

Responsible Party Contact Info:________________________________ Employer:____________________________

Reason For Referral: ____

____

____

NT ______ PT _____ Therapy ______ EducT ______ DOA: ________________________ LOC [ ] Yes [ ] No

Outpatient: ________ Inpatient: _____________________________ Room #: _____________ Records Req?: [ ] Yes [ ] No

Accident?: [ ] Yes [ ] NO - DOI: _________ WC?: [ ] Yes [ ] NO - DOA: _______ Attorney: _________________________

Primary Insurance: ____________________________ ID: _____________________________ Phone #: ________________

Address: ____ Contact: __________________________

Mental Health Carrier (If Different): _____________________________________ Phone#: __________________________

Mental Health Carrier Address: ____ Effective Date: ____________________

Policy Holder Name: _______________________________________ Rel to Pt: ______________ Group#:_______________

Policy Holder D. O. B. ___________________________ Policy Holder Other Info _________________________

Deduct: _________ Met?: ________ Copay/Coinsurance.: ________ Preauth Req?: _______ OTR Req?: _______

Preauth # DI: _________________ Preauth # Test: _________________ Preauth # Therapy: _________________

Notes: ____

____

____

Secondary Insurance: ___________________________ ID: ___________________________ Phone #: __________________

Address: ____ Contact: ___________________

Mental Health Carrier (If Different): ____________________________________ Phone#: __________________

Policy Holder Name: ____ Effective Date: _______________

Deduct: _________ Met?: ________ Copay Visit/Unit: _______ PreAuth Req?: ________ OTR Req?: _________

Preauth # DI: __________________ Preauth # Test: _________________ Preauth # Ther.: __________________

Appointment Date: _________________________ Confirmed Appt w/__ ______ on__________by ______

Appointment Date: _________________________ Confirmed Appt w/________on __________by______

Appointment Date: _________________________ Confirmed Appt w/________on __________by______

Client Informed: Copay Amount: _________ 48-hr Notice: _____ Glasses/Med List: _____ D/E Q_____ Rev. 6/26/10

Fig. 13.1 Referral form

NEUROPSYCHOLOGICAL SERVICES OF VIRGINIA, INC.

PATIENT REGISTRATION

First Name:______________________ Middle:__________ Last Name:____________________

Address:__________________________ City:______________ State:______ ZIP:_________

Home Phone: (______)________-____________ SSN:______/______/_______ Sex: [ ] Male [ ] Female

DOB:______/______/______ AGE:______ Referred by:______________________________

Were you injured while working? (Workers' Comp) [ ] NO [ ] YES-->Date of Injury: ______/______/______

Accident? [ ] NO [ ] YES-->Motor Vehicle? [ ] YES [ ] Other _____________ Date of Accident _____/_____/_____

Are you represented by an attorney? [ ] NO [ ] YES-->Attorney Name ______________________________

Have you been seen at NSV previously? [ ] YES [ ] NO Are you here on an emergency basis? [ ] YES [ ] NO

Are you covered by insurance health plan(s)? [ ] YES [ ] NO If YES, we need to make a copy of your insurance card(s).

Primary Ins. ____________________________ Secondary Ins. ____________________________

Vocational Status:

[ ] full-time student
[ ] part-time student
[ ] homemaker
[ ] retired
[ ] full-time employed
[ ] part-time employed
[ ] unemployed
[ ] disabled
[ ] other __________

Education:________Years Completed Degree:________

Handedness: [ ] right [ ] left [ ] ambidextrous

Occupation:_________________________
Employer:_________________________
Work Phone:_________________________
Cell Phone:_________________________

Marital Status: [ ] Single [ ] Separated [ ] Divorced [ ] Married [ ] Widowed

Medication	Dosage (mg)	# per day	Medication	Dosage (mg)	# per day
1)			4)		
2)			5)		
3)			6)		

Responsible Party, if other than patient: (who is responsible for payment of all costs incurred)

First Name:____________________ Middle:__________ Last Name:________________________

Address:__________________________ City:______________ State:_______ ZIP:_________

Home Phone: (______)__________-__________
Employer:____________________________________ Work Phone: (______)__________-____________

Responsible party's relationship to patient: [ ] Spouse [ ] Child [ ] Parent Other ____________________

Note: Fees are posted at the receptionist's window.

Fig. 13.2 Patient registration form

Neuropsychological Services of Virginia, Inc.

GUARANTEE OF PAYMENT AND ASSIGNMENT OF INSURANCE BENEFITS: For value received, the undersigned guarantor and/or patient (hereinafter the "Responsible Party") promises to pay to Neuropsychological Services of Virginia, Inc. (hereinafter "NSV") all charges incurred for services rendered to the Responsible Party. The Responsible Party understands that NSV will process the paperwork to complete insurance claim(s) but only as a courtesy to the Responsible Party, and the Responsible Party authorizes NSV to release any and all medical information necessary to complete insurance claim(s) and assigns any monies due and owing under the insurance contract to NSV. **It is, however, understood and agreed that the Responsible Party is responsible for all monies due and owing for services rendered by NSV in the event insurance does not pay for these services.** It is acknowledged that the ultimate completing and following-up of any insurance claims is the responsibility of the Responsible Party. It is further agreed by the Responsible Party, that in the event any monies received by NSV from the insurance carrier which are at any time after their receipt withdrawn from NSV by the insurance carrier, the Responsible Party will be responsible for those monies then due and owing, and waives any defense for payment the Responsible Party may have against NSV. In the event this account is turned over to an attorney for collection, the Responsible Party hereby agrees to pay all costs of collection including, but not limited to, court costs and 33 1/3% attorney's fees. The Responsible Party authorizes use of this form on all insurance claim submissions. Release of records to referral sources is also authorized. The Responsible Party agrees to be bound by the terms and conditions of this account with NSV.

A minimum of 48 hours weekday / 2 business days notice is required for cancellation of appointments. If this notice is not received, the Responsible Party may be charged a fee for the amount of time which was reserved for the appointment at the rates posted in the offices of NSV. See page 3 for details. This also applies to Medicare patients. Insurance will not be billed for missed/canceled appointments. Your copay is expected at the time of service. We will file the Responsible Party's initial insurance claim(s) and provide documentation necessary for insurance reimbursement. We do not, however, guarantee that each service will be covered or what percentage will be covered. The Responsible Party may incur extra charges for refiling of insurance claims.

In the event that the Patient's/Responsible Party's insurance does not cover our services (or any portion thereof), NSV will work with the Responsible Party regarding payment (e.g., setting up a payment plan). NSV expects full payment within thirty (30) days of the date of service. **The Responsible Party hereby agrees that accounts not paid within thirty (30) days will be charged a late fee of $15.00 and will accrue interest at the rate of 1.5% per month (18% A.P.R. - a minimum of $1.00 will apply).** The Responsible Party bears ultimate financial responsibility for all services rendered to the Patient/Responsible Party, including workers' compensation claims and personal injury cases, regardless of the outcome of litigation. In the event that coverage is denied under workers' compensation, the Responsible Party will pay any unpaid balance, notwithstanding any appeal of such denial. With respect to personal injury cases, the Responsible Party is responsible for fees incurred, NSV may not be able to seek payment from third parties, and NSV cannot wait on the outcome of pending litigation for payments. NSV does not accept contingency fee arrangements. If there is any remaining balance(s) due at the time of settlement, the Responsible Party hereby authorizes their attorney to clear the Responsible Party's outstanding accounts. In the event the Responsible Party has **"medpay"** available and health insurance, NSV considers medpay to be the primary insurer. The Responsible Party's signature also constitutes the irrevocable agreement to a waiver permitting payment of medpay insurance claims directly to NSV prior to claimant receiving such funds.

Responding to Forensic/Medical Legal requests, conferences and telephone calls with attorneys involve additional time and record keeping. The Responsible Party is responsible for all direct costs and expenses associated with NSV and its attorney responding to discovery requests (including depositions and subpoena duces tecum time and labor costs) and with conferences including, but not limited to court appearances, preparation of reports, photocopying, faxes, long-distance telephone calls, out of office travel, overnight delivery and courier services. These expenses are billed to the Responsible Party and to the Patient's/Responsible Party's Attorney. The Responsible party, however, remains responsible for payment of these charges if not paid in full within sixty (60) days. The above noted direct cost and expenses are understood and accepted to be in addition to any published federal and/or state statutes which may otherwise apply.

NOTE: Testing includes time for (1) administering and (2) scoring the tests, and (3) preparing the report. In nonforensic/nonmedical-legal cases, this will typically add 1-3 hours to the actual testing time. Forensic/medical-legal cases typically require even more time and may include record review and consultation(s) with attorney(s), etc. In certain cases (such as, but not limited to, medical-legal cases), a more comprehensive and time-consuming assessment may be needed than what may be approved under your insurance plan [for example, when an insurance plan covers up to 3 hours of testing/report preparation but your clinician feels that your case requires additional hours of testing/record review/report preparation/etc]. The responsible party as noted below accepts responsibility for these charges.

If you have any questions, please speak with a member of our Management team. Your signature indicates that you have read the above and agree to the terms contained therein. These agreements are irrevocable.

Signature: ______________________________ Responsible Party: ______________________________

Date: ____________ Date: ____________

****If patient is a minor, are you her/his legal guardian?** [ ] YES [ ] NO If **NO**, please notify our Management team regarding this matter.

Rev. 4/12/2011

Fig. 13.2 (continued)

Neuropsychological Services of Virginia, Inc.

Insurance & Appointment No Show Information Notice

From: The Clinicians & Staff at NSV

It has come to our attention that, despite every reasonable effort undertaken by *you* and by our clinicians and highly trained office staff to obtain specific and accurate information/confirmation from your insurance company regarding:

1. Whether our clinicians and/or NSV is an approved provider of services under your health care plan;

2. What are the insurance approved services requested in your case;

3. What is the time limited extent of services which may be provided per appointment;

4. What is the insurance company stated allowed amount of patient copay and/or the allowed amount of insurance payment to be made to NSV;

5. The specific preauthorization and preauthorization number for the requested services;

6. Other information which documents the insurance company's responsibility to pay the patient's claim.

Unfortunately, some insurance companies may provide NSV with the information needed to appropriately process and reimburse NSV for professional services rendered, but then (after we perform the requested services) they inform us that the insurance information which they gave us is incorrect and/or incomplete. Your insurance company then may inform the clinicians and NSV that they are not responsible for payment for the otherwise agreed upon services. Your insurance company may delay and/or defer their reimbursement for previously authorized services. The clinicians and NSV thereby inform the responsible party noted below that: first, this type of situation may develop in your situation despite your/our best efforts to prevent such an event; second, that the responsible party assumes responsibility for making the insurance company take appropriate responsibility for their actions; third, that the responsible party agrees to pay NSV the appropriate payment which is otherwise due from the insurance company while the responsible party seeks to make the insurance company live up to their agreed upon financial obligations to the patient.

7. *Missed/Broken appointments:* A minimum of 48 hours weekday/business days advance notice is required for the cancellation of appointments without incurring a missed/broken appointment penalty. This is strictly enforced. If this notice is not received, the Responsible Party may be charged:

(a) $75.00 for a missed 1 hour Psychotherapy and or Office Feedback appointment and
(b) $75.00 *per hour* for a missed Testing appointment. This may involve 3 – 8 hours of lost time.
(c) $15.00 for a missed 10 minute Telephone Feedback/Conference appointments.
(d) Please see the 2011 rate schedule posted in the office of NSV for further information.

If you have any questions, please speak with a member of our Management team. Your signature indicates that you have read the above and agree to the terms contained therein.

Signature: ______________________________ Date: ______________

Fig. 13.2 (continued)

A. Notifier:

B. Patient Name: **C. Identification Number:**

Advance Beneficiary Notice of Noncoverage (ABN)

NOTE: If Medicare doesn't pay for **D.** ____________ below, you may have to pay.

Medicare does not pay for everything, even some care that you or your health care provider have good reason to think you need. We expect Medicare may not pay for the **D.** ________ below.

D.	E. Reason Medicare May Not Pay:	F. Estimated Cost

WHAT YOU NEED TO DO NOW:

- Read this notice, so you can make an informed decision about your care.
- Ask us any questions that you may have after you finish reading.
- Choose an option below about whether to receive the **D.** ____________ listed above.

  Note: If you choose Option 1 or 2, we may help you to use any other insurance that you might have, but Medicare cannot require us to do this.

G. OPTIONS: Check only one box. We cannot choose a box for you.

☐ **OPTION 1.** I want the **D.** ____________ listed above. You may ask to be paid now, but I also want Medicare billed for an official decision on payment, which is sent to me on a Medicare Summary Notice (MSN). I understand that if Medicare doesn't pay, I am responsible for payment, but **I can appeal to Medicare** by following the directions on the MSN. If Medicare does pay, you will refund any payments I made to you, less co-pays or deductibles.

☐ **OPTION 2.** I want the **D.** ____________ listed above, but do not bill Medicare. You may ask to be paid now as I am responsible for payment. **I cannot appeal if Medicare is not billed.**

☐ **OPTION 3.** I don't want the **D.** ____________ listed above. I understand with this choice I am **not** responsible for payment, and **I cannot appeal to see if Medicare would pay.**

H. Additional Information:

This notice gives our opinion, not an official Medicare decision. If you have other questions on this notice or Medicare billing, call **1-800-MEDICARE** (1-800-633-4227/**TTY:** 1-877-486-2048).

Signing below means that you have received and understand this notice. You also receive a copy.

I. Signature:	J. Date:

According to the Paperwork Reduction Act of 1995, no persons are required to respond to a collection of information unless it displays a valid OMB control number. The valid OMB control number for this information collection is 0938-0566. The time required to complete this information collection is estimated to average 7 minutes per response, including the time to review instructions, search existing data resources, gather the data needed, and complete and review the information collection. If you have comments concerning the accuracy of the time estimate or suggestions for improving this form, please write to: CMS, 7500 Security Boulevard, Attn: PRA Reports Clearance Officer, Baltimore, Maryland 21244-1850.

Form CMS-R-131 (03/11) Form Approved OMB No. 0938-0566

Fig. 13.3 Medicare noncovered service form

necessary by Medicare. In many situations, federal rules still require the provider to submit the claim, even though they have good reason to believe in advance that the service, e.g., forensic issues, is not going to meet the accepted standard of medical necessity. This signed waiver allows the provider to bill the enrollee for the service instead of having to write off the claim. For further information regarding this complex issue, please refer to the website of your state's Medicare Part B carrier.

Medicare and Neuropsychology: A Look Forward to the Abyss or to Eden? What Will Our Business Management Practices Look Like in the Future?

(a) We expect to see per unit reimbursement levels continue to decline over the next 10 years. We also expect to see the upper limit of allowable testing units decline as Medicare increases the demand for computerized testing.
(b) These changes will result in an even greater reliance on forensic and other professional services where fee structures are less regulated. This will also "make up" some of the lost revenue for those who continue to see Medicare patients.
(c) We also envision more neuropsychologists choosing to "opt out" of Medicare and work solely on a private contract arrangement with patients.
(d) Many of the "a la carte" options typically offered to patients for free or little cost will need to become full fee expenses. These items include (1) forms that the patient wants completed and (2) letters to document some element of care or diagnosis. Other services, which may not be billed to Medicare.
(e) Once Medicare and other insurance companies allow for services where the professional is not actually physically present on-site with the patient, the entire question of in-office testing will become moot. The patient will not have to come to the neuropsychologist's office if they can go to another site such as the PCP's office and be interviewed and then accessed via Internet-based video connection (e.g., Skype-type service).
(f) As Medicare moves toward its uncertain future, Congress will explore other mechanisms to rein in the costs of caring for a growing Medicare population. We, as a profession, must work together to create a qualitative and quantitative value proposition. Neuropsychology can and should play a key role in caring for Medicare patients. If they are unable to make a strong case for such, we run the risk of neuropsychology being pushed to the sidelines of patient care.
(g) As electronic medical records become more widespread, private practice neuropsychologists will adopt such technology in greater numbers. There will be many reasons, but simply being able to maintain record access from referral sources, and to provide quick transmission and access of our reports to other sources will become more critical. If we do not stay on an EMR technology par with our MD referral sources, then the MD will see the cost of their office having to copy or fax records to us as a financial disincentive for a referral.

It is therefore incumbent to focus on the "value" of the services we offer. Even as many of our tests become computerized, we must continue to demonstrate the value of the personal interaction between neuropsychologist and patient. We must be able to demonstrate how the information we provide is better and more accurate than "shortcut" software-based neuropsychological testing being sold to (and used by) other medical professions who do not have our training and expertise. We must be able to show how our care creates better patient outcomes. To the extent we can do this, our future is much brighter.

Clinical Pearls

- Know what constitutes a medically necessary service and agree to bill Medicare for such service and the patient for services that are not medically necessary according to Medicare.
- Do not hesitate to educate the patient as to what is a medically necessary service and what is not

medically necessary. The patient should have a say in their health-care delivery choices. This includes accepting financial responsibility for nonmedically necessary services.

- Document time and service provided to the patient properly the first time, according to documentation standards, and you will reduce the risk of audit problems in the future.
- Know what your cost of practice is and use that information properly in your clinical care decisions.
- Do not forget the rules you knew yesterday may have changed overnight. Keep up to date at sites such as http://www.cms.gov/mlnmattersarticles/downloads/SE0816.pdf and other Medicare websites [13, 14].
- Be clear and consistent with patients about collecting co-pays and deductibles.
- One cannot provide "Luxury car quality care at used car rates of reimbursement."
- We enjoy helping people or we would not work in this field. We feel that our professional time has value and that the business arrangements that we make are reasonable and appropriate to providing care to our patients. We cannot provide quality services if we cannot meet our financial obligations.
- The next time you visit your doctor, read the sign next to the receptionist's window. Typically, it will state that "Co-pays are expected at time of service" and that "the doctor cannot see you without your HMO authorization number." Treat your patients appropriately and in the same manner you are treated when you are the patient at the receptionist window.

References

1. http://www.kff.org/medicare/timeline/pf_intro.htm. Accessed 29 May 2011.
2. President Richard M. Nixon. Health care: requests for action on three programs (1972, March 2), message to Congress on Health Care, Congressional Quarterly Almanac 1972. Washington, DC: Congressional Quarterly Books; 1972. p. 43A.
3. http://www.managedcaremuseum.com. Accessed 25 May 2011.
4. Medicare and Medicaid statistical supplement (2010 Edition). Centers for Medicare and Medicaid Services; 2010.
5. Peck EA. Business aspects of private practice in clinical neuropsychology. In: Lamberty GJ, Courtney JC, Heilbronner RL, editors. The practice of clinical neuropsychology: a survey of practices and settings. Lisse: Swets & Zeitlinger; 2003.
6. The long-term outlook for Medicare, Medicaid, and total health care spending. In: Chapter 2, The long-term budget outlook. Congressional Budget Office; 2010.
7. Transmittal 1279. Change request 5613, Pub 100-04 for Medicare claims processing. Department of Health & Human Services, Centers for Medicare & Medicaid Services. http://www.cms.gov//transmittals/downloads/R1279CP.pdf. 29 Jun 2007.
8. Medicare participation options for physicians. The American Medical Association; 2010.
9. Lucien W Roberts III. Preparing Your Practice for 5010. In: Physicians practice pearls (weekly e-publication of Physicians Practice); 2010.
10. http://www.ssa.gov/OP_Home/ssact/title18/1862.htm. Accessed 25 May 2011.
11. http://oig.hhs.gov/fraud/docs/alertsandbulletins/121994.html. Accessed 25 May 2011.
12. https://www.cms.gov/bni/. Accessed 25 May 2011.
13. http://www.cms.gov/mlnmattersarticles/downloads/SE0816.pdf. Accessed 25 May 2011.
14. Medicare Learning Network Centers for Medicare and Medicaid Services. 2011. http://www.cms.gov/mlnmattersarticles. Accessed 25 May 2011.

Professional Competence as the Foundation for Ethical Neuropsychological Practice with Older Adults

14

Arthur C. Russo, Shane S. Bush, and Donna Rasin-Waters

Abstract

This chapter provides practical guidelines for the neuropsychologist contemplating a transition into the professional and ethical practice of geriatric neuropsychology. The focus is pragmatic, with an emphasis on advanced preparation. The chapter uses a top-down structure, with each section identifying the relevant core biomedical ethical principles, followed by an elaboration of the relevant ethical requirements as defined by the American Psychological Association's Code of Ethics. Each section then ends with pragmatic suggestions for translating the core ethical principles and relevant ethical requirements into action so that the ethical standards are met at the highest standard. Topics covered include (a) acquiring professional competence, (b) guidelines and resources, (c) what aspiring geriatric neuropsychologists need to know, and (d) recommendations for promoting professional competence in geriatric neuropsychology.

Keywords

Ethics • Geriatrics • Older adults • Neuropsychological • Assessment • Evaluation

> We do not act rightly because we have virtue or excellence, but rather we have those because we have acted rightly. We are what we repeatedly do. Excellence, then, is not an act but a habit.
>
> Durant paraphrasing Aristotle (1926)

Geriatric neuropsychology is facing a dilemma with ethical implications that are fueled by two divergent trends—the increasingly large number of older adults, and the relatively small number of professionals trained to assess them. The proportion of older adults has steadily increased since the turn of the last century, with projections that it will continue to increase. According to the

A.C. Russo, Ph.D. (✉)
Psychology Department, VA New York Harbor Healthcare System, 800 Poly Place, Room 16-209H, Brooklyn, NY 11209, USA

Fordham University, New York, NY, USA
e-mail: arthur.russo@va.gov

S.S. Bush, Ph.D., ABPP (CN, RP)., ABN.
D. Rasin-Waters, Ph.D.
VA New York Harbor Healthcare System, New York, NY, USA
e-mail: drbush@gmail.com; donna.rasin-waters@va.gov

L.D. Ravdin and H.L. Katzen (eds.), *Handbook on the Neuropsychology of Aging and Dementia*, Clinical Handbooks in Neuropsychology, DOI 10.1007/978-1-4614-3106-0_14,

US Census Bureau [1], Americans 65 years of age or older made up 12% of the population in 2000. That number is projected to increase to 16% in 2020 and increase again to 20% in 2040. Among older adults, the fastest growing segment is expected to be in the oldest age group, those 85 years of age or older, with a US Census Bureau projected increase of 233% in the same 40-year period. By 2050, persons 85 years of age and older are expected to number 19 million [2].

At the same time that the population is aging, neuropsychology is experiencing a current and projected shortage of professionals trained to service the older adult [3,4]. A 2002 survey of practicing psychologists found that fewer than 30% had any graduate coursework in geropsychology and fewer than 20% had any supervised practicum or internship experience with older adults; over half of the respondents reported that they needed further training [5]. Packard [6] noted that although 70% of psychologists have older adults as patients, only 3% have formal geropsychology training. This disparity poses an ethical dilemma due to the increasing likelihood that psychologists will be servicing a population for whom they have had little training.

The purpose of this chapter is to examine the ethical issues and challenges for neuropsychologists contemplating a career in, or transition into, the practice of geriatric neuropsychology. The focus is pragmatic with an emphasis on preparation, consistent with a proactive approach to ethics [7–9]. A proactive approach assumes that mandated professional standards represent only a minimum requirement that the ethical professional uses as a starting point in the pursuit of practicing at the highest ethical level possible [10]. A proactive ethical approach recognizes that preparing in advance for anticipated ethical challenges is always a better course than remediating the ethical impact of poor preparation. We will use a top-down structure, describing the relevant core biomedical ethical principles [11], followed by an elaboration of the relevant ethical requirements as defined by the American Psychological Association [12] *Ethical Principles of Psychologists and Code of Conduct*. In the conclusion, we will offer pragmatic suggestions for translating the core ethical principles and relevant ethical requirements into action so that professional practice is conducted at the highest ethical level.

Preparing to Transition into Geriatric Neuropsychology: Acquiring Professional Competence

Developing and maintaining proficiency in clinical specialties are fundamental to ethical practice. Well before clinical contact with older patients, neuropsychologists transitioning into the field of geriatric neuropsychology should insure that they are competent to provide the service. A core competence in clinical neuropsychology is a prerequisite to the practice of geriatric neuropsychology and in some clinical contexts suffices. As the APA [13] noted in its *Guidelines for Psychological Practice with Older Adults*, some problems of older adults are essentially the same as those of other ages, and clinicians working with older adult patients can generally respond with the same skill set for which all professional psychologists have generic training. However, for many problems facing older adults, a generic competence in neuropsychology is simply not enough.

The core biomedical ethical principles relevant for professional competence are (a) promotion of patient welfare (beneficence) and (b) avoidance of harm (nonmaleficence); together these constitute the first general principle of the APA Ethics Code (see also [11]). The APA [12] Ethics Code further details these core ethical principles in several standards. Ethical Standard 2.01 (Boundaries of Competence) states that psychologists only provide services with populations and in areas "within the boundaries of their competence, based on education, training, supervised experience, consultation, study or professional experience." Ethical Standard 2.03 (Maintaining Competence) requires psychologists to develop and maintain competence through ongoing efforts. Ethical Standard 3.04 (Avoiding Harm) echoes the bioethical principle of nonmaleficence in stating that psychologists "take reasonable steps to avoid harming their clients... and to minimize harm where it is foreseeable and unavoidable." Standard 9.07 (Assessment by Unqualified Persons) specifies that "psychologists do not promote the use of psychological assessment techniques by unqualified persons," except for training purposes.

To maximize the probability of promoting patient welfare while minimizing the potential for patients to be harmed by the service, geriatric neuropsychologists must possess the required specialized knowledge base and skill set to perform assessments with this population. This specialized knowledge and skill set goes beyond a generic competence in neuropsychology.

Guidelines and Resources

Fortunately, excellent resources are now readily available to promote ethical practice and facilitate ethical decision making. APA's [13] *Guidelines for Psychological Practice with Older Adults* provides a resource for self-assessment of current knowledge and skills; it is a good starting point for neuropsychologists who want to transition to clinical assessment of older persons. In addition, the American Bar Association Commission on Law and Aging—American Psychological Association [14] *Assessment of Older Adults with Diminished Capacity: A Handbook for Psychologists* provides general approaches to assessment of the frail elderly with specific recommendations for assessment of various capacities related to cognitive and functional ability within the legal system.

The most recent and comprehensive guidelines are derived from the Pikes Peak model for training in clinical geropsychology that evolved out of the 2006 National Conference on Training in Professional Geropsychology [15]. These comprehensive competencies emphasize self-evaluation and supervisee rating in core knowledge and skill areas, including clinical assessment, intervention, consultation, and other professional services for older persons. Experience with older adults across a wide range of care settings and demographic and sociocultural diversity are emphasized. In addition, resources relating to ethical practice are also available at the national, state, and local levels and include national professional associations, state licensing and ethics boards, liability insurance carriers, institutional ethical guidelines and ethics committees, and an increasingly large number of scholarly books and articles. The study of sentinel or paradigm cases helps prepare a foundation for sound ethical judgment.

The integration of core competencies in clinical neuropsychology combined with the knowledge and skills in geropsychology advocated by the above resources provides the foundation for competent practice of geriatric neuropsychology [8]. At all times, geriatric neuropsychologists are well served by developing familiarity with these guidelines and resources before they are needed, preparation being one of the hallmarks of a proactive ethical approach.

A Nonexhaustive List of What Aspiring Geriatric Neuropsychologists Need to Know

Knowledge of gerontology complements neuropsychological competence in multiple ways. It is particularly valuable for clinicians to consider (1) late adulthood as a distinct developmental stage, (2) medical aspects of aging, (3) psychopathology and neuropathology in older adults, (4) family and social systems, (5) cohort effects, (6) cultural issues, and (7) unique ethical and legal requirements.

Late Adulthood as a Distinct Developmental Stage

The professional and ethical practice of geriatric neuropsychology requires a knowledge base consisting of the theory and research in aging, with an in-depth understanding of expected life span development. Competent geriatric neuropsychologists have a developmental perspective and an understanding of successful aging, as well as the common changes in cognition over time. Cognitive abilities change at different rates, with some abilities more vulnerable to aging than others [16,17].

Without this knowledge, clinicians may be more at risk of misinterpreting normative age-related decline as pathological deterioration. Not only does cognition change over time, but that change is differentially impacted by life experience. For example, although research has found that short-term memory often declines with age, short-term memory related to one's expertise, which Horn described as expertise-wide span memory, is more robust and may increase with age [17,18].

Medical Status

An understanding of biological and health-related aspects of aging contributes to patient care. Therefore, geriatric neuropsychologists pay particular attention to gathering a thorough medical history, including determining the older person's functional status. Over 80% of older adults have at least one chronic health condition, with 75-year-olds averaging three chronic conditions and five prescriptions [19,20]. The aging process affects how the body metabolizes medication, with older adults at risk for being given medication or dosages that are inappropriate [19]. This interplay of chronic medical condition and medications poses a particular challenge to geriatric neuropsychology because of its potential impact on cognition and the possibility of confusing a permanent with a medically based reversible cognitive impairment.

Sensory abilities must be taken into account because sensory deficits disproportionately impact older adults. Surveys find that 37% of those 65 years of age and older have hearing impairment and 30% have impaired vision [21]. Peripheral sensory deficits can impact performance on neurocognitive tests and may be confused with cortical impairments [22]. For example, the older adult may be mistakenly diagnosed with memory impairment due to an apparent inability to learn new information when the real problem is sensory loss that interferes with the reception of new information. Potter and Attix [23] suggested additional considerations for issues of motor function, fatigue, literacy, rapport, and motivation. They recommend practical adaptations for each potential deficit, including tests available in large print or orally presented versions with norms, and shortened batteries to prevent fatigue.

Psychopathology and Neuropathology

Competent geriatric neuropsychologists understand pathological changes in personality and cognition, and how such changes manifest in the older patient. For example, late-life depression may coexist with cognitive impairment and may manifest without an obvious display of sadness. Other problems, such as dementia due to degenerative brain disease and stroke, are rarely seen among the young but find an increasing rate of incidence among an older population [13]. Without a competent grounding in geriatric neuropsychological pathology, clinicians may fail to accurately differentiate normal from abnormal changes or fail to accurately differentiate among disease categories such as dementias due to stroke, frontal-temporal conditions, or Alzheimer's disease, leading to compromised treatment recommendations [24,25].

Family and Social Systems

The impact of family and social systems on patient functioning and independence has age-related aspects. As questions of independent functioning arise, the reliance on family and non-family support systems comes to the fore. In addition, issues surrounding loss increasingly surface. Not only are older adults more likely to have experienced loss, but they may find themselves the only surviving member of their family or peer group [26]. Often the issues of loss become intertwined with the challenge of recreating a meaningful identity and social world. With issues such as dementia, the patient and caregivers can benefit from the support and knowledge of local and national resources. The aspiring geriatric neuropsychologist should develop working knowledge of these resources prior to serving the older person.

Cohort Effects

Because each generation is in part the product of unique historic circumstances, the practitioner needs to understand cohort or generational effects. For example, disruption of education was common among older adults coming of age during the Depression Era and WWII. Differences in attitudes toward test taking and familiarity with computers and multiple choice items may vary. And finally, the stigma of seeing a psychologist/neuropsychologist who handles "mental health"-related issues can often carry a stigma for many older persons. Sensitivity to such issues is important in the development of rapport and interpretation of behavior during the assessment.

Cultural Considerations

Cultural issues must be taken into account. An understanding of variables such as ethnicity, acculturation, quality of education, and racial socialization is important in the interpretation of assessment results [27] (See Chap. 3 in this volume).

Ethical and Legal Requirements

Aspiring geriatric neuropsychologists must develop knowledge of the ethical and legal issues related to geriatric neuropsychology, such as decision-making capacity, competence, confidentiality, informed consent, and managing the potential conflicts of interests inherent in dealing with family and nonfamily caretakers, health care systems, and other entities.

Developing Professional Competence

Despite the availability of numerous resources for establishing professional competence, we believe, like Packard [6], that these resources are at best a partial and piecemeal solution. Qualls (as cited in [6]) presented a similar argument, stating "I think people are getting this training in informal ways, but we need something that's more systematic" (p. 34).

From a proactive ethical approach, the best pathway toward competence is one that is structured, comprehensive, and supervised. Competent professional and ethical practice does not happen by chance [9], nor is it best left to the subjective judgment of the person seeking competence. Some obvious limitations to self-assessment and self-study are that they lack informative feedback, and that they are unable to identify and correct those blind spots which by definition are outside the person's awareness. The development of expertise requires deliberative, repetitive practice presented at an appropriate level of difficulty, for which the person receives informative and corrective feedback [28,29]. Some clinicians achieve the needed additional education and training from a postdoctoral or respecialization program. For those unable to pursue a formal specialization training program, guided study and supervised clinical experience under the direction of an expert mentor may suffice.

Recommendations for Promoting Professional Competence in Geriatric Neuropsychology

Preparation is *the* hallmark of a proactive ethical approach to geriatric neuropsychology. For neuropsychologists aspiring to serve older adults, preparation starts with acquiring the specialized knowledge and skill set of geriatric neuropsychology with appropriate consultation of guidelines, best practices, and supervision prior to serving this population. A proactive ethical approach recognizes that preparing in advance for ethical challenges is always a better choice than remediating the ethical impact of poor preparation. Clinicians who invest the time and effort to establish and maintain competence in neuropsychological practice with older adults will find themselves well positioned to provide valuable services to others while increasing the likelihood of having a personally and professionally rewarding career.

Clinical Pearls

- Enlist the aid of a competent geriatric neuropsychologist to serve as a mentor to guide your skill development.
- Do a self-assessment using the APA's [13] *Guidelines for Psychological Practice with Older Adults* and Knight et al.'s [15] Pikes Peak model for training in professional geropsychology to identify the areas of competence you need to develop. Review this with your mentor for accuracy to identify blind spots.
- Consider utilizing resources from the Council of Professional Geropsychology Training Programs (CoPGTP; available at http://www.uccs.edu/~cpgtp/). The CoPGTP was an unexpected outgrowth from the Pikes Peak conference and offers multiple resources for programs as well as individuals for all levels of training in clinical geropsychology [30].
- With your mentor, create a course of study which addresses any weaknesses discovered during the self-assessment. Include supervised practice in geriatric neuropsychology as needed.

References

1. US Census Bureau. Projections of the population by selected age groups and sex for the United States: 2010 to 2050 (NP2008-T12). 2008. www.census.gov/population/www/projections/summarytables.html. Retrieved 24 Jul 2010.
2. Vincent GK, Velkoff VA. The next four decades. The older population in the United States: 2010 to 2050. In: Current population reports. Washington, DC: U.S. 2010 Census Bureau; 2010. p. 25–1138. www.census.gov/prod/2010pubs/p25-1138.pdf. Retrieved 24 Jul 2010.
3. Clay R. Geropsychology grants in peril: seven geropsychology training efforts have lost funding they receive through the Federal Graduate Psychology Education (GPE) Program. Monitor Psychol. 2006;37:46.
4. Rosen AL. Testimony to the Policy Committee of the White House Conference on Aging. The shortage of an adequately trained geriatric mental health workforce. 2005. www.whcoa.gov/about/policy/meetings/Jan_24/Rosen%20WHCOA%20testimony.pdf. Retrieved 26 May 2010.
5. Qualls S, Qualls SH, Segal DL, Norman S, Niederehe G, Gallagher-Thompson D. Psychologists in practice with older adults: current patterns, sources of training, and need for continuing education. Prof Psychol Res Pract. 2002;33:435–42.
6. Packard E. Polishing those golden years. APA Monitor. 2007;38:34.
7. Bush SS. Ethical decision making in clinical neuropsychology. New York: Oxford University Press; 2007.
8. Bush SS. Geriatric mental health ethics: a casebook. New York: Springer; 2009.
9. Martin T, Bush S. Ethical considerations in geriatric neuropsychology. NeuroRehabilitation. 2008;23: 447–54.
10. Knapp SJ, Vandecreek LD. Practical ethics for psychologists: a positive approach. Washington, DC: American Psychological Association; 2006.
11. Beauchamp TL, Childress JF. Principles of biomedical ethics. 5th ed. New York: Oxford University Press; 2001.
12. American Psychological Association. Ethical principles of psychologists and code of conduct. Washington, DC: American Psychological Association; 2002.
13. American Psychological Association. Guidelines for psychological practice with older adults. Am Psychol. 2004;59:236–60.
14. American Bar Association Commission on Law and Aging, American Psychological Association. Assessment of older adults with diminished capacity: a handbook for psychologists. 2008. www.apa.org/pi/aging/programs/assessment/capacity-psychologist-handbook.pdf. Retrieved 1 Feb 2011.
15. Knight B, Karel M, Hinrichsen G, Qualls S, Duffy M. Pikes Peak model for training in professional geropsychology. Am Psychol. 2009;64(3):205–14.
16. Horn JL, Noll J. Human cognitive abilities: Gf-Gc theory. In: Flanagan DP, Genshaft JL, Harrison PL, editors. Contemporary intellectual assessment: theories, tests, and issues. New York: Guilford Press; 1997. p. 53–91.
17. Horn JL, Blankson N. Foundations for better understanding of cognitive abilities. In: Flanagan D, Harrison P, editors. Contemporary intellectual assessment. New York: Guilford Press; 2005. p. 41–60.
18. Horn JL, Masunaga H. On the emergence of wisdom: expertise development. In: Brown W, editor. Understanding wisdom: source, science and society. Philadelphia, PA: Templeton Foundation Press; 2000. p. 245–76.
19. Merck Institute of Aging and Health. The state of aging and health in America. Washington, DC: Merck Institute of Aging and Health; 2004.
20. National Academy on an Aging Society. Chronic conditions: a challenge for the 21st century, Challenges for the 21st century: chronic and disabling conditions, vol. 1. Washington, DC: National Academy on an Aging Society; 1999.
21. Desai M, Pratt LA, Lentzner H, Robinson KN. Trends in vision and hearing among older Americans. Aging trends, No. 2.. Hyattsville, MD: National Center for Health Statistics; 2001.
22. Baltes PB, Lindenberger U. Emergence of a powerful connection between sensory and cognitive

functions across the adult life span: a new window to the study of cognitive aging? Psychol Aging. 1997;12:12–21.
23. Potter G, Attix D. An integrated model for geriatric neuropsychological assessment. In: Attix DK, Welsh-Bohmer KA, editors. Geriatric neuropsychology: assessment and intervention. New York: The Guilford Press; 2006. p. 5–26.
24. American Psychiatric Association. Practice guidelines for the treatment of patients with Alzheimer' disease and other dementias of late life. Am J Psychiatry. 1997;154(5 Suppl):1–39.
25. American Psychological Association. Guidelines for the evaluation of dementia and age related cognitive decline. Am Psychol. 1998;53:1298–303.
26. Kastenbaum R. Counseling the dying patient. In: Molinari V, editor. Professional psychology in long term care: a comprehensive guide. New York: Hatherleigh Press; 2000. p. 201–26.
27. Manly JJ. Cultural issues. In: Attix DK, Welsh-Bohmer KA, editors. Geriatric neuropsychology: assessment and intervention. New York: Guilford Press; 2006. p. 198–222.
28. Ericsson K. The road to excellence: the acquisition of expert performance in the arts and sciences, sports, and games. Mahwah, NJ: Erlbaum; 1996.
29. Sternberg RJ, Grigorenko EL, editors. The psychology of abilities, competencies, and expertise. New York: Cambridge University Press; 2003.
30. Karel MJ, Emery EE, Molinari V, the CoPGTP Task Force on the Assessment of Geropsychology Competencies. Development of a tool to evaluate geropsychology knowledge and skill competencies. Int Psychogeriatr. 2010;22:886–96.

Ethical Considerations in the Neuropsychological Assessment of Older Adults

15

Arthur C. Russo, Shane S. Bush, and Donna Rasin-Waters

Abstract

Translating core ethical principles and relevant ethical requirements into pragmatic action often presents its own set of challenges for geriatric neuropsychologists aspiring to practice at the highest ethical level. The purpose of this chapter is to provide pragmatic suggestions with an emphasis on preparation. Topics include (a) preparing the older adult and concerned others for what to expect from the assessment, (b) preparing all for potentially distressing results, (c) technical test preparation as seen in the thoughtful selection of instruments that are sufficiently comprehensive, adequately normed, and well grounded in current theory and research, and (d) ethically preparing the feedback session.

Keywords

Ethics • Geriatrics • Older adults • Neuropsychological • Assessment • Evaluation

> In theory there is no difference between theory and practice.
> In practice there is.
>
> Jan van de Snepscheut/Yogi Bera

Translating core ethical principles and relevant ethical requirements into pragmatic action often presents its own set of challenges for geriatric neuropsychologists aspiring to practice at the highest ethical level. The purpose of this chapter is to provide pragmatic suggestions with an emphasis on preparation, consistent with the proactive approach to ethics espoused earlier (see chap. 14, also [1–3]).

A.C. Russo, Ph.D. (✉)
Psychology Department, VA New York Harbor Healthcare System, 800 Poly Place, Room 16-209H, Brooklyn, NY 11209, USA

Fordham University, New York, NY, USA
e-mail: arthur.russo@va.gov

S.S. Bush, Ph.D. • D. Rasin-Waters, Ph.D.
VA New York Harbor Healthcare System, New York, NY, USA
e-mail: drbush@gmail.com; donna.rasin-waters@va.gov

L.D. Ravdin and H.L. Katzen (eds.), *Handbook on the Neuropsychology of Aging and Dementia*, Clinical Handbooks in Neuropsychology, DOI 10.1007/978-1-4614-3106-0_15,

Preparing the Patient and Concerned Others Prior to Performing the Neuropsychological Assessment

Prior to conducting the neuropsychological assessment, the geriatric neuropsychologist ensures that the examinee, and any concerned third-party participants, thoroughly understands the parameters of the evaluation, including who the client is, what the service entails, who has access to the report, and how it will be used, as well as other considerations detailed in this chapter. Many of the ethical pitfalls facing aspiring geriatric neuropsychologists stem from a failure to properly prepare the older adult and any concerned third-party individuals and institutions for the assessment. Often this failure in preparation is due to the clinician's lack of clarity regarding the relevant ethical requirements and guidelines and a lack of experience in translating the relevant requirements into pragmatic actions.

At the core of principle-based ethics are four general bioethical principles: respect for patient autonomy, beneficence, nonmaleficence, and justice [4]. Although all four principles are important to geriatric neuropsychology, respect for autonomy assumes a primary role in the preparation of patients and other involved parties for the neuropsychological assessment. The principle of respect for autonomy is often used to emphasize the freedom to make choices, with freedom understood as being free from interference. This aspect of autonomy recognizes the basic right of competent adults not to be interfered with against their wishes and supports the fundamental human rights of privacy, dignity, and freedom of self-determination [5]. When it comes to seeking professional services, freedom of self-determination implies the freedom to make knowledgeable choices and underlies the importance of informed consent.

In many instances, the same considerations regarding privacy and informed consent that hold for the general practice of neuropsychology also hold for the more specialized practice of geriatric neuropsychology. The American Psychological Association Ethics Code addresses these considerations in several standards, such as 3.10 (Informed Consent), 9.03 (Informed Consent in Assessments), 4.04 (Minimizing Intrusions on Privacy), 3.07 (Third-Party Requests for Services), and 6.04 (Fees and Financial Arrangements) [6]. The basic idea is that the person contemplating a professional service has a right to (a) certain information before consenting to the service, (b) have this information provided in language he or she can understand, and (c) ask questions and receive answers to these questions prior to giving consent. Although there may be adverse consequences in some contexts for doing so, the person also has the right to decline the service.

In terms of specific content, the person has a right to know (a) the nature and purpose of the service, (b) who will receive a report, (c) who will have access to the information obtained, (d) how the information may be used, (e) the possible impact the service may have on his or her life, (f) the limits of confidentiality, (g) the involvement of third parties, and (h) the fee. The person also has the right to refuse the service even after it is underway. In addition, the person consenting to a professional service maintains the right to privacy, so the patient decides how much information may be communicated to others; the neuropsychologist is obligated to share only as much information as is needed to fulfill the terms of the service. There are some exceptions. When the service is court mandated, prior consent is usually not required. But even here the person has a right to know that the service is court mandated and what the service will entail, and the person may refuse the service if the consequence for doing so is preferable to the person. Rather than "informed consent," the examinee in such instances is provided "notification of purpose." In addition, if elder abuse is discovered, or the older person poses a danger to self or others, the neuropsychologist may be required to report that information to help promote safety.

In addition to these common ethical practices, geriatric neuropsychologists often confront less common ethical concerns regarding privacy and confidentiality due to the nature of the population served and the specialized preparation required for informed consent. These aspects of preparation include (a) preparing the competent older person who has compromised functioning; (b) preparing the incompetent older person and the legal surrogate or guardian; (c) preparing family members, caretakers, and third-party systems; and (d) preparing the older person and relevant caretakers for potentially distressing and unwelcomed results.

Preparing the Competent Older Adult with Assumed Compromised Functioning

Capacity and competence are sometimes confused. Capacity is the *clinical* term that refers to the ability to make rational and informed decisions. Competence is the *legal* term that refers to the ability to make rational and informed decisions. Only a court can make a determination of incompetence; until then, adults are considered competent.

Although geriatric neuropsychologists assume older adults are legally competent, unless a court rules otherwise, they should not necessarily assume older adults have full capacity for informed consent. Cognitive abilities differentially decline with age. For example, an older person with otherwise sound mind may show compromised cognitive efficiency as processing speed and working memory decline with age. Sensory impairment may compromise the person's ability to understand. Medical, psychological, or pharmacological factors may impact capacity temporarily or in a fluctuating manner, with the older adult having better and worse days. Simple factors such as fatigue and rest may impact capacity. A person may lack sufficient capacity to make a decision in the evening when tired but show quite adequate capacity to make the same decision the following morning when rested [7].

Consistent with a positive, proactive ethical approach [8], geriatric neuropsychologists exercise care to ensure that older adult patients are well prepared to understand all information necessary to provide informed consent. This process may require the clinician to speak slower and present fewer items for consideration at a time, thus giving the older adult the necessary extra time to process the information without being overwhelmed. Sensory impairment may require compensatory sensory aids, as well as presenting information via more intact sensory channels. The older adult with compromised hearing might have material presented at a higher volume at the same time it is presented visually. Oftentimes, the way the person is approached and spoken to has a direct bearing on the older person's decision-making capacity, with infantilizing "elder speak" undermining the process [7].

Additionally, a diagnosis of dementia does not mean the person lacks all capacity or is incompetent. Until the disease advances, the older adult with a diagnosis of dementia often remains competent and can provide consent if remedial steps are first taken. Even with the progression of dementia, many who cannot give consent can still assent to the service (Ethical Standard 3.10, Informed Consent).

If the older person has fluctuating levels of capacity, the clinician defers discussing informed consent until the older person is more likely to have sufficient capacity to consider it. Some older persons do better with select others present, so the clinician may wait until the person can discuss consent in the company of a trusted, supportive family member or caretaker whose presence brings out the best in the person. But regardless of the particulars, ethical geriatric neuropsychologists strive to ensure that patients are at their cognitive best when discussing consent. See Chap. 31 in this volume for more information about evaluating capacity in older adults.

Preparing the Incompetent Older Adult and the Legal Surrogate or Guardian

When working with incompetent older adults, geriatric neuropsychologists have specific regulatory ethical requirements to both the older adults and to the legal surrogates or guardians. With incompetent older adults, clinicians inform the patients to the extent possible of the nature and purpose of the service, using language that is reasonably understandable. Clinicians answer any questions and concerns, seek assent, and protect patient rights and welfare ([6]; Ethical Standards 3.10, Informed Consent, and 9.03, Informed Consent in Assessments). For clients with a legal surrogate or guardian, the responsible person must also be fully informed of all the issues in order to provide consent for the assessment of the older adult.

From a proactive ethical approach, geriatric neuropsychologists are well served by carefully considering the concept of autonomy. Traditionally, autonomy is given an individualistic emphasis with the value placed on freedom from interference. However, the concept of autonomy as "no interference" can be too limiting, especially when applied to the incapacitated older adult. This traditional concept of autonomy fails to take into account that people are inherently relational and find their autonomy and dignity enhanced and supported by caring relationships. This position was taken by the Nuffield Council on Bioethics [7]: ("…most adults simply do not make autonomous decision in isolation: rather they come to those decisions supported by those close to them and in light of those relationships" (p. 8). Mackenzie and Stoljar [9] used the phrase "relational autonomy" to reflect this enhanced definition.

From a proactive ethical approach, geriatric neuropsychologists embrace the values of both individualistic and relational concepts of autonomy. With the former, ethical clinicians are obligated to protect cognitively compromised older adult patients from harmful interference. With the latter, ethical clinicians recognize that as older adults become more dependent on others due to dementia or other cognitive impairment, they also become more dependent on others for help in retaining their autonomy and sense of self [10]. So, clinicians strive to identify and enlist those caring relationships the older adult finds necessary to support and enhance autonomy and dignity. Patients typically benefit when clinicians encourage joint decision-making, to the extent possible, regarding assessment and treatment.

Molinari et al. [11] noted that joint decision-making may help older adults during that intervening period between the time they possess full capacity and the time they are deemed incompetent. We extend this emphasis on shared decision-making and suggest that even after older adults are declared incompetent, geriatric neuropsychologists make every effort to uncover the capacity that remains and the ways the person might still be encouraged to actively participate in any care decision. When compromised older adults lack the capacity to make major decisions, they may nonetheless have sufficient capacity to make other decisions or at least indicate some preference [7]. The experienced geriatric neuropsychologist realizes that regardless of the older adult's competence, it is unproductive to attempt an evaluation without the person's cooperation.

Preparing Family Members, Caretakers, and Third-Party Systems

Family members, caretakers, and third-party entities (e.g., residential homes and inpatient settings) often pose ethical dilemmas for aspiring geriatric neuropsychologists because of the conflicting agendas and pressure they may bring to bear to obtain confidential information or sway clinical opinions. In some cases, the problem is due to conflicts between individualistic and relational concepts of autonomy. In such cases, caretakers want to help the aging family members retain as much autonomous functioning and dignity as possible, despite cognitive decline and evidence of increasing functional impairment. Oftentimes, they anxiously seek information to make sense of the deterioration they suspect and fear. Caretakers want information regarding which capacities are impaired and which remain, and they want to know what to expect over time, say that they can plan care options.

Sometimes family members and caretakers believe they are entitled to information because of the investment in time, labor, and money made toward the older adult. Many caretakers are intimately involved in maintaining the older family member at home. Almost 80% of people needing long-term care live at home or in a community setting [12]. In some instances, family members pay for the neuropsychological service, oftentimes with the expectation that they will or should have access to the obtained information. Occasionally, family members, caretakers, and third-party systems have agendas that are not in the best interest of the older adult.

Geriatric neuropsychologists prepare involved third-party members and institutions in advance.

When services are provided at the request of third parties, geriatric neuropsychologists are ethically obligated to clarify beforehand the role of the clinician, who the client is or clients are, how the obtained information is likely to be used, and possible limits of confidentiality (Standards 3.07, Third-Party Requests for Services, and 4.01, Maintaining Confidentiality). When the demands of an organization conflict with the APA Ethics Code, the clinician clarifies the conflict in advance and, when possible, resolves it to the satisfaction of all parties (Standard 1.03, Conflicts between Ethics and Organizational Demands; see the 2010 amendments to the APA Ethics Code, [13]).

Pragmatically, geriatric neuropsychologists and their older adult patients both benefit from the information and support that family members, caregivers, and other third-party members provide. Oftentimes, families provide details about the older adult's previous levels of functioning, current capacities, and the onset of cognitive decline. Caretakers can provide information on whether the impairment is transient, fluctuating, or chronic. These contributions by family members become increasingly important as memory impairment becomes part of the clinical presentation. Institutional staff can help ensure that neuropsychological assessments are conducted in appropriate private settings free from interruptions that could undermine the assessment process and results (see also Ethical Standard 3.09, Cooperation with Other Professionals).

Preparing Older Adult Patients and Relevant Others for Potentially Distressing and Unwelcome Results

Ethical geriatric neuropsychologists begin to prepare older adult patients and relevant others for potentially distressing results well in advance of the actual feedback session. From the proactive approach advocated here, the possibility of unwelcome results is addressed during the informed consent process because such information relates to the anticipated risks of the assessment process. This preparation is consistent with APA Ethical Standard 3.04 (Avoiding Harm), which obligates clinicians to minimize harm, including emotional harm caused by distressing test results, where it is foreseeable and unavoidable.

Experience suggests that the assessment results with the greatest potential to provoke marked distress concern those pertaining to loss of functioning, autonomy, and personhood. Geriatric neuropsychological evaluations are often deficit-focused, with referral sources seeking to know if, and to what extent, older adults have lost cognitive functioning and if previously held capacities remain. The older adult may no longer be able to manage a household unassisted, manage complex finances, or safely drive, and, as the impairment progresses, may lose the right to make legal decisions such as making or altering a will or providing informed consent.

A diagnosis of dementia can be particularly devastating. Historically, dementia has been a taboo subject, with many families unwilling to acknowledge that a loved one had been diagnosed with the disorder or even unwilling to discuss the topic in general [14]. Survey data suggests that older adults are more concerned with a diagnosis of dementia than they are about cancer, heart disease, or stroke [15].

Faced with a potential loss of functioning, autonomy, or personhood, it is not unusual for older adults to react with depression or despair, interpreting the results as evidence of personal dishonor or disgrace [7]. Some may react by feeling stigmatized. Thompsell [16] poignantly related how one woman saw her diagnosis of dementia as being "certified as a nonperson." Unfortunately, the diagnosis of dementia or determination of declining capacity may lead some older adults to keep this information secret, thus losing out on the opportunity for social support when it is most needed.

Discussing the benefits of an early diagnosis is helpful, especially if dementia is suspected. For example, knowing the diagnosis may reduce the fear of the unknown, allow for a better understanding of the changes in cognition and functioning over time, and provide time to make plans and to form supportive relationships with professionals and other support groups before the condition is advanced.

Ideally, all parties will reach an agreement about who will attend the feedback session, what information will be disclosed, what information may have to be disclosed, and the possible consequences of disclosing the obtained information. However, if the competent older adult refuses to have anyone attend the feedback session or refuses to have information disclosed, this preference must be honored, except where permitted or mandated by law (APA Ethical Standard 4.05, Disclosures).

Recommendations for Preparing the Patient and Concerned Others Prior to Performing the Assessment

1. Inform patients and their families or other caregivers during the informed consent process of the nature and purpose of the feedback session. Inform them that the information provided will include a discussion of the older adult's strengths and weaknesses, an explanation for any changes in cognitive functioning to the extent possible, and a probable diagnosis or the reasons why a diagnosis is not possible.
2. Encourage older adult patients and their family members to discuss any feared results, including possible limitations to autonomy and freedom. Manage the discussion so that it is done in a sensitive and measured manner that signals an openness to discuss distressing material.
3. Tactfully elicit how the older adult and family members typically react to distressing information. Identify the coping strategies and social supports the patient and family employ to manage difficult information, and enlist these strategies and supports in the event of adverse neuropsychological findings.
4. Encourage the older adult to attend the feedback session with a trusted and supportive family member, preferable the same member or members who attended the pre-assessment session. Having the same family members at both sessions reduces the potential confusion due to differing accounts of the person's past or current functioning [17]. Encourage all involved family members and caretakers to attend the feedback session to avoid later problems with disclosure.
5. Assess the degree to which the older adult and family are involved in social systems that offer support, education, and referral information. This information provides the clinician an estimate of the additional information and resources that may be needed at the time of the feedback session.
6. Carefully document the above process and information, including all agreements and disagreements.

Preparing the Assessment

Geriatric neuropsychological evaluations include a clinical interview of the older adult, a review of the available biographical and medical information, behavioral observations, and neuropsychological testing. Relevant family members and caretakers are often interviewed. This section of the chapter is limited to the ethical issues surrounding the testing of the older adult.

The informing bioethical principles [4] include nonmaleficence and beneficence. Ethical geriatric neuropsychologists use assessment techniques and instruments that are psychometrically sound, supported by research, and appropriate for use with older adults (Ethical Standard 9.02, Use of Assessments), to the extent that such measures exist for a given patient or patient population.

The selection of appropriate tests follows current theory and research. When selecting tests normed during different decades, knowledgeable clinicians consider differences in sample composition and take into account Flynn or cohort effects. Newer tests or revisions of tests may not provide the best assessment of a given construct for certain patient populations [18]. Ethical geriatric neuropsychologists consider the current research on best practices in cross battery test selection [19].

Ethical geriatric neuropsychologists choose assessment measures to address several purposes typically encountered in the assessment of the older adult. The primary focus invariably concerns the purpose of the assessment. For older adults, referral questions are often a mix of descriptive and diagnostic concerns [20]. Descriptive referral questions seek information about level of cognitive capacity relative to the patient's peers. Often older adults or their family members notice a decline in cognition and want to know to what extent such decline is an age-expected decline or something more ominous. With diagnostic referral questions, clinicians are tasked with determining whether there is a disease process and deriving a differential diagnosis. Often the question is whether the person has dementia and, if so, what kind.

The basis upon which to make these judgments differs. Descriptive interpretations are based on normative data and depend on where patients rank compared to age-related peers. Diagnostic interpretations are based on some criteria of ability and pathology. Ethical problems may result from confusing the two types of referral questions. For example, if the average 75-year-old has three chronic health problems, a particular 75-year-old with two is fairing relatively better. This is a descriptive statistic based on the normative average of three. However, it would be erroneous to use this norm to say that the 75-year-old is therefore enjoying above-average health. Unfortunately, more serious examples are sometimes seen in the reports of diagnosed dementia based solely on a standard score cutoff score, without any reference to previous premorbid functioning (see also [21]).

Geriatric neuropsychologists determine which assessment instruments are appropriate to answer specific referral questions for each older adult patient. The selected instruments must assess the relevant abilities and have acceptable levels of validity and reliability for the person's age range. This selection process requires discernment. For example, some instruments provide both a global score and several subscores, but only the global score has reliability adequate for interpretation. Many instruments have inadequate or missing norms for older adults. Norms for the frail elderly who are often seen at bedside are scarce. Some normative studies lack adequate inclusion and exclusion criteria. In the selection of appropriate norms, the quality of the patient's education, as opposed to years of education, may be the most important consideration [22]. When an instrument's validity or reliability is in question, clinicians need to account for such limitations when interpreting and reporting the results.

The test measures or batteries chosen for evaluations should be comprehensive enough to both adequately assess the referral question and rule out possible conflicting hypotheses. To address the referral question, an adequate sampling of the relevant constructs is important. Popular screening measures by themselves are typically inadequate [23] and may lead to over diagnosis of dementia among some ethnic minority groups. Screening measures can also be insensitive to subtle cognitive changes in high-functioning patients. Because memory complaints are often the presenting problems, a thorough assessment of various forms of memory is commonly required.

Capacity evaluations pose a unique problem because they require both a professional competence in geriatric neuropsychology as well as specialized competencies in four areas: (a) knowing the relevant and state-specific legal standards pertaining to capacity, (b) performing risk analysis to determine the older person's risk of harm and need for supervision, (c) assessing decision-making capacity, and (d) assessing executional capacity or the ability to implement or carry out plans once decided upon [24].

In addition, the concept of capacity is still evolving. Earlier conceptualizations focused almost solely on the presence of a disabling condition with the assumption that impaired capacity was monolithic, and either present or not [25]. More current conceptualizations are more likely to emphasize functional impairment, with the understanding that a lack of capacity in one area does not imply a lack of capacity in another [25,26]. Elderly persons unable to drive may still be able to manage a household or consent to medical care.

Ethical geriatric neuropsychologists use a multidimensional assessment approach that includes weighing evidence and information from multiple sources in order to determine the extent to which elderly persons are able to (1) understand relevant information, (2) make a decision or convey a preference, (3) understand the implications and likely consequences of their decisions, and (4) skillfully carry out the actions needed to implement their decision [27]. This assessment approach also includes the assessment of basic activities of daily living (ADLs), such as eating, dressing, and mobility, as well as the assessment of more complex instrumental activities of daily living (IADLs), such as management of money, home, and transportation [28]. Given the need to balance legal, medical, familial, and psychological considerations, geriatric neuropsychologists aspiring to provide ethical capacity evaluations prepare in advance by seeking training, supervision, and knowledge of the literature (see [24] for a useful framework).

Finally, ethical geriatric neuropsychologists anticipate and prepare for the possible confounding impact of non-neurological variables on cognitive functioning, including cultural factors, sensory and motor deficits, fatigue, emotional state, motivation, physical pain and other acute medical conditions, medications, hunger, and environmental conditions. Older adults with little exposure to standardized testing may need more preparation and considerable encouragement to feel at ease with the test demands. This exposure factor becomes more apparent when computer applications are part of the assessment procedure, and the patient has had little experience using a mouse or keyboard [29,30].

Sensory and motor limitations may force the clinician to employ a nonstandardized administration [31–33]. Arthritis may impact the use of manipulables, decreasing performance on motor-dependent tasks such as block design and other construction tasks. The older adults may need additional rest breaks or an assessment spaced over several shorter sessions rather than fewer longer ones. Morning sessions may find the person better rested, with the increased likelihood that the clinician will be assessing best performance. Multiple sessions control for changes over time and allow for the discovery of fluctuating cognitive performance. It is also wise for clinicians to note the medications the person took prior to the exam, as well as whether the current medications are a recent change in type or dosage, which may account for variable performance across testing sessions.

Recommendations for Preparing the Assessment

1. Use assessment techniques and instruments that are psychometrically sound, supported by research, and appropriate for use with the particular older adult being evaluated. Be mindful of inadequate or missing norms.
2. Tailor the assessment to answer the referral question while at least briefly covering all neuropsychological domains. When the answer sought is more descriptive, adequacy of the normative data is imperative. When the answer sought is more diagnostic, criteria of ability and an understanding of pathology become more crucial.
3. Choose combinations of tests or batteries that are sufficiently comprehensive to assess the cognitive functions in question and to rule out conflicting hypotheses. Consider the best practices in cross battery selection.
4. Acquire the additional specialized competencies if aspiring to perform capacity evaluations.
5. Anticipate and prepare for possible confounding non-neurological factors.

Preparing the Feedback Session

The neuropsychological feedback session can be a unique opportunity to provide older adults and their family members with much needed information, guidance, and support. Often neuropsychological feedback sessions are the first time that older adult patients and their families are presented with a detailed understanding of the patient's condition, leaving clinicians the role of introducing patients and family members to the available resources, supports, and care systems. When this opportunity is missed, older adult patients and their family members may be left confused, anxious, and frightened. The Nuffield Council on Bioethics [7] stated:

"There is ample evidence that, in many cases, people are presented with a diagnosis of dementia and simply told to come back in a year's time. It was argued forcefully in one of our fact-finding meetings with people in front-line dementia care that such a lack of information and support in the immediate aftermath of diagnosis is simply morally wrong. We agree. (p. 46)."

The aspiring geriatric neuropsychologist can prevent such failure to educate patients and families by maintaining adequate preparation and a sensitive approach to the feedback session. The stance taken by clinicians during feedback supports the older adult's autonomy and dignity and recognizes that autonomy and dignity are often best preserved within a caring interpersonal matrix. The informing bioethical principles include respect for patient autonomy, nonmaleficence, and beneficence. The APA Ethics Code (3.04, Avoiding Harm) obligates psychologists to take reasonable steps to avoid harming their clients and "to minimize harm where it is foreseeable and unavoidable."

Neuropsychologists typically explain the assessment results to the patients or their designated representatives, although there are some exceptions (Ethical Standard 9.10, Explaining Assessment Results). Consistent with a proactive ethical approach, geriatric neuropsychologists will have prepared the older adult and family in advance and will have previously obtained consent to disclose the information to those present. Results should be presented at the level of detail the older adult and family can receive. Some family members want and can understand precise details about their loved one's strengths and weaknesses and the predicted course of the condition. Other patients or family members may, due to anxiety or other factors, benefit from less detailed information or need time to digest basic information.

Occasionally, caretakers may attempt to limit the discussion due to the belief that a diagnosis of dementia will so distress the older adult that there is no benefit receiving it. However, research shows that the vast majority of older adults with mild dementia want to be informed about their condition and that fears to the contrary are unfounded [34,35].

The content of the feedback session will be influenced by the extent to which older adult patients and their family members are already embedded in a system of care. For example, those under the care of a multidisciplinary team of geriatric specialists often need less information, guidance, and support from the geriatric neuropsychologist. Those not involved in a system of supportive care will typically need more guidance on how to access information and support; the ethical geriatric neuropsychologist comes prepared to the feedback session with handouts of useful information and contact information for local, state, and national resources.

Finally, the way information is conveyed is at least as important as what is conveyed. Respect for the autonomy and dignity of patients is reflected in an emphasis on strengths, and ways to support the person's capacities and opportunities to act, and to find continued enjoyment and meaning.

Recommendations for Preparing the Feedback Session

1. Establish a warm, supportive environment. When the feedback session is conducted in an institutional facility, prepare in advance to ensure that the session will be conducted in an uninterrupted, private setting.
2. Offer a diagnostic formulation and prognosis that takes into account the degree of confidence that can be placed in the diagnosis. For some assessments, clinicians have considerable information, such as history, test results, and radiological reports that converge on a single diagnosis. However, for many assessments, the diagnosis is uncertain, and the results serve

as a baseline against which to compare later evaluations. It can also be informative to describe alternative diagnoses that have been ruled out.

3. Anticipate the need to provide resources for local, state, and national information and support services, and have written handouts available.
4. Maintain focus on the importance of patient autonomy and dignity and take steps to promote both, such as describing ways to modify the patient's environment to maximize independence and quality of life.

Conclusions

Preparation remains *the* hallmark of a proactive ethical approach as geriatric neuropsychologists move from consideration of ethical principles to pragmatic assessment application. Ethical assessment preparation starts and ends with preparing older adults and concerned others for what to expect from the assessment and for potentially distressing results, and includes the information and support they might need to manage potentially troubling diagnoses. This preparation takes into account the non-neuropsychological variables that may impact older adults. Technical assessment preparation then logically follows in the thoughtful selection of instruments that are sufficiently comprehensive, adequately normed, and well grounded in current theory and research. The patients and their loved ones benefit from the preparation.

References

1. Bush SS. Ethical decision making in clinical neuropsychology. New York: Oxford University; 2007.
2. Bush SS. Geriatric mental health ethics: a casebook. New York: Springer; 2009.
3. Martin T, Bush S. Ethical considerations in geriatric neuropsychology. NeuroRehabilitation. 2008;23:447–54.
4. Beauchamp TL, Childress JF. Principles of biomedical ethics. 5th ed. New York: Oxford University; 2001.
5. Koocher GP, Keith-Spiegel PC. Ethics in psychology: Professional standards and cases. 2nd ed. New York: Oxford University; 1998.
6. American Psychological Association. Ethical principles of psychologists and code of conduct. Washington, DC: American Psychological Association; 2002.
7. Nuffield Council on Bioethics. Dementia: ethical issues. London: Author; 2009.
8. Knapp SJ, Vandecreek LD. Practical ethics for psychologists: a positive approach. Washington, DC: American Psychological Association; 2006.
9. Mackenzie C, Stoljar N. Relational autonomy: feminist essays on autonomy, agency and the social self. New York: Oxford University; 2000.
10. Agich G. Dependence and autonomy in old age: an ethical framework for long-term care. Cambridge, England: Cambridge University; 2003.
11. Molinari V, McCullough LB, Coverdale JH, Workman R. Principles and practice of geriatric assent. Aging Ment Health. 2006;10:48–54.
12. Merck Institute of Aging and Health. The state of aging and health in America. Washington, DC: Author; 2004.
13. American Psychological Association. Ethical principles of psychologists and code of conduct: 2010 amendments. Retrieved 2/17/11 from www.apa.org/ethics/code/index.aspx (2010).
14. Corner L, Bond J. Being at risk of dementia: Fears and anxieties of older adults. J Aging Stud. 2004;18:143–55.
15. Foundation MetLife. Alzheimer's survey: what America thinks. New York: Author; 2006.
16. Thompsell A. Life worth living. J Dementia Care. 2008;16:5.
17. Green J. Neuropsychological evaluation of the older adult. New York: Academic; 2000.
18. Bush SS. Determining whether or when to adopt new versions of psychological and neuropsychological tests. Clin Neuropsychol. 2010;24:7–16.
19. Flanagan DP, Ortiz SO. Essentials of cross-battery assessment. 2nd ed. New York: John Wiley & Sons; 2007.
20. Jamora C, Ruff RM, Connor BB. Geriatric neuropsychology: implications for front line clinicians. NeuroRehabilitation. 2008;23:381–94.
21. American Psychological Association. Guidelines for the evaluation of dementia and age related cognitive decline. Am Psychol. 1998;53:1298–303.
22. Manly JJ. Cultural issues. In: Attix DK, Welsh-Bohmer KA, editors. Geriatric neuropsychology: assessment and intervention. New York, NY: Guilford; 2006. p. 198–222.
23. Spann PE, Raaijmakers JG, Jonker C. Early assessments of dementia: the contribution of different memory components. Neuropsychology. 2005;19:629–40.
24. American Bar Association and American Psychological Association. Assessment of older adults with diminished capacity: a handbook for psychologists. Washington, DC: American Bar Association Commission on Law and Aging – American Psychological Association; 2008.
25. Smyer M. Aging and decision-making capacity: an overview. In: Qualis S, Smyer M, editors.

Decision-making capacity in older adults: assessment and intervention. New York: John Wiley & Sons; 2007. p. 3–24.
26. Zarit S, Zarit J. Mental disorders in older adults: fundamentals of assessment and treatment. 2nd ed. New York: Guilford; 2007.
27. Moye J. Assessment of competency and decision making capacity. In: Lichtenberg P, editor. Handbook of assessment in clinical gerontology. New York: John Wiley & Sons; 1999. p. 488–528.
28. Grisso T. Evaluating competencies. New York: John Wiley & Sons Plenum; 1986.
29. Byrd DA, Manly JJ. Cultural considerations in neuropsychological assessment of older adults. In: Bush SS, Martin TA, editors. Geriatric neuropsychology: practice essentials. New York: Psychology; 2005. p. 115–40.
30. Schatz P. Applications of technology to assessment and intervention with older adults. In: Bush SS, Martin TA, editors. Geriatric neuropsychology: practice essentials. New York: Psychology; 2005. p. 85–96.
31. Caplan B, Schecter JA. Test accommodations in geriatric neuropsychology. In: Bush SS, Martin TA, editors. Geriatric neuropsychology: practice essentials. New York: Psychology; 2005. p. 97–114.
32. Morgan J. Ethical issues in the practice of geriatric neuropsychology. In: Bush SS, Drexler ML, editors. Ethical issues in clinical neuropsychology. Lisse, NL: Swets & Zeitlinger Publishers; 2002. p. 87–101.
33. Morgan JE (2005). Ethical challenges in geriatric neuropsychology, part II. In: Bush SS, editor. A casebook of ethical challenges in neuropsychology. New York. pp. 153–158.
34. Carpenter BD, Xiong C, Poresnky EK, Lee MM, Brown PJ, Coats M, et al. Reaction to a dementia diagnosis in individuals with Alzheimer's disease and mild cognitive impairment. J Am Geriatr Soc. 2008;56:405–12.
35. Pinner G, Bouman WP. Attitudes of patients with mild dementia and their carers towards disclosure of the diagnosis. Int Psychogeriatr. 2003;15:279–88.

Part II

Late Life Cognitive Disorders

Mild Cognitive Impairment and Normal Aging

16

Lauren A. Rog and Joseph W. Fink

Abstract

Mild cognitive impairment (MCI) represents an intermediate zone of neurocognitive functioning that falls between normal age-appropriate functioning and dementia. During the past decade, research and clinical interest in MCI has burgeoned. Delineating the cusp between normal aging and MCI is of critical importance not only for accurate diagnosis but also for determining the earliest appropriate time-point to implement early interventions. This chapter will focus on a pragmatic approach to differentiating MCI from normal aging.

Keywords

Mild cognitive impairment • Normal cognitive aging • Neuropsychological assessment/evaluation • Older adults • Cognitive aging theories

Background

Normal Cognitive Aging

As people live longer, scientists are given greater opportunity to improve their knowledge of the structure and function of the aging brain. In the United States, the current life expectancy at birth is 76 years for men and 81 years for women, and approximately 13% of US citizens are 65 years and older [1, 2]. The US Census Bureau's projections estimate that about one in five citizens will be seniors by the year 2030 and the oldest old (85 years and older) is the fastest growing segment of the population. Given these statistics, there is a great need for clinical services and research focusing on normal and pathological cognitive aging.

It is generally accepted that some degree of cognitive decline associated with aging is inevitable, with a great deal of variability as to when these changes begin [3]. Interindividual variation in cognitive performance in areas such as memory and fluid intelligence increases with age.

L.A. Rog, Ph.D. (✉)
Illinois Institute of Technology, Chicago, IL, USA
e-mail: laurenarog@gmail.com

J.W. Fink, Ph.D.
Department of Psychiatry and Behavioral Neuroscience, Neuropsychology Service, University of Chicago, MC-3077, 5841 S. Maryland Ave, Chicago, IL 60637, USA
e-mail: finkjoseph@gmail.com

L.D. Ravdin and H.L. Katzen (eds.), *Handbook on the Neuropsychology of Aging and Dementia*, Clinical Handbooks in Neuropsychology, DOI 10.1007/978-1-4614-3106-0_16,

Thus, with advancing age, there becomes an increase in the proportion of elderly persons who show normative age-associated cognitive decline [4–7]. It can become difficult to parse out "normal" cognitive aging versus pathological cognitive decline in the absence of neuropsychological testing with normative comparison data.

Some aspects of cognition remain relatively intact with normal aging, including implicit memory, vocabulary, and storage of general knowledge [4, 7, 8]. The cognitive decline that typically accompanies normal cognitive aging involves decreased efficiency in information processing in several areas, including speed of processing, reaction time, working memory capacity, short-term memory, executive control (e.g., inhibitory functions), and verbal fluency [4, 9–11]. Visuoperception, visuoconstruction, and spatial orientation also decline with age [12, 13].

Slowed processing speed is a key cognitive change in the aging brain. It has been widely found, for example, that visual-motor tracking, sequencing, and set shifting slow with age [14–16]. Reduced processing speed is suspected to mediate cognitive efficiency by restricting the speed at which cognitive processes can be executed [8, 10, 17, 18]. Reduced processing can also affect the quality and accuracy of performance due to the decreased quantity of information processed that is necessary for completion of the task [18]. Further, products of earlier processing may be lost by the time later processing occurs, rendering integration of relevant information difficult or impossible. The consequences of reduced processing include decreased working memory capacity because less information can be processed within a given time, as well as impaired higher-order cognitive functions such as abstraction or elaboration, because the relevant information is no longer available in working memory or storage [18].

Age-related changes in working memory are likely due to reduced inhibitory mechanisms of selective attention [19]. That is, older adults show decreased ability to effectively suppress the processing of irrelevant, or marginally relevant, stimuli and thoughts. This leads to a generalized attentional dysregulation that is also thought to account for age-related deficits in various aspects of executive performance, including shifting cognitive set, suppressing responses, and response competition [8]. Cognitive aging is also associated with poorer effortful or controlled processing, while automatic processing remains relatively intact [20]. Older adults retain relatively good memory for "gist" or familiar stimuli, while source memory and recollection of contextual details decline [11].

Normal age-related changes in language function include increased inefficiency in phonological retrieval, resulting in word-finding difficulties that are often referred to as the "tip of the tongue" phenomenon [21]. The literature shows that confrontation naming performance declines with age, with the rate of decline accelerating in older age groups [22–24]. Semantic fluency or the ability to retrieve words associated with a particular category also declines with age, as does lexical fluency (i.e., the ability to retrieve words from declarative memory that begin with a particular letter or sound) [25]. However, it is suspected that the age-related decline in verbal fluency is at least partly due to the substantial contributions of auditory attention and verbal memory abilities to the tasks, rather than simply a primary degradation of semantic or lexical networks [26].

Structural Brain Changes

Numerous changes in brain structure accompany normal aging, including volumetric shrinkage, decreased white matter density, loss of dopaminergic receptors, and the emergence of neurofibrillary plaques and tangles. The greatest degree of cortical thinning and volumetric brain shrinkage across the lifespan occurs in the hippocampus, caudate, cerebellum, and calcarine (i.e., occipital) and prefrontal areas [27, 28]. Ventricular volume also increases in old age [29]. Decreases in white matter density and other white matter abnormalities are particularly evident in the frontal and occipital regions of the brain [30, 31]. White matter changes may be the primary culprit for age-related cognitive slowing, as their main function is to transport signals to and from different areas of the brain via myelinated axons. As myelin integrity degrades with age, so does the speed of cognitive processing. Together with findings on cortical volume and thinning, studies on age-associated white matter changes point to significant alterations in frontal networks [30, 31].

Loss of dopaminergic receptors occurs with age and is thought to contribute to the attentional dysregulation, executive dysfunction, and difficulty with contextual processing that accompanies normal cognitive aging [32–34]. It has been proposed that context processing involves using internally represented task-relevant information in a way that influences processing in the pathways responsible for task performance [35]. For example, performance on the Stroop task is dependent upon the ability to use the context of task instructions (i.e., inhibit reading color-named words while saying the printed ink color) in order to maintain attention toward ink color rather than the printed word. Braver and Barch (2002) postulated that contextual representations are housed within the dorsolateral prefrontal cortex and are regulated by dopamine projections to this area. The mechanism of context processing subserves cognitive functions such as attention, working memory, and inhibition by affecting the selection, maintenance, and suppression of information relevant (or irrelevant) to the task, accounting for the decline in these abilities with age [35].

An autopsy study on clinically nondemented oldest old (age ≥ 85 at death; $n = 9$) found neurofibrillary tangles (NFTs) in one or more limbic regions in all study participants [36]. The most affected regions included the entorhinal cortex, amygdala, subiculum, CA1 field of the hippocampus, and inferior temporal regions. Midfrontal, orbitofrontal, and parietal regions were less affected, and occipital regions were minimally affected in clinically nondemented persons. Senile plaque (SP) formation also was observed in this group and was found to affect all brain regions equally, with the exception of relative sparing of the occipital cortex. Participants who were clinically nondemented at death showed significantly less NFTs and SPs than participants with mild cognitive impairment (MCI) and dementia. Pathological lesion density was significantly related to cognitive status. However, two of nine participants who were nondemented in the few months prior to death met *pathological* criteria for Alzheimer's disease, suggesting individual variability in the relationship between brain pathology and cognitive presentation. One explanation for this variability is the notion of cognitive reserve, a hypothesized degree of protection against disease or injury whereby one is behaviorally unaffected by pathology sufficient to cause dementia in someone with less cognitive reserve. The construct of cognitive reserve is discussed more fully elsewhere in this volume (see Chap. 2).

Functional imaging techniques such as positron emission tomography (PET) and functional magnetic resonance imaging (fMRI) allow for the examination of blood flow and oxygenation to particular brain structures, in participants as they engage in cognitive tasks. Comparisons of older and younger adults reveal an increase in bilateral activation with age, whereby tasks associated with focal, unilateral activation in younger adults (e.g., verbal memory) become associated with bilateral activation in older adults [37, 38]. Further, bilateral activation in older adults is associated with *better* performance on cognitive tasks, including working memory, semantic learning, and perception [39–42]. This suggests that the older brain engages in more widely distributed compensatory processing by activating the contralateral hemisphere to achieve greater cognitive benefits [8].

Theories of Aging

In a process termed "dedifferentiation," sensory function (i.e., visual acuity and audition) has been shown to predict performance on a wide range of cognitive tasks in older, but not younger, adults [43, 44]. It has been proposed that abilities that are relatively independent earlier in life, such as sensory ability and cognition, become more interrelated with old age. Functionally, this can be thought of as a decrease in neural specificity, whereby regions that respond selectively in younger adults change to respond to a wider array of inputs in older adults. Similarly, in older adults, increased prefrontal activation is associated with decreased parahippocampal activation and hippocampal volume shrinkage [45, 46]. Whereas activation in the parahippocampal regions is associated with learning new material in younger and middle-aged adults, increased prefrontal activation is instead observed in older adults, suggesting greater frontal activity may be a compensatory mechanism for decreased mesiotemporal activation [8, 45].

Salthouse proposed the processing-speed theory of cognitive aging, which assumes that a wide range of cognitive task performances are limited by the imposed constraints on the speed of processing [18]. Slow processing speed dampens cognition in two ways: (1) cognitive operations are executed too slowly to be successfully completed in the available time and (2) the amount of simultaneously available information, necessary for higher-level processing, is reduced, as early processing is no longer available when new processing occurs. Complex operations are most affected by slow processing speed since they are dependent on the products of simpler (and earlier) operations, and often, the accuracy of performance is dependent on the number of operations that can be carried out in a given time period (e.g., associations, rehearsals). The amount of simultaneously available information may also be reduced due to disruptions in the synchronization of neural signals and activation patterns [18].

The *scaffolding theory* of aging and cognition proposes that structural brain changes associated with aging are accompanied by effort on the part of neural networks to maintain homeostatic cognitive functioning in the face of these changes [8]. This leads to changes in brain function through "strengthening of existing connections, formation of new connections, and disuse of connections that have become weak or faulty" (p. 175). Scaffolding is described as the brain's "normal response to challenge" (p. 183), and the theory can be used to explain the process of acquiring a novel skill. The initially engaged neural networks shift from broad and dispersed to a specific and honed circuit of neural regions. While the more specific regions assume dominant control over functions, the initial broad networks continue to be minimally active, suggesting that they remain available for compensatory processing [45]. In the aging brain, scaffolding is thought to maintain healthy cognitive function in the face of neural degradation. These circuits can provide supplementary, complementary, or alternative ways to complete a cognitive task and are thought to reside largely within the prefrontal cortex, consistent with findings on overactivation of frontal networks with age [8]. Scaffolded networks, however, are less efficient and more prone to error than honed circuits, which are highly functionally interconnected. According to scaffolding theory, this results in the observable and measurable cognitive decline seen in older adults. The need for compensatory scaffolding exceeds the available networks, resulting in a more profound decline in functioning in the oldest old.

Individual Factors in Cognitive Aging

Given the considerable variation in cognitive performance in older persons, particularly in the oldest old, examination of individual difference factors related to the cognitive aging process is warranted [4, 5]. Factors shown to contribute to cognitive reserve or to be related to cognitive decline in clinical studies include education, occupational complexity, physical health, and diet [47]. It is suspected that cognitive reserve is represented biologically by a number of processes, including (1) richer interconnectivity and organization of neural circuits; (2) alterations in synaptic efficiency, marked by changes in neurotransmitter release, receptor density, and receptor affinity; (3) and changes in intracellular signaling pathways [47].

Physical health status is arguably one of the more important factors to consider when predicting performances on cognitive assessment in noncognitively impaired elderly. Clinical and subclinical medical disorders have been found to be better predictors of neuropsychological performance than chronological age, and these disorders include hypertension, hypercholesterolemia, obesity, and white matter lesions [48]. Cardiac arrhythmias [49], sensory loss [50], pulmonary function [51], and other measures of biological age [52] have also been associated with poorer cognitive functioning.

Higher education has been associated with preserved cognitive performance over time (i.e., less decline) in aging adults [53, 54], though not all research has supported this outcome [55]. Occupational complexity is shown to be related to relatively better cognitive functioning with age, above and beyond the benefits afforded by higher levels of education [56]. More specifically, cognitive ability in older adults was found to be related to the degree of complexity of one's work with people but not to occupational complexity with data or things [56]. In particular, participants who held jobs with high complexity of work with people demonstrated better cognitive performance on measures of verbal skills, spatial skills, and processing speed than participants with low occupational complexity with people. No differences in memory performances were found. The cognitive benefit received from high occupational complexity ceased following retirement, suggesting that once these occupational skills are no longer being practiced, they fail to retain their effectiveness in bolstering cognitive ability.

Mild Cognitive Impairment

Defining Mild Cognitive Impairment

Neuropsychological referrals are often made on the basis of a patient's or their family's perceived (i.e., subjective) report of a decline in cognitive ability. An integral part of the neuropsychologist's role is to determine whether a patient's complaints or their family's observations of cognitive decline are due to the normal cognitive aging process or if they instead represent an objective impairment in cognitive functioning relative to the patient's same-age peers. The construct of MCI represents a decline in cognitive performance greater than would be expected for the person's age but not sufficient to meet criteria for a diagnosis of dementia. [57] Petersen described MCI as interposed between normal cognitive changes associated with aging and the very early stages of a dementing process [58]. It is therefore conceptualized as a pathological condition and not merely a manifestation of the normal aging process. Incidence and prevalence rates vary as a consequence of study details, including diagnostic criteria, assessment procedures, and sample characteristics (e.g., community versus clinic, age, education, gender, race, health comorbidities). Within the general population, prevalence rates have been found to range from 1 to 19% [59].

The original criteria for MCI proposed by Petersen et al. [57] are as follows:

1. Presence of a memory complaint
2. Normal activities of daily living
3. Normal general cognitive function
4. Abnormal memory for age
5. Not demented

These criteria are particularly useful for patients who have impairment in the memory domain but intact cognitive performance and functioning in all other domains. Such patients would be labeled as having amnesic MCI (a-MCI). Revised criteria were proposed by a multidisciplinary, international group of experts, in light of the heterogeneity of MCI clinical presentations reflected in the literature [60]. For example, some patients have a primary impairment in the memory domain only, whereas others have memory impairment in addition to other domain impairment(s). Still others have impairments in single or multiple nonmemory cognitive domains. These heterogenous clinical presentations may have multiple etiologies, including degenerative, vascular, metabolic, traumatic, psychiatric, etc. [58, 60].

The most updated clinical diagnostic criteria for MCI are recommended by the National Institute on Aging and Alzheimer's Association workgroup [61]. The diagnostic criteria for MCI in a clinical setting are as follows:

1. Concern regarding change in cognition: There is evidence of concern for change in the patient's cognitive status as compared to his/her previous level. This concern may be on the part of the patient, an informant who knows the patient well, or from a skilled clinician who has observed the patient.
2. Impairment in one or more cognitive domains: There is evidence of lower performance in one or more cognitive domains that is greater than

what would be expected for the patient's age and educational background. Impairment may be in a variety of domains, including memory, attention, language, executive function, and visuospatial skills.

3. Preservation of independence in functional abilities: The patient generally maintains his/her independence of function in daily life without considerable aids or assistance. However, patients may have mild problems performing complex functional tasks (e.g., paying bills, preparing meals, shopping), whereby they may be less efficient, take more time, and make more errors than in the past.
4. Not demented: These cognitive changes are sufficiently mild so that there is no evidence of significant impairment in social or occupational functioning. A diagnosis of MCI requires evidence of intraindividual change. If the patient has been evaluated only once, change will be inferred from the history and/or evidence that cognitive performance is impaired beyond what is expected for that patient. Practical application of these criteria will be considered below in the Assessment section.

Subtypes

We have already mentioned *single-domain amnesic MCI (a-MCI)*, which is a useful category for patients who have impairment in memory but intact cognitive performance in all other domains and in daily functioning. As research on MCI has advanced to include cognitive impairment in domains other than memory, several other subtypes of MCI have been proposed. [58] Some patients display impairment in a single nonmemory cognitive domain (e.g., executive function) but perform normally in other domains, including memory. These patients would be given labels of single-domain non-amnesic MCI (na-MCI). Still other patients present with impairments in multiple domains while continuing to display relatively intact activities of daily living (ADLs) and general cognitive functioning; these patients would be classified generally as having multiple-domain MCI. More specifically, in the event that a deficit in memory is present, a patient is given a diagnosis of multiple-domain MCI with amnesia (md-MCI+a); if memory impairment is not evident, then a diagnosis of multiple-domain MCI without amnesia (md-MCI-a) is appropriate.

Etiology and Prognosis

In addition to different subtypes, there also are multiple etiologies for MCI. Petersen suggested four main etiologies: (1) degenerative (e.g., Alzheimer's disease), (2) vascular (e.g., cerebrovascular disease), (3) psychiatric (e.g., depression), and/or (4) traumatic (e.g., head injury) [58]. Of course, a host of other potential etiologies should always be considered in the differential diagnosis, including medication side effects and other toxic factors, metabolic factors (e.g., thyroid dysfunction, vitamin B12 deficiency), or infection. Particular subtypes of MCI are reported to be more commonly associated with certain etiologies. For example, patients with a-MCI are more likely to convert to Alzheimer's disease than patients with na-MCI [57, 62–64]. An impairment in episodic memory, i.e., the ability to learn and retain new information, is most commonly seen in MCI patients who later convert to Alzheimer's disease [61]. Additionally, a longitudinal decline in cognition provides additional evidence for a likely etiology of Alzheimer's disease [61]. Those with impairments in nonmemory domains such as executive function and visuospatial skills may be more likely to convert to dementia with Lewy bodies [58]. Persons with na-MCI in one study were least likely to convert to any form of dementia [61].

Follow-up data from the initial Petersen et al. study on MCI using patients ($N = 220$) from the Mayo Alzheimer's Disease Center/Alzheimer's Disease Patient Registry (ADC/ADPR) demonstrated a rate of progression from MCI to dementia of 12% per year [57, 58]. At a 6-year follow-up, approximately 80% of MCI patients in the same study were reported to have progressed to dementia. Other studies have found conversion rates of 10–19% per year from MCI to Alzheimer's disease [63, 65]. In comparison, 1–2% of the general population develop Alzheimer's disease per year, providing evidence that MCI places one at increased risk for future dementia above the rate that is expected for a person's age [57]. Persons diagnosed with a-MCI were found in one study to have a fourfold greater risk than noncognitively impaired individuals to develop Alzheimer's disease over a 2-year follow-up period [66]. When considering a general diagnosis of MCI (i.e., not taking into account subtype), patients are found to have a three times greater risk of developing Alzheimer's disease (average follow-up of 4.5 years) [67].

At the same time, however, many persons with MCI remain stable with this diagnosis or revert to normal. For example, in a clinical sample, 41% remained stable over an average 3.5-year follow-up and 17% returned to normal cognitive status [68]. These data suggest that for some patients, MCI represents an intermediate point on the continuum from normal cognition to dementia, while for others, MCI is a transient period of cognitive decline that resolves with time. The latter may be seen in patients with reversible causes of cognitive dysfunction, such as metabolic abnormalities or substance use. Those with na-MCI are most likely to revert to normal or improve their cognitive status over time [62].

Pathophysiology and Neurodiagnostic Findings

Neuroimaging data lends further support for MCI as a unique diagnostic entity, separate from both normal cognitive functioning and dementia states. Retention of Pittsburgh compound B (PIB), used to image beta-amyloid plaques in neuronal tissue, has been examined using positron emission tomography (PET) in persons with normal cognition, MCI, and Alzheimer's disease (AD) [69]. In their study, Forsberg et al. found that PIB retention in MCI patients is higher than that of normal controls but lower than in AD patients. Additionally, the MCI patients who converted to AD within the 2–16-month follow-up period had higher mean PIB retention than the MCI patients who remained stable during follow-up periods. Magnetic resonance imaging (MRI) has been used to examine trajectories of volumetric brain loss in a healthy aging sample over a 15-year period [29]. Ventricular expansion was found to be faster in persons developing MCI years prior to the emergence of clinical symptoms. An increasingly rapid expansion occurred approximately 2 years prior to the clinical diagnosis of MCI.

Neuroimaging studies show that subjects who progressed to AD within an 18-month follow-up period had greater volume loss than a stable MCI group and a control group in areas consistent with volume loss in AD (i.e., medial and inferior temporal lobes, temporoparietal neocortex, posterior and anterior cingulate, precuneus, and frontal lobes). [70] Autopsy studies reveal that subjects who died with a classification of a-MCI showed the early pathologic changes seen in subjects diagnosed with AD prior to death [71, 72]. Annual increase in ventricular volume as assessed by serial MRI has revealed the greatest volume increase in AD subjects, followed by an intermediate increase in a-MCI subjects, and the smallest change in cognitive normals. Further, a-MCI and AD subjects with APOE-ε4 genotype show the greatest increase in ventricular volume. These findings also correlate clinically with concurrent change in cognitive and functional status [73]. Specific and distinguishing MRI abnormalities also have been identified in MCI subjects who ultimately convert to AD, vascular dementia, and Lewy body dementia, lending support for MCI as a prodrome to multiple dementing processes [74].

Assessment

Referrals

Referrals for neuropsychological evaluation when MCI is a diagnostic consideration may come from a variety of sources. Neurologists are likely to be one of the most common referral sources, along with primary care physicians, psychiatrists, and self-referral (initiated either by

Table 16.1 MCI differential diagnosis

Common differential diagnoses associated with MCI
Normal cognitive aging
Dementia (e.g., Alzheimer's, vascular, frontotemporal dementia, Parkinson's plus syndromes)
Depression/"pseudodementia" Delirium
Other reversible causes for cognitive dysfunction (e.g., metabolic abnormalities, substance use, obstructive sleep apnea)

the patient or a family member). One study of male patients with MCI receiving care at a Veterans Affairs hospital found that generally, either patients or their families prompted the consultation for memory loss [75]. In many cases, patients may be seen first by neurologists who then provide a neuropsychological referral for a more comprehensive cognitive evaluation. Most typical referral questions from other medical professionals in the context of an evaluation for MCI will pertain to differential diagnosis and etiology. Typical differentials will include normal cognitive aging versus MCI versus dementia, as well as depression or "pseudodementia" versus MCI or dementia. Etiology of cognitive impairment also is a common referring question and usually involves a question of Alzheimer's disease pathology versus other causes such as vascular cognitive impairment, frontotemporal dementia, a Parkinson's plus syndrome (e.g., Lewy body dementia, multiple system atrophy, progressive supranuclear palsy, corticobasal degeneration), or metabolic causes. Table 16.1 shows a list of common differential diagnoses for MCI. There are other associated issues that may be relevant to referring physicians, such as beginning an appropriate cognitive enhancing medication or psychotropic drugs for treatment of mood disorders. The neuropsychological evaluation is often requested to serve as a baseline for subsequent serial evaluations in order to track the trajectory of cognitive decline or improvement following treatment. Assessment of functional independence may be requested based on cognitive testing, such as whether the patient is completely independent or requires in-home assistance as part of their daily functioning. Cognitive testing may also help form an opinion as to whether the patient may require a formal driving evaluation. Assessment of driving abilities is detailed elsewhere in this volume (see Chap. 10).

Clinical Interview

An important component of the clinical interview when assessing patients with MCI involves obtaining an accurate picture of the emergence of cognitive symptoms and any functional difficulties. For this reason, it is ideal to have a collateral informant present at the interview to provide his or her insight into the patient's behaviors and functional status. The informant is typically a spouse, child, sibling, or other close family member or friend who is knowledgeable about the patient's history and can provide information about changes in cognitive and functional status.

One of the diagnostic criteria of MCI is the presence of a subjective cognitive complaint. Patient complaints may be corroborated by the collateral informant, whereas in some cases, the friend or family member's report is the only evidence for subjective cognitive change. This may occur in cases where the patient has little to no insight into their cognitive changes. It is important to obtain a thorough history of the emergence of cognitive symptoms, including examples of cognitive problems the patient is experiencing in everyday life. For example, the early and prominent emergence of language symptoms may be indicative of a primarily aphasic dementing process, whereas early memory difficulties may signal mesial temporal lobe involvement, the area initially and primarily affected in Alzheimer's disease. Evaluating functional abilities also is essential when considering a diagnosis of MCI. Functional independence is the key factor in the differential diagnosis of MCI or early dementia. Patients with MCI are considered to have intact basic activities of daily living (ADLs), with predominantly intact instrumental ADLs. An assessment of functioning should include questions about the patient's ability to care for his or her basic needs, such as hygiene, dressing, and feeding oneself, as well as his or her more instrumental needs, such as making and keeping appointments, financial management, driving abilities, and medication management.

The patient and his or her informant should also be questioned about changes in behavior or personality, which are often early indicators of a primarily behavioral dementing process, such as frontotemporal dementia. Behaviors to consider include those indicative of apathy, disinhibition, perseveration, or behaviors that are out of the ordinary for the person. In addition, irritability often accompanies symptoms of cognitive decline. Patients should be questioned about emotional symptoms and psychiatric history to assess for the presence or increase in symptoms of depression, anxiety, or other salient psychological problems. This is particularly important because approximately 35–75% of patients with MCI endorse at least one neuropsychiatric symptom at a prevalence rate that is higher than same-age non-MCI peers [76–79]. The most commonly endorsed symptoms include depression/dysphoria, apathy, anxiety, and agitation [80, 81]. Commonly reported symptoms of depression in MCI include poor concentration, inner tension, pessimistic thoughts, lassitude, reduced sleep, thoughts of death, inability to feel, and reduced appetite [82]. There is some evidence for higher rates of depression in a-MCI versus na-MCI and in multiple-domain MCI versus single-domain MCI patients [76, 80]. Given evidence for elevated rates of mood symptoms in persons with MCI, it is imperative that patients are screened for clinical and subclinical symptoms of depression, anxiety, apathy, and irritability.

The clinician should obtain a thorough medical history and assessment of the patient's current health status. Results should be obtained from any completed neurodiagnostic studies (e.g., MRI, CT, EEG) for consideration in the differential diagnosis. Evaluating the presence of vascular risk factors such as hypertension, hypercholesterolemia, and diabetes is essential when considering etiology of cognitive decline. An assessment of the patient's sleep quality is important, including whether he or she has been diagnosed with sleep apnea, which has known effects on executive cognitive functioning [83]. A review of the patient's current and recent medications is also critical in order to consider medication-induced cognitive changes. It is important to obtain not only a list of the patient's medications but also a careful chronology of when each potentially psychoactive medication was introduced in relation to the chronology of cognitive symptom emergence. A review of the patient's use of recreational substances is necessary to rule out preventable causes for cognitive changes. Finally, family history of dementia should be assessed, including approximate age of onset of cognitive difficulties in family members.

Functional Impairment

In assessing whether ability to carry out activities of daily living (ADLs) is essentially normal (a diagnostic criterion for MCI), a thorough history from the patient (and ideally an informant) should be obtained. Self-report or clinician-administered ADL scales can also be employed but do not replace a careful detailed interview, since many of the ADL scales do not pick up on subtle changes in functioning. Petersen noted that minor inconveniences in a patient's daily functioning may be present, but they are not sufficient in severity to constitute a major disability in functioning [58]. Patients with MCI tend to report some degree of decline in their ability to handle daily tasks, whereby they feel they are more forgetful, are less able to multitask, and have difficulties with planning and organization [84]. These inefficiencies can manifest in a variety of ways, such as problems remembering where one has placed objects, forgetting new names, difficulty completing two tasks at once, and trouble remembering shopping items, recalling conversations, or prioritizing tasks by importance. It is often the ability to learn, retain new information and perform higher-order executive skills that is dampened in persons with MCI, resulting in somewhat less efficient daily functioning [84–86]. Persons with MCI tend to make errors in performing tasks accurately and efficiently while still remaining able to complete tasks [87]. This is in contrast to dementia patients, who tend to also make these errors in addition to omitting major portions of tasks.

Poorer memory performance on cognitive testing has been found to predict future difficulties in financial management in patients with MCI, and impaired memory and psychomotor speed are the cognitive domains most strongly related to functional abilities [88]. Other research suggests that attention and executive functioning, but not memory, are associated with difficulties managing multiple-step financial tasks, such as bill payment and preparation and management of bank statements [89]. Persons with MCI tend to show subtle functional declines in driving abilities when compared to noncognitively impaired persons, though their overall performances are not at the level of frank driving impairments [90]. Instead, they are less likely than their cognitively normal peers to perform certain driving routines seamlessly (e.g., left-hand turns, maintaining lane control), and their performances are more often rated as "less than optimal." Although some dampening in functioning is observed in MCI patients, it is much less severe than the functional decline seen in patients with dementia. MCI patients tend to perform functionally on a level intermediate between persons with normal cognition and dementia patients [87]. MCI patients are still able to function independently, albeit perhaps less efficiently and with the use of compensatory strategies.

Cognitive Impairment

Criteria for diagnosing MCI include not only self- or family report of cognitive decline but also objective measurements of deficits in cognitive functioning. An exact cutoff for what constitutes "mild" impairment has not been set in stone, but traditionally, a cutoff score of 1.5 SD below age norms has been used based on Petersen et al.'s original study [57]. In that study, the MCI group performed, on average, 1.5 SD below age-matched controls. However, Petersen emphasizes that this was not intended to serve as a cutoff score and that it is ultimately left up to clinician judgment whether or not a patient displays objective memory impairment relative to his or her baseline [58]. The most recent consensus criteria notes that scores on cognitive tests for patients with MCI are typically 1–1.5 SD below the mean for age and education matched peers on culturally appropriate normative data [61]. It is emphasized that these ranges are to be used as guidelines and not cutoff scores.

Selecting neuropsychological instruments for evaluating MCI should include an evaluation of the patient's performance in all major cognitive domains (i.e., memory, attention, processing speed, language, executive functioning, visuospatial skills, motor functioning) in order to ensure a comprehensive assessment. Typically, a dementia screening measure is also administered and ideally an estimate of premorbid functioning (e.g., word reading). A comprehensive assessment approach that employs detailed neuropsychological assessment is advocated to improve the reliability and stability of the MCI diagnosis [91]. Although all major neurocognitive domains should be validly sampled, it is of particular importance to obtain multiple measures of memory, as this domain is typically the presenting subjective complaint and is essential for differential diagnosis. Because there are multiple possible etiologies of MCI, it would be inappropriate to focus only on memory testing and a global screening measure. Assessment of other areas, including executive, attentional, and motor abilities in assessing for a vascular etiology, as well as visuospatial functioning in assessing for Lewy body pathology, allows for the most comprehensive approach to determining etiology, a common referral question. Careful examination of memory profile patterns is also helpful in this regard. Given that a significant proportion of MCI patients present with neuropsychiatric symptoms, it is important to also include self-report measures of mood functioning, such as assessments of depression and anxiety symptoms. Table 16.2 provides a sample test battery for a comprehensive neuropsychological evaluation when MCI is con-

Table 16.2 Sample core neuropsychological battery for assessment in MCI

Mini-Mental State Exam [106]
Repeatable Battery for the Assessment of Neuropsychological Status [107]
Wechsler Adult Intelligence Scale IV [108] or Wechsler Abbreviated Scale of Intelligence [109]
Wide Range Achievement Test 4 (Reading subtest) [110]
Trail Making Test A & B [111]
Stroop Color Word Test [112]
California Verbal Learning Test II [113] or Hopkins Verbal Learning Test—Revised [114]
Rey Complex Figure Test [115, 116] or Brief Visuospatial Memory Test—Revised [117]
Wechsler Memory Scale III (Logical Memory) [118]
Boston Naming Test [119]
Controlled Oral Word Association [120] and Semantic Fluency (i.e., Animal Fluency) [121]
Wisconsin Card Sorting Test [122]
Clock Drawing and Copy [123]
Finger Tapping Test [124]
Grooved Pegboard [125]
Geriatric Depression Scale [126] *or* Beck Depression Inventory, Second Edition [127]
State-Trait Anxiety Inventory [128]

sidered in the differential diagnosis. Other measures and test batteries may be chosen, but the guiding principles of test selection should be comprehensive sampling of cognitive domains, appropriate norms for age and other patient demographic factors, and wide range of measurement between the floor and ceiling captured by the measures, and whenever possible, measures with alternate forms for retesting over time should be used.

Common Neurocognitive Deficits

The most common neuropsychological impairment seen in MCI patients who ultimately convert to Alzheimer's disease is a decline in episodic learning and memory early in the disease process [92, 93]. This is thought to be consistent with early involvement of structures in the medial temporal lobes (e.g., hippocampus, entorhinal cortex) in the progression to Alzheimer's disease (AD). Memory profile patterns in a-MCI tend to display reduced learning, rapid forgetting, poor recognition discrimination, and elevated intrusion errors [92, 94].

In terms of overall cognitive profiles, MCI patients have been found to show clearly defined memory impairments with only mild impairments in other domains, such as executive functioning [95, 96]. While a-MCI patients may show some difficulty in planning and problem solving, md-MCI patients show the most severe impairments [97]. It is unclear whether md-MCI patients' cognitive profiles are more impaired due to different disease etiology (e.g., vascular) or whether differences are due to md-MCI patients being further along in the disease process.

Although visual confrontation naming impairment is a hallmark symptom of AD, patients with a-MCI have not been found to differ from controls on such tasks, suggesting that the breakdown in semantic knowledge does not typically occur at the MCI stage [98]. At the same time, however, MCI patients have been shown to have poorer performance than controls on tasks of semantic memory, receive less benefit than controls when semantically cued on memory tasks, and use less semantic clustering strategies on verbal learning tasks [67, 99, 100]. It may be the case that these deficits in semantically related learning are due at least in part to dampened executive functioning processes that affect categorization or semantic organization [101].

In the attention domain, MCI patients who ultimately convert to AD demonstrate poorer immediate serial recall and divided attention than their MCI counterparts who remain cognitively stable [102]. This subgroup demonstrates the early stages of attentional impairment seen in AD, suggesting that such attentional impairments slowly decline over the course of the disease.

Vascular MCI has been less extensively studied in the research literature, though data suggest that patients with vascular disease or significant vascular risk factors demonstrate poorer attention, executive function, visuospatial performance, and slower processing speed than patients without vascular risk factors [103, 104].

Diagnosing MCI Subtypes

Once a diagnosis of MCI is established based on diagnostic criteria, selecting an MCI subtype is based on the results of the neurocognitive profile. In amnesic MCI (a-MCI), there is a single deficit in the learning and memory domain with preserved cognitive functioning in all other domains. Other patients have impaired learning and memory in addition to impairment in another domain (oftentimes, executive functioning, but any other domain is possible), and these patients would receive a diagnosis of multiple-domain amnesic-MCI (md-MCI+a). Patients who have a single nonmemory domain impairment (again, often executive dysfunction or attention/processing speed) are given the diagnosis of non-amnesic MCI (na-MCI). A subset of patients demonstrates impairment in two or more nonmemory domains and would be diagnosed with multiple-domain non-amnesic MCI (md-MCI-a).

Feedback and Recommendations

When reporting a diagnosis of MCI to a patient and possibly his or her family members, it is important that the clinician clearly explain the nature of the MCI diagnosis. Important information to highlight includes the degree of cognitive impairment associated with the diagnosis (i.e., greater than normal for the patient's age but not severe enough to warrant a diagnosis of dementia). Equally important to convey sensitively is the patient's increased risk for converting to dementia in the future, particularly for patients given an amnesic MCI diagnosis (single or multiple domain), which has the greatest association with future conversion to dementia, typically Alzheimer's disease [62, 66]. Patients should be made aware of their particular areas of difficulty (e.g., memory, executive functioning) and the real-world implications for these deficits. At the same time, cognitive and other personal strengths should be highlighted in the context of developing compensatory strategies for dealing with objective cognitive deficits and the functional difficulties that often accompany such deficits. If a-MCI is diagnosed, given its heightened association with a progression to Alzheimer's dementia, retesting may be recommended in 1 year. For other types of MCI, it may be more appropriate to recommend retesting as clinically warranted, if further cognitive changes are suspected by the patient, family, or referring clinician.

Useful information for clinicians disclosing an MCI diagnosis, including the meaning and impact for the patient, can be gleaned from a unique analysis of qualitative interview data from a small clinical sample of MCI patients ($N = 12$, diagnosed 3 to 6 months prior) [105]. The authors examined patient's experiences of living with and making sense of an MCI diagnosis. Interestingly, over 40% ($n = 5$) of their sample used positively valenced words to depict their emotional reactions to the diagnosis. Narrative accounts typically revealed satisfaction in finding professional validation for their subjective symptoms, as well as relief associated with a negative dementia diagnosis. Given evidence that MCI often is a precursor for dementia, this raises the issue of whether patients with MCI are adequately explained their increased risk of developing dementia in the future. Only 2 of 12 participants expressed a negative reaction to their diagnosis, and this occurred in the context of a perceived looming dementia diagnosis. Several participants did mention awareness of the possibility of further decline in cognitive status, often in the context of being unsure whether a decline would occur. Oftentimes, a current state of relief occurred simultaneously with tension surrounding an uncertain dementia prognosis. Around half of the participants related MCI as part of the normal aging process. Taken together, these findings suggest that there are varying interpretations of an MCI diagnosis, which the investigators pointed out have the potential to impact health behaviors, including returning for follow-up cognitive testing or planning for future states of decisional incapacity.

Recommendations for patients diagnosed with MCI may include follow-up with the patient's neurologist or psychiatrist to discuss potentially beginning a trial of anti-dementia medication, such as an acetylcholinesterase inhibitor. If the patient does not already have established medical care within these specialties, an appropriate referral should be made, particularly if baseline neurodiagnostic studies (e.g., MRI, EEG) have not yet been completed. Management of risk factors associated with cognitive decline, such as medical comorbidities (e.g., vascular risk factors such as hypertension, diabetes, hyperlipidemia, sleep apnea, metabolic levels) should be recommended. Similarly, patients should be encouraged to participate in a physician-approved exercise regimen and maintain a healthful diet. Given that mood factors can exacerbate symptoms of cognitive impairment, appropriate monitoring of depression, anxiety, or other psychological factors is necessary. In some cases, a psychiatric or psychotherapy referral is warranted to assist in managing symptoms pharmacologically or cognitively/behaviorally. Patients should be encouraged to remain cognitively and socially active and to continue to complete daily tasks as independently as possible.

In terms of functional abilities, it is important for patients and their families to continuously monitor functional status, particularly with regard to potentially dangerous tasks such as driving. A change in functional status may be the simplest way for families of patients with MCI to recognize advancing cognitive decline, and they should be encouraged to assist the patient in monitoring instrumental activities of daily living (IADLs) such as financial management, driving, medication management, and higher-level organizational abilities. A decline in the ability to manage and perform IADLs is likely to represent a concordant decline in cognitive status and may alert the patient and family that neuropsychological reevaluation is warranted to assess for progression to a dementia syndrome.

With regard to neuropsychological retesting, it is difficult to establish a universally appropriate time for follow-up evaluation. Whereas a significant proportion of MCI patients will ultimately convert to dementia, many will also remain stable with the diagnosis or will revert to normal, depending on etiology. In those patients who ultimately receive a dementia diagnosis, the course of cognitive decline may be quite variable, with some patients remaining in the MCI category for years after initial evaluation and others converting to dementia rather rapidly. Patients present for their initial neuropsychological evaluation at various points on the continuum, further complicating an estimate for possible dementia conversion. Two points of reference can be helpful in determining a follow-up evaluation: (1) the severity and number of domains impaired and (2) the patient's functional status. It is likely that patients with relatively more severe cognitive impairments are further along in their disease progression and patients with multiple impaired domains may reach a dementia diagnosis sooner. Similarly, patients who show relatively greater impairment in daily functioning may be closer to a dementia diagnosis. Perhaps the safest benchmark for retesting is a 1-year follow-up period, in conjunction with the recommendation that the patient return for testing earlier should he or she (or family members) notice a significant decline in cognitive ability or functional status prior to the 1-year mark.

In conclusion, accurate clinical discrimination between normal cognitive aging and MCI is an important diagnostic challenge. This discrimination will become increasingly critical as new interventions are developed to target the very earliest manifestations of incipient brain disease.

Clinical Pearls

- A significant proportion of MCI patients will ultimately convert to dementia, although many will remain stable or will revert to normal, depending on the etiology of the cognitive disturbance.
- The most recent consensus criteria indicate MCI is associated with cognitive test scores that are typically 1–1.5 SD below the mean for age and education matched peers; it is emphasized that these ranges are to be used as guidelines, *not cutoff scores*.
- Although memory complaints of some kind are typically the most common presenting reason for evaluation, it is important to carefully assess the nature of the complaint since other

aspects of cognition may actually underlie the perceived deficit.

- Memory complains such as forgetting what you went into a room for or difficulty recalling names are common in older adults and may not be clinically significant. However, collateral reports suggesting repetitive speech/questioning or trouble navigating a familiar environment are more likely to be clinically relevant.
- Assessment of mood/personality functioning is critical since subjective memory complaints tend to be more strongly correlated with negative affect than with objective memory performance.
- The examiner should get the patient's consent to obtain collateral information from a well-known source. The congruence, or lack thereof, between patient self-report and collateral report is clinically informative in terms of lack of insight/awareness of deficits or a tendency to amplify complaints.
- Assessing impact on activities of daily living (ADLs) requires careful clinical judgment. Be certain to clarify how ADLs are impaired by *cognitive* factors as opposed to physical or emotional factors. Ask the collateral source if the patient would still be *capable* of performing activities (e.g., driving, managing finances) that other family members are conducting.
- In addition to taking a general medical history, be sure to inquire about pain, sleep, and substance use in the context of the cognitive complaints.

References

1. World Health Organization. World health statistics 2010. Geneva, Switzerland: WHO Press; 2010.
2. US Census Bureau. Annual estimates of the resident population by sex and five-year age groups for the United States: April 1, 2000 to July 1, 2009. Retrieved October 15, 2010 from http://www.census.gov/popest/national/asrh/NC-EST2009-sa.htmlv.
3. Christensen H. What cognitive changes can be expected with normal aging? Aust N Z J Psychiatry. 2001;35:768–75.
4. Christensen H, Mackinnon A, Jorm AF, Henderson AS, Scott LR, Korten AE. Age differences and inter-individual variation in cognition in community-dwelling elderly. Psychol Aging. 1994;9:381–90.
5. Der G, Allerhand M, Starr JM, Hofer SM, Deary IJ. Age-related changes in memory and fluid reasoning in a sample of healthy old people. Aging, Neuropsychol Cognition. 2009;17:55–70.
6. Lindenberger U, Baltes PB. Intellectual functioning in old and very old age: Cross-sectional results from the Berlin Aging Study. Psychol Aging. 1997;12:410–32.
7. Rabbit PMA, McInnes L, Diggle P, Holland F, Bent N, Abson V, Horan M. The University of Manchester longitudinal study of cognition in normal healthy old age, 1983 through 2003. Aging NeuropsycholCognition. 2004;11:245–79.
8. Park DC, Reuter-Lorenz P. The adaptive brain: Aging and neurocognitive scaffolding. Annu Rev Psychol. 2009;60:173–96.
9. Gunstad J, Paul RH, Brickman AM, Cohen RA, Arns M, Roe D, Gordon E. Patterns of cognitive performance in middle-aged and older adults: A cluster analytic examination. J Geriatr Psychiatry Neurol. 2006;19:59–64.
10. Park DC, Lautenschlager G, Hedden T, Davidson NS, Smith AD, Smith PK. Models of visuospatial and verbal memory across the adult life span. Psychol Aging. 2002;17:299–320.
11. Rush BK, Barch DM, Braver TS. Accounting for cognitive aging: Context processing, inhibition, or processing speed? Aging, Neuropsychol Cognition. 2006;13:588–610.
12. Howieson D, Holm L, Kaye J, Oken B. Neurologic function in the optimally healthy oldest old: Neuropsychological evaluation. Neurology. 1993;43:1882–6.
13. Woodard J, Benedict R, Roberts V, Goldstein F. Short-form alternatives to the Judgment of Line Orientation Test. J Clin Exp Neuropsychol. 1996;18:898–904.
14. Giovagnoli AR, Del Pesce M, Mascheroni S, Simoncelli M, Laiacona M, Capitani E. Trail Making Test: Normative values from 287 normal adult controls. Ital J Neurol Sci. 1996;17:305–9.
15. Goul WR, Brown M. Effects of age and intelligence on Trail Making Test performance and validity. Percept Mot Skills. 1970;30:319–26.
16. Kennedy KJ. Age effects on Trail Making Test performance. Percept Mot Skills. 1981;52:671–5.
17. Clay OJ, Edwards JD, Ross LA, Okonkwo O, Wadley VG, Roth DL, Ball KK. Visual function and cognitive speed of processing mediate age-related decline in memory span and fluid intelligence. J Aging Health. 2009;21:547–66.
18. Salthouse TA. The processing speed theory of adult age differences in cognition. Psychol Rev. 1996;103:403–28.
19. Kane MJ, Hasher L, Stoltzfus ER, Zacks RT, Connelly SL. Inhibitory attention mechanisms and aging. Psychol Aging. 1994;9:103–12.
20. Jennings JM, Jacoby LL. Automatic versus intentional uses of memory: Aging, attention, and control. Psychol Aging. 1993;8:283–93.

21. Shafto MA, Burker DM, Stamatakis EA, Tam PP, Tyler LK. On the tip-of-the-tongue: Neural correlates of increased word-finding failures in normal aging. J Cogn Neurosci. 2007;19:2060–70.
22. Au R, Joung P, Nicholas M, Obler L. Naming ability across the adult life span. Aging Cognition. 1995;2:300–11.
23. Randolph C, Lansing AE, Ivnik RJ, Cullum CM, Hermann BP. Determinants of confrontation naming performance. Arch Clin Neuropsychol. 1999;6:489–96.
24. Ross TP, Lichtenberg PA. Effects of age and education on neuropsychological test performance: A comparison of normal versus cognitively impaired geriatric medical patients. Aging, Neuropsychol Cognition. 1997;4:74–80.
25. Kempler D, Tang E, Dick M, Taussig I, Davis D. The effects of age, education, and ethnicity on verbal fluency. J Int Neuropsychol Soc. 1998;4:531–8.
26. Ruff RM, Light RH, Parker SB, Levin HS. The psychological construct of word fluency. Brain Lang. 1997;57:394–405.
27. Raz N, Lindenberger U, Rodrigue KM, Kennedy KM, Head D, Williamson A, Acker JD. Regional brain changes in aging healthy adults: General trends, individual differences, and modifiers. Cereb Cortex. 2005;15:1676–89.
28. Salat DH, Buckner RL, Snyder AZ, Greve DN, Desikan RSR, Busa E, Fischl B. Thinning of the cerebral cortex in aging. Cereb Cortex. 2004;14:721–30.
29. Carlson NE, Moore MM, Dame A, Howieson D, Silbert LC, Quinn JF, Kaye JA. Trajectories of brain loss in aging and the development of cognitive impairment. Neurology. 2008;70:828–33.
30. Head D, Buckner RL, Shimony JS, Williams LE, Akbudak E, Conturo TE, Snyder AZ. Differential vulnerability of anterior white matter in nondemented aging with minimal acceleration in dementia of the Alzheimer type: Evidence from diffusion tensor imaging. Cereb Cortex. 2004;14:410–23.
31. Wen W, Sachdev P. The topography of white matter hyperintensities on brain MRI in healthy 60- to 64-year-old individuals. Neuroimage. 2004;22:144–54.
32. Backman L, Ginovart N, Dixon RA, Robins Wahlin TB, Wahlin A, Halldin C, Farde L. Age-related cognitive deficits mediated by changes in the striatal dopamine system. Am J Psychiatry. 2000;157:635–7.
33. Backman L, Nyberg L, Lindenberger U, Li S, Farde L. The correlative triad among aging, dopamine, and cognition: Current status and future prospects. Neurosci Biobehav Rev. 2006;30:791–807.
34. Li S, Lindenberger U, Sikstrom S. Aging cognition: From neuromodulation to representation. Trends Cogn Sci. 2001;5:479–86.
35. Braver TS, Barch DM. A theory of cognitive control, aging cognition, and neuromodulation. Neurosci Biobehav Rev. 2002;26:809–17.
36. Green MS, Kaye JA, Ball MJ. The Oregon Brain Aging Study: Neuropathology accompanying healthy aging in the oldest old. Neurology. 2000;54:105–13.
37. Cabeza R, Grady CL, Nyberg L, McIntosh AR, Tulving E, Kapur S, Craik FIM. Age-related differences in neural activity during memory encoding and retrieval: A positron emission tomography study. J Neurosci. 1997;17:391–400.
38. Grady CL, McIntosh AR, Rajah MN, Beig S, Craik FI. The effects of age on the neural correlates of episodic encoding. Cereb Cortex. 1999;9:805–14.
39. Cherry BJ, Adamson M, Duclos A, Hellige JB. Aging and individual variation in interhemispheric collaboration and hemispheric asymmetry. Aging, Neuropsychol Cognition. 2005;12:316–39.
40. Fera F, Weickert TW, Goldberg TE, Tessitore A, Hariri A, Das S, Mattay VS. Neural mechanisms underlying probabilistic category learning in normal aging. J Neurosci. 2005;25:11340–8.
41. Reuter-Lorenz PA, Marshuetz C, Jonides J, Smith EE, Hartley A, Koeppe R. Neurocognitive ageing of storage and executive processes. Eur J Cognit Psychol. 2001;13:257–78.
42. Rypma B, D'Esposito M. Age-related changes in brain-behaviour relationships: Evidence from event-related functional MRI studies. Eur J Cognit Psychol. 2001;13:235–56.
43. Baltes PB, Lindenberger U. Emergence of a powerful connection between sensory and cognitive functions across the adult life span: A new window to the study of cognitive aging? Psychol Aging. 1997;12:12–21.
44. Lindenberger U, Baltes PB. Sensory functioning and intelligence in old age: A strong connection. Psychol Aging. 1994;9:339–55.
45. Gutchess AH, Welsch RC, Hedden T, Bangert A, Minear M, Liu LL, Park DC. Aging and the neural correlates of successful picture encoding: Frontal activations compensate for decreased medial-temporal activity. J Cogn Neurosci. 2005;17:84–96.
46. Persson J, Nyberg L, Lind J, Larsson A, Nilsson L, Ingvar M, Buckner RL. Structure-function correlates of cognitive decline in aging. Cereb Cortex. 2006;16:907–15.
47. Whalley LJ, Deary IJ, Appleton CL, Starr JM. Cognitive reserve and the neurobiology of cognitive aging. Ageing Res Rev. 2004;3:369–82.
48. Bergman I, Blomberg M, Almkvist O. The important of impaired physical health and age in normal cognitive aging. Scandanavian J Psychol. 2007;48:115–25.
49. Kilander L, Andren B, Nyman H, Lind L, Boberg M, Lithell H. Atrial fibrillation is an independent determinant of low cognitive function: A cross-sectional study in older men. Stroke. 1998;29:1816–20.
50. Anstey KJ, Smith GA. Interrelationships among biological markers of aging, health, activity, acculturation, and cognitive performance in late adulthood. Psychol Aging. 1999;14:605–18.

51. Moss M, Franks M, Briggs P, Kennedy D, Scholey A. Compromised arterial oxygen saturation in elderly asthma sufferers results in selective cognitive impairment. J Clin Exp Neuropsychol. 2005;27:139–50.
52. Wahlin A, MacDonald SWS, deFrias CM, Nilsson L, Dixon RA. How do health and biological age influence chronological age and sex differences in cognitive aging: Moderating, mediating, or both? Psychol Aging. 2006;21:318–32.
53. Johnson W, Deary IJ, McGue M, Christensen K. Genetic and environmental transactions linking cognitive ability, physical fitness, and education in late life. Psychol Aging. 2009;24:48–62.
54. Yaffe K, Fiocco AJ, Lindquist K, Vittinghoff E, Simonsick EM, Newman AB, Harris TB. Predictors of maintaining cognitive function in older adults: The Health ABC Study. Neurology. 2009;72: 2029–35.
55. Van Dijk KRA, Van Gerven PWM, Van Boxtel MPJ, Van der Elst W, Jolles J. No protective effects of education during normal cognitive aging: Results from the 6-year follow-up of the Maastricht Aging Study. Psychol Aging. 2008;23:119–30.
56. Finkel D, Andel R, Gatz M, Pedersen NL. The role of occupational complexity in trajectories of cognitive aging before and after retirement. Psychol Aging. 2009;24:563–73.
57. Petersen RC, Smith GE, Waring SC, Ivnik RJ, Tangalos EG, Kokmen E. Mild cognitive impairment: Clinical characterization and outcome. Arch Neurol. 1999;56:303–8.
58. Petersen RC. Mild cognitive impairment as a diagnostic entity. J Intern Med. 2004;256:193–4.
59. Panza F, D'Introno A, Colacicco AM, Capurso C, Del Parigi A, Caselli RJ, Solfrizzi V. Current epidemiology of mild cognitive impairment and other predementia syndromes. Am J Geriatr Psychiatry. 2005;13:633–44.
60. Winblad B, Palmer K, Kivipelto M, Jelic V, Fratiglioni L, Wahlund L-O, Petersen RC. Mild cognitive impairment - beyond controversies, towards a consensus: Report of the International Working Group on Mild Cognitive Impairment. J Intern Med. 2004;56:240–6.
61. Albert MS, DeKosky ST, Dickson D, Dubois B, Feldman HH, Fox NC, Phelps CH (2011). The diagnosis of mild cognitive impairment due to Alzheimer's disease: Recommendations from the National Institute on Aging and Alzheimer's Association workgroup. Alzheimer's & Dementia, 7: in press.
62. Busse A, Hensel A, Guhne U, Angermeyer MC, Riedel-Heller SG. Mild cognitive impairment: long-term course of four clinical subtypes. Neurology. 2006;67:2176–85.
63. Fischer P, Jungwirth S, Zehetmayer S, Weissgram S, Hoeningschnabl S, Gelpi E, Tragl KH. Conversion from subtypes of mild cognitive impairment to Alzheimer dementia. Neurology. 2007;68:288–91.
64. Taber MH, Manly JJ, Liu X, Pelton GH, Rosenblum S, Jacobs M, Devanand DP, et al. Neuropsychological prediction of conversion to Alzheimer disease in patients with mild cognitive impairment. Arch Gen Psychiatry. 2006;63:916–24.
65. Fleisher AS, Sowell BB, Taylor C, Gamst AC, Petersen RC, Thal LJ. Clinical predictors of progression to Alzheimer's disease in amnestic mild cognitive impairment. Neurology. 2007;68:1588–95.
66. Ganguli M, Dodge HH, Shen C, DeKosky ST. Mild cognitive impairment, amnestic type: an epidemiologic study. Neurology. 2004;63:115–21.
67. Bennett DA, Wilson RS, Schneider JA, Evans DA, Beckett LA, Aggarwal NT, Bach J. Natural History of mild cognitive impairment in older persons. Neurology. 2002;59:198–205.
68. Alexopolous P, Grimmer T, Perneczky R, Domes G, Kurz A. Do all patients with mild cognitive impairment progress to dementia? J Am Geriatr Soc. 2006;54:1008–10.
69. Forsberg A, Engler H, Almkvist O, Blomquist G, Hagman H, Wall A, Nordberg A. PET imaging of amyloid deposition in patients with mild cognitive impairment. 2007.
70. Whitwell JL, Shiung MM, Przybelski SA, Weigand SD, Knopman DS, Boeve BF, Jack CR. MRI patterns of atrophy associated with progression to AD in amnestic mild cognitive impairment. Neurology. 2008;70:512–20.
71. Makesbery WR, Schmitt FA, Kryscio RJ, Davis DG, Smith CD, Wekstein DR. Neuropathologic substrate of mild cognitive impairment. Arch Neurol. 2006;63:38–46.
72. Petersen RC, Parisi JE, Dickson DW, Johnson KA, Knopman DS, Boeve BF, Kokmen E, et al. Neuropathologic features of amnestic mild cognitive impairment. Arch Neurol. 2006;63:665–72.
73. Vemuri P, Wiste HJ, Weigand SD, Knopman DS, Trojanowski JQ, Shaw LM, Jack CR. Serial MRI and CSF biomarkers in normal aging, MCI, and AD. Neurology. 2010;75:143–51.
74. Meyer JS, Huang J, Chowdhury MH. MRI confirms mild cognitive impairments prodromal for Alzheimer's, vascular, and Parkinson-Lewy body dementias. J Neurol Sci. 2007;257:97–104.
75. Prodan CI, Monnot M, Brumback RA, Ross ED. Initiating referral in mild cognitive impairment: Who rings the bell? J Am Geriatr Soc. 2007;55:1147–9.
76. Apostolova LG, Cummings JL. Neuropsychiatric manifestations in mild cognitive impairment: A systematic review of the literature. Dement Geriatr Cogn Disord. 2008;25:115–26.
77. Chan D, Kasper JD, Black BS, Rabins PV. Prevalence and correlates of behavioral and psychiatric symptoms in community-dwelling elders with dementia or mild cognitive impairment: The Memory and Medical Care Study. Int J Geriatr Psychiatry. 2003;18:174–82.
78. Geda YE, Roberts RO, Knopman DS, Petersen RC, Christianson TJH, Pankratz VS, Rocca WA.

Prevalence of neuropsychiatric symptoms in mild cognitive impairment and normal cognitive aging: Population-based study. Arch Gen Psychiatry. 2008;65:1193–8.
79. Lyketsos CG, Sheppard JE, Steinberg M, Tschanz JT, Norton MC, Steffens DC, et al. Neuropsychiatric disturbance in Alzheimer's disease clusters into three groups: The Cache County study. Int J Geriatr Psychiatry. 2001;16:1043–53.
80. Ellison JM, Harper DG, Berlow Y, Zeranski L. Beyond the "C" in MCI: Noncognitive symptoms in amnestic and non-amnestic mild cognitive impairment. CNS Spectr. 2008;13:66–72.
81. Hwang TJ, Masterman DL, Ortiz F, Fairbanks LA, Cummings JL. Mild cognitive impairment is associated with characteristic neuropsychiatric symptoms. Alzheimer Dis Assoc Disord. 2004;18:17–21.
82. Gabryelewicz T, Styczynska M, Pfeffer A, Wasiak B, Barczak A, Luczywek E, et al. Prevalence of major and minor depression in elderly persons with mild cognitive impairment: MADRS factor analysis. Int J Geriatr Psychiatry. 2004;19:1168–72.
83. Beebe DW, Gozal D. Obstructive sleep apnea and the prefrontal cortex: Towards a comprehensive model linking noctural upper airway obstruction to daytime cognitive and behavioral deficits. J Sleep Res. 2002;11:1–16.
84. Farias ST, Mungas D, Reed BR, Harvey D, Cahn-Weiner D, DeCarli C. MCI is associated with deficits in everyday functioning. Alzheimer Dis Assoc Disord. 2006;20:217–33.
85. Royall DR, Palmer R, Chiodo LK, Polk MJ. Executive control mediates memory's association with change in instrumental activities of daily living: The Freedom House Study. J Am Geriatr Soc. 2005;53:11–7.
86. Schmitter-Edgecombe M, Woo E, Greeley DR. Characterizing multiple memory deficits and their relation to everyday functioning in individuals with mild cognitive impairment. Neuropsychology. 2009;23:168–77.
87. Giovannetti T, Bettcher BM, Brennan L, Libon DJ, Burke M, Duey K, Wambach D. Characterization of everyday functioning in mild cognitive impairment: A direct assessment approach. Dement Geriatr Cogn Disord. 2008;25:359–65.
88. Tuokko H, Morris C, Ebert P. Mild cognitive impairment and every day functioning in older adults. Neurocase. 2005;11:40–7.
89. Okonkwo OC, Wadley VG, Griffith HR, Ball K, Marson DC. Cognitive correlates of financial abilities in mild cognitive impairment. J Am Geriatr Soc. 2006;54:1745–50.
90. Wadley VG, Okonkwo O, Crowe M, Vance DE, Elgin JM, Ball KK, Owsley C. Mild cognitive impairment and every day function: an investigation of driving performance. J Geriatr Psychiatry Neurol. 2009;22:87–94.
91. Bondi MW, Jak AJ, Delano-Wood L, Jacobson MW, Delis DC, Salmon DP. Neuropsychological contributions to the early identification of Alzheimer's disease. Neuropsychol Rev. 2008;18:73–90.
92. Bondi MW, Salmon DP, Galasko D, Thomas RG, Thal LJ. Neuropsychological function and apolipoprotein E genotype in the preclinical detection of Alzheimer's disease. Psychol Aging. 1999;14: 295–303.
93. Collie A, Maruff P. The neuropsychology of preclinical Alzheimer's disease and mild cognitive impairment. Neurosci Biobehav Rev. 2000;24:365–74.
94. Greenaway MC, Lacritz LH, Binegar D, Weiner MF, Lipton A, Cullum CM. Patterns of verbal memory performance in mild cognitive impairment, Alzheimer disease, and normal aging. Cogn Behav Neurol. 2006;19:79–84.
95. Crowell TA, Luis CA, Vanderploeg RD, Schinka JA, Mullan M. Memory patterns and executive functioning in mild cognitive impairment and Alzheimer's disease. Aging Neuropsychol Cognition. 2002;9:288–97.
96. Grundman M, Petersen RC, Ferris SH, Thomas RG, Aisen PS, Bennett DA, Thal LJ. Mild cognitive impairment can be distinguished from Alzheimer's disease and normal aging for clinical trials. Arch Neurol. 2004;61:59–66.
97. Brandt J, Aretouli E, Neijstrom E, Samek J, Manning K, Albert MS, Bandeen-Roche K. Selectivity of executive function deficits in mild cognitive impairment. Neuropsychology. 2009;23:607–18.
98. Balthazar MLF, Cendes F, Damasceno BP. Semantic error patterns on the Boston Naming Test in normal aging, amnestic mild cognitive impairment, and mild Alzheimer's disease: Is there semantic disruption? Neuropsychology. 2008;22:703–9.
99. Ribeiro F, Guerreiro M, De Mendonca A. Verbal learning and memory deficits in mild cognitive impairment. J Clin Exp Neuropsychol. 2007;29:187–97.
100. Spaan PEJ, Raaijmakers JGW, Jonker C. Early assessment of dementia: the contribution of different memory components. Neuropsychology. 2005;19: 629–40.
101. Taler V, Phillips NA. Language performance in Alzheimer's disease and mild cognitive impairment: a comparative review. J Clin Exp Neuropsychol. 2008;30:501–56.
102. Belleville S, Chertkow H, Gauthier S. Working memory and control of attention in persons with Alzheimer's disease and mild cognitive impairment. Neuropsychology. 2007;21:458–69.
103. Gainotti G, Ferraccioli M, Vita M, Marra C. Patterns of neuropsychological impairment in MCI patients with small subcortical infarcts or hippocampal atrophy. J Int Neuropsychol Soc. 2008;14:611–9.
104. Norlund A, Rolstad S, Klang O, Lind K, Hansen S, Wallin A. Cognitive profiles of mild cognitive impairment with and without vascular disease. Neuropsychology. 2007;21:706–12.
105. Lingler JH, Nightingale MC, Erlen JA, Kane AL, Reynolds CF, Schulz R, DeKosky ST. Making sense of mild cognitive impairment: a qualitative

exploration of the patient's experience. Gerontologist. 2006;46:791–800.
106. Folstein MF, Folstein SE, McHugh PR. Mini-mental state. A practical method for grading the cognitive state of patients for the clinician. J Psychiatr Res. 1975;12:189–98.
107. Randolph C, Tierney MC, Mohr E, Chase TN. The Repeatable Battery for the Assessment of Neuropsychological Status (RBANS): Preliminary clinical validity. J Clin Exp Neuropsychol. 1998;20:310–9.
108. Wechsler D. Wechsler Adult Intelligence Scale, Fourth Edition administration and scoring manual. San Antonio, TX: Pearson; 2008.
109. Wechsler D. Wechsler Abbreviated Scale of Intelligence (WASI) manual. San Antonio, TX: Pearson; 1999.
110. Wilkinson GS, Robertson GJ. Wide Range Achievement Test-4 professional manual. Lutz, FL: Psychological Assessment Resources; 2006.
111. Reitan RM. Validity of the Trail Making Test as an indicator of organic brain damage. Percept Mot Skills. 1958;8:271–6.
112. Golden CJ. Stroop Color and Word Test: a manual for clinical and experimental uses. Chicago, IL: Skoelting; 1978.
113. Delis DC, Kramer JH, Kaplan E, Ober BA. California Verbal Learning Test. 2nd ed. San Antonio, TX: Psychological Corporation; 2000.
114. Brandt J, Benedict RHB. Hopkins Verbal Learning Test-Revised. Lutz, FL: Psychological Assessment Resources; 2001.
115. Rey A. L'examen psychologique dans les cas d'encéphalopathie traumatic. Arch Psychol. 1941;28:286–340.
116. Osterrieth PA. Le test de copie d'une figure complexe. Arch Psychol. 1944;30:206–356.
117. Benedict RH. Brief Visuospatial Memory Test—Revised. Odessa, FL: Psychological Assessment Resources, Inc.; 1997.
118. Wechsler D. WAIS-III/WMS-III technical manual. San Antonio: The Psychological Corporation; 1997.
119. Kaplan E, Goodglass H, Weintraub S. The Boston Naming Test. Philadelphia, PA: Lea and Febiger; 1983.
120. Benton AL, Hamsher K, Sivan AB. Multilingual Aphasia Examination. 3rd ed. Iowa City, IA: AJA Associates; 1994.
121. Tombaugh T, Kazak J, Rees L. Normative data stratified by age and education for two measures of verbal fluency: FAS and animal naming. Arch Clin Neuropsychol. 1999;14:167–77.
122. Heaton RK, Chelune GJ, Talley JL, Kay GG, Curtis G. Wisconsin Card Sorting Test (WCST) manual, revised and expanded. Odessa, TX: Psychological Assessment Resources, Inc.; 1993.
123. Goodglass H, Kaplan E. The assessment of aphasia and related disorders. 2nd ed. Philadelphia, PA: Lea & Febiger; 1982.
124. Halstead WC. Brain and intelligence. A quantitative study of the frontal lobes. Chicago: University of Chicago; 1947.
125. Heaton RK, Grant I, Matthews CG. Comprehensive norms for an expanded Halstead-Reitan battery. Odessa, FL: Psychological Assessment Resources; 1992.
126. Yesavage JA, Brink TL, Rose TL, Lum O, Huang V, Adey M, Leirer VO. Development and validation of a geriatric depression screening scale: A preliminary report. J Psychiatr Res. 1983;17:37–49.
127. Beck AT, Steer RA, Brown GK. Manual for Beck Depression Inventory II (BDI-II). San Antonio, TX: Psychology Corporation; 1996.
128. Spielberger CD, Gorsuch RL, Lushene PR, Vagg PR, Jacobs AG. Manual for the State-Trait Anxiety Inventory (form Y). Palo Alto, CA: Consulting Psychologists Press, Inc.; 1983.

Differential Diagnosis of Depression and Dementia

17

Linas A. Bieliauskas and Lauren L. Drag

Abstract

Cognitive complaints and depressive symptoms are common in older adults. While depressive symptoms may represent a primary mood disorder, they may also reflect the early signs of a dementia. Depression and dementia often differ in terms of their cognitive profile as well as the phenomenology of the depressive symptoms. Neuropsychologists can play an important role in making diagnostic decisions by providing objective assessment of both cognitive and psychological functioning. This chapter reviews considerations for differential diagnosis and provides practical tips for the clinician.

Keywords

Depression • Aging • Dementia • Pseudodementia • Diagnosis

Depression in older adults has prevalence rates estimated to be between 3 and 14% in the community-dwelling population [1–3]. Approximately 1 in 15 older adults may experience major depression over the course of 1 year [2]. Late-life depression has been associated with negative outcomes such as functional impairment and disability, increased medical symptoms, negative rehabilitation outcomes, and increased utilization of health care services [4–6]. Depression can also have significant economic costs. Due to unexplained somatic complaints and functional impairments, older adults with depression tend to use more medical services. Katon et al. [7] found that depressed older adults incurred approximately 50% higher medical costs than their non-depressed counterparts, even when taking chronic medical illness into account. Only a small part of these costs went to mental health care; the majority of costs were associated with primary care visits, diagnostic visits, emergency room visits, and pharmacy costs. Thus, late-life depression

L.A. Bieliauskas, Ph.D. (✉)
Mental Health Service, Ann Arbor VA Healthcare System, Neuropsychology Section, Department of Psychiatry, University of Michigan Healthcare System, 2101 Commonwealth Blvd, Suite C, Ann Arbor, MI 48105, USA
e-mail: linas@med.umich.edu

L.L. Drag, Ph.D.
Neuropsychology Section, Department of Psychiatry, University of Michigan Healthcare System, Ann Arbor, MI, USA
e-mail: laurenldrag@gmail.com

L.D. Ravdin and H.L. Katzen (eds.), *Handbook on the Neuropsychology of Aging and Dementia*, Clinical Handbooks in Neuropsychology, DOI 10.1007/978-1-4614-3106-0_17,

can place a significant burden on patients, their caregivers, and the health-care system, illustrating the importance of adequately assessing, managing, and treating this disorder.

Depression-Related Cognitive Impairment or "Pseudodementia"

In addition to negative clinical outcomes, late-life depression can be accompanied by significant cognitive impairments. These depression-related changes are often similar to those associated with dementia. Historically, a psychiatric illness that mimicked dementia symptoms was referred to as "pseudodementia." The cognitive symptoms of pseudodementia were assumed to be related to transient mood symptoms and therefore reversible with adequate psychiatric treatment. Therefore, the term "reversible dementia" was also used to describe depression-induced cognitive impairments. One of the early clinicians to popularize this term, Wells [8], provided a detailed characterization of pseudodementia based on his own clinical observations. He noted that individuals with pseudodementia typically had complaints of memory loss that were not apparent to the examiner. They tended to highlight their failures and emphasize their disability; however, their functional deficits were often incongruent with the typically mild nature of their cognitive deficits. This was in stark contrast to patients with dementia, who often lacked insight into the extent and severity of their dysfunction and therefore tended to minimize their symptoms. Wells also reported that patients with pseudodementia often provided "don't know" responses to close-ended questions despite being able to provide coherent and detailed responses to open-ended questions. In addition, patients with depression-related deficits typically had equally severe recent and remote memory deficits (compared to the temporally graded memory deficits typically seen in degenerative dementia), a clear onset of cognitive symptoms, and limited symptoms of sundowning. According to Wells, demented individuals also often tried to rely on notes and calendars, whereas depressed individuals did not make attempts to compensate for their difficulties.

Despite the initial popularity of "pseudodementia" amongst clinicians, there has been debate about the use of this term and it has generally fallen out of favor in current practice. The term has been of historical importance in that it encouraged clinicians to evaluate every patient carefully and look for alternate causes of cognitive decline other than dementia. However, as Reifler [9] has pointed out, there were some drawbacks to using this term. Pseudodementia implies a mutually exclusive process, which can lead a clinician to focus on whether a patient is depressed or demented at the exclusion of the possibility that both conditions could be present. The term also implies complete reversibility and a lack of organic pathology without taking into account that there may be both reversible and irreversible components to the illness. Several more recent studies have confirmed that the cognitive deficits associated with "reversible dementias" may not actually be truly reversible. For example, Fretter and colleagues [10] examined individuals with dementia and found that of the 45 individuals with potentially reversible causes (e.g., depression, alcohol abuse, vitamin deficiencies), only seven individuals (16%) showed improvement of their cognitive symptoms following successful treatment. Similarly, Butters and colleagues [11] found that in some older adults with depression and cognitive impairment, executive functioning did improve following successful antidepressant treatment but failed to reach normal levels of performance. Finally, Alexopoulos and colleagues [12] followed older adults with depression who showed a pattern of "reversible dementia" as demonstrated by cognitive impairment at baseline followed by improvement in cognitive symptoms subsequent to treatment for their depression. However, at follow-up 1 year later, individuals with reversible dementia were five times more likely than depressed individuals without cognitive impairment to develop a true dementia syndrome. Although the treatment of depression may initially lead to improvements in dementia-related symptoms, follow-up over time suggests that true reversibility of such dementia is an uncommon occurrence [13]. The term "pseudodementia" is discussed in the Diagnostic and Statistical Manual of Mental Disorders (DSM) III, [14] but is no longer used in more current revisions of the DSM.

Depression as a Symptom of Dementia

Although late-life depression can sometimes reflect a primary psychiatric disorder, it is often the case that depressive symptoms are in fact early manifestations of an underlying progressive dementing illness. High rates of depression and psychiatric symptoms in general are found across various neurodegenerative disorders, including Alzheimer's disease (AD), vascular dementia, Lewy body dementia, multiple system atrophy, and Parkinson's disease [15–20]. Okura and colleagues [21] found that approximately half of all individuals with cognitive impairment or diagnosed with dementia exhibited at least one psychiatric symptom. Depression was the most common psychiatric symptom in individuals with cognitive impairment or mild dementia. In a study of nursing home residents, Verkaik and colleagues [22] demonstrated a depression prevalence rate of 19% amongst residents with dementia, with depressed mood, irritability, and fatigue being the most frequently endorsed symptoms. Similarly, Starkstein and colleagues [23] examined 670 patients with probable AD and found that approximately half of these individuals had significant symptoms of depression. Thus, depressive symptoms appear to be highly prevalent in individuals with dementia. It is not likely that depression can be attributed solely to a reaction to the disease itself as awareness of deficits has not clearly been linked to the development of depressive symptoms [24]. There has also not been strong support for an association between severity of dementia and depression; depressive symptoms have been shown to be equally prevalent across disease stages [22, 25].

While this cross-sectional research illustrates the high comorbidity between depression and dementia, longitudinal research has demonstrated that depressive symptoms may actually be an early sign or risk factor for subsequent cognitive impairment and dementia [26]. Modrego and Ferrández [27] followed individuals with amnesic mild cognitive impairment over 3 years and found that those individuals with baseline depression were more than twice as likely to develop dementia compared to their nondepressed counterparts and also more likely to develop dementia earlier. Similarly, Rosenberg and colleagues [28] followed a large sample of 436 older women over a 9-year period and found that baseline depressive symptoms were associated with increased rates of incident impairments on cognitive tests across multiple domains. Although it may be that depression is a risk factor for dementia (possibly through neuronal loss via dysregulation of glucocorticoids), it is just as likely that depression is a behavioral manifestation of the dementia process itself [29]. Further research is needed to better elucidate the possible causal relationships between depressive symptoms and subsequent cognitive impairment.

Clinical Assessment

Neuropsychologists play an important role in the assessment and treatment of both depression and dementia. Various clinicians such as primary care practitioners, psychologists, psychiatrists, or neurologists often refer older adults for neuropsychological evaluation to better clarify a patient's cognitive and psychiatric complaints. Neuropsychological evaluation can have significant contributions to diagnosis, management, and treatment of these symptoms through an objective characterization of cognitive and psychiatric profiles, identification of areas of weakness that can lead to functional impairments or be addressed through interventions, and follow-up assessments that can track the extent to which symptoms improve, worsen, or remain stable in response to interventions or time [30].

Assessment of Geriatric Depression

An important part of a neuropsychological evaluation of a patient with depressive symptoms is to gain both a qualitative and quantitative understanding of these symptoms. However, depression is often difficult to assess in older adults for a number of reasons. Symptoms of depression are easily confounded by the effects of age and medical disorders. Changes in weight, appetite, and libido; psychomotor retardation or agitation; and a loss of interest in activities are common to medical illnesses, physical effects of aging, and age-related lifestyle changes, as well as depression. For instance, a patient may endorse a decline in social activities, but upon further prompting, clarify that he or she can no longer drive and do not have many friends or family members who live nearby. Similarly, it may be that a preference to stay home reflects fatigue related to medical conditions rather than a symptom such as anhedonia.

Older adults may also be more likely to underestimate their depressive symptoms. They may have lower functional expectations for themselves due to their increasing age (e.g., they may believe that their fatigue is a normal part of the aging process) and therefore dismiss their depressive symptoms as a common response to life stressors or normal aging. This is a common misconception; depression is not a normal part of aging (Table 17.1). While older adults may be prone to depressive symptoms due to declining health and functioning, the aging process itself does not confer an increased risk for depression [31].

Further complicating matters, older adults are less likely to report dysphoric mood than their younger counterparts. Rather, they tend to present with vague symptoms such as sleep disturbances or fatigue [32]. Given that older adults may not endorse prominent dysphoria, clinicians need to be aware of the more subtle indicators of depression. These can include frequent office visits or use of medical services, persistent reports of pain, fatigue, insomnia, headaches, changes in sleep or appetite, unexplained GI symptoms, social isolation, increased dependency, delayed recovery from medical or surgical procedures, and refusal of treatment [33].

Table 17.1 Instruments commonly used to assess depression in older adults

For use in both adults and older adults
Beck Depression Inventory-II [35]
Center for Epidemiological Studies Depression Scale (CES-D) [94]
Zung Depression Rating Scale [95]
DSM-IV Depression Checklist [96]
Hamilton Depression Rating Scale [36]
For use in older adults
Geriatric Depression Scale [37]
Geriatric Depression Scale (short form) [97]
For use in patients with dementia
Cornell Scale for Depression in Dementia [98]
Dementia Mood Assessment Scale [99]
Depression Sign Scale [100]
Neuropsychiatric Inventory [101]
CERAD Behavior Rating Scale [102]

Patients may be referred for a neuropsychological assessment for subjective cognitive complaints, and only after detailed questioning will evidence of possible depression emerge. Older adults with depression are more likely to initially present to their primary care physician rather than to a specialist such as a psychiatrist [34] and may report only vague physical symptoms. Therefore, depression may go undetected in some patients unless a careful evaluation is performed. This suggests that all older adults complaining of cognitive problems should be screened for depression, regardless of the referral question.

Several psychometric instruments have been developed to screen for depression (Table 17.1). Popular instruments include the Beck Depression Inventory-II (BDI-II) [35] and the Hamilton Depression Rating Scale (HDRS) [36]. The Geriatric Depression Scale (GDS) [37] specifically targets symptoms common to depression in older adults. Several rating scales have also been developed specifically for use in patients with dementia. Table 17.1 provides a list of psychometric instruments that are commonly used to assess depression in older adults. These inventories can be useful to quantify and monitor depressive symptoms over time, yet they should be used as a supplement to a clinical interview. Individuals with cognitive impairment may endorse depressive symptoms, but further prompting may be required to tease apart primary depression from possible secondary effects of cognitive symptoms. Cognitive impairment can limit a person's ability (but not necessarily desire) to be involved and engaged with activities. For example, individuals with cognitive impairment may be unable to drive or have difficulty keeping up with social activities (e.g., playing complex card games) like they used to. On questionnaires such as the GDS, which probes for symptoms such as a decrease in activities or boredom, further discussion is warranted to determine whether these symptoms reflect a true underlying depression rather than situational factors.

Considerations for Differential Diagnosis

When a patient presents with reported changes in both mood and cognitive functioning, there are several potential rule-out diagnoses to consider. Table 17.2 provides a list of disorders that have been associated with both cognitive and psychiatric symptoms in older adults. Primary psychiatric disorders such as depression, anxiety, and bipolar disorder should be considered, although an initial onset of psychiatric symptoms in late adulthood is unusual. Psychiatric symptoms such as depression, irritability, and apathy are also common across many of the dementia subtypes, including AD, Lewy body dementia, frontotemporal dementia, and vascular dementia. Whether symptoms primarily represent depression or a dementing condition is typically considered a major consideration, and a more detailed discussion of the differential diagnosis between primary depression and dementia is provided below. Changes in mood and cognition can also be associated with strokes, particularly those affecting frontal regions or frontostriatal circuits. In addition, many medications commonly used to treat medical illness in older adults can cause depression-like symptoms [38]. For example, calcium channel blockers, beta-blockers, levodopa, corticosteroids, and even certain antibiotics can affect both mood and cognitive functioning. While depression can be the direct physiological sequelae of some medical conditions such as hypothyroidism or vitamin deficiencies, clinicians should also consider that depression may be a secondary reaction to a chronic medical illness. Digestive disorders, respiratory ailments, and heart disease in particular have been associated with an increased rate of depressive symptoms, most likely due to functional limitations associated with the disorder and a lack of perceived control over medical symptoms [39].

Table 17.2 Common differential diagnoses to consider for older adults with psychiatric symptoms and cognitive complaints

Dementias
Alzheimer's disease
Frontotemporal dementia
Lewy body dementia
Vascular dementia/stroke
Dementia associated with Parkinson's disease
Psychiatric disorders
Depression
Bipolar disorder
Anxiety
Other potential causes
Medications (e.g., beta-blockers, calcium channel blockers)
Vitamin deficiencies (e.g., vitamin D, vitamin B12, thiamine)
Hormonal conditions (e.g., hypothyroidism, menopause)
Substance abuse
Brain tumor
Normal pressure hydrocephalus

Differences Between Depression and Dementia

Cognitive and psychiatric symptoms associated with a primary depression can differ from those associated with a dementia process. Depression is typically associated with a more acute onset of symptoms (e.g., days to weeks), whereas the impairments associated with dementia can progress over the course of years. Therefore, a gradual onset and progression of cognitive and mood symptoms is more likely to reflect an underlying dementing process, whereas a more acute onset is typically associated with depression. In addition, depression is often accompanied by significant subjective cognitive complaints [40, 41]. Older adults with depression are more likely to complain more about their cognitive difficulties than individuals with dementia [42], and these cognitive complaints may be out of proportion to an individual's actual level of functioning. For example, a patient may complain of severe memory deficits yet continue to independently manage his or her medications and finances. In contrast, a lack of insight into symptoms is common in dementia, particularly AD, making these individuals more likely to minimize their cognitive difficulties.

The presence of apathetic symptoms can also have clinical indications when differentiating between depression and dementia. Apathy is typically defined as a loss of motivation and can manifest as diminished initiation, lack of interest, low social engagement, and a blunted emotional response. While apathy can be a principal symptom of depression, it can also reflect an independent syndrome, distinct from the dysphoria typically associated with depression. Apathy is often characterized by indifference, and dysphoric symptoms are better characterized by sadness, guilt, self-criticism, hopelessness, and helplessness. Bieliauskas [43] suggests that true primary depression significantly includes a loss of self-esteem and that, in the absence of this loss, depressive symptoms likely reflect neurological change. Apathy is a prominent feature in various neurodegenerative disorders, including AD, frontotemporal dementia, and Parkinson's disease [44, 45]. In AD in particular, apathy symptoms are more prevalent than dysphoric symptoms [46, 47] and older adults who present with apathetic symptoms are more likely to develop AD than those with either no depression or depression without apathy [48, 49]. This affirms that mood symptoms in the early stages of dementia are better characterized by an apathetic syndrome rather than dysphoric mood. Therefore, apathy, particularly in the context of cognitive changes, may be an early marker of preclinical AD, whereas dysphoric mood may be more indicative of a primary depressive disorder [50, 51].

When assessing apathy in patients with cognitive impairments, it is important that clinicians focus on the behaviors for which a patient is still capable of performing, as cognitive impairments can limit a person's ability to engage with their environment independent of motivational factors. Structured measures have been designed to specifically measure symptoms of apathy, including the Neuropsychiatric Inventory [52] and the Apathy Evaluation Scale [53]. The Irritability/Apathy Scale has been used to measure apathy in patients with dementia [54].

In addition to apathy, depressive symptoms associated with dementia may be characterized by fewer and less prominent symptoms compared to a primary depression, with salient features of social withdrawal and irritability [55]. Because depressive profiles can differ between primary depression and dementia, a new set of diagnostic criteria has been proposed specifically for depression in the context of AD [56]. These new criteria require the presence of three symptoms (compared to the five required for a diagnosis of major depressive disorder). Symptoms are similar to those in major depressive disorder with the addition of social isolation and irritability. A depressed mood or decreased positive affect or pleasure in response to social contacts or usual activities is required. Given that depressive symptoms in AD are less prominent compared to those associated with a primary depression, symptoms are not required to be present nearly every day.

The age of onset of depressive symptoms should also be taken into consideration. There are significant differences both phenomenologically and etiologically between early-onset and late-onset depression, suggesting that these may be distinct psychiatric entities. The median age of onset in depression is 32 years of age with 50% of individuals reporting onset between ages 19 and 44 [57]. Late-onset depression is typically defined as depression with a first onset between 45 and 60 years of age. It is likely that there are stronger pathogenetic contributions from brain degenerative changes in late-onset depression compared to early-onset depression [58, 59]. Bieliauskas [43] suggested that when older patients present cognitive difficulties associated with an initial onset of depression, these are most likely based on neurological disease. Lamberty and Bieliauskas [60] reviewed a number of studies showing high correlations between cognitive changes with depression and positive findings on neuroimaging. In a later review of neuroimaging findings, Kumar, Bilker Jin, and Udupa [61] suggest that atrophy and high-intensity lesions may represent relatively independent pathways to late-life major depression. The underlying neurological basis for depressive symptoms has been recently explored by Langenecker et al. [62], not only for depression with onset in late life, but for a neuroanatomical network impacted in the majority of individuals with mood disorders.

Loss of interest is also greater in late-onset depression [61, 63], which is consistent with the findings that apathy may be an indicator of a progressive dementing process. Similarly, in patients with both depression and dementia, age of onset was later than in patients with depression alone [64]. Again, depression with a late age of onset is more likely to be associated with underlying neuropathology or the early stages of dementia [65].

Depression and dementia can also differ with regard to sleep, although the clinical utility sleep patterns in differential diagnosis is uncertain. AD is typically associated with poor sleep efficiency with frequent night awakenings. Phase delays are prominent, meaning that the onset of sleep is later and accompanied by difficulty awakening in the morning [66]. While older adults with depression also have frequent night awakenings, impaired sleep continuity, and difficulty falling asleep, early morning awakenings are a prominent feature of depression [67]. Individuals with depression have difficulty staying asleep in the morning, whereas those with dementia are more likely to have difficulty waking up. In addition, when directly compared to individuals with AD, individuals with depression had a higher number of night awakenings [68]. Increased REM sleep may also be a specific to depression and helpful in distinguishing depression from dementia (which is associated with reduced REM); however, this type of detailed sleep data is typically not available to clinicians without requesting a formal sleep study [67].

In sum, the phenomenology of a depressive syndrome can differ between primary depression and dementia. Depression is associated with an earlier age of onset of symptoms; subjective reporting of significant cognitive symptoms; an acute onset of cognitive deficits; the presence of dysphoria, including loss of self-esteem, rather than apathy; and early morning awakenings. This is in contrast to dementia-related symptoms that are associated with a later age of onset of symptoms, a lack of insight into cognitive symptoms, a gradual onset of cognitive deficits, the presence of apathy rather than dysphoria, and difficulty waking in the morning. Although these patterns can be useful as a heuristic in combination with other observations and objective testing, caution needs to be taken when applying findings using group differences to a single individual given the significant variability across individuals.

Neuropsychological Profiles of Depression and Dementia

Differences in symptom presentation between depression and dementia can be informative; however, a neuropsychologist's unique contribution to differential diagnosis is the ability to provide an objective assessment of cognitive functioning. As discussed previously, older adults with depression are more likely to report subjective cognitive difficulties than patients with dementia. However, as these complaints are not always indicative of true impairments [69, 70]; the importance of objective neuropsychological testing is highlighted.

In general, the cognitive changes associated with dementia tend to be more severe than those associated with depression [71–73]. Aside from differences in severity, research also suggests that there are qualitative differences between the two disorders with regard to neuropsychological profiles. Cognitive symptoms associated with neurodegenerative disorders are progressive, whereas cognitive deficits related to depression should generally stabilize or even improve with adequate management of psychiatric symptoms. Thus, repeat neuropsychological evaluations can be helpful to monitor cognitive changes over time. In addition, the cognitive changes that accompany depression are also generally thought to reflect deficits in effortful processing, leading to difficulty on tasks that require a high degree of cognitive resources. According to this hypothesis, performance is generally adequate on tasks that are more automatic and require less effort to complete [74]. In contrast, the deficits found in dementia are associated with decrements in ability rather than effort, and therefore, impairments are apparent independent of the degree of effortful processing required. While this effortful-automatic hypothesis can be a useful heuristic, it may be overly generalized and has not consistently been supported by research.

Late-life depression is typically associated with cognitive deficits primarily in the domains of memory, executive functioning, and attention [75–78]. In general, executive functioning difficulties are most prominent in depression and can mediate the cognitive difficulties found in other domains, such as memory [79]. In contrast, AD is typified by prominent memory deficits. With regard to memory, although depression and dementia can both impact performance on immediate and delayed memory tasks, delayed retrieval tasks can be useful for differentiating between the groups [73]. AD is associated with rapid forgetting of information, which results in poor delayed recall and recognition performance. Therefore, patients with AD do not benefit significantly when given mnemonic support such as cues at retrieval, as information has not adequately been retained in memory. This difficulty with the retention of information in memory is not surprising given that AD pathology affects the hippocampus and surrounding regions and areas critical to memory encoding and storage. In contrast, depressed individuals may struggle with delayed recall, but performance can improve significantly when given cues. This is because in depression, memory difficulties are associated with deficits in executive functioning and strategic processing. When there is a reduced demand on strategic processing, as is the case when cues or organization are already provided, memory abilities are better. For example, Elderkin-Thompson and colleagues [79] demonstrated that older adults with depression performed poorly on list learning tasks, but when given semantic cues, memory significantly improved to normal levels. Thus, it appears that depressed patients derive more benefit from cuing than AD patients. This is consistent with multiple studies comparing individuals with AD and depression that have found an AD-specific deficit in cued recall tasks [80–83]. This suggests that this cued recall tasks may be effective in distinguishing AD from depression. Suggestions for cued recall tasks that can be included in a neuropsychological battery include Verbal Paired Associates from the Wechsler Memory Scale-IV [84], Paired Associates Learning from the CANTAB [85], and Cued Recall from the California Verbal Learning Test-II [86].

Recognition performance is another way to differentiate between memory difficulties associated with dementia versus depression. Given that recognition tasks minimize the need for effortful and strategic retrieval, depressed individuals typically show adequate performance on these tasks. In contrast, patients with AD tend to show impairments given that information is often not encoded or retained in memory and therefore even recognition of this information is deficient. In addition, there are also differences in how individuals with depression and dementia approach recognition tasks. Whereas depressed individuals tend to take a more conservative approach, leading to "I don't know" answers and false-negative errors, individuals with AD tend to adopt a more liberal response bias, leading to a high number of false-positive errors [87]. Suggestions for memory tasks with a recognition component include Logical Memory, Visual Reproduction, and Verbal Paired Associates from the Wechsler Memory Scale-IV, the Hopkins Verbal Learning

Test-Revised [88], the California Verbal Learning Test, the Brief Visuospatial Memory Test-Revised [89], the Rey Auditory Verbal Learning Test [90], and the Recognition Memory Test [91].

Analysis of serial position effects can also be informative. Foldi [92] found that patients with AD showed poorer overall recall of a word list compared to depressed individuals. Moreover, AD was associated with an advantage of recency over primacy (i.e., individuals recalled words from the end of the list better than those at the beginning), which is consistent with difficulty retaining information in memory over time. In contrast, individuals with depression showed both a strong primacy and recency effect with poorer recall of words in the middle of the list. This poor middle-list performance distinguished depressed patients from healthy controls. Therefore, recall abilities in individuals with AD across a word list can reflect an upward-sloping line (with better performance at the end of the word list), whereas the performance of individuals with depression may be better characterized by a U-shaped function (with better performance at the beginning and end of the word list).

Patients with depression and AD can also differ on other nonmemory tasks. For example, Kaschel and colleagues [93] found that even when memory performance was equated, AD patients had more difficulty compared to depressed patients on tasks requiring dual-tasking. In addition, compared to depression, dementia is more associated with impairments on tasks of naming, visuoperceptual processing (e.g., right-left orientation), and ideomotor and ideational praxis [71, 72, 81].

Overall, depression and dementia can differ in both the quantity and quality of cognitive deficits. The cognitive profile associated with AD is most reflective of a cortical dementia, typified by a prominent memory disturbance and additional deficits in language and praxis. In contrast, depression is better represented by a frontally mediated (or subcortical) pattern leading to executive functioning deficits that can affect other cognitive domains due to the lack of initiation of strategic or effortful processing.

Conclusions

Depressive symptoms and cognitive complaints are common in older adults. While depressive symptoms may reflect a primary depressive disorder, they may also represent the early signs of a dementing process. Depression and dementia can differ in terms of their cognitive profile as well as the phenomenology of the depressive symptoms. Table 17.3 presents differential features of depression and AD that can be used as a general guideline in clinical practice. Accurate differential diagnosis has significant clinical implications as treatment approaches and prognosis vary significantly depending on etiology. Neuropsychologists can play an important role in differential diagnosis by providing an objective assessment of an individual's cognitive and psychological functioning.

Table 17.3 Differential features of depression and AD

	Depression	AD
Onset of depressive symptoms	Early	Late
Prior psychiatric history	Present	Absent
Family psychiatric history	Present	Absent
Sleep	Frequent night and morning awakenings; increased REM	Delayed sleep onset, difficulty waking in morning
Onset of cognitive symptoms	Acute	Gradual
Severity of cognitive symptoms	Less impaired	More impaired
Severity of mood symptoms	More severe	Less severe
Prominent mood symptom	Dysphoria	Apathy

(continued)

Table 17.3 Continued

	Depression	AD
Temporal relationship between cognitive and mood symptoms	Mood symptoms precede or concurrent with cognitive symptoms	Mood symptoms precede, equal to, or follow cognitive symptoms
Insight into cognitive deficits	Exaggerated complaints	Poor insight
Memory		
Serial position curve	Intact primacy and recency, reduced middle	Impaired primacy, intact recency
Cued recall	Intact	Impaired
Immediate recall	Impaired	Impaired
Delayed recall	Impaired	Substantially impaired
Recognition	Generally intact	Impaired
Language (naming)	Intact	Impaired
Response biases	"I don't know" answers False negatives	Prone to guessing False positives
Praxis	Intact	Impaired
Retention	Adequate	Rapid forgetting
Orientation	Adequate	Can be impaired
Copying	Intact	Impaired
Dual-tasking	Intact	Impaired
Effortful processing	Impaired	Depends on task
Automatic processing	Intact	Depends on task
Primary area of cognitive impairment	Executive functioning	Memory
Pattern of cognitive deficits	Subcortical	Cortical

Clinical Pearls

- Depressive symptoms of apathy tend to be associated with neurologic disorders as compared to the dysphoria (especially with a loss of self-esteem) that is more often associated with primary depressive disorders.
- Significant subjective complaints, in particular those that are disproportionate to objective findings, are more often associated with primary depression rather than a neurologic etiology.
- Symptoms of sadness, misery, and a feeling of being abandoned by others are not uncommon with older age, failing health, and loss of close friends and older relatives. They represent losses that lead more to expressions of grief and are *not* equivalent to depression.
- If the onset is gradual, there is more likely an underlying neurological basis than an affective one.
- Pharmacological intervention will often be associated with some improvements in cognitive weaknesses. If the underlying cause is neurologic, the patient may feel better after pharmacological intervention, but cognitive efficiency will not improve.

References

1. Beekman AT, Copeland JR, Prince MJ. Review of community prevalence of depression in later life. Br J Psychiatry. 1999;174:307–11.
2. Mojtabai R, Olfson M. Major depression in community-dwelling middle-aged and older adults: prevalence and 2- and 4-year follow-up symptoms. Psychol Med. 2004;34(4):623–34.
3. Steffens DC, Fisher GG, Langa KM, Potter GG, Plassman BL. Prevalence of depression among older Americans: the Aging, Demographics and Memory Study. Int Psychogeriatr. 2009;21(5):879–88.
4. Alexopoulos G. Depression in the elderly. Lancet. 2005;365(9475):1961–70.
5. Baldwin RC, Gallagley A, Gourlay M, Jackson A, Burns A. Prognosis of late life depression: a three-year cohort study of outcome and potential predictors. Int J Geriatr Psychiatry. 2006;21(1):57–63.
6. Katz IR, Streim J, Parmelee P. Prevention of depression, recurrences, and complications in late life. Prev Med. 1994;23(5):743–50.

7. Katon WJ, Lin E, Russo J, Unutzer J. Increased medical costs of a population-based sample of depressed elderly patients. Arch Gen Psychiatry. 2003;60(9):897–903.
8. Wells CE. Pseudodementia. Am J Psychiatry. 1979;136(7):895–900.
9. Reifler BV. Arguments for abandoning the term pseudodementia. J Am Geriatr Soc. 1982;30(10): 665–8.
10. Fretter S, Bergman H, Gold S, Chertkow H, Clarfield aM. Prevalence of potentially reversible dementias and actual reversibility in a memory clinic cohort. Can Med Assoc J. 1998;159(6):657–62.
11. Butters MA, Becker JT, Nebes RD, Zmuda MD, Mulsant BH, Pollock BG, et al. Changes in cognitive functioning following treatment of late-life depression. Am J Psychiatry. 2000;157(12): 1949–54.
12. Alexopoulos GS, Meyers BS, Young RC, Mattis S, Kakuma T. The course of geriatric depression with "reversible dementia": a controlled study. Am J Psychiatry. 1993;150(11):1693–9.
13. Clarfield AM. The decreasing prevalence of reversible dementias: an updated meta-analysis. Arch Intern Med. 2003;163(18):2219–29.
14. American Psychiatric Association. Diagnostic and statistical manual of mental disorders. 3rd ed. Washington, DC: American Psychiatric Association; 1980.
15. Becker C, Brobert GP, Johansson S, Jick SS, Meier CR. Risk of incident depression in patients with Parkinson disease in the UK. Eur J Neurol. 2010; (17):1–6.
16. Josephs KA, Whitwell JL. Parkinson disease and down in the dumps: pumped or stumped? Neurology. 2010;75(10):846–7.
17. Kao AW, Racine CA, Quitania LC, Kramer JH, Christine CW, Miller BL. Cognitive and neuropsychiatric profile of the synucleinopathies: Parkinson disease, dementia with Lewy bodies, and multiple system atrophy. Alzheimer Dis Assoc Disord. 2009;23(4):365–70.
18. Newman SC. The prevalence of depression in Alzheimer's disease and vascular dementia in a population sample. J Affect Disord. 1999;52(1–3):169–76.
19. Payne JL, Lyketsos CG, Steele C, Baker L, Galik E, Kopunek S, et al. Relationship of cognitive and functional impairment to depressive features in Alzheimer's disease and other dementias. J Neuropsychiatr. 1998;10(4):440–7.
20. Spalletta G, Musicco M, Padovani A, Rozzini L, Perri R, Fadda L, et al. Neuropsychiatric symptoms and syndromes in a large cohort of newly diagnosed, untreated patients with Alzheimer disease. Am J Geriatr Psychiatry. 2010;18(11):1026–35.
21. Okura T, Plassman BL, Steffens DC, Llewellyn DJ, Potter GG, Langa KM. Prevalence of neuropsychiatric symptoms and their association with functional limitations in older adults in the United States: the aging, demographics, and memory study. J Am Geriatr Soc. 2010;58(2):330–7.
22. Verkaik R, Francke AL, van Meijel B, Ribbe MW, Bensing JM. Comorbid depression in dementia on psychogeriatric nursing home wards: which symptoms are prominent? Am J Geriatr Psychiatry. 2009;17(7):565–73.
23. Starkstein SE, Jorge R, Mizrahi R, Robinson RG. The construct of minor and major depression in Alzheimer's disease. Am J Psychiatry. 2005;162(11): 2086–93.
24. Verhey FRJ, Rozendaal N, Ponds RWHM, Jolles J. Dementia, awareness and depression. Int J Geriatr Psychiatry. 1993;8(10):851–6.
25. Verkaik R, Nuyen J, Francke A. The relationship between severity of Alzheimer's Disease and prevalence of comorbid depressive symptoms and depression: a systematic review. Int J Geriatr Psychiatry. 2007;22(11):1063–86.
26. Modrego PJ, Ferrández J. Depression in patients with mild cognitive impairment increases the risk of developing dementia of Alzheimer type: a prospective cohort study. Arch Neurol. 2004;61(8): 1290–3.
27. Jorm AF. Is depression a risk factor for dementia or cognitive decline? A review. Gerontology. 2000;46(4):219–27.
28. Rosenberg PB, Mielke MM, Xue Q-L, Carlson MC. Depressive symptoms predict incident cognitive impairment in cognitive healthy older women. Am J Geriatr Psychiatry. 2010;18(3):204–11.
29. Pfennig A, Littmann E, Bauer M. Neurocognitive impairment and dementia in mood disorders. J Neuropsychiatry Clin Neurosci. 2007;19(4):373–82.
30. Steffens DC, Potter GG. Geriatric depression and cognitive impairment. Psychol Med. 2008;38(2): 163–75.
31. Roberts RE, Kaplan GA, Shema SJ, Strawbridge WJ. Does growing old increase the risk for depression? Am J Psychiatry. 1997;154(10): 1384–90.
32. Gallo JJ, Anthony JC, Muthén BO. Age differences in the symptoms of depression: a latent trait analysis. J Gerontol. 1994;49(6):251–64.
33. Birrer RB, Vemuri SP. Depression in later life: a diagnostic and therapeutic challenge. Am Fam Physician. 2004;69(10):2375–82.
34. Boswell EB, Stoudemire A. Major depression in the primary care setting. Am J Med. 1996;101(6A): 3S–9S.
35. Beck AT, Steer RA, Brown GK. Manual for the beck depression inventory-II. San Antonio, TX: Psychological Corporation; 1996.
36. Hamilton M. A rating scale for depression. J Neurol Neurosurg Psychiatry. 1960;23:56–62.
37. Yesavage JA, Brink TL, Rose TL, Lum O, Huang V, Adey M, et al. Development and validation of a geriatric depression screening scale: A preliminary report. J Psychiatr Res. 1982;17(1):37–49.
38. Kotlyar M, Dysken M, Adson DE. Update on drug-induced depression in the elderly. Am J Geriatr Pharmacother. 2005;3(4):288–300.

39. Mills TL. Comorbid depressive symptomatology: isolating the effects of chronic medical conditions on self-reported depressive symptoms among community-dwelling older adults. Soc Sci Med. 2001;53(5): 569–78.
40. Ginó S, Mendes T, Maroco J, Ribeiro F, Schmand BA, de Mendonça A, et al. Memory complaints are frequent but qualitatively different in young and elderly healthy people. Gerontology. 2010;56(3): 272–7.
41. Jessen F, Wiese B, Cvetanovska G, Fuchs A, Kaduszkiewicz H, Kölsch H, et al. Patterns of subjective memory impairment in the elderly: association with memory performance. Psychol Med. 2007;37(12):1753–62.
42. Siu AL. Screening for dementia and investigating its causes. Ann Intern Med. 1991;115(2):122–32.
43. Bieliauskas LA. Depressed or not depressed? That is the question. J Clin Exp Neuropsychol. 1993;15: 119–34.
44. Chase, TN. Apathy in neuropsychiatric disease: diagnosis, pathophysiology, and treatment. Neurotox Res. 2010, epub ahead of print.
45. Zgaljardic DJ, Borod JC, Foldi NS, Rocco M, Mattis PJ, Gordon MF, et al. Relationship between self-reported apathy and executive dysfunction in nondemented patients with Parkinson disease. Cogn Behav Neurol. 2007;20(3):184–92.
46. Clarke DE, van Reekum R, Simard M, Streiner DL, Conn D, Cohen T, et al. Apathy in dementia: clinical and sociodemographic correlates. J Neuropsychiatry Clin Neurosci. 2008;20(3):337–47.
47. Landes AM, DP, Sperry SD, Strauss ME. Prevalence of apathy, dysphoria, and depression in relation to dementia severity in Alzheimer's disease. *J Neuropsychiatry & Clinical Neurosciences*. 2005;17: 342–9.
48. Berger AK, Fratiglioni L, Forsell Y, Winblad B, Bäckman L. The occurrence of depressive symptoms in the preclinical phase of AD: a population-based study. Neurology. 1999;53(9):1998–2002.
49. Robert PH, Berr C, Volteau M, Bertogliati C, Benoit M, Sarazin M, et al. Apathy in patients with mild cognitive impairment and the risk of developing dementia of Alzheimer's disease: a one-year follow-up study. Clin Neurol Neurosurg. 2006;108(8): 733–6.
50. Hattori H, Yoshiyama K, Miura R, Fujie S. Clinical psychological tests useful for differentiating depressive state with Alzheimer's disease from major depression of the elderly. Psychogeriatrics. 2010;10(1):29–33.
51. Landes AM, Sperry SD, Strauss ME, Geldmacher DS. Apathy in Alzheimer's disease. J Am Geriatr Soc. 2001;49(12):1700–7.
52. Cummings JL, Mega M, Gray K, Rosenberg-Thompson S, Carusi DA, Gornbein J. The Neuropsychiatric Inventory: comprehensive assessment of psychopathology in dementia. Neurology. 1994;44(12):2308–14.
53. Marin RS, Biedrzycki RC, Firinciogullari S. Reliability and validity of the apathy evaluation scale. Psychiatry Res. 1991;38(2):143–62.
54. Burns A, Folstein S, Brandt J, Folstein M. Clinical assessment of irritability, aggression, and apathy in Huntington and Alzheimer disease. J Nerv Ment Dis. 1990;178(1):20–6.
55. Zubenko GS, Zubenko WN, McPherson S, Spoor E, Marin DB, Farlow MR, et al. A collaborative study of the emergence and clinical features of the major depressive syndrome of Alzheimer's disease. Am J Psychiatry. 2003;160(5):857–66.
56. Olin JT, Katz IR, Meyers BS, Schneider LS, Lebowitz BD. Provisional diagnostic criteria for depression of Alzheimer disease: rationale and background. Am J Geriatr Psychiatry. 2002;10(2): 129–41.
57. Kessler RC, Angermeyer M, Anthony JC, de Graaf R, Demyttenaere K, Gasquet I, et al. Lifetime prevalence and age-of-onset distributions of mental disorders in the World Health Organization's World Mental Health Survey Initiative. World Psychiatry. 2007; 6(3):168–76.
58. Alexopoulos GS, Young RC, Meyers BS, Abrams RC, Shamoian CA. Late-onset depression. Psychiatr Clin North Am. 1988;11(1):101–15.
59. Brodaty H, Luscombe G, Parker G, Wilhelm K, Hickie I, Austin MP, et al. Early and late onset depression in old age: different aetiologies, same phenomenology. J Affect Disord. 2001;66(2–3): 225–36.
60. Lamberty GJ, Bieliauskas LA. Distinguishing between depression and dementia in the elderly: A review of neuropsychological findings. Arch Clin Neuropsychol. 1993;8:149–70.
61. Kumar A, Bilker W, Jin Z, Udupa J. Neuropsychopharmacology. 2000;22:264–74.
62. Langenecker SA, Lee HJ, Bieliauskas LA. Neuropsychology of depression and related mood disorders. In: Grant I, Adams KM, editors. Neuropsychological assessment of neuropsychiatric and neuromedical disorders, 3rd ed. New York: Oxford, 2009;523–59.
63. Krishnan KR, Hays JC, Tupler LA, George LK, Blazer DG. Clinical and phenomenological comparisons of late-onset and early-onset depression. Am J Psychiatry. 1995;152(5):785–8.
64. Alexopoulos GS, Young RC, Meyers BS. Geriatric depression: age of onset and dementia. Biol Psychiatry. 1993;34(3):141–5.
65. van Reekum R, Simard M, Clarke D, Binns MA, Conn D. Late-life depression as a possible predictor of dementia: cross-sectional and short-term follow-up results. Am J Geriatr Psychiatry. 1999;7(2):151–9.
66. Song Y, Dowling GA, Wallhagen MI, Lee KA, Strawbridge WJ. Sleep in older adults with Alzheimer's disease. Neuroscience. 2010;42(4):190–8.
67. Buysse DJ. Insomnia, depression and aging. Assessing sleep and mood interactions in older adults. Geriatrics. 2004;59(2):47–51.

68. Dykierek P, Stadtmuller G, Schramma P, Bahro M, Vancalker D, Braus D, et al. The value of REM sleep parameters in differentiating Alzheimer's disease from old-age depression and normal aging. J Psychiatr Res. 1998;32(1):1–9.
69. Gallassi R, Oppi F, Poda R, Scortichini S, Stanzani Maserati M, Marano G, et al. Are subjective cognitive complaints a risk factor for dementia? Neurol Sci. 2010;31(3):327–36.
70. Reid LM, Maclullich AMJ. Subjective memory complaints and cognitive impairment in older people. Dement Geriatr Cogn Disord. 2006;22(5–6):471–85.
71. Crowe SF, Hoogenraad K. Differentiation of dementia of the Alzheimer's type from depression with cognitive impairment on the basis of a cortical versus subcortical pattern of cognitive deficit. Arch Clin Neuropsychol. 2000;15(1):9–19.
72. King DA, Caine ED, Conwell Y, Cox C. The neuropsychology of depression in the elderly: a comparative study of normal aging and Alzheimer's disease. J Neuropsychiatry Clin Neurosci. 1991;3(2):163–8.
73. Lachner G, Engel RR. Differentiation of dementia and depression by memory tests. A meta-analysis. J Nerv Mental Dis. 1994;182(1):34–9.
74. Hartlage S, Alloy LB, Vázquez C, Dykman B. Automatic and effortful processing in depression. Psychol Bull. 1993;113(2):247–78.
75. Butters MA, Whyte EM, Nebes RD, Begley AE, Dew MA, Mulsant BH, et al. The nature and determinants of neuropsychological functioning in late-life depression. Arch Gen Psychiatry. 2004;61(6):587–95.
76. Hickie I, Naismith S, Ward PB, Turner K, Scott E, Mitchell P, et al. Reduced hippocampal volumes and memory loss in patients with early- and late-onset depression. Br J Psychiatry. 2005;186:197–202.
77. Lockwood KA, Alexopoulos GS, Kakuma T, Van Gorp WG. Subtypes of cognitive impairment in depressed older adults. Am J Geriatr Psychiatry. 2000;8(3):201–8.
78. Salloway S, Malloy P, Kohn R, Gillard E, Duffy J, Rogg J, et al. MRI and neuropsychological differences in early- and late-life-onset geriatric depression. Neurology. 1996;46(6):1567–74.
79. Elderkin-Thompson V, Mintz J, Haroon E, Lavretsky H, Kumar A. Executive dysfunction and memory in older patients with major and minor depression. Arch Clin Neuropsychol. 2007;22(2):261–70.
80. Blackwell AD, Sahakian BJ, Vesey R, Semple JM, Robbins TW, Hodges JR, Dementia & Geriatric Cognitive Disorders. 2004;17(1-2):42–8.
81. Christensen H, Griffiths K, Mackinnon A. A quantitative review of cognitive deficits in depression and Alzheimer-type dementia Selection of Studies. J Int Neuropsychol Soc. 1997;3(6):631–51.
82. Dierckx E, Engelborghs S, De Raedt R, De Deyn PP, Ponjaert-Kristoffersen I. Differentiation between mild cognitive impairment, Alzheimer's disease and depression by means of cued recall. Psychol Med. 2007;37(5):747–55.
83. Swainson R, Hodges JR, Galton CJ, Semple J, Michael A, Dunn BD, et al. Early Detection and Differential Diagnosis of Alzheimer's Disease and Depression with Neuropsychological Tasks. Dement Geriatr Cogn Disord. 2001;12(4):265–80.
84. Wecshler D. Wechsler memory scale: fourth edition technical and interpretive manual. San Antonio: Pearson; 2009. p. 2009.
85. Sahakian BJ, Morris RG, Evenden JL, Heald A, Levy R, Philpot M, et al. A comparative study of visuospatial memory and learning in Alzheimer-type dementia and Parkinson's disease. Brain. 1988;111:695–718.
86. Delis DC, Kramer JH, Kaplan E, Ober BA. The California Verbal Learning Test. 2nd ed. San Antonio: The Psychological Corporation; 2000.
87. Gainotti G, Marra C. Some aspects of memory disorders clearly distinguish dementia of the Alzheimer's type from depressive pseudo-dementia. J Clin Exp Neuropsychol. 1994;16(1):65–78.
88. Shapiro AM, Benedict RH, Schretlen D, Brandt J. Construct and concurrent validity of the Hopkins Verbal Learning Test-revised. Clin Neuropsychol. 1999;13(3):348–58.
89. Benedict RHB, Schretlen D, Groninger L, Dobraski M, Shpritz B. Revision of the Brief Visuospatial Memory Test: Studies of normal performance, reliability, and validity. Psychol Assess. 1996;8(2):145–53.
90. Rey A. L'examen clinique en psychologie. Paris: Presses Universitaires de France; 1964.
91. Warrington EK. Recognition Memory Test manual. Windsor, England: NFER-Nelson; 1984.
92. Foldi N. Distinct serial position profiles and neuropsychological measures differentiate late life depression from normal aging and Alzheimer's disease. Psychiatry Res. 2003;120(1):71–84.
93. Kaschel R, Logie RH, Kazén M, Della Sala S. Alzheimer's disease, but not ageing or depression, affects dual-tasking. J Neurol. 2009;256(11):1860–8.
94. Radloff LS. 'The CES-D scale: A self report depression scale for research in the general population'. *Applied Psychological Measurement*. 1977; 1:385–401.
95. Zung WW. "A self-rating depression scale". *Archives of General Psychiatry*. 1965;12:63–70.
96. Kashani J, McKnew D, & Cytryn L. Symptom checklist for major depressive disorders (*Adapted*). Psychopharmacology Bulletin, 1985;21:957–958.
97. Sheikh JI, Yesavage JA. Geriatric Depression Scale (GDS): recent evidence and development of a shorter version. *Clin Gerontol*. 1986;June;5(1/2):165–173.
98. Alexopoulos GA, Abrams RC, Young RC & Shamoian CA: Cornell scale for depression in dementia. Biol Psych, 1988;23:271–284.
99. Trey Sunderland and Marcia Minichiello. Dementia Mood Assessment Scale. International Psychogeriatrics, 1997;8:329–331.

100. Hammond MF, O'Keeffe ST, Barer DH. Development and validation of a brief observerrated screening scale for depression in elderly medical patients. Age Ageing. 2000;Nov;29(6):511–5
101. Cummings JL, Mega M, Gray K, Rosenberg-Thompson S, Carusi DA, Gornbein J. The Neuropsychiatric Inventory: comprehensive assessment of psychopathology in dementia. Neurology 1994;44: 2308–2314.
102. Mack, J.L., & Patterson, M.B. (1993). *CERAD Behavioral Rating Scale for Dementia. CERAD.* [Unpublished; Center for Mental Health Services Research, Washington University in St. Louis].

Assessment of Alzheimer's Disease 18

David Loewenstein

Abstract

Alzheimer's disease (AD) is a devastating illness, affecting over 5.5 million adults in the United States and costing over 170 billion dollars annually. In addition, there is growing recognition that mild cognitive impairment (MCI) constitutes a risk factor for AD and other neurodegenerative disorders. In this chapter, we describe the clinical manifestations of early AD and other neurogenerative brain disorders and describe the appropriate neuropsychological measures that tap the important cognitive domains that should be assessed in these conditions. A summary of useful clinical tips as well as future directions in the field are addressed.

Keywords

Cognitive assessment • Alzheimer's • MCI diagnosis • Early Alzheimer's disease

The Diagnosis of Alzheimer's Disease

Alzheimer's disease (AD) is a devastating illness, affecting over 5.5 million adults in the United States and costing over 170 billion dollars annually [1, 3]. With a growing aging population and the fact that age is the greatest risk factor for AD, this disorder could reach epidemic proportions. Alzheimer's disease (AD) was first discovered in 1906, but the causes of this devastating disorder were not known until recently. The characteristic neuropathology of AD is the presence of senile plaques and neurofibrillary tangles upon autopsy. It is thought that plaque formation in AD begins with the abnormal misfolding of a protein called beta amyloid (A-beta) that causes toxic amyloid fibrils as many as 20–30 years before any clinical symptoms of the disease are manifested. These abnormal proteins continue to aggregate, particularly in the frontal lobes, anterior cingulate, posterior cingulate, precuneas and striatum. Eventually, a cascade effect occurs in which there

D. Loewenstein, Ph.D. (✉)
Department of Psychiatry and Behavioral Sciences, Miller School of Medicine, University of Miami Miller School of Medicine, Mental Health Building, 1695 NW 9th Avenue, Suite 3208G, Miami, FL 33136, USA
e-mail: dloewenstein@att.net

L.D. Ravdin and H.L. Katzen (eds.), *Handbook on the Neuropsychology of Aging and Dementia*, Clinical Handbooks in Neuropsychology, DOI 10.1007/978-1-4614-3106-0_18,

are difficulties with the phosphorylation of the microtubule-associated protein (MAP) tau which results in neurofibrillary degeneration [4] and is seen as neurofibrillary tangles. These changes lead to synaptic disruption and neurodegeneration of structures such as the hippocampus and the entorhinal cortex, and these changes can eventually be visualized on structural magnetic resonance imaging (MRI).

Because of early neurodegeneration in medial temporal lobe structures, the first clinical manifestations of AD are typically seen as the disruption of short-term memories. As the disease progresses, there are typically more pronounced memory difficulties evidenced by misplacing possessions, forgetting appointments, repetitive conversations, and worsening ability to recall recent events. The patient may begin to have difficulties with word finding, may get lost while driving, and begin to exhibit problems with judgment. This reflects the increasing involvement of the cortical regions of the brain such as the frontal, temporal, and parietal lobes. Over time, the patient becomes less able to manage their affairs and loses the ability to perform activities of daily living. The progression of the illness is quite variable from several years to as many as 20 years, but eventually leads to total disability and eventual death [1].

The clinical diagnosis of probable AD by the National Institute of Neurologic, Communicative Disorders and Stroke–AD and Related Disorders Association (NINCDS–ADRDA) [5] criteria requires (a) memory impairment and impairment in at least one other cognitive domain, (b) impairment in social and/or occupational function, and (c) ruling out any other possible causes of the dementia syndrome. In short, a clinical diagnosis of probable AD is a diagnosis of exclusion, which can only be rendered after all other causes for the dementia have been ruled out. Neuropsychological assessment is recommended as a means of confirming the presence and quantifying the degree of different cognitive deficits. Typical presentations of AD with gradual onset of memory decline and progressive course are typically referred to as probable AD, while atypical presentations when other etiologies may affect cognitive impairment are generally referred to as possible AD. While the accuracy of the clinical criteria for probable AD generally exceeds 85% in most specialized memory disorders centers, a final diagnosis of the disorder can only be rendered upon examination of the density of senile plaques and neurofibrillary tangles upon autopsy (see [7]). Recently, the National Institutes on Aging and the Alzheimer's Association workgroup recommended a revision in the proposed guidelines for the clinical diagnosis of AD [6]. They refined the diagnosis of probable AD to include nonamnesic presentations of the illness (i.e., language presentation, visuospatial presentation, and executive presentation). Possible AD would represent a case meeting all clinical core criteria for AD dementia but would present with an atypical course or insufficient evidence of cognitive decline. An important feature of these new proposed criteria is the addition of biomarkers which strengthen the certainty of diagnoses, such as positive positron emission tomography (PET), amyloid imaging, low AB42 in the cerebrospinal fluid, as well as downstream neuronal markers of injury including decreased fluorodeoxyglucose (FDG) uptake on PET scan in the temporoparietal cortex; disproportionate atrophy in the medial, basal, and lateral temporal lobe and medial parietal cortex on structural MRI; or CSF elevation of tau or p-tau proteins. These recommendations usher in an era where the clinical diagnosis of AD is no longer a diagnosis of exclusion and where clinical criteria for the diagnosis are strengthened by the presence of beta amyloid in the brain and specific patterns of neuronal degeneration on neuroimaging.

In diagnosing AD, there is nothing more important than establishing the presence or absence of cognitive impairment, which is related to the integrity of specific brain systems. In cases where an individual is moderately or severely impaired, the clinician is provided with ample information to arrive at a clinical impression. However, there are a significant number of cases where the cognitive deficits can be quite mild and even difficult to detect by experienced clinicians. Persons with high cognitive reserve can employ other cognitive and brain resources to mask any overt deficits. It is not uncommon to see family members completely unaware of the substantial cognitive deficits that are only uncovered with a comprehensive neuropsychological evaluation.

At the present time, there is a reluctance by some to seek early evaluation given that current treatments for Alzheimer's disease, such as the cholinesterase inhibitors, are merely palliative and do not treat the underlying pathology of AD. However, a recent advance in knowledge suggests that emerging treatments will be most effective in the earliest stages of AD, before the advent of multisystem degeneration [7]. Moreover, accurate diagnosis can ensure that the patient and family receive proper counseling and advice to better help manage their lives and to plan for the future. Conversely, neuropsychological methods can help reassure persons with unimpaired cognitive function and can provide a valuable baseline to compare future results for those at risk. Finally, there are a number of conditions that may mimic the symptoms of AD where neuropsychological assessment can be an important part of differential diagnosis.

Mild Cognitive Impairment

It has been increasingly recognized that the clinical manifestations of Alzheimer's disease (AD) occur well before the manifestation of a dementia syndrome [48] and a clinical diagnosis of the disorder. Petersen [8, 9] coined the term mild cognitive impairment (MCI) as an intermediary state between a normal cognitive state and dementia. The criteria for MCI are as follows:

(a) Subjective memory complaint by the patient or preferably by a knowledgeable informant.
(b) Objective evidence of memory impairment confirmed by neuropsychological testing, typically 1.5 SD below expected levels.
(c) Intact intellectual function and global mental status as defined by an MMSE score of 24 or above.
(d) Not sufficient cognitive impairment to cause significant impairment in social and/or occupational function.

Implicit to this characterization was the notion that amnesic difficulties do not represent a static state of affairs, but reflect a decline from premorbid levels of function that heightens the probability of progression to probable AD [9]. Indeed, a number of studies have suggested that impairment of episodic memory may be the best cognitive marker of AD in its predementia state, [10–12] even among asymptomatic, community-dwelling elders [13]. In clinical settings, the rate of progression from amnesic MCI to dementia was 10–15% per year [8, 9, 14], while 100% of subjects diagnosed with MCI progressed to dementia over a 9.5-year period, and 84% received a neuropathological diagnosis of probable AD [15]. In contrast, the progression to dementia among subjects with MCI is considerably less in community settings where the base rates of MCI is lower [7, 16].

Subsequently, Petersen [17] proposed that MCI did not have to be confined to only an amnesic impairment, but could also be defined by nonmemory impairments. Different types of MCI included amnesic MCI single domain, amnesic MCI multiple domains, nonamnesic MCI single domain, and nonamnesic MCI multiple domains. The degree of impairment on both amnesic as well as nonamnesic measures is associated with the likelihood that individuals with MCI will progress to dementia versus reverting to a normal state over time [18]. Alexopolous et al. [19] found that 25% of subjects with amnesic MCI, 38% of subjects with nonamnesic MCI, and 54% of individuals with mixed amnesic and nonamnesic impairment progressed to dementia over a 3.5-year follow-up period. Roundtree et al. [20] found no differences in the rates of progression between those with amnesic MCI (56%) versus those with nonamnesic MCI (52%) over a 4-year follow-up. Manley and associates found that impairment in more than one cognitive domain was most predictive of progression to dementia over a 4.5-year period. In a more recent study, Loewenstein and associates [18] showed that those with multiple memory impairments, multiple nonmemory impairments, or a combination of nonmemory impairments have a much greater likelihood of stability or worsening of their deficits over a 2- to 3-year period. The greatest likelihood of progression to dementia was in the multiple memory impairment group followed by the mixed memory and nonmemory group. Subsequent studies have also shown that individuals with multiple-domain MCI have a much greater likelihood of progression to dementia upon longitudinal follow-up [21, 22]. The National Institute on Aging and the Alzheimer's Association recently published guidelines that guide research criteria for MCI related to AD, recognizing the changes to the brain occur well before the manifestation of dementia symptoms. These criteria allow for incorporation of biomarkers such as amyloid imaging of the brain by PET or lower CSF levels AB42 as well as evidence of neuronal degeneration characteristic of AD by FDG PET, MRI, or elevated CSF tau. These criteria address the question of whether the individual with MCI has an AD or non-AD etiology. Further research is required to determine applicability to clinical practice [47].

The Clinical Interview

An important part of a comprehensive neuropsychological assessment is a detailed clinical interview with the patient and a collateral informant who is very familiar with the patient's activities of daily living. This is especially true when evaluating older adults with cognitive impairment. It is generally most effective to interview the patient and the caregiver separately so that they feel free to speak honestly about their concerns. Many informants, particularly spouses and children, are reluctant to share sensitive information about cognitive and functional deterioration in front of their loved ones. The informant may be particularly reluctant to disclose information in front of a patient who is in denial about their symptoms or who tends to react negatively to any suggestion of memory loss.

During the clinical interview, it is important to initially gather information about the current cognitive difficulties experienced by the patient. It is especially helpful to determine whether the primary symptoms reported are primarily those associated with memory or whether they also represent language, executive, attention, or visuospatial disturbance. Most individuals with early Alzheimer's disease have recent memory deficits while still able to recall information from the recent past. This is related to medial temporal lobe deficits, specifically in the hippocampus and entorhinal cortex, which interfere with the storage and consolidation of new information.

While memory impairment is a hallmark feature of the disease, individuals may initially present with language deficits, visuospatial disturbance, or problems with executive function. Sometimes, the cognitive symptoms of AD will first become apparent in the face of stressful life events which tax an individual's cognitive reserve (e.g., the loss of a loved one, a taxing physical illness, depression). These underlying symptoms may abate after time as the person marshals the cognitive resources to compensate for these deficits or these stressors are no longer present. Unfortunately, the neurodegenerative process continues until the individual progresses to the point where successful compensation is no longer possible.

Occasionally, the first deficits exhibited by patients with Alzheimer's (particularly those who are 70 years or younger) will be characterized by a language disturbance such as the inability to retrieve words. Some patients present with primary deficits with reasoning, judgment, and other aspects of executive function. In younger patients, when the predominant symptoms are language and executive dysfunction (such as disinhibition), the clinician must consider the possibility of a frontotemporal dementia versus AD. On the other hand, diffuse Lewy body disease must be considered if there are predominant concerns with attention, cognitive slowing, executive and visuospatial disturbance particularly in the presence of Parkinsonian features, psychiatric disturbances such as visual hallucinations, and rapid eye movement REM behavior sleep disorders. REM behavior sleep disorders are evidenced by difficulties in sleeping and dream-enacting behaviors such as punching, kicking, or jumping from the bed.

It is important to determine whether there has been a sudden onset of cognitive symptoms (often observed in vascular or other non-AD neurological disorders) or whether the cognitive disorder has a slowly progressive course with a gradual worsening of symptoms such as is typically seen in AD. While the clinical interview often starts as open ended so that the clinician can obtain as much information in the patient's and caregiver's own words, there are often a follow-up series of questions (see Table 18.1) that can be helpful in elucidating the exact nature of cognitive symptoms.

The clinical interview allows the examiner to ascertain the premorbid function of the patient, to determine the nature and extent of cognitive decline, and to determine the extent to which observed deficits interfere with social or occupational function. It also provides an opportunity to determine the effects of anxiety and depression on function and to assess the effects of current medical conditions as well as current medications on cognition. The clinical interview also provides an opportunity to determine the effects of premorbid factors such as learning disabilities, attention deficit disorder, a lack of formal education, and previous as well as current difficulties such as alcohol and drug abuse might have on cognitive performance.

The importance of the clinical interview is that it provides a context in which to view and interpret neuropsychological findings.

Table 18.1 Questions that help elucidate cognitive symptoms

(1) Are there increasing difficulties with remembering recent events (i.e., conversations, activities)?
(2) Are there problems with misplacing possessions?
(3) Are there issues with remembering the names of familiar persons or changes in the ability to remember persons one has just met?
(4) Are there difficulties getting lost driving, losing one's way in a public place, or getting lost in the neighborhood?
(5) Is there repetitive questioning?
(6) Is there a decline in the ability to drive, to operate a computer, or to use household objects?
(7) Are there difficulties with finding the correct word or words in free speech?
(8) Is there a decline in the ability to understand what one has read in a newspaper, magazine, or book?
(9) Are there difficulties remembering what one has seen on television or the movies?
(10) Has the person withdrawn from activities such as work, playing cards, or social clubs as a result of cognitive changes?
(11) Has there been any changes in the ability of the person to manage finances (i.e., write a check, balancing a checkbook)
(12) Has the person shown increasingly poor judgment in work and social situations?
(13) Has there been a change in personality (disinhibition, ability, apathy)?

Overview of Neuropsychological Assessment

The most sophisticated neuropsychological batteries assess different aspects of neuropsychological function at baseline and ensure that their measurements have sufficient range to track changes in different cognitive domains longitudinally. The optimal neuropsychological battery assesses (1) learning and retentive memory, (2) executive function, (3) language, and (4) visuospatial skills. It is also beneficial to have measures of both attention and processing speed, as these are frequently impaired by a variety of brain disorders and may serve as a more general marker of impairment.

Assessment of Memory

There are a plethora of validated measures for the assessment of memory. In evaluating an individual for the presence of MCI or early dementia, the most important memory measure is a list learning task. The advantage of such an assessment is that it provides an assessment of learning over several trials that can evaluate the effects of proactive and retroactive interference and provide measures of delayed recall. Recognition memory or cued recall can also be assessed. Each of these components is important in the evaluation of AD. Difficulties with delayed recall and rate of forgetting are seen as hallmark features of AD [23, 24], but there is evidence that not all AD patients exhibit these deficits [25]. Difficulties with learning and a flat learning curve may be among the most prominent deficits in AD patients

Table 18.2 List learning and other memory tests for the assessment of AD

California Verbal Learning Test (CVLT-II: [27])
Hopkins Verbal Learning Test—Revised (HVLT-R: [30])
Rey Auditory Verbal Learning Test [28, 29]
Modified Fuld Object Memory Evaluation [31, 32]
Semantic Interference Test [26]
Logical Memory for Passages (Wechsler Memory Scale—4th Edition: [34])
Visual Reproduction (Wechsler Memory Scale—4th Edition; 2008)
Paired Associates (Wechsler Memory Scale—4th Edition; 2008)
Brief Visual Memory Test-Revised (BVMT-R) [35]

[26]. A list of commonly used list learning measures is presented in Table 18.2.

The choice of memory test depends on the circumstances of the evaluation. The California Verbal Learning Test—Second Edition (CVLT-II: [27]) is the most comprehensive test, presenting the older adult with 16 items representing four semantic categories. The patient has five trials to learn the to-be-remembered targets, and a second list of 16 items is then administered to assess the potential effects of proactive interference (old learning interfering with new learning), retroactive interference (presentation of the new list interfering with learning from the old list), and the use of semantic cues to facilitate recall. There is a delayed free and cued recall after a 20-min period as well a recognition memory test. Even though there is the availability of shorter CVLT-II lists for older adults, the standard edition is typically preferable for the evaluation of early patients. There are numerous indices for learning and memory that can be very helpful in diagnostic determination. An alternative to the CVLT-II is the Rey Auditory Verbal Learning Test (AVLT: [28, 29]) which is similar to the CVLT-II but does not make use of semantic cues or different semantic categories. For subjects that are depressed or anxious, a list learning task across five learning trials can be sometimes experienced as overwhelming and are relatively lengthy to give. An excellent alternative is the Hopkins Verbal Learning Test—Revised (HVLT-R: [30]), which requires the older participant to learn 12 words across only 3 learning trials. When issues such as very low education or significant hearing deficits are an issue, a modified Three-Trial Fuld Object Memory Evaluation [31, 32] can be quite useful. This requires the individual to select ten common objects from a bag and to recall the objects after a verbal fluency distracter task. The participant is then selectively reminded of those items not recalled and then another distracter task is administered followed by the real objects for a total of three recall trials. Loewenstein et al. [26] modified the Three-Trial Fuld Object Memory Evaluation paradigm by having subjects recall a second list of items that are all semantically similar to the original to-be-remembered targets (i.e., ring versus bracelet). Reduced recall for the second list compared to the first list was thought to be due to competition from the previously presented targets on the first list (proactive interference), while reduced recall for the first list after recall of the second list was thought to be related to retroactive interference. The Semantic Interference Test (SIT: [26]) evidenced high sensitivity and specificity in distinguishing normal elderly subjects from subjects with MCI and early dementia. Moreover, vulnerability to proactive interference was most associated with those MCI subjects who progressed to dementia over a 2- to 3-year period [33].

There are also a number of memory tasks that tap other aspects of memory function including measures such as logical memory for story passages, paired-associate learning, and immediate and delayed recall of simple and increasingly complex geometric designs. Some of the memory tests that we have found useful in our clinical laboratory are listed in Table 18.2.

In our laboratory, we typically like to augment a list learning test with a nonverbal test of immediate and delayed visual reproduction and immediate and delayed logical memory for two story passages. Other memory measures can be administered as the need arises.

Assessment of Nonmemory Functions

The assessment of *language function* includes both an evaluation of expressive and receptive language skills. Confrontation naming and word retrieval skills can be assessed by measures such as the Boston Naming Test [36]. Access from semantic lexicon can be evaluated using a category fluency test for animals, fruits, and vegetables [37]. In contrast, letter fluency is a more orthographic memory task that requires retrieval from phonological stores and is sensitive to frontal lobe dysfunction (see [38]). We also obtain a brief reading sample, a writing sample, as well as repetition of phrases. Receptive language can be assessed by having the subject perform simple and more complex commands or performing the Token Test [39, 44].

Common elements of *executive function* tests are the ability to plan, solve problems, engage in concept formation, and shift cognitive sets. One of the most sensitive measures for executive dysfunction is the Wisconsin Card Sorting Test [40], which provides an excellent measure of concept formation, perseverations, and the ability to shift cognitive sets. Unfortunately, since this is a test of novel learning, this is not an optimal measure for repeated testing. The Trail-Making Test [41, 42], a test of simple visual scanning abilities which requires alternation between numbers and letters and shifting cognitive sets, is widely thought to be an executive function task. Since there are so many cognitive processes required for this test of complex visual scanning abilities, Trails B is very sensitive to cerebral dysfunction in general, although observed deficits may not be specific to dysexecutive impairments and can also be highly influenced by motor skills and speed. *Visuospatial disturbances and constructional praxis* can be ascertained by constructional tasks such as the Block Design Subtest of the Wechsler Adult Intelligence Scale (WAIS-IV; [43]). When it is important to distinguish between a perceptual disturbance from the inability to construct figures based on that perception, tests such as Judgment of Line Orientation [44] or Hooper Visual Organization Test [45] may be useful. Praxis is the ability to perform skilled motor movements. Simple tests of ideational praxis may be to have the patient prepare a letter for mailing while simple tests of ideomotor praxis are to show how to use scissors, use a hammer, or blow out a match.

Attention may be assessed by tests of digit span or continuous performance tasks that require vigilance and a response when certain stimuli flash across a computer screen. *Psychomotor speed* may be assessed by Trails A in which a patient connects numbers spread out across a page as quickly as possible, employing tests of simple or choice reaction time on the computer or manual finger tapping.

When Should Neuropsychological Tests Be Administered

Neuropsychological testing should be administered to any older adult in which it is important to establish the presence, or absence of cognitive deficits or where the clinician is unsure about the nature and the extent of cognitive deficits. Examining different patterns of neuropsychological deficits may also help the clinician in diagnostic formulation and provide an objective baseline in which to monitor progression and response to treatment. Finally, neuropsychological test results can highlight patterns of strengths and weaknesses that can be helpful in patient management.

Consider the example of an 85-year-old woman born in Lithuania with a fifth grade education, presenting with significant depression in an outpatient setting. On her mental status evaluation, she gave the wrong day of the week and recalled two of three objects. One of her sisters insisted that she had cognitive decline, whereas another sister insisted that there had been no change in cognitive function. In this case, the clinician was unsure of the diagnosis and ordered a neuropsychological evaluation. The neuropsychologist can test memory, language, executive function, attention, and language and by using objective normative data appropriate to the patient's age, education, and background as well as comparing test results in different domains. This data can greatly assist with determining the presence or absence of cognitive impairment in patients such as the one described above, and can contribute greatly to the diagnostic determination.

There are some cases that will remain equivocal even with the most sensitive neuropsychological assessment. In these instances, the neuropsychologist may conduct serial assessments in 6–9 months to track progression. Sometimes, the neuropsychologist will use parallel forms when available to reduce the possibility of practice effects. The CVLT-II, HVLT-Revised, and AVLT are all examples of memory tests with alternate forms. The neuropsychologist may also use reliable change indices to determine the extent to which changes on certain other tests reflect true differences, rather than resulting from chance or practice effects. It should be noted that neuropsychological test results provide a snapshot of a person's performance at one point in time, but that longitudinal assessment may be required to more accurately define the parameters of a particular condition.

Summary and Future Trends in Neuropsychological Assessment

Neuropsychological assessment has an important role in distinguishing between the cognitive effects of normal aging versus deficits related to cerebral dysfunction. The objective nature of the tests, the ability to relate results to appropriate normative data, and the comparison of patterns of strengths and weaknesses all contribute important information that can improve clinical decision making. As efforts are made to detect AD in its earliest stages, it will become even more important for the field of neuropsychology to develop tests that are sensitive to specific deficits in utilizing semantic cues, the effects of semantic interference, and evidence of subtle executive dysfunction. With the increased reliance on biomarkers for early detection of AD, there will also be a need to develop algorithms that incorporate both cognitive variables and biomarkers. To this point, a recent investigation has revealed that measures of episodic memory and combined FDG-PET scans together predicted progression from MCI to AD better than either measure alone [46]. The diagnosis of early AD is strengthened by evidence of amyloid deposition in the brain by PET imaging, CSF evidence of amyloid or tau levels suggestive of AD, atrophy of the hippocampus, entorhinal cortex and other medial temporal structures on MRI, or being homozygous for the APOE-ε4 allele. Despite these advances in technology that will aid in early detection of AD, assessment of memory and other cognitive deficits will always be essential in characterizing the disease, monitoring progression over time, and helping to evaluate the effectiveness of treatment strategies. Finally, as new treatments are developed, cognitive and functional measures will be at the forefront as a means to measure outcome.

Clinical Pearls

- The hallmark features of Alzheimer's disease (AD) are deficits in delayed recall and rate of forgetting. However, some AD patients will evidence their greatest deficits in learning information across multiple trials.
- List learning tests are optimal for assessment of AD in that they test the ability to learn new information across multiple trials and also assess delayed recall and rate of forgetting.
- It is desirable to assess memory for verbal as well as nonverbal information (i.e., immediate and delayed visual reproduction).
- The AD patient may on occasion present with primary impairments in executive dysfunction, language, or visuospatial function. Therefore, it is important to assess these domains.
- Amnesic mild cognitive impairment (aMCI) is a risk factor for Alzheimer's disease and memory disorders. In specialty memory disorders clinics, the rate of progression to dementia and a diagnosis of probable AD is 12–15% per year while the rate of progression in other settings where the base rates may be lower are considerably less.
- The clinical diagnosis of probable AD requires a dementia syndrome by DSM-IV criteria, and cognitive impairment must be sufficiently severe to interfere with social and/or occupational function.

- A new diagnosis of dementia cannot be made in the presence of a delirium.
- A clinical diagnosis of AD is greatly strengthened by evidence of medial temporal lobe atrophy on MRI (particularly in the hippocampus and entorhinal cortex), CSF findings of Aβ-42/Aβ-40 ratios or Aβ-42/tau40 ratio suggestive of AD, blood tests showing two APOE-ε4 alleles, positron emission tomography (PET) scans showing abnormal beta amyloid imaging on PET imaging, or hypometabolism in temporal and parietal cortices.
- Parkinsonian signs and symptoms, REM sleep behavioral disturbance, fluctuating attention, memory, executive and visuospatial deficits should raise the possibility of diffuse Lewy body disease.
- Early language disturbances or predominant changes in personality (i.e., disinhibition) and an earlier onset of symptoms should raise the possibility of frontotemporal dementia (FTD). These individuals typically have predominant frontal temporal atrophy on structural MRI, high levels of executive dysfunction and characteristic patterns of frontal and temporal lobe decreased metabolism or blood flow, and functional neuroimaging such as PET or SPECT.
- Serial testing is recommended in cases where the presence or the extent of cognitive deficits is unclear or when it is important to monitor potential improvement or worsening over time.
- Denial of symptoms is commonly observed in AD, yet some early AD patients are aware of changes, which may lead to significant levels of depression and anxiety. Although pseudodementia is relatively uncommon in outpatient settings, the clinician should be aware of the effects of anxiety and depression in depressing performance on neuropsychological tests.

References

1. Alzheimer's Association. Alzheimer's disease facts and figures. Alzheimers Dement. 2010;6:158–94.
2. Park D, Schwartz N. Cognitive aging: a primer. Philadelphia: Taylor and Francis (Psychology Press); 2000.
3. Hebert LE, Scherr PA, Bienias JL, Bennett DA, Evans DA. Alzheimer's disease in the U.S. population: prevalence estimates using the 2000 census. Arch Neurol. 2003;60:1119–22.
4. Iqbal K, Liu F, Gong CX, Alonso Adel C, Grundke-Iqbal I. Mechanisms of tau induced neurodegeneration. Acta Neuropathol. 2009;118(1):53–69.
5. McKhann G, Drachman D, Folstein M, Katzman R, Price D, Stadlan E. Clinical diagnosis of Alzheimer's disease: report of the NINCDS-ADRDA work group under the auspices of department of health and human services task force on Alzheimer's disease. Neurology. 1984;34:939–44.
6. McKhann G, Knopman D, Chertkow H, Hyman BT, Jack CR, Kawas KH, Klunk WE, Koroshetz WJ, Manley JJ, Mayeux R, Mohs RC, Morris JC, et al. The diagnosis of dementia due to Alzheimer's disease: recommendations from the National Institutes on Aging-Alzheimer's Association workgroup on diagnostic guidelines for Alzheimer's disease. Alzheimers Dement. 2011;7(3):263–9.
7. Brooks LG, Loewenstein DA. Assessing the progression of mild cognitive impairment (MCI) to Alzheimer's disease: current trends and future directions. Alzheimers Res Ther. 2010;2:28.
8. Petersen RC, Smith GE, Waring SC, Ivnik RJ, Tangalos EG, Kokmen E. Mild cognitive impairment: clinical characterization and outcome. Arch Neurol. 1999;56:303–8.
9. Petersen RC. Mild cognitive impairment: transition between aging and Alzheimer's disease. Neurologia. 2000;15:93–101.
10. Grober E, Lipton RB, Hall C, et al. Memory impairment on free and cued selective reminding predicts dementia. Neurology. 2000;54:827–32.
11. Howieson DB, Dame A, Camicioli R, et al. Cognitive markers preceding Alzheimer's dementia in the healthy oldest old. J Am Geriatr Soc. 1997;45:584–9.
12. Small BJ, Mobly JL, Laukka EJ, Jones S, Backman L. Cognitive deficits in preclinical Alzheimer's disease. Acta Neurol Scand Suppl. 2003;179:29–33.
13. Assal F, Cummings JL. Neuropsychiatric symptoms in the dementias. Curr Opin Neurol. 2002;15:445–50.
14. Luis CA, Loewenstein DA, Acevedo A, Barker WW, Duara R. Mild cognitive impairment: directions for future research. Neurology. 2003;61:438–44.
15. Morris JC, Storandt M, Miller JP, McKeel DW, Price JL, Rubin EH, Berg L. Mild cognitive impairment represents early-stage Alzheimer's disease. Arch Neurol. 2001;58(3):397–405.
16. Larrieu S, Letenneur L, Orgogozo JM, Fabrigoule C, Amieva H, Le Carret N, Barberger-Gateau P, Dartigues JF. Incidence and outcome of mild cognitive impairment in a population-based prospective cohort. Neurology. 2002;59:1594–9.
17. Petersen R. Mild cognitive impairment. J Intern Med. 2004;256:183–94.
18. Loewenstein DA, Amarilis Acevedo A, Small BJ, Agron J, Crocco E, Duara R. Stability of different

subtypes of mild cognitive impairment among the elderly over a two to three year follow-up period. Dement Geriatr Cogn Disord. 2009;17(5):437–40.
19. Alexopoulos P, Grimmer T, Perneczky R, Domes G, Kurz A. Progression to dementia in clinical subtypes of mild cognitive impairment. Dement Geriatr Cogn Disord. 2006;22:27–34.
20. Rountree SD, Waring SC, Chan WC, Lupo PJ, Darby EJ, Doody RS. Importance of subtle amnestic and nonamnestic deficits in mild cognitive impairment: prognosis and conversion to dementia. Dement Geriatr Cogn Disord. 2007;24:476–82.
21. Manly JJ, Tang MX, Schupf N, Stern Y, Vonsattel JP, Mayeux R. Frequency and course of mild cognitive impairment in a multiethnic community. Ann Neurol. 2008;63:494–506.
22. Ritchie LJ, Tuokko H. Patterns of cognitive decline, conversion rates, and predictive validity for 3 models of MCI. Am J Alzheimers Dis Other Demen. 2010;25(7):592–603.
23. Locasio JJ, Growdon JH, Corkin S. Cognitive test performance in detecting, staging, and tracking Alzheimer'sdisease. Arch Neurol. 1995;52:1087–99.
24. Tröster AI, Butters N, Salmon D, Cullum CM, Jacobs D, Brandt J, White RF. The diagnostic utility of savings scores: differentiating Alzheimer's and Huntington's disease with the logical memory and visual reproduction tests. J Clin Exp Neuropsychol. 1993;5:773–88.
25. Christensen H, Kopelman MD, Stanhope N, Lorentz L, Owen P. Rates of forgetting in Alzheimer dementia. Neuropsychologia. 1998;36:547–57.
26. Loewenstein DA, Acevedo A, Luis CA, Crum T, Barker WW, Duara R. Semantic interference deficits and the detection of mild Alzheimer's disease and mild cognitive impairment without dementia. J Int Neuropsychol Soc. 2004;1:91–100.
27. Delis DC, Kramer JH, Kaplan E, Ober BA. California verbal learning test- second edition. San Antonio: The Psychological Corporation; 2000.
28. Rey A. L'examen Clinique en psychologie. Paris: Presses Universitaries de France; 1964.
29. Lezak MD. Neuropsychological assessment. New York: Oxford University Press; 1998.
30. Benedict R, Schretlen D, Groninger L, et al. Hopkins Verbal Learning Test—Revised: normative data and analysis of inter-form and test-retest reliability. Clin Neuropsychol. 1998;12:43–55.
31. Fuld PA. Fuld object-memory evaluation. Chicago: Stoelting Co; 1981.
32. Loewenstein DA, Arguelles T, Barker WW, et al. The utility of a modified Object Memory Test in distinguishing between three different age groups of Alzheimer's disease patients and normal controls. J Mental Health Aging. 2001;7:317–24.
33. Loewenstein DA, Acevedo A, Agron J, Duara R. Vulnerability to proactive semantic interference and progression to dementia older adults with mild cognitive impairment (MCI). Dement Geriatr Cogn Disord. 2007;24(5):363–8.
34. Wechsler D. The Wechsler Memory Scale. 4th ed. San Antonio: The Psychological Corporation; 2008.
35. Benedict R. Brief Visual Memory Test. Odessa: Psychological Assessment Resources; 1996.
36. Goodglass H, Kaplan E, Weintraub S. The Boston Naming Test. Philadelphia: Lea and Febiger; 1983.
37. Monsch AY, Bondi MW, Butters N, Salmon DP, Katzman R, Thal L. Comparison of verbal fluency tasks in the detection of dementia of the Alzheimer's type. Arch Neurol. 1992;49(12):1253–8.
38. Spreen O, Strauss E. A compendium of neuropsychological tests: administration, norms, and commentary. 2nd ed. New York: Oxford University Press; 1998.
39. Benton A, des Hamsher K, Sivan AB. Multilingual aphasia examination. Iowa City: AJA Associates; 1994.
40. Heaton RK, Chelune GJ, Talley JL, Kay GG, Curtiss G. Wisconsin Card Sorting Test manual: revised and expanded. Odessa: Psychological Assessment Resources; 1993.
41. War Department Adjutant General's Office. Army Individual Test Battery. Manual of directions and scoring. Washington, DC: War Department Adjutant General's Office; 1944.
42. Reitan RM, Wolfson D. The Halstead-Reitan neuropsychological test battery: theory and clinical interpretation. 2nd ed. Tucson: Neuropsychology Press; 1993.
43. Wechsler D. The Wechsler Adult Intelligence Scale. 4th ed. San Antonio: The Psychological Corporation; 2008.
44. Benton A, Sivan AG, des Hamsher K, Varney NR, Spreen O. Contributions to neuropsychological assessment: a clinical manual. 2nd ed. Oxford: London; 1994.
45. Hooper HE. Hooper Visual Organization Test (VOT). Los Angeles: Western Psychological Services; 1983.
46. Landau SM, Harvey D, Madison CM, Reiman EM, Foster NL, Aisen PS, Petersen RC, Shaw LM, Trojanowski JQ, Jack Jr CR, Weiner MW, Jagust WJ. Comparing predictors of conversion and decline in mild cognitive impairment. Neurology. 2010;75:230–8.
47. Albert MS, Dekosky ST, Dicksen D, Dubois B, Feldman HH, Fox N, Gamst A, Holtzman D, Jagust WJ, Petersen R. The diagnosis of mild cognitive impairment due to Alzheimer's disease: Recommendations from the National Institute on Aging and Alzheimer's Association workgroup. Alzheimer's & Dementia; 2011. p. 1–10.
48. American Psychiatric Association. Task force on DSM-IV: diagnostic and statistical manual of mental disorders: DSM-IV. 4th ed. Washington, DC: American Psychiatric Association; 1994.

Vascular Cognitive Impairment

19

Robert Paul, Elizabeth Lane, and Angela Jefferson

Abstract

The risk of cerebrovascular disease increases with advanced age, with almost two thirds of individuals over 70 exhibiting vascular lesions on MRI. Cognitive presentations vary from little or no no cognitive impairment to clinical dementia, and the extent of cognitive impairment is not necessarily correlated with lesion size or burden. The term vascular cognitive impairment (VCI) describes all forms of cognitive impairment caused by cerebrovascular disease. Early identification of vascular disease is critical since many risk factors are modifiable, and the neuropsychologist can play an important role in characterizing the extent of cognitive and behavioral change. This chapter provides an overview of the clinical guidelines to consider when evaluating older adults with possible VCI and includes an illustrative case example and useful recommendations for the clinician.

Keywords

Vascular dementia • Dementia • Stroke • Neuropsychology

R. Paul, Ph.D. (✉) • Elizabeth Lane, Ph.D.
University of Missouri, St. Louis, MO, USA

Department of Psychology, Division of Behavioral Neurosciences, 1 University Blvd, St. Louis, MO 63121, USA
e-mail: paulro@umsl.edu; emlane@umsl.edu

A. Jefferson, Ph.D.
Vanderbilt Memory & Alzheimer's Center, Department of Neurology, Vanderbilt University Medical Center, A0118 Medical Center North, Nashville, TN 37232, USA
e-mail: angela.jefferson@vanderbilt.edu

L.D. Ravdin and H.L. Katzen (eds.), *Handbook on the Neuropsychology of Aging and Dementia*, Clinical Handbooks in Neuropsychology, DOI 10.1007/978-1-4614-3106-0_19,

The risk of cerebrovascular disease increases as individuals age, with as many as 70% of individuals over the age of 70 exhibiting evidence of vascular lesions on MRI [1]. Such lesions can yield different clinical profiles, with some smaller lesions resulting in little to no cognitive impairment and other lesions severe enough to result in clinical dementia. The term vascular cognitive impairment (VCI) was introduced to describe all forms of cognitive impairment caused by cerebrovascular disease. The type of impairment associated with VCI can be variable depending on the location and amount of damaged tissue, which in turn influences the severity of cognitive, behavioral, and psychiatric features. Early identification of vascular disease is critical since many of the risk factors for VaD are modifiable, yet it is not known exactly how much damage is necessary to produce clinical impairment.

At the mildest stage, VCI is referred to as vascular cognitive impairment no dementia (VCIND) and is often secondary to small vessel ischemic disease. At the more severe clinical end, VCI is referred to as vascular dementia (VaD) and is believed to represent one of the more common types of dementia among older adults after AD. About one-third of individuals will develop dementia within 1 year after a stroke [1]. When a stroke is strategically located (e.g., in Broca's area) or affects a very large vessel, the clinical result is likely consistent with the traditional concept of dementia due to stroke (i.e., a sudden loss of cognitive function and a stepwise pattern of cognitive deterioration). However, clinical symptoms associated with stroke are highly variable and depend upon the area impacted. Table 19.1 lists common stroke sites and corresponding deficits, which can be viewed on structural brain imaging as cortical or lacunar infarcts. While impairment due to strategic or large vessel stroke is most commonly tied to the concept of VaD, it is not the most common expression of the disease. As discussed in more detail below, VaD more often has an insidious onset with a slow and gradual decline. Additionally, mixed dementia between VCI and AD is common and argued by some to share neuropathogenic mechanisms [2], though this position is controversial in the field. Even though the diagnosis of VCI can be complicated by several factors, there appears to be a general cognitive pattern associated with the type of deficits found in this disorder.

Table 19.1 Common stroke sites and corresponding clinical features

Stroke site	Clinical features
Middle cerebral artery	Hemiplegia, aphasia, homonymous, hemianopia, hemianesthesia contralateral
Anterior cerebral artery	Paraplegia, incontinence, abulia, executive dysfunction, personality changes
Posterior cerebral artery	Homonymous hemianopia, alexia with or without agraphia, visual agnosias, color anomia, Balint syndrome, prosopagnosia

Clinical Presentation

In the case of VCI, clinical preconceptions of disease expression and progression are often not realized, as heterogeneity is the rule. As discussed in greater detail below, patterns of abrupt onset and stepwise decline in function are less common than a slow and progressive disease course [3]. Further, while a pattern of executive dysfunction may predominate, the neuropsychological presentation will be driven by the extent of focal and diffuse vascular injuries in the brain. Below, clinical concepts on the VCI spectrum are described in more detail.

Vascular Cognitive Impairment: No Dementia

VCIND refers to vascular lesions evident on MRI that cause impairment too mild to impact activities of daily living. The most common types of lesions associated with VCIND are visualized on MRI as lacunes (i.e., small cerebrospinal filled cavities in the white matter) and subcortical hyperintensities (SH; i.e., areas of bright white on neuroimaging that represent vascular-related damage). However, it is not uncommon for an individual to have this type of vascular damage and exhibit normal neuropsychological abilities. These "silent" infarcts may not be truly silent, as they represent vascular damage that may be a core determinant of what is considered normal age-related cognitive decline. As such, not all patients with MRI lesions will exhibit neuropsychological impairment in part because the clinical norms likely included older individuals with age-related infarcts as well.

Most importantly, VCIND may be a prodromal stage for VaD, and as such, modifiable risk factors may be important in reducing the progression of the disease. A longitudinal study by Wentzel et al. [4] revealed that half of the VCIND cases progressed to dementia over a 5-year period of time. Further, individuals with VCIND and evidence of frontal white matter hyperintensities are less likely to revert back to normal cognitive function after 1 year as compared to individuals with VCIND who do not have frontal white matter hyperintensities [5]. Modifiable risk factors, such as hypertension, may play an important role in determining the progression of VCIND to VaD. Notably, current pharmacological treatment options for VaD are comparable to AD treatment options (i.e., relatively ineffective at arresting disease progression) [6], emphasizing the need for early identification and clinical intervention.

Though there does not appear to be a consistent neuropsychological profile that is predictive of advancement from VCIND to VaD [7], individuals with VCIND often display poor performance on tests of cognitive flexibility and verbal retrieval [8], learning [9], and psychomotor speed [9]. Additionally, VCIND may increase the incidence of depression, although it is unknown if vascular damage is the cause of depression or a result of perceived deficits [9].

Vascular Dementia

VaD is the result of extensive white matter lesions and lacunar infarcts due to small vessel disease [10], the result of one or more strokes to the main cerebral arteries, or some combination of the two. Executive function, learning, and delayed memory, with intact recognition memory are the most consistently impaired domains of function in VaD [11]. Deficits in executive function are most typically found on tests of verbal fluency, mental flexibility, and response inhibition [10]. Episodic memory deficits are typically found on tests of list learning and recall, but recognition may remain intact particularly if the structures of the medial temporal lobe are spared of vascular damage. These patterns of impairment are useful in distinguishing VaD from strategic stroke and AD. Physical symptoms of VaD include extrapyramidal symptoms, bilateral pyramidal symptoms, positive masseter reflex, imbalance, incontinence, dysarthria, and dysphagia [12].

Depression is the most common behavioral feature associated with stroke. About 20% of individuals with stroke also exhibit depression [13]. The strongest predictor of depression is reduction in the ability to carry out activities of daily living [13], which may be confounded by stroke severity. Additionally, increased depression is associated with greater cognitive impairment and increased mortality. Of note, the cognitive deficits found in patients with VaD cannot be explained by the depression, as they persist even when the depressive symptoms are statistically controlled [10].

Several diagnostic criteria have been proposed for VaD. The three most commonly used diagnostic criteria include the Diagnostic and Statistical Manual, Fourth Edition [14] (DSM-IV; see Table 19.2), the State of California Alzheimer's Disease Diagnostic and Treatment Centers criteria [15] (ADDTC), and the National Institute of Neurological Disorders and Stroke-Association Internationale pour la Recherche et L'Enseignement en Neurosciences [16] (NINDS-AIREN) criteria. The most commonly used criteria in the clinical setting are the DSM-IV given that third-party insurance reimbursement is tied to the DSM-IV (and ICD). The DSM-IV criteria are based on symptoms similar to AD and require memory deficits as a prominent feature. This requirement presents a diagnostic conundrum since core aspects

Table 19.2 DSM-IV criteria for VaD

A. The development of multiple cognitive deficits manifested by both
1. Memory impairment (impaired ability to learn new information or to recall previously learned information)
2. One (or more) of the following cognitive disturbances:
(a) Aphasia (language disturbance)
(b) Apraxia (impaired ability to carry out motor activities despite intact motor function)
(c) Agnosia (failure to recognize or identify objects despite intact sensory function)
(d) Disturbance in executive functioning (i.e., planning, organizing, sequencing, abstracting)
B. The cognitive deficits in criteria A1 and A2 each cause significant impairment in social or occupational functioning and represent a significant decline from a previous level of functioning
C. Focal neurological signs and symptoms (e.g., exaggeration of deep tendon reflexes, extensor plantar response, pseudobulbar palsy, gait abnormalities, weakness of an extremity) or laboratory evidence indicative of cerebrovascular disease (e.g., multiple infarctions involving cortex and underlying white matter) that are judged to be etiologically related to the disturbance
D. The deficits do not occur exclusively during the course of a delirium

of episodic memory can remain intact in the context of vascular disease, and memory impairment may not be the primary feature of the disease. Additionally, the DSM-IV criteria do not require neuroimaging evidence of cerebrovascular disease, increasing the likelihood that an individual may be misdiagnosed.

Both the ADDTC and NINDS-AIREN criteria are used most often in research settings. Both sets of criteria allow for the diagnosis of possible, probable, and definite VaD, and both require neuroimaging evidence of cerebrovascular disease for a probable diagnosis. However, the NINDS-AIREN criteria are still modeled after the diagnostic criteria for AD and require episodic memory impairment for the diagnosis, yielding misdiagnosis issues consistent with the DMS-IV criteria. The ADDTC criteria are the most flexible with regard to the neuropsychological pattern of impairment, allowing for diagnosis even when memory is not the prominent area of cognitive impairment. For a more detailed review on VaD diagnostic criteria convergence and divergence, the reader is referred to Cosentino et al. [17].

VCI Risk Factors

There are a number of variables associated with increased risk for stroke. Though stroke occurs in younger cohorts, such as sickle cell anemia in very young children, it is most common among older individuals. In fact, the greatest risk factor associated with VCI is age. Additional unmodifiable risk factors for stroke include male sex, low birth weight, atrial fibrillation, race (i.e., African American), and ethnicity (i.e., Latino) [18]. Additionally, there are several deterministic and susceptibility genetic factors that increase an individuals' risk of vascular disease, including cerebral autosomal dominant arteriopathy with subcortical infarcts leukoencephalopathy (CADASIL) as a deterministic factor and angiotensinogen as susceptibility factor.

CADASIL, a rare autosomal dominant disease, is associated with a Notch3 defect that causes infarcts in the deep white matter, basal ganglia, and brain stem. The average age of onset for stroke is age 45, although many individuals with CADASIL will experience migraine with aura with an average onset at age 30 years. Individuals with CADASIL typically develop dementia by the sixth decade of life with death in the seventh decade. Cognitive deficits associated with CADASIL typically follow a subcortical pattern impacting executive function, organization abilities, and attention [19]. In contrast to the deterministic nature of CADASIL, one major susceptibility gene for vascular disease that has been identified is angiotensinogen. Studies have shown that angiotensinogen may be involved in abnormal vascular responsivity and the development of subcortical ischemic disease [20].

Since cerebrovascular disease is the underlying cause of VCI, the risk factors related to the development of VCI overlap with those related to cardiovascular disease. Not surprisingly, improvement in risk factors underlying overall cardiovascular health lowers the risk of stroke. Specifically, studies have demonstrated that successful lowering of hypertension and cessation of smoking result in reduced stroke risk in advanced age [19]. Other modifiable factors include control of diabetes mellitus, hypertension, and dyslipidemia.

VCI Differential Diagnosis

Diagnostic considerations that will challenge the clinician when evaluating older adults for VCI might include Lewy body dementia, AD, frontotemporal dementias, and normal pressure hydrocephalus (NPH). NPH can clinically present very similarly to VCI as both conditions share frontal symptoms [21]; however, NPH more frequently includes urinary urgency (or urinary frequency/incontinence) and gait disturbance [22]. The combination of gait disturbance and urinary symptoms greatly increases the likelihood of NPH as the appropriate diagnosis even when executive dysfunction is present. Of course, evidence of MRI abnormalities characteristic of either NPH (i.e., grossly enlarged lateral ventricles) or VCI (e.g., lacunar infarcts, white matter hyperintensities) will provide more definitive information regarding the differential diagnosis. Frontotemporal dementia typically presents with more unique symptoms than VCI, such as significant aphasia or personality abnormalities. Furthermore, the age of onset for VCI is often, but not always, older than what is typical for frontotemporal dementia with behavioral disturbances present before age 65.

Ruling out AD or diagnosing mixed dementia (i.e., AD and VCI) is definitely more challenging for the clinician. Historically, the course of decline and neuropsychological patterns seen in AD versus VCI were believed to be disease specific, but more recent research has challenged this position. Autopsy evidence suggests that AD and vascular neuropathology frequently coexist; therefore, many patients likely exhibit some degree of shared disease presentation in vivo. It remains unclear, however, whether both conditions develop independently or whether the development of one condition precipitates the development or progression of the other. Regardless of the temporal association or causation of these two pathologies, the clinician is challenged with sorting through the possible diagnostic entities using a combination of clinical interview data, neuropsychological outcomes, and neuroimaging results. More details regarding best strategies for clinically evaluating patients and interpreting relevant data are provided below.

Clinical Evaluation

Perhaps more so than other neurodegenerative conditions, the model of vascular-mediated brain injury has evolved over the last few decades. Historical beliefs regarding the course of decline, the neuropsychological pattern, and the utility or necessity of MRI-defined vascular burden have shifted the approach and accuracy of the neuropsychological evaluation. To effectively navigate these challenges, the clinical evaluation of vascular-mediated cognitive impairment should follow a traditional hypothesis-driven, patient-oriented approach. Further, the integration of personal, medical (including laboratory and MRI data), and neuropsychological information is necessary to reach a sound conceptualization and clinical diagnosis. Below we describe clinical evaluation guidelines along with some of the common hurdles that clinicians face in the process of integrating this information (see Paul et al. [23] for a more complete review of these clinical concerns).

Clinical Interview and History

The clinical interview is an important area of neuropsychological assessment for vascular disease. Patients may have very good insight into the nature of their cognitive difficulties, though it would be incorrect to presume that insight is fully intact for all patients. Attention is needed to review signs and symptoms with patients and to ensure that descriptions of stroke-related terms and MRI findings are communicated accurately. Oftentimes, patients will confuse concepts such as transient ischemic attack (or TIA) with stroke, or they will misinterpret the MRI report regarding subcortical versus cortical vascular disease. Obviously, access to medical records will clarify these issues, but for some clinicians working in independent practice, the records may arrive after the patient has been evaluated (as in the clinical case provided below), or they may never arrive.

The interview can also provide an excellent opportunity to observe language skills and the potential for various aphasic abnormalities. Solicitation of responses during the interview process and probing of specific areas represents an excellent opportunity to informally characterize the pattern of memory impairments as individuals recall personal and medical-related information. Patients may describe memory failures as "tip of the tongue" phenomena rather than outright amnesic failure (e.g., "I cannot remember the word"). Finally, mood and apathy are relevant constructs to extract from the interview process. While neither may be particularly affected in cases of small vessel ischemic involvement, large vessel stroke is a predictor of depression and apathy [13].

One common hurdle that clinicians face during the clinical interview and conceptualization of VCI is differentiating between a stepwise versus progressive decline. Historically, the VCI literature has characterized the decline in cognitive and physical status associated with stroke as "stepwise," which contrasted the insidious and progressive decline characterizing AD. If the patient or family described a repetitive pattern of sharp decline followed by stabilization, the stepwise pattern was confirmed and a diagnosis of vascular etiology would be considered more likely than a diagnosis of AD. Such a description of decline was, and still is, appropriate for large vessel infarcts (e.g., middle cerebral, anterior cerebral, or posterior cerebral arteries) or very strategic small vessel strokes (e.g., thalamic infarct), but the pattern does not hold for small vessel disease where the microvasculature degrades slowly over a period of time, especially when isolated to the subcortical white matter. Such small vessel infarcts are now recognized as the most common form of stroke associated with age (compared to large vessel strokes) [24], and functional status (associated with such small vessel infarcts) deteriorates along a slow and progressive course that is similar to AD. In short, clinicians cannot rely on the course of decline as a pathogenic sign of vascular disease, and detailed review of both neuropsychological data and neuroimaging results are critical to reach a solid and accurate case conceptualization.

In some instances, family members may attribute the slow insidious changes in function caused by small vessel disease as "normal aging." It is not until the patient suffers a sharp decline in function due to a strategic stroke or large vessel stroke that the family (or primary care physician) initiates a clinical evaluation. In our studies of VaD, all patients with large vessel infarcts also exhibited significant, concomitant microvascular disease in the subcortical white matter, emphasizing that small vessel disease is more the norm than the exception. The combination of cortical or strategic infarcts *and* small vessel ischemic damage in the white matter significantly complicates the clinical picture owning to the presence of mixed symptoms, and in turn, this clinical presentation almost always complicates the description of disease course by family members.

Neuropsychological Assessment

Neuropsychological evaluation of VCI requires sufficient breadth and coverage. Screening measures, such as the mini mental state exam, lack sensitivity to vascular-related cognitive impairment [25, 26]. More recently, the Montreal Cognitive Assessment (MoCA) was introduced to provide greater coverage of executive processes in the screening of dementia [27]. Studies indicate that the MoCA has greater sensitivity to more subtle cognitive impairment and early AD than the MMSE [27]. However, the MoCA was not

Table 19.3 Neuropsychological protocol recommendations

Domain	Harmonization 30-min protocol[a]	Harmonization 60-min protocol[a]	Authors' recommended protocol[b]
Global	MMSE	MMSE	MoCA
Executive function/ activation	Animal fluency	Animal fluency	Animal fluency
	Letter fluency	Letter fluency	Letter fluency
	Digit Symbol Coding	Digit Symbol Coding	Digit Symbol Coding
		Trail Making	Trail Making
			Letter-Number Sequencing
			Stroop Test
Psychomotor speed			Grooved Pegboard Test
Language		Boston Naming Test	Boston Naming Test
Attention/reaction time		Simple and Choice RT	Digit Span
Visuospatial skill		Rey Complex Figure Test	Rey Complex Figure Test
Memory	Hopkins Verbal Learning Test—Revised	Hopkins Verbal Learning Test—Revised or California Verbal Learning Test-II	Hopkins Verbal Learning Test—Revised or California Verbal Learning Test-II
			Brief Visual Memory Test—Revised
Neuropsychiatric/ depressive symptoms	Mood questionnaire	Neuropsychiatric Inventory Mood questionnaire (BDI II, CES-D)	Mood questionnaire

MoCA Montreal Cognitive Assessment, *BDI II* Beck Depression Inventory II
[a]Adapted from NINDS and Canadian Stroke Harmonization Network Protocol Recommendations (Hachinski et al.)
[b]Recommended by Robert Paul, Liz Lane, and Angela Jefferson (Note, animal fluency is recommended by the authors as a measure of language rather than executive function/activation)

developed specifically for VCI, and it is unclear whether the limited task demands adequately capture mild to moderate cognitive impairments associated with cerebrovascular disease. Overall, studies to date do not suggest that brief screening measures offer sufficient neuropsychological coverage for detecting milder forms of VCI.

In 2006, the NINDS and Canadian Stroke Harmonization Network [28] recommended a brief 30-min and a more comprehensive 60-min neuropsychological battery for VCI, which are summarized in Table 19.3. As evident from the table, the 30-min battery is limited to verbal memory, psychomotor speed, and verbal fluency. By contrast, the 60-min battery was designed to represent all major cognitive systems, including attention, processing speed, working memory, multiple aspects of executive function, verbal and visual learning and memory, psychomotor speed, language, visuospatial skill, and mood. In terms of memory assessment, it is critical to include measures that capture learning efficiency across trials, delayed retention, and recognition. This assessment strategy will help to differentiate the amnesic pattern of AD from the inefficient learning pattern common in, but not necessarily pathognomonic of, vascular disease. Similarly, it is recommended that measures of both lexical (letter) and semantic (category) fluency are administered, as vascular pathology tends to result in poorer performance on lexical than semantic tasks. The opposite pattern is more characteristic of AD, though this differential pattern remains only a heuristic and not an algorithm [29, 30].

Finally, as evident from Table 19.3, there is a heavy weighting on the heterogeneous aspects of executive dysfunction, including working memory, response inhibition, cognitive flexibility, planning, and organization. Comprehensive coverage of executive function skills is important, as vascular disease purportedly interrupts frontal-subcortical circuits that mediate executive difficulties commonly associated with VCI [31, 32], and performance on executive function tasks is a critical determinant of ADL completion, which is directly tied to diagnostic criteria for dementia. While it is not recommended that one make assumptions about ADL independence based on performance in this domain, there are times clinically when vascular patients report no difficulties in their abilities to perform ADLs, yet they exhibit striking impairments across multiple executive function measures. In these instances, it is important to communicate to families that while the patient may be independent today with instrumental activities that facilitate independence (e.g., cooking, driving, medication, and financial management), this independence is likely to change. Such changes or decline cannot be predicted, and an unfortunate accident may result before some intervention is initiated.

Neuroimaging Corroboration

It can be tempting to rely too heavily on neuropsychological data alone to determine the etiology of cognitive impairment with any clinical referral, and reliance on the cognitive data can be most problematic to the clinician in the case of VCI. A pattern of executive dysfunction in the absence of amnesic episodic memory impairment and/or anomic aphasia can lead clinicians toward a vascular conceptualization. This conceptualization is even more likely when patients present with significant vascular risk factors (e.g., high blood pressure, high cholesterol, diabetes) in the absence of other obvious rule outs, such as NPH or cortical dementias (e.g., frontotemporal dementia). However, in the absence of a known "fingerprint" of neuropsychological impairment for VCI, it is absolutely critical that neuroimaging results are integrated into the case conceptualization to reach a more complete diagnostic formulation.

Neuroimaging abnormalities associated with stroke are most readily identified on high-powered MRI (e.g., 3T) using fluid-attenuated inversion recovery (FLAIR) scans [33]. Imaging abnormalities are also evident at lower field strengths (e.g., 1.5T), but recent data suggests that abnormalities on 3T may not be readily visible at 1.5T [34, 35]. Most often, vascular disease on FLAIR images is characterized by lacunes in subcortical gray and white matter, white matter hyperintensities, and/or periventricular capping along the perimeter of the lateral ventricles (see Fig. 19.1). Neuropsychologists are not routinely trained to review films

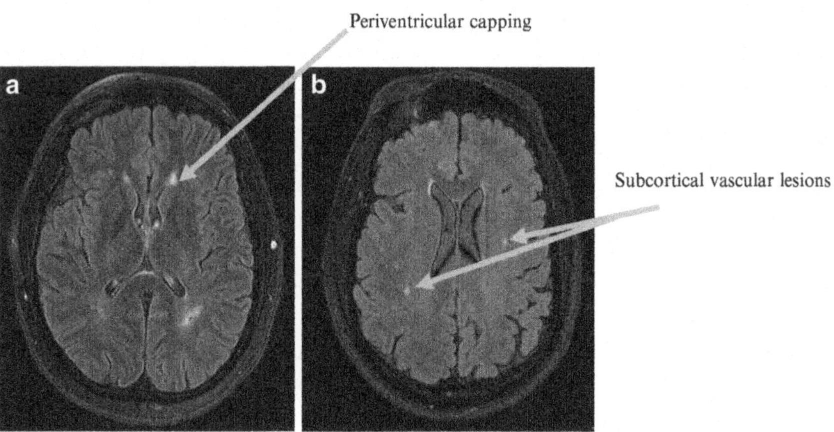

Fig. 19.1 Evidence of vascular disease using 3T MRI. (**a**) Example of periventricular capping in a "healthy" older adult. (**b**) Evidence of periventricular capping and subcortical lesions in a mildly impaired older adult with ischemic vascular disease

independently, so the degree of vascular burden must be gleaned from the radiologist's report. This situation is an unfortunate reality because the field of radiology, unlike the field of neuropsychology, does not utilize a standard metric system for determining the level of pathologic burden. That is, the semantic labels often included in radiology reports to describe the extent of vascular damage (e.g., "age-related," "mild," "severe") reflect the training and personal nuances of a particular radiologist rather than a standardized measure of variance from "normal" (e.g., evidence that 25% of the white matter is affected with hyperintensities [36]). Complicating the picture further is that cerebrovascular disease is common among the general population after age 65 years [37, 38]. Collectively, the key question is not whether or not the MRI report included any reference to vascular disease, but rather whether or not the amount of vascular burden is sufficient to account for the cognitive difficulties.

So, how does a neuropsychologist incorporate neuroimaging data into a clinical evaluation? First, if there is no MRI report available, then the diagnosis of VCI can only be described as a possibility pending a subsequent MRI. Second, if an MRI has been conducted and there is no mention of vascular disease, it is unlikely that a person's cognitive impairment is driven largely (solely) by vascular mechanisms. Third, if the radiology report describes some degree of vascular disease (e.g., "mild ischemic vascular disease is noted…" or "age-appropriate ischemic vascular disease"), then the possibility of a vascular etiology (at least in part) exists but is not necessarily confirmed (i.e., necessary but not sufficient). Descriptors such as "extensive vascular disease" or strategic lacunar infarcts are plausibly related to cognitive status. Further, while debated across various groups, we believe it is appropriate to conclude that descriptors, such as "extensive vascular disease," are etiologically relevant regardless of other comorbid conditions. That is, even if the final diagnosis appears consistent with AD, the vascular burden likely contributes to the overall clinical picture in some form.

Clinical Case Example

A case example is included below that incorporates the necessary elements of a clinical evaluation for illustration purposes. The case involves a baseline and 12-month follow-up neuropsychological evaluation that required the integration of clinical history, neuropsychological data, and neuroimaging findings. As is often the case in general private practice settings, the MRI report was not available at the time of the initial evaluation. Similarly, while corroboration of the clinical history from family is always important, the patient's husband was in poor health and could not participate in the clinical interview in person or by phone, which further limited the information available for the clinical interview. The case example was extracted from a clinical file and modified to remove personal identification.

Background and History

Mrs. Smith (fictional name) is a 71-year-old, right-handed, married woman who was referred for neuropsychological evaluation by her neurologist for concern regarding cognitive difficulties. During the interview, Mrs. Smith reported a history of TIAs, "stroke," and memory loss that began 5 years prior to the evaluation, but she exhibited some difficulty describing the chronology of these events. Mrs. Smith experienced a TIA-like event in 2003 followed by an episode of electrolyte depletion and "stroke." She was unable to provide any details regarding the "stroke." However, she stopped driving in 2004 due to recurrent sensory episodes that involved tingling in her hands.

Since 2004, Mrs. Smith described problems with short-term memory, including frequently repeating herself and difficulty remembering the names of people she has recently met (though she has no difficulty remembering the names of people well known to her). She remains independent in terms of medication management and other aspects of activities of daily living. She denied hallucinations, fluctuating symptoms, urinary incontinence/urgency/frequency, significant visuospatial abnormalities, or any changes in personality.

Mrs. Smith's medical history includes high cholesterol, high blood pressure, TIAs as described above, and possible seizures secondary to vascular injury (insert relative time frame). Psychiatric history is unremarkable. Mrs. Smith completed college with a degree in business education, and she worked as a high school business teacher for many years. Mrs. Smith and her husband now live in an independent senior community where they enjoy a very active lifestyle; as noted above, her husband was unavailable for corroboration of the clinical history. She does not smoke cigarettes or drink alcohol. She reported no family history of dementia. A brain MRI report dated 3 weeks prior to the neuropsychological evaluation was remarkable for "periventricular white matter low attenuation related to chronic small vessel ischemia" and "findings consistent with generalized age-related cerebral volume loss." No other abnormalities were noted, and the original scans were not available for visual inspection.

No clear disturbances in gait, posture, physical asymmetries, or evidence of tremor or rigidity were noted. Mrs. Smith was oriented to person, time, and place. Her conversational speech was fluent and goal directed. She exhibited appropriate prosody, and there was no evidence of paraphasias. Mild word-finding difficulties were noted in conversational speech, and she exhibited some confusion in the chronology of her recent medical and cognitive histories as noted above. Receptive speech was generally intact, and Mrs. Smith exhibited no difficulty comprehending simple or complex material. She was very friendly and cooperative. Her mood was euthymic, and she remained engaged throughout the evaluation.

Baseline Neuropsychological Test Results

Baseline neuropsychological data are presented in Table 19.4. Mrs. Smith recalled 23 words across three learning trials on a verbal learning and measure (HVLT-R). After a brief delay, she recalled 6 out of 12 target words (low average performance). Her performance was less strong on a recognition trial, as she tended to endorse semantically related foils. It is of interest that she appeared a bit more confused on this aspect of the test compared to the free recall portions of the task. On a test of learning and memory of prose passages, Mrs. Smith exhibited generally intact learning and retention of information, and she performed one standard deviation above average on the delayed trial, suggesting no rapid loss of information. Further, her recognition memory was adequate. Performance on a test of visual learning and memory (BVMT-R) was significantly impaired in terms of learning and retention, though her recognition memory was intact. Mrs. Smith's performance on the learning trial was severely impaired, and while she retained what she learned on the delayed trial, her overall performances were low on both trials.

On a measure of semantic (animal) fluency, Mrs. Smith performed within expectations for her age with 17 animals named within 1 min. By contrast, on the lexical (FAS) fluency test, she produced only 20 words across all three-letter cues (i.e., 3 min), resulting in a below-average performance. Mrs. Smith also correctly named only 47/60 items on the Boston Naming Test (below-average performance), and the incorrect items included both high- and low-frequency test items. Her copy reconstruction of a Rey Complex Figure was very impaired. She did not appear to grasp the gestalt of the overall design, and her placement of details was poorly planned and organized.

Mrs. Smith's ability to repeat a string of digits forward was intact suggesting adequate simple attention. Her performance on a test of visual scanning and psychomotor speed (Trail Making Test, Part A) was moderately impaired. Though she successfully completed the practice trial of Trail Making Test, Part B, she became very confused on the test trial, which she was unable to complete, suggesting significant problems with cognitive flexibility. Similarly, she exhibited significant impairment on the Stroop interference

Table 19.4 Baseline and 12-month follow-up neuropsychological data for case example

Test	Baseline (raw)	12-month evaluation (raw)	Outcome
Attention			
WAIS III Digit Span	14	10	**Decline**
Executive function			
Trail Making B	Timed out[a]	Unable to complete due to confusion[b]	**Decline**
Clock	Unable to draw accurately	Concrete setting	Stable
WAIS III Digit Symbol	25[a]	27[a]	Stable
Psychomotor speed			
Trail Making A	77[a]	141[b]	**Decline**
WAIS III Symbol Search	12[a]	11[a]	Stable
Pegs dominant	145	155[b]	**Decline**
Pegs nondominant	123	133[a]	**Decline**
Activation/language			
Semantic fluency	17	17	Stable
Letter fluency	20[a]	16[b]	**Decline**
Boston Naming Test	47[a]	48[a]	Stable
Visuospatial			
Rey Copy	15.5[a]	18.5 (more disorganized)[a]	**Decline**
Memory			
HVLT-R learning	23	17[a]	**Decline**
HVLT-R delay	6	6	Stable
HVLT-R recognition	6[b]	9	**Improve**
BVMT-R learning	10[b]	16[a]	**Improve**
BVMT-R delay	3[b]	7	**Improve**
BVMTR recognition	100%	100%	Stable
WMS III LM I	40	36	Stable
WMS III LM II	26	24	Stable
Beck Depression	4	3	Stable

[a]Mild impairment
[b]Moderate impairment

test (i.e., a test of response inhibition). Mild to moderate difficulties were noted on tests of psychomotor speed and visual scanning (i.e., Digit Symbol and Symbol Search). When asked to construct a clock and set the hands to a specified time, she drew a clock with the numbers in the reverse order on two separate efforts. When a clock was drawn for her and she was then asked to set the hands of the clock to a specified time, she was unable to complete the task.

Psychomotor speed performance on the Grooved Pegboard Test was moderately impaired for the dominant (right) hand, but her performance on the nondominant (left) hand was stronger, with a score in the borderline normal range. Mrs. Smith's total score on the Beck Depression Inventory-II was not suggestive of current depressive symptoms.

Based on the comprehensive neuropsychological test results, clinical history, and neuroimaging data, the evaluation suggests that the etiology of cognitive difficulties is consistent with cerebrovascular disease. Based on this initial evaluation, diagnostically, it appeared that Mrs. Smith met criteria for mild cognitive impairment, single-domain (executive function).

Repeat Neuropsychological Evaluation

One year later, Mrs. Smith returned for a follow-up examination, which yielded little change in her neuropsychological profile. As evident in the data provided in Table 19.4, the predominant change in function was isolated to domains of executive function and processing speed. Performance on a test of learning efficiency mildly declined, but performance on a test of visual learning improved, and there was no decline on either test of verbal retention. Overall, the lack of decline in retention of newly learned information argues against a change in diagnostic formulation for this patient, suggesting that the original clinical diagnosis of a vascular etiology was accurate. Her MRI report dated 11 months after the first MRI revealed "Mild to moderate diffuse punctuate T2 and FLAIR hyperintensities within the left and right frontal parietal periventricular subcortical white matter and more confluent increased T2 and FLAIR signal within the left and right parietal periventricular white matter are again identified without change suggesting mild to moderate small vessel ischemic changes. There may be mild diffuse cortical atrophy with prominent sulci bilateral cerebral hemispheres."

Case Summary

The case above exemplifies several common issues in the evaluation of VCI. First, the patient's age and medical history places VCI high in the list of differential diagnoses. Second, the patient's own description of her medical history and vascular injuries was limited, and there was no available informant to corroborate the patient's history. Third, the neuropsychological pattern was fairly typical of a "subcortical" pattern with impairment in learning, executive function, and motor skills; however, performances were also low in other cognitive domains, such as language. Also, this patient performed poorly on the recognition trial of a verbal serial list learning test, but it is unlikely that such poor performance was due to an amnesic form of memory impairment, since the patient's score on the retention trial demonstrated no appreciable loss of information. Finally, her brain MRIs were congruent with her history and neuropsychological patterns.

Clinical Pearls

As a summary, there are a number of clinical guidelines to consider when evaluating older adults with cognitive difficulties that have possible VCI. We outline a few of these take-home messages below:

- The course of decline associated with VCI can be abrupt with stepwise decline or slow, insidious, and progressive, resembling the course for age-related neurodegenerative diseases, such as AD or frontotemporal dementia. The presence of an insidious course should not be used to differentiate between VCI and primary dementing disorders.
- The pattern of neuropsychological deficits associated with vascular burden is heterogeneous and dependent on the location of the cerebrovascular damage. Executive impairment may be dominant but not universal and not necessary for the diagnosis.
- Integration of structural brain MRI results is critical for the diagnosis of VCI.
- The progression of VCI can be influenced by healthy lifestyle interventions. Early diagnosis is critical.

References

1. O'Brien JT, Erkinjuntti T, Reisberg B, et al. Vascular cognitive impairment. Lancet Neurol. 2003;2:89–98.
2. Sadowski M, Pankiewicz J, Sholtzava H, et al. Links between the pathology of Alzheimer's disease and vascular dementia. Neurochem Res. 2004;29(6):1257–66.
3. Hachinski VC, Lliff D, Zihlka E, et al. Cerebral blood flow in dementia. Arch Neurol. 1975;32(9):632–7.
4. Wentzel C, Rockwood K, MacKnight C, et al. Progression of impairment in patients with vascular cognitive impairment without dementia. Neurology. 2001;57(4):714–6.
5. Williamson JB, Nyenhuis DL, Pedelty L, et al. Baseline differences between vascular cognitive impairment reverters and nonreverters. J Neurol Neurosurg Psychiatry. 2008;79(11):1208–14.
6. Williams M. Progress in Alzheimer's disease drug discovery: an update. Curr Opin Investig Drugs. 2009;10(1):23–34.
7. Ingles JL, Wentzel C, Fisk JD, Rockwood K. Neuropsychological predictors of incident dementia

in patients with vascular cognitive impairment, no dementia. Stroke. 2002;33:1999–2002.

8. Garrett KD, Browndyke JN, Whelihan W, Paul RH, DiCarlo M, Moser DJ, et al. The neuropsychological profile of vascular cognitive impairment—no dementia: comparisons to patients at risk for cerebrovascular disease and vascular dementia. Arch Clin Neuropsychol. 2004;19:745–57.
9. Nyenhuis DL, Gorelick PB, Geenen EJ, et al. The pattern of neuropsychological deficits in vascular cognitive impairment—no dementia (Vascular CIND). Clin Neuropsychol. 2004;18(1):41–9.
10. Jokinen H, Kalska H, Mantyla R, et al. Cognitive profile of subcortical ischaemic vascular disease. J Neurol Neurosurg Psychiatry. 2006;77:28–33.
11. Traykov L, Baudic S, Rauox N, et al. Patterns of memory impairment and perseverative behavior discriminate early Alzheimer's disease from subcortical vascular dementia. J Neurol Sci. 2005;229–230: 75–9.
12. Wallin A, Milos V, Sjogren M, Pantoni L, Erkinjuntti T. Classification and subtypes of vascular dementia. Int Psychogeriatr. 2003;15(1):27–37.
13. Robinson RG, Spalleta G. Poststroke depression: a review. Can J Psychiatry. 2010;55(6):341–9.
14. American Psychiatric Association Committee on Nomenclature and Statistics. Diagnostic and statistical manual of mental disorders (DSM-IV). 4th ed. Washington, DC: American Psychiatric Association; 1994.
15. Chui HC, Victoroff JI, Margolin D, Jagust W, Shankle R, Katzman R. Criteria for the diagnosis of ischemic vascular dementia proposed by the state of California Alzheimer's Disease Diagnostic and Treatment Centers. Neurology. 1992;42:473–80.
16. Roman GC, Tatemichi TK, Erkinjuntti T, et al. Vascular dementia: diagnostic criteria for research studies: report of the NINDS-AIREN International Workshop. Neurology. 1993;43:250–60.
17. Cosentino SA, Jefferson AL, Carey ME, et al. The clinical diagnosis of vascular dementia: a comparison among four classification systems and a proposal for a new paradigm. Clin Neuropsychol. 2004; 18(1):6–21.
18. Goldstein LB, Bushnell CD, Adams RJ, et al. Guidelines for the primary prevention of stroke: a guideline for healthcare professionals from the American Heart Association/American Stroke Association. Stroke. 2011;42:1–68.
19. Guidetti D, Casali B, Mazzei RL, Dotti MT. Cerebral autosomal dominant arteriopathy with subcortical infarcts and leukoencephalopathy. Clin Exp Hypertens. 2006;28:271–7.
20. Hajjar I, Sorond F, Hsu Y-H, Galica A, Cupples LA, Lipsitz LA. Renin angiotensin system gene polymorphisms and cerebral blood flow regulation: the MOBILIZE Boston study. Stroke. 2010;41:635–40.
21. Ogino A, Kazui H, Miyoshi N, et al. Cognitive impairment in patients with idiopathic normal pressure hydrocephalus. Dement Geriatr Cogn Disord. 2006;21(2):113–9.
22. Factora R, Luciano M. When to consider normal pressure hydrocephalus in the patient with gait disturbance. Geriatrics. 2008;63(2):32–7.
23. Paul R, Garrett K, Cohen R. Vascular dementia: a diagnostic conundrum for the clinical neuropsychologist. Appl Neuropsychol. 2003;10(3):129–36.
24. Chui H, Gontheir R. Natural history of vascular dementia. Alzheimer Dis Assoc Disord. 1999;13:S124–30.
25. O'Sullivan M, Morris RG, Markus HS. Brief cognitive assessment for patients with cerebral small vessel disease. J Neurol Neurosurg Psychiatry. 2005;76(8): 1140–5.
26. Pachet A, Astner K, Brown L. Clinical utility of the mini-mental status examination when assessing decision-making capacity. J Geriatr Psychiatry Neurol. 2010;23(1):3–8.
27. Nasreddine ZS, Phillips NA, Bédirian V, et al. The Montreal Cognitive Assessment, MoCA: a brief screening tool for mild cognitive impairment. J Am Geriatr Soc. 2005;53(4):695–9.
28. Hachinski V, Iadecola C, Petersen RC, et al. National Institute of Neurological Disorders and Stroke-Canadian Stroke Network vascular cognitive impairment harmonization standards. Stroke. 2006;37(9):2220–41.
29. Canning SJ, Leach L, Stuss D, Ngo L, Black SE. Diagnostic utility of abbreviated fluency measures in Alzheimer disease and vascular dementia. Neurology. 2004;62(4):556–62.
30. Henry JD, Crawford JR, Phillips LH. Verbal fluency performance in dementia of the Alzheimer's type: a meta-analysis. Neuropsychologia. 2004;42(9): 1212–22.
31. Jefferson AL, Cahn-Weiner D, Boyle P, Paul RH, Gordon N, Moser D, Cohen RA. Cognitive predictors of changes in activities of daily living among patients with vascular dementia. Int J Geriatr Psychiatry. 2006;21(8):752–4.
32. Jefferson AL, Paul RH, Ozonoff A, Cohen RA. Evaluating elements of executive functioning as predictors of instrumental activities of daily living (IADLs). Arch Clin Neuropsychol. 2006;21(4): 311–20.
33. De Coene B, Hajnal JV, Gatehouse P, et al. MR of the brain using fluid-attenuated inversion recovery (FLAIR) pulse sequences. Am J Neuroradiol. 1992;13(6):1555–64.
34. Kamada K, Kakeda S, Ohnari N, Moriya J, Sato T, Korogi Y. Signal intensity of motor and sensory cortices on T2-weighted and FLAIR images: intraindividual comparison of 1.5T and 3T MRI. Eur Radiol. 2008;18(12):2949–55. Epub 2008 Jul 19.
35. Stankiewicz JM, Glanz BI, Healy BC, et al. Brain MRI lesion load at 1.5T and 3T versus clinical status in multiple sclerosis. J Neuroimaging. 2011;21(2): e50–6.
36. Price CC, Jefferson AL, Merino JG, Heilman KM, Libon DJ. Subcortical vascular dementia: integrating

neuropsychological and neuroradiological data. Neurology. 2005;65(3):376–82.
37. Boone KB, Miller BL, Lesser IM, et al. Neuropsychological correlates of white matter lesions in healthy elderly subjects: a threshold effect. Arch Neurol. 1992;49:549–54.
38. Seno H, Ishino H, Inagaki T, Yamamori C, Miyaoaka T. Comparison between multiple lacunar infarcted patients with and without dementia in nursing homes in shimane prefecture, Japan. Dement Geriatr Cogn Disord. 2000;11:161–5.

Assessment in Acute Stroke Rehabilitation*

20

George M. Cuesta

Abstract

Stroke is the third leading cause of death in the United States, preceded by cancer and heart disease. Stroke is the primary cause of adult disability in the USA according to the Centers for Disease Control and Prevention, and stroke survivors represent the largest diagnostic category of referrals to rehabilitation hospitals. Neuropsychologists who work in acute stroke rehabilitation settings require a broad range of skills. They must be knowledgeable and competent in neuropsychology, rehabilitation psychology, and health psychology in order to provide effective assistance to their three principal constituencies: stroke patients, their family caregivers, and the stroke rehabilitation treatment team. Neuropsychologists assist these constituencies by managing the physical, cognitive, behavioral, emotional, social, sexual, and vocational consequences of stroke. This chapter provides a primer on stroke and suggestions are provided for effective neuropsychological practice in the acute rehabilitation hospital setting.

Keywords

Acute stroke • Cerebrovascular disease • Rehabilitation • Recovery • Cognitive remediation

*The views expressed in this chapter are those of the author and do not reflect the official policy of the Department of Veterans Affairs or the US Government.

G.M. Cuesta, Ph.D. (✉)
United States Department of Veterans Affairs,
Manhattan Vet Center, Readjustment Counseling Service,
Veterans Health Administration, 32 Broadway, Suite 200,
Manhattan, NY 10004, USA
e-mail: george.cuesta@va.gov

L.D. Ravdin and H.L. Katzen (eds.), *Handbook on the Neuropsychology of Aging and Dementia*, Clinical Handbooks in Neuropsychology, DOI 10.1007/978-1-4614-3106-0_20,

Stroke is the third leading cause of death in the United States, preceded by cancer and heart disease. As of December 31, 2009, there were an estimated 616,067 deaths due to heart disease and 562,875 deaths due to cancer in the USA; the death toll for stroke (cerebrovascular disease) was 135,952 (Centers for Disease Control and Prevention, CDC/National Center for Health Statistics). Stroke is the primary cause of adult disability in the USA according to the Centers for Disease Control and Prevention, and stroke survivors represent the largest diagnostic category of referrals to rehabilitation hospitals [1]. As a consequence of the accelerated aging of the US population, stroke will remain a public health problem with adverse personal, societal, and economic implications. According to Caplan, rehabilitation services for stroke patients are typically provided to those in the middle range of impairment [2]. While those with milder strokes are frequently discharged directly to home with outpatient therapy or home care, those with more severe strokes who cannot tolerate inpatient rehabilitation are discharged to a long-term care facility with limited rehabilitation therapy services.

Introduction and Brief Literature Review

Stroke is the third leading cause of death in the USA, preceded by cancer and heart disease. As of December 31, 2009, there were an estimated 616,067 deaths due to heart disease and 562,875 deaths due to cancer in the USA; the death toll for stroke (cerebrovascular disease) was 135,952 (Centers for Disease Control and Prevention, CDC/National Center for Health Statistics). Stroke is the primary cause of adult disability in the USA according to the Centers for Disease Control and Prevention, and stroke survivors represent the largest diagnostic category of referrals to rehabilitation hospitals [1]. As a consequence of the accelerated aging of the US population, stroke will remain a public health problem with adverse personal, societal, and economic implications. According to Caplan [2], rehabilitation services for stroke patients are typically provided to those in the middle range of impairment. While those with milder strokes are frequently discharged directly to home with outpatient therapy or home care, those with more severe strokes who cannot tolerate inpatient rehabilitation are discharged to a long-term care facility with limited rehabilitation therapy services.

Neuropsychologists who work in acute stroke rehabilitation settings will find that providing assessment and intervention to this patient population demands a broad range of skills. They must be knowledgeable and competent in neuropsychology, rehabilitation psychology, and health psychology in order to provide effective assistance to their three principal constituencies: stroke patients, their family caregivers, and the stroke rehabilitation treatment team. Neuropsychologists assist these constituencies by managing the physical, cognitive, behavioral, emotional, social, sexual, and vocational consequences of stroke.

Prevalence

An estimated 6,400,000 Americans, 20 years of age and older, have had a stroke (extrapolated to 2006 using National Center for Health Statistics/National Health and Nutrition Examination Survey 2003–2006 data). Overall stroke prevalence during the period from 2003 to 2006 was estimated at 2.9% [3]. According to data from the 2005 Behavioral Risk Factor Surveillance System of the Centers for Disease Control and Prevention, 2.7% of men and 2.5% of women age 18 and greater had a history of stroke. Among these, 2.3% were non-Hispanic white, 4.0% were non-Hispanic black, 1.6% Asian/Pacific Islanders, 2.6% were Hispanic of any race, 6.0% were Native American Indian/Alaska Native, and 4.6% were admixed [4].

Incidence

On average, every 40 seconds, someone in the USA has a stroke. In the USA alone, more than

700,000 people suffer a stroke each year, and about 2/3 of these individuals survive and require rehabilitation [5]. The most recent data from the Heart Disease and Stroke Statistics 2010 Update, a report from the American Heart Association [6], indicated that each year, about 795,000 people experience a new or recurrent stroke. About 610,000 of these are first attacks, and 185,000 are recurrent attacks. The age-adjusted incidence of first ischemic stroke per 100,000 was 88 in whites, 191 in blacks, and 149 in Hispanics, according to the data from the Northern Manhattan Study [7]. The stroke incidence rate is higher for men compared with women at younger ages but not at older ages. The male-to-female incidence ratio was 1.25 in those 55–64 years of age, 1.50 in those 65–74 years of age, 1.07 in those 75–84 years of age, and 0.76 in those 85 years of age or greater [6].

On average, every four minutes, someone dies of a stroke. Mortality data from 2006 indicated that stroke accounted for approximately 1 of every 18 deaths in the USA. In the decade from 1996 to 2006, the stroke death rate fell 33.5%, and the actual number of stroke deaths declined to 18.4%. More women than men die of stroke each year due to the larger number of elderly women. Women accounted for 60.6% of stroke deaths in the USA in 2006. The 2006 overall death rate for stroke was 43.6 per 100,000. Death rates were 41.7 for white males, 67.1 for black males, 41.1 for white females, and 57.0 for black females [8].

Prognosis

In 2009, there were 135,952 Americans who died as a result of stroke. However, mortality rates are declining. During the first year, over 75% of patients survive a first stroke and over half survive beyond 5 years [9]. Those patients who suffer ischemic strokes have a much better chance of survival than those with hemorrhagic strokes. Among the ischemic stroke categories, embolic strokes pose the greatest threat to survival, followed by thrombotic and lacunar strokes. Hemorrhagic strokes destroy brain cells and pose other threats to survival like increased pressure on the brain or spasms in the blood vessels; both of these conditions can be very dangerous for the patient. However, studies suggest that those patients with hemorrhagic stroke have a greater chance for recovering function than those patients with ischemic stroke [10].

It is estimated that between 50% and 70% of patients recover functional independence after a stroke. However, between 15% and 30% of patients who survive either an ischemic or hemorrhagic stroke remain with some permanent disability [10]. The National Institutes of Health (NIH) devised a scoring system that helps predict stroke severity and outcome by scoring the following 11 factors: levels of consciousness, gaze, visual fields, facial movement, motor functions in the upper and lower extremities, coordination, sensory loss, problems with language, inability to articulate, and attention. In addition to use of the NIH Stroke Scale (NIHSS), described above, measurement of brain injury using magnetic resonance imaging (MRI) and time (in hours) since onset of stroke symptoms to the time of the MRI brain scan are two additional factors used to predict stroke severity and outcome [10]. Up to 70% of patients with ischemic strokes who score less than 10 on the NIHSS have favorable outcome after 1 year. Only between 4% and 16% of patients have favorable outcome if their NIHSS score is more than 20 [10].

One question neuropsychologists frequently get from stroke patients and their families is, "What are my chances of having another stroke?" The literature points out that the risk for recurrent stroke is highest within the first few weeks and months. Risk for recurrent stroke is approximately 14% in the first year and about 5% thereafter. Specific risk factors for early recurrence include the following: older age, evidence of blocked arteries (i.e., history of coronary artery disease, peripheral artery disease, ischemic stroke, or transient ischemic attack), hemorrhagic or embolic stroke, diabetes, alcoholism, valvular heart disease, and atrial fibrillation [10]. When patients and their families are being educated about stroke recurrence, neuropsychologists can emphasize that preventive measures be instituted as soon as possible. These measures include encouraging patient compliance with medication for hypertension, hypercholesterolemia, diabetes, and heart disease. Preventive measures also include encouraging the patient to make and maintain lifestyle choices like quitting smoking, reducing alcohol consumption, eating a more healthy diet, and getting more aerobic exercise. However, these behaviors are more challenging to change and some may be physically impossible (e.g., exercise) for some patients to change after a devastating stroke.

Definition of Stroke

A *stroke* occurs when brain cells die as a consequence of inadequate blood perfusion. When blood flow is interrupted, brain cells are robbed of vital supplies of oxygen and nutrients. Approximately 80% of strokes are caused by blockage of an artery in the neck or brain. These are referred to as *ischemic strokes*. In ischemic strokes, blood flow is insufficient to maintain neurologic function, and infarction occurs when ischemia reaches a threshold to produce cell death. The remaining 20% of strokes are caused by a blood vessel that bursts in the brain and causes bleeding into or around the brain. These are called *hemorrhagic strokes*. A *transient ischemic attack* is an acute transient neurological deficit that typically lasts less than 1 hour and is without persistent neurological abnormality or evidence of acute infarction on neuroimaging [11]. A *silent stroke* is a brain injury of vascular origin that is appreciated on neuroimaging but is not associated with symptoms. Silent strokes are frequently found during diagnostic neuroimaging of an acute stroke in patients with no known history of a prior stroke. A *lacunar infarct* is a small cavity caused by a small deep cerebral infarct and is most often associated with arterial hypertension. These appear predominantly in the basal ganglia, thalamus, and white matter of the internal capsule and the pons [11].

Risk Factors

Some risk factors for stroke are modifiable (e.g., hypertension, diabetes mellitus, atrial fibrillation, alcohol use, smoking) and are subject to external control by changes in lifestyle. Manipulation of modifiable risk factors may have dramatic effects on the incidence, prevalence, economic effects, and personal costs of stroke. Devasenapathy and Hachinski [12] asserted that up to 75% of all strokes are preventable. Other researchers have asserted that nearly 379,000 strokes could be prevented each year through treatment of atrial fibrillation, cigarette smoking, hypertension, heavy alcohol consumption, and physical inactivity [13].

However, some of the risk factors for stroke are not modifiable. These include prior stroke, age, gender, race, ethnicity, and heredity. Stroke risk increases with age. For example, the lifetime risk for stroke in adults over the age of 55 is greater than 1 in 6 and doubles with each successive decade after age 55 [14].

Clinical Signs and Symptoms of Stroke

In general, onset of stroke symptoms is acute. According to the National Institute of Neurological Disorders and Stroke (NINDS), common presenting neurological symptoms include [15]:

1. Sudden numbness or weakness of the face, arm, or leg on one side of the body,
2. Sudden confusion, trouble speaking, or understanding,
3. Sudden trouble seeing in one or both eyes,
4. Sudden trouble walking, dizziness, and loss of balance or coordination, and
5. Sudden severe headache with no known cause.

Pathophysiology

There are many different types of strokes, each having a different cause. The two main types of stroke are *ischemic* stroke and *hemorrhagic* stroke. The following is a basic description of these stroke types and the four most common causes of stroke (two of which are ischemic and two of which are hemorrhagic). For a more detailed description of the pathophysiology of stroke, the interested reader is referred to Barnett et al. [16].

The pathophysiology of *ischemic* strokes is widely known. They are the most common type of stroke, contributing to more than 80% of all stroke cases. They are caused by plaque buildup and blood clots that subsequently deprive parts of the brain from adequate perfusion or blood flow, oxygen, and nutrients; this results in damage and death of brain cells, tissue, and stroke. There are many factors that affect the buildup of a blood clot that results in stroke. The most common cause of ischemia and the infarction that follows it is *atherosclerosis,* a noninflammatory progressive disease that begins in childhood, peaks between the ages of 50 and 70, and can affect any artery in the body. Fatty deposits accumulate on the arterial wall. These deposits produce a *thrombus* that over time gradually narrows the arterial passage until the blood vessel becomes sufficiently occluded to produce a stroke. Permanent damage generally ensues with complete deprivation of blood flow beyond several minutes [2]. The likelihood of a stroke is largely affected by several factors including age, family history, systolic blood pressure, smoking, alcohol use/abuse, diet, myocardial disease, diabetes, and atrial fibrillation. Of these, age and systolic blood pressure are the most influential factors in ischemic strokes.

Another type of ischemic event is the *lacunar stroke* that occurs when small penetrating branches of the major cerebral arteries become clogged and result in a thrombotic infarction. These types of strokes frequently affect the basal ganglia, internal capsule, thalamus, and the pons. Location-specific syndromes can result from lacunar infarcts. These include pure motor or sensory stroke, dysarthric stroke, and hemiparesis with ataxia [2].

The *embolic stroke* is produced by an abrupt interruption of blood supply by pieces of thrombus that have broken loose from one part of the blood vessel system and later lodged in a narrower vessel downstream. This type of stroke mechanism causes rapid focal onset symptoms with little opportunity for compensation by collateral blood supply routes [2, 16].

Hemorrhagic strokes are caused by a blood vessel that bursts either within the brain or just outside it. These strokes frequently result in dramatic onset of symptoms. Hemorrhagic strokes are typically classified according to the anatomical location of the bleeding. The main causes of hemorrhagic strokes are systolic blood pressure, age, and anticoagulation. High blood pressure is the main cause of both hemorrhagic and ischemic strokes. Less common causes include cranial trauma, tumors, hypertensive hemorrhages, and vasculitides, all of which lead to accumulation of blood around the brain causing hemorrhagic stroke.

The third most common cause of stroke after thrombotic and embolic strokes is the *primary intracerebral hemorrhage.* This hemorrhagic stroke results from degeneration and rupture of a penetrating cerebral artery, often due to hypertension. The blood rarely reaches the surface of the cortex but enters the cerebrospinal fluid in about 90% of the cases. Significant compression of the brain stem structures can be fatal [2, 16].

The fourth most common cause of stroke is the *subarachnoid hemorrhage* (SAH). This hemorrhagic stroke results from rupture of a saccular aneurysm. An aneurysm is a ballooning of an arterial wall due to congenital weakness in its structure. The ballooning further weakens the blood vessel's arterial wall, making it prone to rupture and hemorrhage. In this type of hemorrhagic stroke, blood leaks into the subarachnoid space between the external surface of the brain and the arachnoid meningeal layer. This type of stroke announces itself in an acute or gradual manner depending on the size of the affected blood vessel and the rupture itself. When onset is rapid, the consequences are often severe and life-threatening. The patient complains of a sudden and severe headache, and intracranial pressure dramatically elevates as a consequence of the injection of blood into the brain from the ruptured vessel [2, 16].

Table 20.1 Most common symptoms and signs of stroke and their reliability [17]

Symptom or sign	Prevalence (%) [18]	Agreement among examiners (Kappa*) [19]
Symptoms		
Acute onset	96	Good (0.63) [19]
Subjective arm weakness[b]	63	Moderate (0.59) [19]
Subjective leg weakness[b]	54	Moderate (0.59) [19]
Self-reported speech disturbance	53	Good (0.64) [19]
Subjective facial weakness	23	–
Arm paresthesia[c]	20	Good (0.62) [19]
Leg paresthesia[c]	17	Good (0.62) [19]
Headache	14	Good (0.65) [19]
Nonorthostatic dizziness	13	–
Signs		
Arm paresis	69	Moderate to excellent (0.42–1.00) [19, 20]
Leg paresis	61	Fair to excellent (0.40–0.84) [19, 20]
Dysphasia or dysarthria	57	Moderate to excellent (0.54–0.84) [19, 20]
		Fair to excellent (0.29–1.00) [19, 20]
Hemiparetic or ataxic gait	53	Excellent (0.91) [20]
Facial paresis	45	Poor to excellent (0.13–1.00) [19, 20]
Eye movement abnormality	27	Fair to excellent (0.33–1.00) [20]
Visual field defect	24	Poor to excellent (0.16–0.81) [19, 20]

[a]Kappa statistic: 0–0.20 = poor agreement; 0.21–0.40 = fair agreement; 0.41–0.60 = moderate agreement; 0.61–0.80 = good agreement; 0.81–1.00 = excellent agreement
[b]Noted as "loss of power" [17]
[c]Noted as "loss of sensation" [17]
Information from references [18–20]

Diagnosis of Stroke

In general, diagnosis of stroke is beyond a neuropsychologist's scope of practice; nevertheless, knowing the decision-making process whereby physicians make a stroke diagnosis can richly inform neuropsychological practice. According to Yew and Cheng [17], the history and physical examination remain the pillars of diagnosing stroke. The most common *historical feature* of an ischemic stroke is acute onset; the most common *physical findings* of ischemic stroke are focal weakness and speech disturbance [18]. The most common and reliable *signs and symptoms* of ischemic stroke are listed in Table 20.1 [17–20]. In a community-based study of diagnostic accuracy, primary care physicians practicing in an emergency setting had 92% sensitivity for diagnosis of transient ischemic attack (TIA) and stroke [21].

Physicians must quickly assess persons with suspected acute ischemic stroke because acute stroke therapies (i.e., thrombolysis) have a narrow time window of effectiveness. One instrument that can assist the physician with rapid diagnosis of stroke is The National Institute of Health Stroke Scale (NIHSS) [22, 23]. The NIHSS is available at http://www.ninds.nih.gov/doctors/NIH_Stroke_Scale.pdf. This scale was designed to be completed within 5–8 min.

The physician must determine the exact time of symptom onset since it is critical for determining eligibility for thrombolysis. However, one community-based study found that clinicians agreed, to the minute, less than 50% of the time [19]. Corroboration time of symptom onset with a known event or from a witness to the symptoms may help to improve this estimate.

Neuroimaging must be completed in order to reliably distinguish between ischemic stroke and intracerebral hemorrhage. Both are characterized by acute onset of focal symptoms. However, patients with intracerebral hemorrhage typically have gradual worsening of symptoms after the abrupt onset. These worsening symptoms reflect the increasing size of the hematoma. Intracerebral hemorrhagic patients may also have decreased level of consciousness.

The primary purpose of neuroimaging in a patient with suspected ischemic stroke is to rule out the presence of other types of central nervous system lesions and to distinguish between ischemic and hemorrhagic stroke. Figure 20.1 provides examples of intracerebral and subarachnoid hemorrhages on computed tomography (CT) scans. CT scans are considered to be sufficiently sensitive at detecting mass lesions (e.g., brain masses or abscesses) as well as detection of acute hemorrhages. They may not, however, be sensitive enough to detect ischemic stroke, especially when the stroke is small, acute, or in the posterior fossa (e.g., brain stem and cerebellum areas) [17, 24]. The purpose of CT scan is to rule out stroke mimics and to detect hemorrhage, however, not to rule in a diagnosis of ischemic stroke. A normal CT scan of the brain does not rule out the diagnosis of ischemic stroke. Multimodal magnetic resonance imaging (MRI) sequences, especially diffusion-weighted imaging, have better resolution than CT and, therefore, have better sensitivity for detecting acute ischemic stroke. Figure 20.2 is a dramatic illustration of this point.

Patients with subarachnoid hemorrhage present differently from intracerebral and ischemic stroke patients. The most common symptom described by the patient is having "the worst headache of my life." According to Suarez et al. [25], other symptoms may include vomiting, seizures, meningismus, and decreased level of consciousness. These patients may not exhibit focal signs given that bleeding occurs outside the brain. An exception to this is when an aneurysm bursts and bleeds into a focal location (e.g., a posterior communicating artery aneurysm that compresses the third cranial nerve).

Current guidelines for classification of early stroke severity recommend the use of the NIHSS [22]; however, no trial data currently exists that demonstrates that its use improves outcomes. It is one of the most common classification tools available and provides a structured neurological examination that has both diagnostic and prognostic values [22]. Yew and Cheng [17] suggested

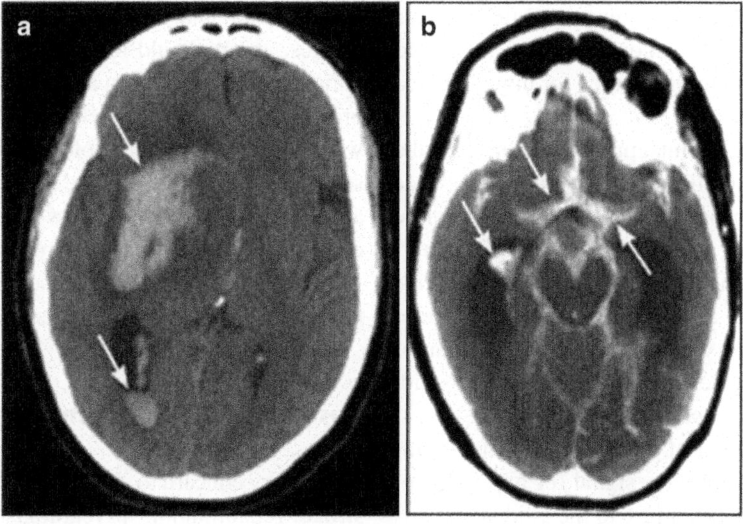

Fig. 20.1 Head computed tomography (CT) scans showing (**a**) intracerebral hemorrhages (*arrows*) and (**b**) subarachnoid hemorrhages (*arrows*). Note that acute hemorrhage appears hyperdense (*white*) on a CT scan

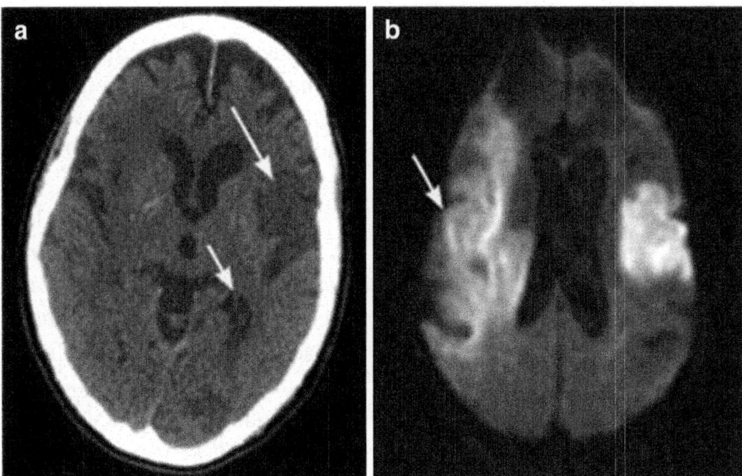

Fig. 20.2 (**a**) Noncontrast computed tomography (CT) scan showing two hypodense regions indicating old infarctions in the distribution of the left-middle cerebral (*long arrow*) and posterior cerebral arteries (*short arrow*). (**b**) Diffusion-weighted magnetic resonance imaging scan obtained shortly after the CT reveals a new extensive infarction (*arrow*) in the right-middle cerebral artery distribution not evident on the CT. Reprinted with permission from MedPix®. Retrieved from http://rad.usuhs.edu/medpix

that, in general, combinations of signs and symptoms are more useful than any single finding. These authors presented a helpful algorithm derived from several consensus sources for the diagnosis of stroke (see Fig. 20.3).

The Internet Stroke Center [27] has an excellent summary of the computed tomography (CT) and magnetic resonance imaging (MRI) criteria for infarction and hemorrhage; the interested reader is referred to that source for more detailed information.

Briefly, in CT imaging of *infarction*, the neuroradiologist will find a focal *hypodense* area in cortical, subcortical, or deep gray or white matter, following the vascular territory or watershed distribution. CT imaging of *hemorrhage* will demonstrate a *hyperdense* image in white or deep gray matter, with or without involvement of the cortical surface. Hematoma refers to a solid, homogeneously *hyperdense* image [27].

In MRI imaging of an acute stroke, the clinician will find subtle low signal (or hypointense) on T1 imaging. According to the guidelines, this is often difficult to see at this stage. There is high signal (or hyperintense) on spin density or T2-weighted and proton density-weighted images starting about 8 hours after onset, and it should follow vascular distribution. Mass effect is usually maximal at about 24 hours and starts about 2 hours after onset even in the absence of parenchymal signal changes. In subacute stroke, defined as 1 week or older, there is low signal on T1-weighted and high signal on T2-weighted images, and it should follow the vascular distribution. Revascularization and blood–brain barrier breakdown may cause parenchymal enhancement with contrast agents. In old stroke, defined as several weeks to years, there is low signal on T1 and high signal on T2. Mass effect disappears usually after one month. There is loss of tissue with large infarcts, and parenchymal enhancement fades after several months [27].

Poststroke Cognitive Impairment

Of primary concern to stroke neuropsychologists, stroke rehabilitation psychologists, and other stroke rehabilitation specialists is the evaluation of cognitive impairment resulting from stroke.

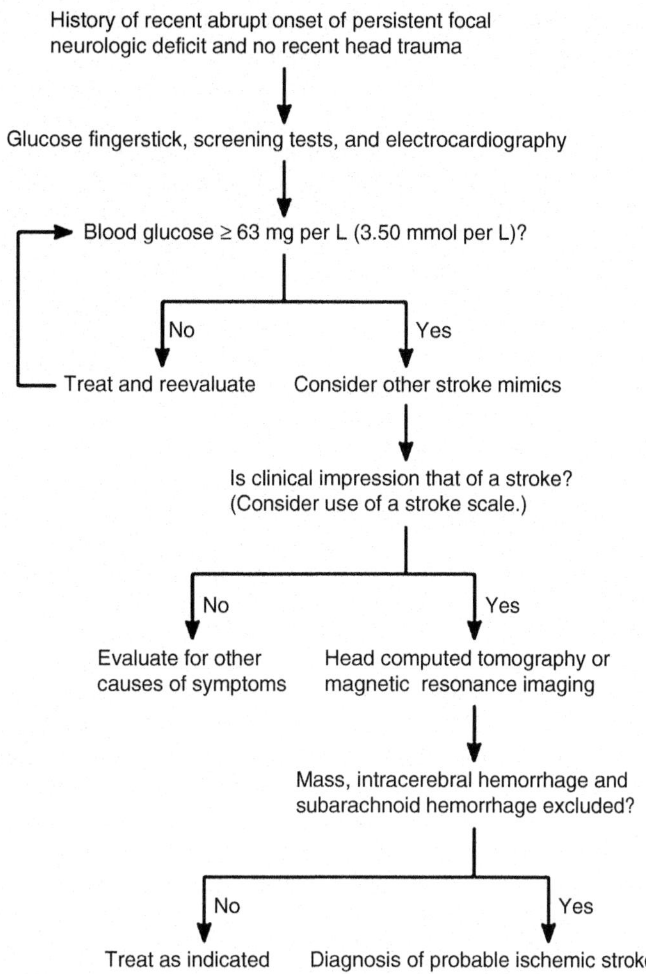

Fig. 20.3 Algorithm for the diagnosis of acute stroke. Information from references [19, 22, 26]

Up to 64% of persons who have a stroke will have some degree of cognitive impairment [28] with up to a third developing frank dementia [29–31]. Cognitive impairment that is caused by or associated with vascular factors has been called vascular cognitive impairment or VCI [32–34].

Prior to 2006, there were no commonly agreed upon standards for identifying and describing stroke patients with cognitive impairments, particularly in the early stages, and especially with cognitive impairment related to vascular factors, or vascular cognitive impairment. In 2006, the National Institute for Neurological Disorders and Stroke (NINDS) and the Canadian Stroke Network (CSN) convened researchers in clinical diagnosis, epidemiology, neuropsychology, brain imaging, neuropathology, experimental models, biomarkers, genetics, and clinical trials to recommend minimum, common, clinical, and research standards for the description and study of vascular cognitive impairment [35]. The Neuropsychology Working Group of this convention was charged with recommending test protocols that could be used in multicenter investigations of potential patients with vascular cognitive impairment (VCI). Three different protocols were developed by the Neuropsychology Working Group to serve three different purposes. One protocol required about 60-minutes of administration time, the second required about 30-minutes, and the third required only 5-minutes of administration time. The 60-minutes protocol was developed for use in research studies. The 30- and 5-minutes protocols were developed with clinical purposes in mind and will be further explained in the next section on Neuropsychological Assessment Techniques. The interested reader is referred to the Hachinski et al. [35] journal article for more detailed information.

Neuropsychological Assessment Techniques and Issues

Diagnosis of acute ischemic stroke is often straightforward. The sudden onset of a focal neurologic deficit in a recognizable vascular distribution with a common presentation, i.e., hemiparesis, facial weakness, and aphasia, identifies a common syndrome of acute stroke. However, there are differential diagnostic problems because there are several subtypes of stroke, and some nonvascular disorders may have clinical pictures that appear identical to strokes. Table 20.2 provides a listing of common conditions that should be considered in the differential diagnosis of stroke as delineated by the Internet Stroke Center.

In an acute rehabilitation setting, by the time the patient arrives at the hospital, the diagnosis of stroke has usually been well established. Typically, the stroke event occurred in the community while the patient was going about his normal everyday activities. The patient is taken to an acute care hospital where diagnosis is made by an emergency room physician or a stroke team, where available, and the patient is medically stabilized. In consultation with the stroke team, a determination is made by family caregivers about whether the patient can manage the significant intensive intervention of an acute rehabilitation program. The patient is transferred to the acute rehabilitation hospital to begin orientation, assessment, and treatment intervention from a team of multidisciplinary professionals. The team typically includes a neurologist or physiatrist, nurses and nursing aides, social workers, occupational therapists, physical therapists, speech and language pathologists, recreational therapists, and a neuropsychologist.

Table 20.2 Differential diagnosis of stroke

Differential diagnosis of stroke
Ischemic stroke
Hemorrhagic stroke
Craniocerebral/cervical trauma
Meningitis/encephalitis
Intracranial mass
Tumor Subdural hematoma
Seizure with persistent neurological signs
Migraine with persistent neurological signs
Metabolic
Hyperglycemia (nonketotic hyperosmolar coma) Hypoglycemia Post-cardiac arrest ischemia Drug/narcotic overdose

Source: American Heart Association. Basic Life Support for Healthcare Providers and Advanced Cardiac Life Support

From: Acute Ischemic Stroke: New Concepts of Care

From the day of admission, frequent anxiety-provoking concerns for family members/caregivers, rehabilitation team members, and clinicians are discharge planning and where the patient will go after they complete the trial of acute rehabilitation. Alternatives include short-term subacute rehabilitation (usually in long-term care facilities), home with homecare services, home with daycare services, or home with outpatient care. Ideally, all of these alternatives share in common varying degrees of frequency and intensity of occupational therapy, physical therapy, and speech therapy. The answer to the discharge placement question depends on the severity of the functional limitations (e.g., physical, cognitive, behavioral) produced by the stroke, the amount of functional recovery the patient makes during acute rehabilitation, and the resources (i.e., time, financial, emotional) available to the family. Neuropsychologists working in an acute rehabilitation setting are frequently consulted to evaluate the cognitive and behavioral limitations of stroke patients.

Common referral questions for the neuropsychologist working with stroke patients in the acute rehabilitation setting include:

1. Determining the cognitive strengths and weaknesses of the patient,
2. Determining capacity to consent to treatment,
3. Consultation regarding behavioral problems, e.g., agitation, aggression, apathy.

Cognitive Assessment

Regarding determination of cognitive strengths and weaknesses, family members and clinicians are frequently concerned about the patient's ability to manage activities of daily living and instrumental activities of daily living at home. The neuropsychologist can provide the rehabilitation team and the patient's caregivers with information from neuropsychological testing about the cognitive abilities that have been spared and the problem areas that remain. Rarely are these cognitive difficulties unaccompanied by behavioral issues. For example, a stroke patient may have impaired attention on neuropsychological testing that may be accounted for by destruction of attention pathways in the brain and exacerbated by the presence of poststroke depression. The neuropsychologist can use any and every source of information available to determine impairments and strengths. Properly administered, scored, and interpreted neuropsychological testing provides valid and reliable quantifiable information. In an acute rehabilitation setting, the neuropsychologist can observe the patient in occupational therapy during a cooking task or a dressing task and make inferences about the patient's attention and memory functioning based upon these observations. Information from these observations can augment neuropsychological testing results. When these observations are consistent with neuropsychological testing results, they add to the ecological validity of the data.

Whenever possible, the neuropsychologist should, first, gather the facts about the stroke patient by reviewing his medical chart and obtain feedback about cognition and behavior from the stroke rehabilitation team and from family caregivers. Additional key information to gather from collateral sources (e.g., family caregivers) includes a history of the patient's premorbid level of functioning (e.g., occupation, education, social support, temperament). Initially, a short visit with the patient might be helpful; in this visit, the neuropsychologist introduces himself, explains the reason for the visit, begins to build rapport, elicits the patient's informed consent for evaluation, and books a time to meet. The evaluation has already begun since the visit provides the opportunity for the neuropsychologist to start gathering preliminary information about the stroke patient's behavior, cognition, abilities, and challenges.

When selecting the instruments he will use, the neuropsychologist takes care to consider the stroke patient's obvious impairments, e.g., right or left hemiparesis/plegia, right or left hemineglect/inattention, and receptive/expressive aphasia. Other patient conditions to be aware of, that can affect cognitive performance, are the patient's energy level and presence of depression.

For the stroke patient unencumbered by aphasia with sufficient energy to withstand about 30 min of sustained cognitive activity, a standard neuropsychological screening assessment can include brief history taking and neuropsychological testing measures such as the one recommended by the Neuropsychology Working Group in Hachinski et al. [35]. The 30-min protocol suggested by the Neuropsychology Working Group included the following neuropsychological test battery: semantic and phonemic fluency [36], Digit Symbol-Coding [37], and the revised Hopkins Verbal Learning Test [38], in addition to the Center for Epidemiologic Studies-Depression Scale (CES-D) developed by the National Institute of Mental Health [39] and Neuropsychiatric Inventory [40]. The Trail Making Test A and B [41] and the Mini Mental State Examination (MMSE) [42] can supplement the battery.

When time is short or the patient is encumbered with decreased energy or short attention span, the neuropsychologist can use the 5-min protocol recommended by the Neuropsychology Working Group in Hachinski et al. [35]. The protocol consists of selected subtests from the Montreal

Cognitive Assessment. This test is available with instructions in 34 different languages and normative data at www.mocatest.org (MoCA) [43]. It includes a five-word immediate and delayed memory test, a six-item orientation task, and a one-letter phonemic fluency test (the letter F). The MoCA may be used without permission, free of charge, for clinical or educational noncommercial purposes (Copyright Ziad Nasreddine, MD).

Medical test results (e.g., computed tomography or magnetic resonance imaging of the brain) are often included in the history and physical report completed by the attending neurologist or physical medicine and rehabilitation physician upon the patient's admission to the acute rehabilitation hospital. These results can be easily included in the neuropsychologist's initial report with reference to their source. Since diagnosis is typically already made by the attending physician, the neuropsychologist can focus on developing hypotheses about patterns of deficits and how they may manifest. Consequently, neuropsychological assessment results can either confirm or refute these hypotheses. These conclusions and, more importantly, their functional implications can be discussed in team meetings and recorded in the patient's evaluation reports.

Family members are a valuable source of information about the patient's premorbid (pre-stroke) functioning. Neuropsychologists can obtain information from reliable family members about the patient's social, academic, and occupational functioning. This information provides the neuropsychologist with a basis of comparison for their current functioning. It is suggested that the neuropsychologist integrate this information into the neuropsychological testing report. A portion of the history section of the report can be devoted to the patient's premorbid functioning with appropriate references.

Capacity Assessment

In acute rehabilitation settings, occasionally, there will be patients who refuse to be treated or insist on going home, i.e., leave the hospital against medical advice. These patients might be depressed, frightened, or confused or might possess characterological features that account for their behavior. Another variable for the neuropsychologist to consider is the energy level of the patient. Acute rehabilitation programs typically require 3 hours a day of occupational therapy and physical therapy. On top of this requirement is about 45–60 minutes of speech therapy. Add to this intense schedule recreational therapy programs, nursing care, meals, visits from the neuropsychologist, and family and friend visits, and you have a regimen that can be very taxing for some patients who are already significantly physically and emotionally compromised by the stroke.

Treatment refusal and the desire to leave the hospital create stress not only for the treatment team but also for the family caregivers who typically want the patient to remain in the acute rehabilitation hospital for treatment. In these cases, the attending neurologist or physiatrist will often request a consult from the neuropsychologist to determine if the patient has the capacity to make treatment decisions for himself or herself. Determining capacity to make treatment decisions can have the beneficial effect of respecting the autonomy of the patient, logically seeking a solution, and documenting the reasonable action taken in response to the problem. The details of how to conduct a formal capacity evaluation go beyond the scope of this chapter but in general include a careful review of the entire available medical record, a directed clinical interview with the patient, or use of formal, structured assessment tools like the Aid to Capacity Evaluation (ACE) [44] and the MacArthur Competence Assessment Tool (MacCAT) [45]. Grisso and Appelbaum [45] developed an excellent formal structured assessment tool to evaluate capacity, and the reader is referred to that source for more detailed information.

In cases where it is determined that the patient has the capacity to make decisions for himself and persists in their desire to leave hospital, then the rehabilitation team will have few options but to concede to these wishes even though it is thought by the team that continued treatment will be in the best interest of the patient. In an acute rehabilitation setting, this usually means the patient leaves the hospital against medical advice or due to lack of motivation for treatment is discharged to home or subacute treatment. In order to increase safety, the neuropsychologist can join with the attending physician, the social worker, and nursing staff in providing the patient and the family caregivers with education about safety in the home, prohibiting driving and use of other mechanical equipment, medication administration/compliance, and prohibiting consumption of alcohol and other illicit drugs. The stroke rehabilitation team will also need to coordinate the assistance (e.g., home health care aide) and equipment (e.g., shower chair, wheel chair) that will be needed at home.

Behavioral Assessment

A common referral question for neuropsychologists working with stroke patients in an acute rehabilitation setting is consultation regarding behavioral problems. Poststroke depression, irritability, agitation, confusion, and aggression are just a few examples. Neuropsychologists are called upon in these settings to provide assessment, treatment, and consultation about these difficult behaviors. One approach to assessment of these behaviors is multimodal. The neuropsychologist can obtain information about the patient's behavior from a number of sources. Feedback about the behaviors can be elicited from each of the stroke rehabilitation team members working with the patient, including the occupational therapist, physical therapist, and speech therapist. Feedback from the patient's family, nursing staff and nursing aides should not be overlooked. Sometimes, there are inconsistencies in the patient's behavior in the therapy gyms vs. on the nursing floor. For example, patients might angrily insist on getting help from, nursing staff for tasks they have demonstrated in the occupational therapy gym they are capable of completing independently. In addition to formal and informal interaction directly with the patient, neuropsychologists can observe the patient's behavior on the nursing floor and in the therapy gyms. A structured mental status examination combined with formal measures like the Beck Depression Inventory Fast Screen for Medical Patients (BDI-FS) [46] or the Beck Anxiety Inventory (BAI) [47] can be used to assess for depression and anxiety, respectively.

One way the neuropsychologist can effectively use his time and the time of the stroke rehabilitation team is by having a once or twice weekly behavioral management team meeting. The team gathers at a specific time and place and discusses the problem behaviors of the patient. The neuropsychologist acts as the facilitator of the meeting and the consultant. Each member of the stroke rehabilitation team working with the patient provides their feedback on the behavioral problems as experienced in their respective disciplines. It is strongly recommended that nursing has representation in these meetings. It has been the author's experience that nursing aides provide valuable information about the patient's behavior since they work with them so intimately in otherwise very private activities such as personal hygiene, eating, bathing, toileting, etc. Each member of the team describes what interventions they have tried to alter the problem behavior. After each of the team members have described problem behaviors and attempted interventions, the neuropsychologist then makes other intervention suggestions based upon established guidelines. The author has found the practical guidelines from the Rehabilitation Institute of Chicago Publication Series to be very helpful [48].

Follow-Up/Recommendations

In terms of follow-up, the neuropsychologist working with stroke patients in an acute rehabilitation setting will typically know the discharge disposition of the patient. Discharge alternatives include home with homecare services, home with outpatient care or therapeutic day care, subacute rehabilitation in a nursing home, or skilled nursing facility. In cases where contact with the patient and family caregivers has been intensive, it is recommended that the neuropsychologist be involved with discharge planning and coordinating of neuropsychological rehabilitation services. For example, during the acute rehabilitation admission, neuropsychological evaluation was completed, a trial of cognitive remediation begun, and psychological readjustment counseling initiated. The neuropsychologist, in cooperation with the social worker, can make recommendations and arrangements for the patient to obtain follow-up neuropsychological evaluation 90 days and 12 months poststroke to monitor progress. The neuropsychologist can also make recommendations and arrangements for continued cognitive remediation and counseling. In some cases, depending on time, third party payment, and logistical constraints, the neuropsychologist may be able to provide these services on an outpatient basis.

Treatment and intervention recommendations in-clude the following: follow-up (at 90 days and 12 months) neuropsychological evaluation to monitor progress made in cognitive and psychological functioning, readjustment counseling to continue to assist the patient with the psychological consequences of stroke, referral to a psychiatrist for prescription and management of psychotropic medication as indicated, and cognitive remediation to assist the patient with learning strategies to compensate for impairments. Specific techniques for remediation of memory have been suggested by Cuesta [49]. Reinforcement of education about stroke and its consequences for both patient and family caregivers, recommendation and referral for respite care, and therapeutic consultation with the family caregivers, are also suggested. Neuropsychologists can be especially influential in improving the care of the patient by attending to the emotional and education needs of the family caregivers.

Case Example

James was a 42-year-old, right-hand dominant, married, employed, domiciled, Caucasian man who was status post a right hemisphere stroke. He had a history of hypertension, hypercholesterolemia, diabetes, and smoking. He also led a somewhat sedentary lifestyle prior to the stroke. One day, while at work as a letter carrier for the post office, he fell ill and collapsed in the mailroom. Coworkers called 911, and he was taken to the emergency department of the local medical center. The emergency physicians in consultation with the acute stroke team diagnosed a right hemisphere ischemic stroke that left James with a left hemiparesis, left visual field neglect, and dysarthria. It was determined that onset of the symptoms of stroke was within 3 hours, and therefore, tissue plasminogen activator (tPA) was initiated to enhance blood flow. He remained in the acute care hospital for about a week and was determined to be a good candidate for acute rehabilitation. Some factors that determined his candidacy were relative youth, absence of aphasia, hemodynamic stability, good social support from his wife and family, and his own positive motivation to get better. Factors that were potential obstacles to progress were suspected onset of poststroke depression and lack of education about stroke and its consequences. He was medically stabilized and transferred to the acute rehabilitation center. James and his wife received orientation to the stroke rehabilitation unit. The first 48 hours at the unit were dedicated to completing evaluations and assessments by the multidisciplinary team. The neuropsychologist met with the patient and his wife and provided orientation to the role of the neuropsychologist on the treatment team. A time was booked for a neuropsychological screening evaluation. When James first came to the office for the appointment, he began to sob uncontrollably. So, therefore, the time was spent focusing on treating his emotional well-being. Once he was able to compose himself, emotional support, encouragement, and education about stroke were provided to the patient. The neuropsychologist queried James about symptoms of depression. The following symptoms of depression were acknowledged: early, middle, and late insomnia; loss of appetite with weight loss of about 10 lb since stroke onset; lethargy; decreased concentration; anhedonia; dysphoric/depressed mood with affective lability; a sense of helplessness; and decreased self-esteem and self-confidence. The BDI-FS and BAI were administered, and he endorsed depression at a moderate level of severity and mild-moderate anxiety. The neuropsychologist recommended, and James agreed, to consider use of antidepressant medication, weekly individual readjustment counseling, weekly stroke education group, and weekly stroke support group. He also agreed to neuropsychological evaluation of his cognitive functioning later in the first week of his admission. His wife was very dedicated to him and was able to be present for the greater part of the treatment day; this support was positively influential in James' progress. She agreed to attend the weekly family/caregiver stroke education and support groups. On neuropsychological evaluation, James was administered the 30-minutes protocol described above. Effort was adequate on testing, and he was motivated to learn about his abilities and difficulties. His intelligence level was estimated to be in the average range. Cognitive impairments (greater than 2 standard deviations below the mean) were in the areas of attention, speed of processing, and visual hemi-inattention to the left side of space. Relative weaknesses (1–2 standard deviations below the mean) were in the areas of delayed recall of verbal and visual information. Cognitive remediation protocol was initiated. He responded well to some of the strategies he learned to compensate for problems with attention and memory. For example, he used external memory aids as described by Cuesta [49]. He was observed to reliably refer to his daily journal and written schedule to help him recall important events and appointments. His depression was monitored, and behavior was discussed in the weekly behavioral management team meeting. During the last week of his 4-week stay, the 30-minutes protocol was readministered to determine progress made since admission. A family meeting was convened with his wife, two young adult children, and his parents to provide them with feedback about functional progress made in rehabilitation and to discuss discharge planning issues. Also, during the last week of his admission, the neuropsychologist made arrangements, in cooperation with the stroke rehabilitation team's social worker, for James to obtain individual psychotherapy for depression from a psychologist in his community. Also, a referral was made to a psychiatrist in the community for antidepressant medication management. Finally, arrangement for referral to a neuropsychologist in the community was made for follow-up neuropsychological evaluation 90 days poststroke.

Summary and Future Directions

Neuropsychology work in an acute rehabilitation setting is challenging, exciting, and meaningful. Neuropsychologists that enjoy interacting with multidisciplinary teams will find the work rich and rewarding. The work requires the clinician to go beyond the comfort zone of the classic role of neuropsychological evaluation and consultation. The successful neuropsychologist employed in an acute rehabilitation setting with stroke patients will learn and implement the competencies of rehabilitation psychology and health psychology.

Some, but by no means exhaustive, directions for future research include more precise determination of the predictive validity of neuropsychological measures. Increased precision in predictive validity of these tests can assist in establishing early prognosis and guiding treatment decisions [2]. Caplan [2] suggested that a post-discharge placement algorithm developed by Ween et al. [50] can be strengthened with the addition of neuropsychological data.

Improving the ecological validity of neuropsychological testing is another important area of future research. Neuropsychological tests with good ecological validity can aid in making reasonable and practical post-discharge recommendations related to functional activities such as driving, handling personal finances, and returning to school and work. Research collaboration with other disciplines like occupational therapy can be especially helpful in this endeavor.

A third important topic for future research is in the area of treatment efficacy for the emotional and behavioral problems associated with stroke, i.e., poststroke depression, anxiety, and other behavioral disturbances that adversely impact on the rehabilitation potential of the patient. Behavioral/psychological treatment can be for individuals or groups and can take the form of psycho-education, skill building classes, and cognitive behavioral interventions.

Neuropsychologists are an important part of the multidisciplinary treatment teams working in acute rehabilitation settings with stroke patients. Awareness and recognition of the importance of the role of the neuropsychologist is increasing as evidenced by the work of a task force of the American Stroke Association [51]. Their report, "Recommendations for the Establishment of Stroke Systems of Care," explicitly recognized the place of neuropsychologists on the stroke rehabilitation team. Neuropsychologists must cultivate evidence that demonstrates that their competencies, skills, knowledge, and abilities are essential to acute rehabilitation multidisciplinary teams working with stroke patients.

What follows are some suggestions for neuropsychologists working with acute rehabilitation teams. These suggestions were lessons learned and developed from the author's own experiences working in an acute rehabilitation setting over the last 13 years.

Clinical Pearls

- Neuropsychologists should not see themselves as having exclusive dominion over the assessment and treatment of the patient's cognitive and behavioral problems. The other members of the team can provide valuable information about the patient's functioning in these domains.
- In addition to assessment of cognitive and emotional functioning, the neuropsychologist on a stroke team can contribute to judgments about the patient's suitability for rehabilitation, capacity to make decisions, psychological and social factors that affect recovery, advising other members of the treatment team about neurobehavioral matters, educating patients and their families about stroke and its consequences, and making post-discharge referrals and recommendations for post-discharge living [2].
- Neuropsychologists in an acute stroke rehabilitation setting should take lead the behavioral management aspect of the acute stroke rehabilitation program. One way to do this is to have frequent, short (e.g., 30 minute) behavioral management meetings with the multidisciplinary team.
- Nursing aides can provide extremely valuable behavioral observations about patients. They work closely and intimately with the patients when they are on the nursing unit, and they can provide unique insights and observations. These patient behaviors might not be demonstrated in the physical therapy gym or occupational therapy gym.
- When maladaptive behaviors are identified and it is determined that the patient can reason and make judgments, it might be effective for the patient to meet with the team so that maladaptive behavior can be communicated in a non-critical manner. Frequent visits to the patient can build rapport and a foundation for future intervention and can ease the transition into rehabilitation.
- The neuropsychologist's interactions with the patient's family are a golden opportunity to obtain collateral information about the patient's cognitive and behavioral functioning. Contact with the family is also an opportunity to alleviate some of their anxieties about the patient's behaviors and functioning and provide education about stroke and recovery.

References

1. Centers for Disease Control. Hospitalizations for stroke among adults aged over 65 years—United States, 2000. J Am Med Assoc. 2003;290:1023–4.
2. Caplan B. Rehabilitation psychology and neuropsychology with stroke survivors. In: Frank RG, Rosenthal M, Caplan B, editors. Handbook of rehabilitation psychology. 2nd ed. Washington, DC: American Psychological Association; 2010. p. 63–94.
3. Lloyd-Jones D, Adams RJ, Brown TM, Carnethon M, Dai S, De Simone G, Ferguson TB, Ford E, Furie K, Gillespie C, Go A, Greenlund K, Haase N, Hailpern S, Ho PM, Howard V, Kissela B, Kittner S, Lackland D, Lisabeth L, Marelli A, McDermott MM, Meigs J, Mozaffarian D, Mussolino M, Nichol G, Roger V,

Rosamond W, Sacco R, Sorlie P, Stafford R, Thom T, Wasserthiel-Smoller S, Wong ND, Wylie-Rosett J and on behalf of the American Heart Association Statistics Committee and Stroke Statistics Subcommittee (2009). Heart disease and stroke statistics 2010 update. A report from the American Heart Association. Circulation. J Am Heart Assoc. doi: 10.1161/CIRCULATIONAHA.109.192667.

4. Centers for Disease Control and Prevention (CDC). Prevalence of stroke: United States, 2005. MMWR Morb Mortal Wkly Rep. 2007;56:469–74.
5. http://ninds.nih.gov/disorders/stroke/poststrokerehab.htm.
6. National Heart, Lung, and Blood Institute. Incidence and Prevalence: 2006 Chart Book on Cardiovascular and Lung Diseases. Bethesda, MD: National Heart, Lung, and Blood Institute; 2006.
7. White H, Boden-Albala B, Wang C, Elkind MS, Rundek T, Wright CB, Sacco RL. Ischemic stroke subtype incidence among whites, blacks, and Hispanics; the Northern Manhattan Study. Circulation. 2005;111:1327–31.
8. National Center for Health Statistics. Health Data Interactive File, 1981–2006. Hyattsville, MD: National Center for Health Statistics; 2006.
9. www.healthcentral.com/heart-disease/stroke-000045_4-145.html. Accessed 16 Dec 2010.
10. Baird AE, Dambrosia J, Janket S, Eichbaum Q, Chaves C, Silver B, Barber PA, Parsons M, Darby D, Davis S, Caplan LR, Edelman RR, Warach S. A three-item scale for the early prediction of stroke recovery. Lancet. 2001;357(9274):2095–9.
11. Festa JR, Lazar RM, Marshall RS. Ischemic stroke and aphasic disorders. In: Morgan JE, Ricker JH, editors. Textbook of clinical neuropsychology. New York: Taylor & Francis; 2008. p. 363–83.
12. Devasenapathy A, Hachinski V. Cerebrovascular disease. In: Rizzo M, Eslinger PJ, editors. Principles and practice of behavioral neurology and neuropsychology. Philadelphia: W.B. Saunders Company; 2004. p. 597–613.
13. Gorelick PB. Stroke prevention: an opportunity for efficient utilization of health care resources during the coming decade. Stroke. 1994;25:220–4.
14. Goldstein LB, Adams R, Becker K, Furberg CD, Gorelick PB, Hademenos G, et al. Primary prevention of ischemic stroke: a statement for healthcare professionals from the Stroke Council of the American Heart Association. Stroke. 2001;32(1):280–99.
15. "Know Stroke. Know the Signs. Act in Time", National Institute of Neurological Disorders and Stroke (NINDS). January 2008. NIH Publication No. 08-4872.
16. Barnett HJM, Stein BM, Mohr JP, Yatsu FM, editors. Stroke. Pathophysiology, diagnosis, and management. 2nd ed. New York: Churchill Livingstone; 1992.
17. Yew KS, Cheng E. Acute stroke diagnosis. Am Fam Physician. 2009;80(1):33–40.
18. Nor AM, Davis J, Sen B, et al. The recognition of stroke in the emergency room (ROSIER) scale: development and validation of a stroke recognition instrument. Lancet Neurol. 2005;4(11):727–34.
19. Hand PJ, Haisma JA, Kwan J, et al. Interobserver agreement for the bedside clinical assessment of suspected stroke. Stroke. 2006;37(3):776–80.
20. Goldstein LB, Simel DL. Is this patient having a stroke? J Am Med Assoc. 2005;293(19):2391–402.
21. Morgenstern LB, Lisabeth LD, Mecozzi AC, et al. A population-based study of acute stroke and TIA diagnosis. Neurology. 2004;62(6):895–900.
22. Adams Jr HP, del Zoppo G, Alberts MJ, et al. Guidelines for the early management of adults with ischemic stroke: a guideline from the American Heart Association/American Stroke Association Stroke Council, Clinical Cardiology Council, Cardiovascular Radiology and Intervention Council, and the Atherosclerotic Peripheral Vascular Disease and Quality of Care Outcomes in Research Interdisciplinary Working Groups: the American Academy of Neurology affirms the value of this guideline as an educational tool for neurologists [published corrections appear in Stroke. 2007;38(6):e38 and Stroke. 2007;38(9):e96]. Stroke. 2007;38(5):1655–711.
23. National Institute of Neurological Disorders and Stroke. NIH Stroke Scale. 2003. http://www.ninds.nih.gov/doctors/NIH_Stroke_Scale.pdf. Accessed 12 Dec 2010.
24. Mullins ME, Schaefer PW, Sorensen AG, et al. CT and conventional and diffusion-weighted MR imaging in acute stroke: study in 691 patients at presentation to the emergency department. Radiology. 2002;224(2):353–60.
25. Suarez JL, Tarr RW, Selman WR. Aneurysmal subarachnoid hemorrhage. N Engl J Med. 2006;354(4):387–96.
26. Adams Jr HP, Bendixen BH, Kappelle LJ, et al. Classification of subtype of acute ischemic stroke. Definitions for use in a multicenter clinical trial. TOAST. Trial of Org 10172 in Acute Stroke Treatment. Stroke. 1993;24(1):35–41.
27. Practice guidelines for the use of imaging in transient ischemic attacks and acute stroke. A report of the Stroke Council, American Heart Association (1997).
28. Jin YP, DiLegge S, Ostbye T, Feightner JW, Hachinski V. The reciprocal risks of stroke and cognitive impairment in an elderly population. Alzheimer's Dement. 2006 1;2(3):171–8.
29. Barba R, Martinez-Espinosa S, Rodriguez-Garcia E, Pondal M, Vivancos J, Del Ser T. Post stroke dementia: clinical features and risk factors. Stroke. 2000;31:1494–501.
30. Pohjasvaara T, Erkinjuntti T, Vataja R, Kaste M. Dementia three months after stroke: baseline frequency and effect of different definitions of dementia in the Helsinki Stroke Aging Memory Study (SAM) cohort. Stroke. 1997;28:785–92.
31. Tatemichi TK, Desmond DW, Stern Y, Sano M, Mayeux R, Andrews H. Prevalence of dementia after

stroke depends on diagnostic criteria. Neurology. 1992;42:413.
32. Hachinski VC, Bowler JV. Vascular dementia. Neurology. 1993;43:2159–60. author reply 2160–2161.
33. Bowler JV, Hachinski VC, editors. Vascular cognitive impairment. Oxford and New York: Oxford University; 2003.
34. Snowdon DA, Greiner LH, Mortimer JA, Riley KP, Greiner PA, Markesbery WR. Brain infarction and the clinical expression of Alzheimer's disease. The Nun Study. J Am Med Assoc. 1997;277:813–7.
35. Hachinski V, Iadecola C, Peterson RC, Breteler MM, Nyenhuis DL, Black SE, Powers WJ, DeCarli C, Merino JG, Kalaria RN, Vinters HV, Holtzman DM, Rosenberg GA, Wallin A, Dichgans M, Marler JR, Leblanc GG. National Institute of Neurological Disorders and Stroke—Canadian Stroke Network vascular cognitive impairment harmonization standards. Stroke. 2006;37:2220–41.
36. Heaton RK, Miller SW, Taylor MJ, Grant I. Revised comprehensive norms for an expanded Halstead-Reitan battery: demographically adjusted neuropsychological norms for African American and Caucasian adults. Lutz, FL: PAR; 2004.
37. The Psychological Corporation. WAIS-III/WMS-III: Updated Technical Manual. San Antonio: The Psychological Corporation; 2002.
38. Brandt J, Benedict RHB. Hopkins Verbal Learning Test—revised. Odessa, FL: PAR; 2001.
39. Parikh RM, Eden DT, Price TR, Robinson RG. The sensitivity and specificity of the center for epidemiologic studies depression scale in screening for post-stroke depression. Int J Psychiatry Med. 1988;18:169–81.
40. Cummings JL, Mega MS, Gray K, Rosemberg-Thompson S, Gornbein T. The neuropsychiatric inventory: comprehensive assessment of psychopathology in dementia. Neurology. 1994;44:2308–14.
41. Army Individual Test Battery: Manual of directions and scoring. Washington, D.C.: War Department, Adjutant General's Office; 1944.
42. Folstein MF, Folstein SE, McHugh PR, Fanjiang G. Mini-Mental State Examination: User's guide. Odessa, FL: PAR; 2001.
43. Nasreddine ZS, Phillips NA, Bedirian V, Charbonneau S, Whitehead V, Collin I, Cummings JL, Chertkow H. The Montreal cognitive assessment, moca: a brief screening tool for mild cognitive impairment. J Am Geriatr Soc. 2005;53:695–9.
44. Etchells E, Sharpe G, Elliott C, Singer PA. Bioethics for clinicians: 3. Capacity. CMAJ. 1996;155:657–61.
45. Grisso T, Appelbaum PS. Assessing competence to consent to treatment: a guide for physicians and other health professionals. New York: Oxford University; 1998.
46. Beck AT, Steer RA, Brown GK. Beck depression inventory-fast screen for medical patients: manual. San Antonio, TX: Psychological Corporation; 2000.
47. Beck AT, Steer RA. Beck anxiety inventory: manual. San Antonio, TX: The Psychological Corporation Harcourt Brace & Company; 1993.
48. Rothke SE, Berquist TF, Schmidt M, Landre NA, Speizman R. Behavioral management strategies for working with persons with brain injury: a practical manual. Chicago: Rehabilitation Institute of Chicago; 1998.
49. Cuesta GM. Cognitive rehabilitation of memory following stroke. Theory, practice, and outcome. In: Barnett HJM, Bogousslavsky J, Meldrum H, editors. Ischemic stroke: advances in neurology, vol. 92. Philadelphia: Lippincott Williams & Wilkins; 2003. p. 415–21.
50. Ween JE, Alexander MP, D'Esposito M, Roberts M. Factors predictive of stroke rehabilitation outcome in a rehabilitation setting. Neurology. 1996;47:388–92.
51. Schwamm LH, Pancioli A, Acker III JE, Goldstein LB, Zorowitz RD, Shephard TJ, et al. Recommendations for the establishment of stroke systems of care: Recommendations from the American Stroke Association's Task Force on the Development of Stroke Systems. Stroke. 2005;36:690–703.

Accurate Assessment of Behavioral Variant Frontotemporal Dementia

21

Amanda K. LaMarre and Joel H. Kramer

Abstract

Behavioral variant Frontotemporal dementia (bvFTD) is a neurodegenerative syndrome characterized by profound changes in personality and behavior, including social disinhibition, loss of empathy, apathy and compulsive behaviors. While cognitive decline does occur (typically beginning with executive dysfunction), these issues tend to emerge mid-disease course, rather than early on. Onset is insidious, typically beginning between ages 45-65 and prevalence is equal to Alzheimer's disease (AD) in individuals under the age of 65. Despite significant advancements in our understanding of bvFTD over the past 12 years, misdiagnosis remains common. For example, a significant subset of individuals with bvFTD initially receive a diagnosis of early-onset AD, or late life psychiatric disturbance. Given their expertise in the assessment of cognition, behavior and emotion, neuropsychologists can play an important role in the differential diagnosis and management of this disease. This chapter begins with an up-to-date discussion of the clinical, neuropathological and genetic features of the disease, and then moves into a review of the neuropsychological literature. A structured discussion of key aspects to cover in a neuropsychological assessment is provided, and a case example of a 'typical' bvFTD patient is presented.

Keywords

Behavioral variant frontotemporal dementia • Diagnostic criteria • Neuropsychological assessment • Emotion • Social behavior • Clinical assessment

---

A.K. LaMarre, Ph.D. (✉) • J.H. Kramer, Psy.D.
Memory and Aging Center, University of California, San Francisco, Box 1207, San Francisco, CA 94143-1207, USA
e-mail: alamarre@memory.ucsf.edu; jkramer@memory.ucsf.edu

L.D. Ravdin and H.L. Katzen (eds.), *Handbook on the Neuropsychology of Aging and Dementia*, Clinical Handbooks in Neuropsychology, DOI 10.1007/978-1-4614-3106-0_21,

Behavioral variant frontotemporal dementia (bvFTD) is one of three neurodegenerative syndromes that are collectively referred to as frontotemporal dementia (FTD). Initially thought to be rare, we now know that it is equally as common as Alzheimer's disease in individuals under the age of 65 [1] and is the third most common dementia after Alzheimer's disease (AD) and dementia with Lewy bodies (DLB) [2]. While estimates of the prevalence of FTD vary, population-based studies in both the United States and United Kingdom estimate a sporadic occurrence at around 3.3–3.5/100,000 in individuals between 45 and 65 years of age [3, 4]. Age of onset is typically in the presenium, though onset ranges considerably from the 30s to 90s [1, 5, 6]. The usual duration of FTD ranges from 8 to 11 years [7].

Clinically, FTD is expressed as three main variants [8]. BvFTD is characterized by profound and early changes in personality and behavior [8]. This phenotype is most common and accounts for approximately 70% of the clinical expression of the disease [9]. As such, bvFTD will be the focus of this chapter. The other two variants are primary progressive aphasic syndromes. The semantic variant (svPPA) is associated with the loss of word knowledge (e.g., semantic structure of language), while the nonfluent variant (nfPPA) is characterized by early disturbances in motor speech output and loss of syntax (e.g., grammatical structure of language) [8, 10]. These two variants account for approximately 15% and 10% of the phenotypic expression of the disease, respectively [9]. Gender distribution tends to vary by clinical syndrome. Many studies find a male bias in bvFTD and svPPA and a female bias in nfPPA [1, 5, 6].

Earliest Signs of bvFTD

The earliest signs of disease in bvFTD are frequently subtle personality and behavioral changes that become increasingly pronounced as time goes on. These symptoms often include apathy or disinhibition, reduced emotional response, changes in personality or beliefs [11], poor judgment, and impairment in personal and social awareness [12–15]. These changes are often dramatic, resulting in the dissolution of the individual's former self, such that partners and families no longer recognize their loved one [11]. For example, individuals may begin to make impulsive decisions or actions, including such behaviors as shoplifting, driving recklessly, or physically assaulting others [12, 14, 16, 17]. They might violate social norms by making inappropriate sexual comments [18] or become emotionally cold and self-centered such that they no longer respond to others' emotional needs or pain [19]. These changes often present in sharp contrast to their cognitive ability, which may remain relatively intact for some time.

Diagnostic Criteria for bvFTD

Until recently, diagnosis of bvFTD has most often been made using the revised version of the Lund–Manchester criteria, which were reformulated by a consensus of specialists in the area of FTD in 1998 [8]. Considerable advancements in our understanding of this disease over the past 12 years has led to development of new criteria by the International bvFTD Criteria Consortium [20] (Table 21.1). With these criteria, diagnosis of possible bvFTD is based solely on clinical presentation. Patients must meet at least three of the six following criteria: (1) early behavioral disinhibition, (2) early apathy/inertia, (3) early loss of sympathy or empathy, (4) early perseverative, stereotyped or compulsive behaviors, (5) hyperorality or dietary changes, and (6) a neuropsychological profile suggesting deficits on tasks of executive function with *relative* sparing of memory and visuospatial function. To meet criteria for probable bvFTD, a patient must meet criteria for possible bvFTD, exhibit significant functional decline, and show evidence of frontal and/or temporal atrophy on structural MRI or CT, or hypometabolism on positron emission tomography (PET). Sensitivity of the new criteria has recently been demonstrated via retrospective chart review of pathologically confirmed cases in a multisite study, and findings suggest that the new criteria

Table 21.1 International consensus criteria for bvFTD [20]

I. Neurodegenerative disease
The following symptom must be present for any FTD clinical syndrome:
A. Shows progressive deterioration of behavior and/or cognition by observation or history (as provided by a knowledgeable informant)
II. Possible bvFTD
Three of the following behavioral/cognitive symptoms [A–F] must be present to meet criteria. These symptoms should occur repeatedly, not just as a single instance
A. Early behavioral disinhibition
a. Socially inappropriate behavior b. Loss of manners or decorum c. Impulsive, rash, or careless actions
B. Early apathy or inertia
a. Apathy: loss of interest, drive, or motivation b. Inertia: decreased initiation of behavior
C. Early loss of sympathy or empathy
a. Diminished response to other people's needs or feelings: positive rating should be based on specific examples that reflect a lack of understanding or indifference to other people's feelings b. Diminished social interest, interrelatedness, or personal warmth: general decrease in social engagement
D. Early perseverative, stereotyped, or compulsive/ritualistic behavior
a. Simple repetitive movements b. Complex, compulsive, or ritualistic behaviors c. Stereotypy of speech
E. Hyperorality and dietary changes
a. Altered food preferences b. Binge eating, increased consumption of alcohol or cigarettes c. Oral exploration or consumption of inedible objects
F. Neuropsychological profile: executive/generation deficits with relative sparing of memory and visuospatial functions
a. Deficits in executive tasks b. Relative sparing of episodic memory (compared to degree of executive dysfunction) c. Relative sparing of visuospatial skills (compared to degree of executive dysfunction)
III. Probable bvFTD
A. Meets criteria for possible bvFTD B. Exhibits significant functional decline (by caregiver report or as evidenced by CDR or FAQ scores) C. Imaging results consistent with bvFTD
a. Frontal and/or anterior temporal atrophy on CT or MRI b. Frontal hypoperfusion or hypometabolism on SPECT or PET
IV. bvFTD with definite FTLD pathology
Criterion A and either Criterion B or C must be present to meet criteria
A. Meets criteria for possible bvFTD B. Histopathological evidence of FTLD on biopsy or at postmortem C. Presence of known pathogenic mutation
V. Exclusion criteria for bvFTD
Criteria A and B must both be answered negatively for any bvFTD diagnosis. Criterion C can be positive for possible bvFTD but must be negative for probable bvFTD
A. Pattern of deficits is better accounted for by other nondegenerative nervous system or medical disorders: e.g., delirium, cerebrovascular disease, cerebellar disorder, systemic disorders (e.g., hypothyroidism), or substance-induced conditions B. Behavioral disturbance is better accounted for by a psychiatric diagnosis, e.g., depression, bipolar disorder, schizophrenia, preexisting personality disorder C. Biomarkers strongly indicative of Alzheimer's disease or other neurodegenerative process (e.g., genetic mutations, extensive PIB finding, CSF markers)

have greater sensitivity to the diagnosis of bvFTD, compared to the previous criteria (0.85 vs. 0.52, respectively) [20].

Neuroanatomy and Pathology of bvFTD

The hallmark symptoms of bvFTD strongly reflect initial areas of neurodegeneration. A recent structural neuroimaging analysis in patients in the earliest stages of bvFTD (Clinical Dementia Rating Scale (CDR) = 0.5; mild dementia) suggests that initial degeneration occurs primarily in paralimbic structures such as the anterior cingulate cortex, frontoinsular region, dorsal anterior insula, and lateral orbitofrontal cortex [21], and disease staging of autopsy-confirmed cases of bvFTD are consistent with this finding [22]. These structures have been widely implicated in human social function and awareness of the self [23] and are part of a neural network thought to play a role in decoding the emotional salience (visceral, homeostatic, hedonic value) of a stimulus in order to facilitate appropriate action [24]. As the disease progresses, neurodegeneration occurs in widespread areas of the frontal and temporal lobes [25–29].

BvFTD is caused by abnormal aggregation of protein in the brain, referred to collectively as frontotemporal lobar degeneration (FTLD). The two most common pathologies associated with bvFTD are FTLD with tau-positive inclusions (FTLD-tau) and FTLD with TDP-43 positive inclusions (FTLD-TDP) [2, 30], with a handful of additional proteins accounting for a very small proportion of bvFTD cases [30]. Under normal conditions, both tau and TDP-43 play important roles in neuronal cell structure and function [31, 32]. Under pathologic conditions, however, these proteins aggregate and accumulate in the cytoplasm of neurons and glial cells and are associated with neuronal death and atrophy [2, 30].

Advancements in our understanding of the underlying pathology of FTD over the last 10 years have also demonstrated links with diseases not historically believed to be associated with changes in cognition and behavior [33–35]. For example, FTLD-tau includes cases fulfilling pathological diagnostic criteria for not only Pick's disease and frontotemporal dementia and parkinsonism linked to chromosome 17 (FTDP-17) but also for motor disorders such as progressive supranuclear palsy (PSP) and corticobasal degeneration (CBD) [36, 37]. Similarly, cases found to have FTLD-TDP may present alone or in combination with motor neuron disease (e.g., amyotrophic lateral sclerosis; ALS) [38, 39]. There is also a growing consensus that the behavioral syndrome of bvFTD can be found in patients with PSP, CBD, and ALS [40–42].

Genetics

While sporadic cases are common in bvFTD, at least 30–40% of all cases appear to be genetic in nature [43], with rates of autosomal dominant pattern of inheritance ranging from 10% to 30% [44, 45]. At this time, genetic mutations known to cause familial FTD have been found on three different chromosomes (three, nine, seventeen) [46–48]. By and large, the greatest proportion of familial cases comes from individuals who have mutations on two independent, but extremely close locations on chromosome 17 [9, 49]. The first was discovered in 1998 and was found to be caused by mutations in the microtubule-associated protein ("MAPT") gene [50]. It is now known that *MAPT* codes for the protein tau, which as mentioned above, is a major pathological subtype of bvFTD [51]. More recently, linkage analysis in the same region of chromosome 17 has shown that mutations in the gene coding for the growth factor progranulin are associated with bvFTD (*PGRN*; [52]). Unlike *MAPT*, these cases display TDP-43 inclusions rather than tau [53], though the mechanistic link between progranulin and TDP-43 has yet to be elucidated. Interestingly, any of the three clinical variants of FTD may occur in familial forms of the disease; however, certain variants are more likely to be expressed than others [9, 49, 54]. For example, *PGRN* mutation carriers tend to develop symptoms characteristic of bvFTD or nfPPA [55].[1]

[1]For a recent review on the genetics of FTD, please read See et al. [58].

Differential Diagnosis

Despite significant advancements in the field, diagnosis of bvFTD remains clinically challenging. BvFTD is commonly misdiagnosed as early onset AD, which is not surprising, given that AD is the most prevalent dementia syndrome. Many symptoms of the two diseases overlap, including neuropsychiatric disturbance and executive dysfunction [56, 57]. Patients with neurodegenerative motor syndromes may also exhibit symptoms consistent with a diagnosis of bvFTD (or an aphasia variant) [40–42]. As such, having a concomitant syndrome such as PSP or ALS should not be considered exclusionary for a diagnosis of bvFTD. Huntington's disease may also mimic many of the behavioral and psychiatric disturbances seen in bvFTD [59].

Patients with bvFTD may also be misdiagnosed with a late-onset psychiatric disturbance. Symptoms of disinhibition, euphoria, and poor judgment can mimic those of mania, while profound apathy and eating disturbance might be misconstrued as depression. Wooley and colleagues [60] completed a retrospective chart review of 252 patients with neurodegenerative disease presenting to our clinic. Of the patients with bvFTD, 51% of patients had received a prior diagnosis of a psychiatric disorder (e.g., major depression, bipolar disorder, schizophrenia) compared to 23% of patients with Alzheimer's disease (e.g., major depression, anxiety), suggesting that the symptoms of bvFTD are particularly misunderstood by mental-health-care providers. A small subset of patients diagnosed with bvFTD have been characterized as "nonprogressive" or "bvFTD phenocopies" due to the presence of a behavioral disturbance in the context of lack of notable atrophy on imaging or cognitive decline over time [61–63]. As these individuals rarely come to autopsy, the etiology of this subset of individuals is unclear. Careful characterization and longitudinal follow-up will be important in understanding how these individuals relate to the progressive form of bvFTD. The importance of accurate differential diagnosis cannot be overstated. Treatments aimed at an alternate diagnosis (i.e., targeting AD) can potentially exacerbate bvFTD symptoms (Table 21.2).

Table 21.2 Disorders that may present with similar neurobehavioral features to bvFTD

Neurodegenerative diseases	Progressive supranuclear palsy
	Corticobasal syndrome
	Amyotrophic lateral sclerosis
	Alzheimer's disease
	Semantic variant primary progressive aphasia
	Huntington's disease
	Lewy body dementia
Psychiatric disorders	Bipolar disorder
	Major depression
	FTD phenocopy
	Psychopathy
Neurologic disorders	Cerebrovascular accident
	Traumatic brain injury

Efforts to develop specific, disease-modifying therapies for FTLD are advancing rapidly, focusing on the major proteins currently known to be involved in the pathogenesis of the disease. Clinical trials aimed at manipulating tau have already begun, while researchers are actively working to develop agents that might modify TDP-43 and PGRN levels. Testing the efficacy of these medications greatly depends upon our ability to ensure homogenous samples in clinical trials. As there are currently no definitive methods for determining pathology prior to autopsy, predicting pathology antemortem remains a key challenge. Researchers are actively working to better understand the clinicopathologic correlations relevant to each protein currently believed to be involved in the development of FTLD.

Review of Neuropsychological Literature

Despite obvious impairment in the patient's behavior and judgment, researchers seeking to characterize a neuropsychological profile specific to bvFTD have not been highly successful. Research is plagued with a number of significant issues that likely contribute to discrepancies in the data, including the lack of universally applied diagnostic criteria, variability in diagnostic terminology, lumping together of all three clinical variants of the disease, small sample sizes, and lack of reporting of disease severity or symptom duration [64]. Issues can also arise due to test selection and interpretation issues, including the possibility that impaired performance on tests are due to factors that are beyond what the test is meant to measure. For example, a study examining qualitative features of performance on neuropsychological testing in bvFTD and AD found that patients with bvFTD tend to perform poorly on tasks of visuoconstructive ability, not due to deficits in visual perceptive ability, but rather, due to perseverations and deficits in organizational ability [65]. Moreover, behavioral manifestations of the disease itself, including poor motivation and distractibility, may contribute to variability in cognitive performance scores.

Our current understanding of the neuropsychology of bvFTD lies largely within the context of research seeking to improve differential diagnosis between neurodegenerative diseases. In most cases, the cognitive profiles of individuals with bvFTD and AD are compared, though efforts to delineate specific tasks or cognitive facets that will reliably differentiate the two have been unsuccessful. As such, *relative test score patterns* between domains appear to be most informative to differential diagnosis.

Memory

Compared to patients with AD who exhibit severe verbal and visuospatial episodic memory deficits [66–69], patients with bvFTD demonstrate a *relative* preservation in their episodic memory [65, 70–72]. The pattern is typically one of attenuated learning with a disorganized or inefficient approach. For example, Glosser and colleagues found that difficulty with serial-order recall was more common in individuals with bvFTD than in those with AD and svPPA [73]. Perhaps the most salient difference between bvFTD and AD is that bvFTD patients tend to retain information over delays, while AD patients exhibit more rapid forgetting. While some studies suggest that bvFTD patients improve considerably with cued recall or recognition [72, 74, 75], data from our center suggest that this effect does not hold up when bvFTD and AD subjects are matched for severity. Visual memory also appears to be relatively spared in bvFTD [70–72]. When both visual and verbal memory are intact, this may help strengthen diagnostic certainty that the patient does not have Alzheimer's disease.

These patterns of memory performance, however, are not specific to bvFTD. Disorders with frontal–subcortical involvement such as Parkinson's disease and PSP may also demonstrate similar patterns [76, 77]. LaMarre and colleagues demonstrated that episodic memory declines longitudinally at the same rate in bvFTD and AD, though mean scores at baseline were significantly different [78]. Nevertheless, relative preservation of episodic memory in bvFTD compared to AD remains one of the most reliable differences between these diseases.

Language

Individuals with bvFTD do not experience the same types of changes in language that accompany PPA variants of FTD; however, speech and language ability may reflect notable changes. There are often reductions in spontaneous speech; decreased verbal output (single words or decreased phrase length) can potentially progress to complete mutism [8, 79–81]. Reiterative speech disorders can also occur, such as palilalia, echolalia, verbal stereotypies, and automatic speech [7, 8]. Despite these changes in verbal output, examination of semantic and syntactical knowledge using measures of confrontation naming, word/picture matching, and sentence comprehension suggest that these aspects of language remain relatively intact in bvFTD [65, 71, 82, 83].

There have been few studies that have directly examined differential language patterns between bvFTD and other diseases [80, 83, 84]. Rascovsky and colleagues [84] studied verbal fluency in pathology-confirmed cases of FTD and AD who were matched on age, education, and dementia severity. When converted to z-scores based on an age-matched control sample, scores on semantic fluency in the AD group were significantly lower than their scores on phonemic fluency, while the FTD patients performed poorly on both semantic and phonemic fluency.

Visuospatial

Although several studies have found that patients with bvFTD have visuoconstructional deficits on par with AD when the figure is very complex [70, 85, 86], the vast majority of research indicates that visuoconstruction and visual perceptual skills are better preserved in patients with bvFTD relative to AD [65, 75, 79, 87, 90]. Difficulties can arise for bvFTD patients when the task relies heavily on top-down control of spatial processing. For example, Possin and colleagues [88] recently demonstrated that figure copy performance was significantly correlated with right parietal cortex volume in patients with AD, but not with right dorsolateral prefrontal cortex (DLPFC) volume. The opposite relationship was demonstrated in patients with bvFTD. We have also examined longitudinal data to show that visuospatial function remains relatively stable in bvFTD and svPPA groups but declines significantly in the AD group [78].

Attention/Executive Functions in bvFTD

While intuitive, the claim that attention and executive functions are broadly and disproportionately impacted in bvFTD lacks strong empirical support. Investigation of this domain using "traditional" tasks of executive function has led to largely conflicting findings. While some studies find impairments in this domain [71, 91–93], others do not [94–96]. One reason for this discrepancy likely relates to stage of disease at which patients are assessed. As neurodegeneration begins in the ventromedial aspect of the frontal lobe and moves dorsolaterally with disease progression [21, 24, 25, 97, 98], we would not expect to see executive deficits manifest until later in the disease. It is now being demonstrated that some pathological subtypes of bvFTD do not necessarily exhibit significant DLPFC degeneration (e.g., TDP-43, Type II) [99]; as such, one might hypothesize that patients with this type of pathology will be less likely to demonstrate executive function deficits.

Another reason why findings have been inconsistent may be due to the fact that executive functions are a poorly defined construct that encompass heterogeneous facets of cognition such as working memory, inhibition, and set shifting [69, 100, 101]. Moreover, they depend heavily on lower-order aspects of cognition such as processing speed and visual perception. It appears that any number of tasks may be subsumed under this umbrella term and are often discussed as if interchangeable. Within the bvFTD neuropsychological literature, there appears to have been little consideration and consistency regarding which component of executive function might be particularly impaired in bvFTD (working memory vs. inhibition), or consistency in the type of task chosen (e.g., Trail Making Test vs. Digit Span).

Overall, it appears that "traditional" clinical measures of executive function are not particularly sensitive early in the disease process. It is possible, however, that experimental measures of executive function may be more sensitive to subtle declines. For example, Krueger et al. [93] administered traditional tasks of executive function, as well as a computerized Flanker task (measuring cognitive control) to patients with bvFTD and healthy control subjects. Patients were dichotomized into those who scored within normal limits on standard tasks of executive function and those who did not, and their scores on the Flanker task were compared. Interestingly, *both* bvFTD patient groups showed a significantly larger congruency effect (e.g., longer latency on incongruent vs. congruent trials) compared to the normal control subjects [93]. These results suggest that even those patients who perform well on standard tasks of executive function may still have subtle, yet perceptible deficits in cognitive control, if measured by the appropriate method.

Another approach to measuring executive functioning in bvFTD has been to measure process-oriented features of performance such as errors. Kramer et al. found that overall error scores on tasks of executive function discriminated between patients with bvFTD and AD [71]. Rule violation errors may also be helpful in discriminating between AD and bvFTD. Carey and colleagues [102] found that despite similar achievement scores on the Delis–Kaplan Executive Function System Tower Task, patients with bvFTD made significantly more rule violations compared to patients with AD and normal controls. Poor "online" detection of errors has also been shown to distinguish between bvFTD, CBS, and PSP [103].

Thompson et al. qualitatively analyzed error types between patients with AD and bvFTD on multiple tasks from several different domains of cognition, including language, memory, visuospatial, and executive function. While several tests were significantly different between the two groups, overall, differences in the types of errors made were best able to distinguish between AD and bvFTD on regression analysis (e.g., spatial errors vs. perseverations on a drawing task) [65].

Examining errors is also important given that some researchers have found that patients with bvFTD often perform faster on measures of executive function (e.g., Stroop Inhibition) than patients with AD, but also make significantly more errors, indicating an imbalance in their ability to accurately make speed/error trade-offs [95, 96].

Social Behavior and Personality

The dorsolateral prefrontal cortex (DLPFC) degenerates in both AD and bvFTD, though this may occur at different stages in disease course [97]. This likely explains why large group differences in executive functioning are not regularly demonstrated between the two diseases [89, 94, 104]. Investigations into social and emotional function have produced more consistent results, likely due to the fact that they are mediated by more anterior and ventral aspects of the prefrontal cortex [105–108], areas that are more selectively involved in bvFTD relative to other neurodegenerative disorders.

Studies examining social behavior in bvFTD have found that these individuals tend to demonstrate flat affect, reduced initiative, and more perseveration than patients with other neurodegenerative diseases [109]. Other studies have also found deficits in social pragmatics during conversation [80] and poor social judgment compared to patients with primary progressive aphasia [110]. Changes in personality facets related to interpersonal function have also been noted to occur in bvFTD. For example, Rankin et al. demonstrated that agreeableness (one of the Big Five personality traits) was not only decreased in bvFTD, but also significantly related to right orbitofrontal cortex volumes [111].

Several researchers have found that patients with bvFTD have significantly less self-awareness regarding their current personality and behavioral deficits [19, 112–114] compared to patients with other neurodegenerative diseases, such as AD. This lack of awareness or concern may be due, in part, to the emotion-processing deficits that have been documented in bvFTD. While basic emotion processing such as the startle reflex has been shown to remain intact in patients with bvFTD [115], there are deficits in more complex forms of emotion such as self-conscious emotion, including embarrassment, [115, 116], emotional downregulation [117], recognition of emotions in others [19, 118–121], and ability to empathize with others [110, 113, 122].

Complex Learning and Decision Making

The ventral and orbital medial regions of the prefrontal cortex are also thought to be involved in self-advantageous decision making and adaptive responses to changing emotional or social demands in the environment [106, 108]. Researchers have begun to create experimental paradigms which are thought to tap these processes, including tasks which measure risk taking via computerized gambling programs (e.g., Iowa Gambling Task) [123] and reversal learning tasks focused on reward and punishment [106].

Several researchers have found impairments on these tasks in patients with bvFTD [92, 124–126]; however, these studies have not directly compared bvFTD to patients with other neurodegenerative diseases, so their utility for differential diagnosis is unclear.

Summary of Neuropsychology Literature

While the "classic" pattern of impaired attention and executive function with relative sparing of memory, language, and visuospatial function can occur in bvFTD, this pattern is not a constant and is just one of six symptoms (the other five being social or behavioral) that define bvFTD. As such, it is imperative that practitioners *do not* use evidence of this neuropsychological pattern as justification for diagnosis of the disease in absence of other symptoms outlined in the International Diagnostic Criteria [20].

Clinical Assessment of bvFTD

A comprehensive evaluation of bvFTD should include a clinical interview, neuropsychological assessment, assessment of social and emotional function, and informant based measures. Given that cognition can be relatively preserved in the early stages of the disease, the history, informant report, and observable behavior seen throughout the assessment will likely be the most helpful information you gather.

Interview

A well-structured clinical interview with a collateral source is critical. The patients typically lack insight into the social, emotional, or behavioral issues that are most germane to their caregivers and tend to deny problems. If the informant does not feel comfortable speaking frankly in front of the patient, one should consider conducting a separate interview. During the interview, important areas to cover include:

Onset and Progression

Has the onset been slow and insidious, or abrupt and explicit? Behavioral variant FTD is an insidious disease that may begin many years before changes become obvious. Moreover, because the age of onset of bvFTD tends to be in the late 50s, the personality and behavior changes are often misinterpreted as "mid-life" troubles. While insidious change is common to most neurodegenerative disease, abrupt onset changes in personality and behavior are less likely to be bvFTD.

Nature of Change

As evidenced in the International Criteria for bvFTD [20], changes in personality, emotionality, and social behavior are the most salient symptoms of bvFTD, and the six major symptoms of the International criteria can be used to structure the interview:

1. *Early behavioral disinhibiton.* Has the person become socially, behaviorally, or cognitively disinhibited? Do they make inappropriate comments or engage in socially unacceptable behaviors (e.g., flatulence, nose picking)? Do they approach strangers and engage them in conversations, or have new-onset gambling or stealing?
2. *Early apathy/inertia.* Does the patient demonstrate a significant loss of interest, drive, or initiation of behavior? For example, those patients who were once hardworking and spontaneous may become passive and indifferent to the surrounding environment. They may also become disengaged in others around them and show little interest in initiating or maintaining conversations.
3. *Early loss of empathy/sympathy.* Does the patient make hurtful or insensitive comments to others (e.g., make disparaging remarks about other's weight or looks), seem not to notice the pain or distress of others, lack emotional warmth?
4. *New-onset compulsive/stereotyped behaviors.* Patients with bvFTD can manifest complex compulsions, such as counting or checking rituals

or hoarding of useless items such as paper napkins. They may also display simple motor or vocal stereotypies such as tapping, picking, lip smacking, and repeating nonsensical phrases.

5. *Hyperorality or dietary changes*. Changes in eating or hyperorality may occur as well, such that a person may begin to consume alcohol in large quantities, take up smoking cigarettes, or prefer to eat only fast food or sweets. Indeed, significant weight gain is common in bvFTD. Eating behaviors can also take on a compulsive or rigid quality such as binge eating, eating only certain foods, or needing to be served meals at a particular time.
6. *Neuropsychological profile (executive deficits with relative preservation of memory and visuospatial function)*: does the patient seem to have trouble completing complex tasks, or doing two things at once, but can still drive, navigate around town, or remember conversations that occurred a few days earlier? As many patients will not have undergone neuropsychological testing prior to your assessment, pointed "real-world" questions regarding attention/executive functions vs. memory and visuospatial function can help get a better understanding of their cognitive profile.

Family History

Approximately 30–40% of all individuals with bvFTD have a strong family history of the disease. Unfortunately, clear family histories are often difficult to elicit. There may be vague recollections that one of their grandparents was "senile" or had been diagnosed with a psychiatric disorder later in life. However, if a history reveals family members who exhibited significant changes in personality and social behavior after the fifth decade or who had symptoms of motor disorder (e.g., ALS, PSP, CBS), these are potential clues that the individual may have a genetic form of the disease.

Neuroimaging

If the patient has had neuroimaging, it will be helpful to obtain the report or review the scan with a neuroradiologist or neurologist. Atrophy is often asymmetric (right > left) and, in the early middle stages, confined to the medial frontal and anterior temporal lobes. With increasing disease severity, more diffuse areas of these brain regions degenerate, and more posterior areas including the parietal cortex become involved [22, 97, 98]. Of note, atrophy of the hippocampus also occurs in bvFTD [21, 22]; therefore, this finding should not be used to support a diagnosis of AD rather than bvFTD. Clinically, structural magnetic resonance imaging (MRI) is best for reviewing these findings, though positron emission tomography (PET) scans may also reveal hypometabolism of the frontal and temporal lobes. While currently available only through research, PET imaging that utilizes Pittsburg Compound B (PIB), a radioligand which binds to amyloid in the brain, has been shown to be negative in bvFTD [97].

Cognitive Assessment

In general, tests of global cognition such as Folstein's Mini Mental Examination (MMSE; [127]), the Blessed-Roth Dementia Rating Scale [128], or the Montreal Cognitive Assessment (MoCA; [129]) can be insensitive to the subtle changes in cognition that occur early in bvFTD. Indeed, some bvFTD patients in our clinic score 30/30 on the MMSE, despite significant behavioral and social deficits. Nevertheless, inclusion of a measure of global cognition is standard practice in dementia assessment. With its greater focus on verbal fluency and executive functions, the MoCA may be better able to pick up on subtle deficits in bvFTD, and is our measure of choice in this population.

We find that a short battery (approximately 1–1.5 h) that examines all major cognitive domains is a quick and useful way to help aid differential diagnosis without overtaxing the patient. While by no means invariable, the relative neuropsychological profile of a patient with bvFTD tends to be one of spared visuospatial and language function and relatively better performance than patients with AD on tests of episodic and semantic memory. Verbal fluency is relatively better categorically than phonemically (though both may be attenuated due to economy of speech). We also recommend executive function tests that elicit and quantify performance errors like rule violations, perseveration, environmental dependency, impulsivity, and distractibility since achievement scores have not been shown to reliably differentiate between bvFTD and AD.

Behavioral Observations

After neuropsychological evaluation, examiners at our center complete a brief behavior-rating scale where patients are rated on a scale ranging from none, mild, moderate, and severe on the following observable behaviors: agitation, stimulus boundedness, perseverations, decreased initiation, motor stereotypies, distractibility, lack of social/emotional engagement, impulsivity, socially inappropriate behavior, and impaired or fluctuating levels of attention. Data from our center suggest that perseverative and inappropriate behaviors and lack of social engagement significantly discriminate between patients with bvFTD and AD. In addition to providing important diagnostic information, quantifying behaviors systematically can also be helpful in interpreting the neuropsychological data (e.g., did the patient fully attend to the task, or were they distracted and disinhibited?).

Informant-Based Measures

The inclusion of informant-based measures in your assessment can yield important information which, for one reason or another, was not gleaned on interview. These scales can provide invaluable information regarding social and emotional deficits experienced by the patient.

Neuropsychiatric Inventory [130]

The Neuropsychiatric Inventory (NPI) is a screening measure that is administered to the patient's informant by the clinician and is a well-validated measure of neuropsychiatric symptoms common in neurodegenerative disease. It was developed as a way to quickly and accurately assess the frequency and severity of 12 different neuropsychiatric behaviors that may occur in the context of dementia (e.g., anxiety, apathy, disinhibition, aberrant motor behavior). The informant is also asked to rate their level of distress by each symptom, which can be useful in helping structure feedback with the family. Extensive research investigating neuropsychiatric symptoms in dementia has been completed with the NPI [130]. Patients with bvFTD tend to have higher overall total scores on the NPI compared to AD, and the domains of apathy, disinhibition, aberrant motor behavior, and appetite/eating changes appear to best differentiate between bvFTD and AD [131–133].

Revised Self-Monitoring Scale [134]

This 13-item questionnaire measures an individual's sensitivity and responsiveness to social cues. While the measure was initially designed for self-report, this questionnaire is easily adapted to an informant-based questionnaire.

Interpersonal Reactivity Index [135]

The empathic concern (EC) and perspective taking (PT) subscales of the Interpersonal Reactivity Index (IRI) were designed to evaluate an individual's ability to empathize with others. The 7-item EC scale specifically measures an individual's emotional response which results from the perception of another's emotional state. The 7-item PT subscale measures an individual's tendency to spontaneously employ perspective taking in their typical social interactions.

Experimental Measures of Emotional/ Social Function

There are a number of commercially available measures of emotional and social function that have been used to study deficits in bvFTD, but we have found that many of these tasks are too long or attentionally demanding for our patients, and do not provide us with reliable information. We have found that the following two measures are well tolerated by our patients and provide diagnostically valuable information. Both tasks are in the final stages of development and will be published shortly. Copies can be obtained from the developer, Dr. Katherine Rankin at the University of California, San Francisco (UCSF; krankin@memory.ucsf.edu).

Dynamic Affect Recognition Test (Rankin et al., personal communication)

This test was designed to assess emotion recognition using dynamic, ecologically valid stimuli. Individuals are asked to watch 12 brief (20 s) vignettes of actors depicting one of six basic emotions (happy, surprised, sad, angry, fearful, and disgusted) with a semantically neutral script and choose the correct emotion. Comparison of performance between patients with AD and bvFTD at our center suggests that those with AD perform comparably to normal controls, while those with bvFTD have significant deficits in their ability to accurately recognize emotions.

Social Norms Questionnaire (Rankin et al., personal communication)

This simple, 22-item yes/no questionnaire was developed as a way to determine the degree to which patients understand and can accurately identify implicit, but widely accepted social boundaries dominant in US culture. The social norms questionnaire (SNQ22) includes both inappropriate (e.g., "Cut in line if you are in a hurry," "Pick your nose in public," and "Wear the same shirt every day") and generally acceptable behaviors (e.g., "Tell a coworker your age," "Blow your nose in public," and "Eat ribs with your fingers"). Data from our center suggests that compared to patients with AD, those with bvFTD rate many behaviors as appropriate that normal adults would say are inappropriate.

Case History

History of Presenting Illness

Mr. R is a 63-year-old, right-handed, retired policeman presenting for evaluation of personality and behavioral changes. While Mr. R denies any changes in his cognition or behavior, his wife and son provided additional clinical history.

Mr. R's symptoms began insidiously around the age of 58. Previously kind and even tempered, Mr. R became progressively more negative and critical of others. His demeanor became sarcastic and socially inappropriate, telling off-color jokes in mixed company, and making loud derogatory remarks about overweight individuals standing nearby. He was more irritable and impatient when driving, lashing out verbally against other drivers for perceived infractions. There were no reported incidents of aggressive or violent behaviors. His family reported an overall emotional blunting, social withdrawal, and detachment from his family, losing all interest in their lives. The patient's wife reported that if she did not plan activities, Mr. R would stand and stare out the window all day. His son noted that his previously strong interest in the upkeep of his car had dissipated over the prior 2 years. In addition, his diet drastically changed from healthy, low-fat foods to primarily junk food, candy, and large quantities of coffee. His family reported a weight gain of over 20 pounds in the past 5 years.

Mr. R's family also reported a significant decline in function, such that he became unable to follow through with paying bills, instead just leaving paperwork in piles around the house. His wife was not aware of this issue until they began receiving a series of notices. While previously handy around the home, Mr. R became unable to complete familiar projects, such as hanging doors, instead starting the job but then leaving it midstream. His family was also aware that Mr. R's job category at the police station changed once or twice in the 2 years before retirement for reasons that were unclear to them, but which they now believe may have had to do with his impairments.

The patient's family noted that Mr. R had begun to engage in compulsive behaviors including emptying the recycling bin at home several times a day, checking the lint trap in the dryer repeatedly, and collecting paper napkins from restaurants. He also engaged in repetitive behaviors such as whistling and tapping his hands on the table for prolonged periods of time. He compulsively scratches himself but no rash has been noted. He continues to display loss of empathy and will laugh when other people get hurt. He will often say repeatedly throughout the day, "everyone has lost their sense of humor!" or "where has your sense of humor gone?" He is restless and often wants to go somewhere; however, upon arriving at a new destination, he quickly wants to go back home. The family did not endorse any significant declines in his episodic memory, language, visuospatial, or motor function.

Mr. R's typical day consists of getting up, showering, and getting dressed. He requires reminders to bathe and groom himself. He will stand at a window for long periods of time and report that his son has gone by or that he is waiting for somebody to arrive. He appears insatiable and will eat for extended periods of time if he is not stopped. Current medications include Lexapro (20 mg/daily) and Simvastatin (20 mg/daily).

Social/Medical History

Mr. R has been married to his wife for 44 years. They have four adult children. He completed a Master's Degree in Sociology. He worked in law enforcement for 30 years. According to his family, he performed his job in an extremely professional manner and was well respected.

Past medical history is significant for a history of hypercholesterolemia. He has never been hospitalized nor had any surgery. He has no history of head trauma, severe febrile illness, or thyroid disease.

Family history is significant for a mother who developed signs of significant cognitive dysfunction around age 85 which was characterized mainly by memory loss and hallucinations. She died in 2007 with a diagnosis of dementia. His father died at age 59 of a heart attack. There is no other known family history of dementia, neurological or neuromuscular disorders, or psychiatric illness.

Neuropsychological Test Summary

Please see Table 21.3

Neuropsychiatric Symptom Assessment

Examination of the NPI subscales indicates that the patient's wife endorsed frequent symptoms of agitation, apathy, disinhibition, aberrant motor behavior, and changes in appetite/eating behavior that cause her significant distress (NPI Total Score: 60).

Functional Evaluation

The patient's Clinical Dementia Rating Scale (CDR) total score was 1.0. His most significant impairments occurred in the domains of judgment and problem solving, home and hobbies and personal care.

Imaging Results (Fig. 21.1)

Impressions and Formulation

Mr. R is a 63-year-old, retired policeman with a 5-year history of significant personality and behavior changes marked by disinhibited and socially inappropriate behavior, irritability, apathy and social withdrawal, poor executive functioning, obsessive–compulsive activities, and hyperorality with a 20-pound weight gain in the past five years.

On neuropsychological testing, his affect was notable for emotional blunting and mild irritability. Overall, Mr. R demonstrated below average performance on free recall measures of verbal and visual episodic memory. Verbal and visual recognition memory were within normal limits. His performance on measures of executive functioning varied, ranging from impaired to average. Of note, he made a total of 22 errors, which is well above average compared to others in his age range. Global cognition, attention/working memory, language, and visuospatial function remain largely intact.

Given his history of significant emotional and behavioral changes, error-prone pattern of performance on measures of executive function and

Table 21.3 Neuropsychological test summary

Domain	Test	Raw score	Range
Global	MMSE	29/30	Within normal limits (WNL)
Attention/working memory	Longest digit span forward	7	WNL
	Longest digit span backward	5	WNL
Memory	CVLT-II-SF trial 1–4 total	23/36	Below average
	CVLT-II-SF 10-min delay	6/9	Below average
	CVLT-II-SF cued recall	7/9	Below average
	CVLT-II-SF recognition	9/9; 1 false positive	WNL
	Figure copy recall	10/17	Below average
	Figure copy recognition	YES	WNL
Language	Abbreviated BNT total	15/15	WNL
	Syntax comprehension	5/5	WNL
	Repetition	5/5	WNL
Visuospatial	Figure copy	15/17	WNL
	Object–number location matching	10/10	WNL
	Face perception	12/12	WNL
	Calculations	4/5	Below average
Executive function	Modified Trail Making Test (time)	64/120	Below average
	Modified Trail Making Test errors	4	–
	Design fluency	11	Average
	Design fluency errors	4	–
	"D" word fluency (60)	3	Impaired
	"D" word errors	3	–
	Animal fluency (60)	14	Below average
	Animal fluency errors	2	–
	Stroop interference total	54	Average
	Stroop interference errors	9	–
	Affect naming	9/16	Impaired

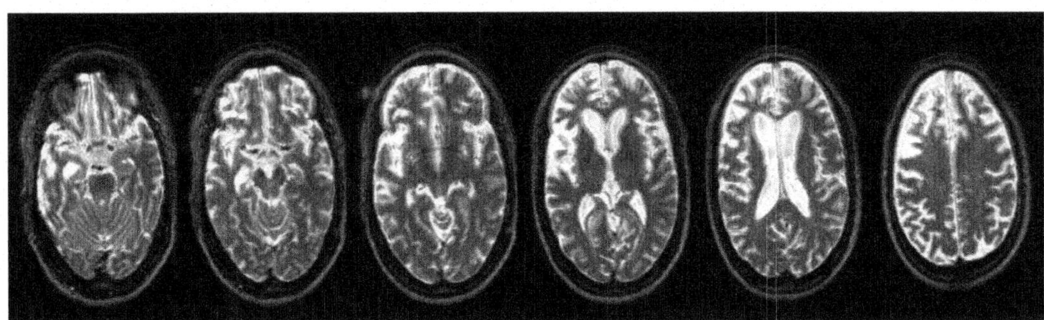

Fig. 21.1 T2-weighted structural magnetic resonance imaging (MRI) of Mr. R's brain. Note the significant volume loss in the frontal and temporal lobes bilaterally, worse on the right compared to left (image is oriented according to radiological convention; e.g., left = right, right = left)

neuroimaging findings of right > left degeneration of paralimbic frontal, temporal, and insular structures, his pattern of findings is most suggestive of a diagnosis of behavioral variant frontotemporal dementia.

In terms of treatment, Mr. R's primary care physician may want to consider prescribing treatment with a selective-serotonin reuptake inhibitor (SSRI) in order to target his obsessive–compulsive behaviors and irritability. However, anticholinesterase agents should not be prescribed, as these have been known to exacerbate the irritability seen in frontotemporal dementia. I also recommend that Mr. R begin a program of vigorous physical activity, as exercise has been shown to have neuroprotective properties. His entire family may want to consider attending a FTD caregiver support group. Finally, despite intact attention and visuospatial skills, it is strongly recommended that Mr. R discontinue driving, in order to avoid the possibility of an untoward event.

Clinical Pearls

- FTD is first and foremost a disease that disrupts behavior and social function.
- Compared to AD, patients with bvFTD tend to have little insight into their condition and are more flat, perseverative, inappropriate, and emotionally dysregulated.
- Due to its pathological heterogeneity, bvFTD can present alone or in combination with other diseases such as PSP, CBD, and ALS.
- BvFTD is often misdiagnosed as late-onset psychiatric disease or early onset AD.
- The presence of executive dysfunction in the absence of other major cognitive impairments is not specific to bvFTD.
- Neuropsychological testing should focus on *relative patterns* of performance vs. domain impairments.
- In the early stages of disease, process-oriented features of performance such as rule-violations and errors appear to best discriminate between bvFTD and AD.
- Integration of history, behavioral observations, imaging, social/emotional function, informant questionnaires, and relative test scores in keeping with the disease are most important in coming to an accurate diagnosis.
- A multidisciplinary team approach, working with a neurologist and other health-care professionals, is most helpful in diagnosing this elusive disease.

References

1. Ratnavalli E, Brayne C, Dawson K, Hodges JR. The prevalence of frontotemporal dementia. Neurology. 2002;58(11):1615–21.
2. Cairns NJ, Bigio EH, Mackenzie IR, Neumann M, Lee VM, Hatanpaa KJ, et al. Neuropathologic diagnostic and nosologic criteria for frontotemporal lobar degeneration: consensus of the consortium for frontotemporal lobar degeneration. Acta Neuropathol. 2007;114(1):5–22.
3. Mercy L, Hodges JR, Dawson K, Barker RA, Brayne C. Incidence of early-onset dementias in Cambridgeshire, United Kingdom. Neurology. 2008;71(19):1496–9.
4. Knopman DS, Petersen RC, Edland SD, Cha RH, Rocca WA. The incidence of frontotemporal lobar degeneration in rochester, minnesota, 1990 through 1994. Neurology. 2004;62(3):506–8.
5. Johnson JK, Diehl J, Mendez MF, Neuhaus J, Shapira JS, Forman M, et al. Frontotemporal lobar degeneration: demographic characteristics of 353 patients. Arch Neurol. 2005;62(6):925–30.
6. Hodges JR, Davies R, Xuereb J, Kril J, Halliday G. Survival in frontotemporal dementia. Neurology. 2003;61(3):349–54.
7. Mendez M, Cummings J. Dementia: a clinical approach. Philadelphia: Butterworth Heinemann; 2003.
8. Neary D, Snowden JS, Gustafson L, Passant U, Stuss D, Black S, et al. Frontotemporal lobar degeneration: a consensus on clinical diagnostic criteria. Neurology. 1998;51(6):1546–54.
9. Pickering-Brown SM. The complex aetiology of frontotemporal lobar degeneration. Exp Neurol. 2007;206(1):1–10.
10. Gorno-Tempini ML, Hillis AE, Weintraub S, Kertesz A, Mendez M, Cappa SF, et al. Classification of primary progressive aphasia and its variants. Neurology. 2011;76(11):1006–14.
11. Miller BL, Seeley WW, Mychack P, Rosen HJ, Mena I, Boone K. Neuroanatomy of the self: evidence from patients with frontotemporal dementia. Neurology. 2001;57(5):817–21.
12. Boxer AL, Miller BL. Clinical features of frontotemporal dementia. Alzheimer Dis Assoc Disord. 2005;19 Suppl 1:S3–6.
13. Liu W, Miller BL, Kramer JH, Rankin K, Wyss-Coray C, Gearhart R, et al. Behavioral disorders in the frontal and temporal variants of frontotemporal dementia. Neurology. 2004;62(5):742–8.
14. Passant U, Elfgren C, Englund E, Gustafson L. Psychiatric symptoms and their psychosocial consequences in frontotemporal dementia. Alzheimer Dis Assoc Disord. 2005;19 Suppl 1:S15–8.

15. Shinagawa S, Ikeda M, Fukuhara R, Tanabe H. Initial symptoms in frontotemporal dementia and semantic dementia compared with Alzheimer's disease. Dement Geriatr Cogn Disord. 2006;21(2):74–80.
16. Mendez MF, Chen AK, Shapira JS, Miller BL. Acquired sociopathy and frontotemporal dementia. Dement Geriatr Cogn Disord. 2005;20(2–3):99–104.
17. Miller BL, Darby A, Benson DF, Cummings JL, Miller MH. Aggressive, socially disruptive and antisocial behaviour associated with fronto-temporal dementia. Br J Psychiatry. 1997;170:150–4.
18. Miller BL, Cummings JL, Villanueva-Meyer J, Boone K, Mehringer CM, Lesser IM, et al. Frontal lobe degeneration: clinical, neuropsychological, and SPECT characteristics. Neurology. 1991;41(9):1374–82.
19. Rankin KP, Baldwin E, Pace-Savitsky C, Kramer JH, Miller BL. Self awareness and personality change in dementia. J Neurol Neurosurg Psychiatry. 2005;76(5):632–9.
20. Rascovsky K, Hodges JR, Knopman D, Mendez MF, Kramer JH, Neuhaus J, et al. Sensitivity of revised diagnostic criteria for the behavioural variant of frontotemporal dementia. Brain. 2011;134(9):2456–77.
21. Seeley WW, Crawford R, Rascovsky K, Kramer JH, Weiner M, Miller BL, et al. Frontal paralimbic network atrophy in very mild behavioral variant frontotemporal dementia. Arch Neurol. 2008;65(2): 249–55.
22. Broe M, Hodges JR, Schofield E, Shepherd CE, Kril JJ, Halliday GM. Staging disease severity in pathologically confirmed cases of frontotemporal dementia. Neurology. 2003;60(6):1005–11.
23. Adolphs R. The social brain: neural basis of social knowledge. Annu Rev Psychol. 2009;60:693–716.
24. Seeley WW, Menon V, Schatzberg AF, Keller J, Glover GH, Kenna H, et al. Dissociable intrinsic connectivity networks for salience processing and executive control. J Neurosci. 2007;27(9):2349–56.
25. Rosen HJ, Gorno-Tempini ML, Goldman WP, Perry RJ, Schuff N, Weiner M, et al. Patterns of brain atrophy in frontotemporal dementia and semantic dementia. Neurology. 2002;58(2):198–208.
26. Perry RJ, Graham A, Williams G, Rosen H, Erzinclioglu S, Weiner M, et al. Patterns of frontal lobe atrophy in frontotemporal dementia: a volumetric MRI study. Dement Geriatr Cogn Disord. 2006;22(4):278–87.
27. Salmon E, Kerrouche N, Herholz K, Perani D, Holthoff V, Beuthien-Baumann B, et al. Decomposition of metabolic brain clusters in the frontal variant of frontotemporal dementia. Neuroimage. 2006;30(3):871–8.
28. Boccardi M, Sabattoli F, Laakso MP, Testa C, Rossi R, Beltramello A, et al. Frontotemporal dementia as a neural system disease. Neurobiol Aging. 2005;26(1):37–44.
29. Varrone A, Pappata S, Caraco C, Soricelli A, Milan G, Quarantelli M, et al. Voxel-based comparison of rCBF SPET images in frontotemporal dementia and Alzheimer's disease highlights the involvement of different cortical networks. Eur J Nucl Med Mol Imaging. 2002;29(11):1447–54.
30. Mackenzie IR, Neumann M, Bigio EH, Cairns NJ, Alafuzoff I, Kril J, et al. Nomenclature and nosology for neuropathologic subtypes of frontotemporal lobar degeneration: an update. Acta Neuropathol. 2010;119(1):1–4.
31. Ballatore C, Lee VM, Trojanowski JQ. Tau-mediated neurodegeneration in Alzheimer's disease and related disorders. Nat Rev Neurosci. 2007;8(9):663–72.
32. Chen-Plotkin AS, Lee VM, Trojanowski JQ. TAR DNA-binding protein 43 in neurodegenerative disease. Nat Rev Neurol. 2010;6(4):211–20.
33. Kertesz A, Martinez-Lage P, Davidson W, Munoz DG. The corticobasal degeneration syndrome overlaps progressive aphasia and frontotemporal dementia. Neurology. 2000;55(9):1368–75.
34. Kertesz A, McMonagle P, Blair M, Davidson W, Munoz DG. The evolution and pathology of frontotemporal dementia. Brain. 2005;128(Pt 9): 1996–2005.
35. Irwin D, Lippa CF, Swearer JM. Cognition and amyotrophic lateral sclerosis (ALS). Am J Alzheimers Dis Other Demen. 2007;22(4):300–12.
36. Tolnay M, Probst A. The neuropathological spectrum of neurodegenerative tauopathies. IUBMB Life. 2003;55(6):299–305.
37. Lee VM, Goedert M, Trojanowski JQ. Neurodegenerative tauopathies. Annu Rev Neurosci. 2001;24:1121–59.
38. Lillo P, Hodges JR. Frontotemporal dementia and motor neurone disease: overlapping clinic-pathological disorders. J Clin Neurosci. 2009;16(9):1131–5.
39. Mackenzie IR. The neuropathology of FTD associated with ALS. Alzheimer Dis Assoc Disord. 2007;21(4):S44–9.
40. Josephs KA, Petersen RC, Knopman DS, Boeve BF, Whitwell JL, Duffy JR, et al. Clinicopathologic analysis of frontotemporal and corticobasal degenerations and PSP. Neurology. 2006;66(1):41–8.
41. Lomen-Hoerth C, Anderson T, Miller B. The overlap of amyotrophic lateral sclerosis and frontotemporal dementia. Neurology. 2002;59(7):1077–9.
42. Strong MJ, Grace GM, Freedman M, Lomen-Hoerth C, Woolley S, Goldstein LH, et al. Consensus criteria for the diagnosis of frontotemporal cognitive and behavioural syndromes in amyotrophic lateral sclerosis. Amyotroph Lateral Scler. 2009;10(3):131–46.
43. Sikkink S, Rollinson S, Pickering-Brown SM. The genetics of frontotemporal lobar degeneration. Curr Opin Neurol. 2007;20(6):693–8.
44. Goldman JS, Farmer JM, Wood EM, Johnson JK, Boxer A, Neuhaus J, et al. Comparison of family histories in FTLD subtypes and related tauopathies. Neurology. 2005;65(11):1817–9.
45. Seelaar H, Kamphorst W, Rosso SM, Azmani A, Masdjedi R, de Koning I, et al. Distinct genetic forms of frontotemporal dementia. Neurology. 2008;71(16):1220–6.
46. Gydesen S, Hagen S, Klinken L, et al. Neuropsychiatric studies in a family with presenile

dementia different from Alzheimer and Pick disease. Acta Psychiatr Scand. 1987;76:276–84.
47. DeJesus-Hernandez M, Mackenzie IR, Boeve BF, Boxer AL, Baker M, Rutherford NJ, et al. Expanded GGGGCC hexanucleotide repeat in noncoding region of C9ORF72 causes chromosome 9p-linked FTD and ALS. Neuron. 2011;72(2):245–56.
48. Sha S, Takada L, Rankin KP, Yokoyama JS, Rutherford NJ, Fong JC, et al. Frontotemporal dementia due to *C9ORF72* mutations: Clinical and imaging features. 2012. Neurology, in press.
49. Kumar-Singh S, Van Broeckhoven C. Frontotemporal lobar degeneration: current concepts in the light of recent advances. Brain Pathol. 2007;17(1):104–14.
50. Hutton M, Lendon CL, Rizzu P, Baker M, Froelich S, Houlden H, et al. Association of missense and 5′-splice-site mutations in tau with the inherited dementia FTDP-17. Nature. 1998;393(6686):702–5.
51. Lynch T, Sano M, Marder KS, Bell KL, Foster NL, Defendini RF, et al. Clinical characteristics of a family with chromosome 17-linked disinhibition-dementia-parkinsonism-amyotrophy complex. Neurology. 1994;44(10):1878–84.
52. Baker M, Mackenzie IR, Pickering-Brown SM, Gass J, Rademakers R, Lindholm C, et al. Mutations in progranulin cause tau-negative frontotemporal dementia linked to chromosome 17. Nature. 2006;442(7105):916–9.
53. Mackenzie IR, Baker M, Pickering-Brown S, Hsiung GY, Lindholm C, Dwosh E, et al. The neuropathology of frontotemporal lobar degeneration caused by mutations in the progranulin gene. Brain. 2006;129(Pt 11):3081–90.
54. Rabinovici GD, Miller BL. Frontotemporal lobar degeneration: epidemiology, pathophysiology, diagnosis and management. CNS Drugs. 2010;24(5):375–98.
55. Snowden JS, Pickering-Brown SM, Mackenzie IR, Richardson AM, Varma A, Neary D, et al. Progranulin gene mutations associated with frontotemporal dementia and progressive non-fluent aphasia. Brain. 2006;129(Pt 11):3091–102.
56. Johnson JK, Head E, Kim R, Starr A, Cotman CW. Clinical and pathological evidence for a frontal variant of Alzheimer disease. Arch Neurol. 1999;56(10): 1233–9.
57. Woodward M, Jacova C, Black SE, Kertesz A, Mackenzie IR, Feldman H, et al. Differentiating the frontal variant of Alzheimer's disease. Int J Geriatr Psychiatry. 2010;25(7):732–8.
58. See TM, LaMarre AK, Lee SE, Miller BL. Genetic causes of frontotemporal degeneration. J Geriatr Psychiatry Neurol. 2010;23(4):260–8.
59. Rosenblatt A. Neuropsychiatry of Huntington's disease. Dialogues Clin Neurosci. 2007;9(2):191–7.
60. Woolley JD, Khan BK, Murthy NK, Miller BL, Rankin KP. The diagnostic challenge of psychiatric symptoms in neurodegenerative disease: rates of and risk factors for prior psychiatric diagnosis in patients with early neurodegenerative disease. J Clin Psychiatry. 2011;72(2):126–33.
61. Kipps CM, Nestor PJ, Fryer TD, Hodges JR. Behavioural variant frontotemporal dementia: not all it seems? Neurocase. 2007;13(4):237–47.
62. Mioshi E, Hodges JR. Rate of change of functional abilities in frontotemporal dementia. Dement Geriatr Cogn Disord. 2009;28(5):419–26.
63. Davies RR, Kipps CM, Mitchell J, Kril JJ, Halliday GM, Hodges JR. Progression in frontotemporal dementia: identifying a benign behavioral variant by magnetic resonance imaging. Arch Neurol. 2006;63(11):1627–31.
64. Wittenberg D, Possin KL, Rascovsky K, Rankin KP, Miller BL, Kramer JH. The early neuropsychological and behavioral characteristics of frontotemporal dementia. Neuropsychol Rev. 2008;18(1):91–102.
65. Thompson JC, Stopford CL, Snowden JS, Neary D. Qualitative neuropsychological performance characteristics in frontotemporal dementia and Alzheimer's disease. J Neurol Neurosurg Psychiatry. 2005;76(7):920–7.
66. McKhann G, Drachman D, Folstein M, Katzman R, Price D, Stadlan EM. Clinical diagnosis of Alzheimer's disease: report of the NINCDS-ADRDA work group under the auspices of department of health and human services task force on Alzheimer's disease. Neurology. 1984;34(7):939–44.
67. Welsh K, Butters N, Hughes J, Mohs R, Heyman A. Detection of abnormal memory decline in mild cases of Alzheimer's disease using CERAD neuropsychological measures. Arch Neurol. 1991;48(3):278–81.
68. Moss MB, Albert MS, Butters N, Payne M. Differential patterns of memory loss among patients with Alzheimer's disease, Huntington's disease, and alcoholic Korsakoff's syndrome. Arch Neurol. 1986;43(3):239–46.
69. Lezak MD, Howieson DB, Loring DW. Neuropsychological assessment. 4th ed. New York: Oxford University Press; 2004.
70. Hodges JR, Patterson K, Ward R, Garrard P, Bak T, Perry R, et al. The differentiation of semantic dementia and frontal lobe dementia (temporal and frontal variants of frontotemporal dementia) from early Alzheimer's disease: a comparative neuropsychological study. Neuropsychology. 1999;13(1):31–40.
71. Kramer JH, Jurik J, Sha SJ, Rankin KP, Rosen HJ, Johnson JK, et al. Distinctive neuropsychological patterns in frontotemporal dementia, semantic dementia, and Alzheimer disease. Cogn Behav Neurol. 2003;16(4):211–8.
72. Wicklund AH, Johnson N, Rademaker A, Weitner BB, Weintraub S. Word list versus story memory in Alzheimer's disease and frontotemporal dementia. Alzheimer Dis Assoc Disord. 2006;20(2):86–92.
73. Glosser G, Gallo JL, Clark CM, Grossman M. Memory encoding and retrieval in frontotemporal dementia and Alzheimer's disease. Neuropsychology. 2002;16(2):190–6.
74. Gregory CA, Serra-Mestres J, Hodges JR. Early diagnosis of the frontal variant of frontotemporal dementia: how sensitive are standard neuroimaging

and neuropsychologic tests? Neuropsychiatry Neuropsychol Behav Neurol. 1999;12(2):128–35.

75. Walker AJ, Meares S, Sachdev PS, Brodaty H. The differentiation of mild frontotemporal dementia from Alzheimer's disease and healthy aging by neuropsychological tests. Int Psychogeriatr. 2005; 17(1): 57–68.
76. Salmon DP, Filoteo JV. Neuropsychology of cortical versus subcortical dementia syndromes. Semin Neurol. 2007;27(1):7–21.
77. Kertesz A, McMonagle P. Behavior and cognition in corticobasal degeneration and progressive supranuclear palsy. J Neurol Sci. 2010;289(1–2):138–43.
78. LaMarre AK, Bostrum A, Miller BL, Kramer JH. Differential rates of cognitive decline in bvFTD, svFTD and AD. Dement Geriatr Cogn Disord. 2010;30(Supp 1):62.
79. Blair M, Marczinski CA, Davis-Faroque N, Kertesz A. A longitudinal study of language decline in Alzheimer's disease and frontotemporal dementia. J Int Neuropsychol Soc. 2007;13(2):237–45.
80. Rousseaux M, Seve A, Vallet M, Pasquier F, Mackowiak-Cordoliani MA. An analysis of communication in conversation in patients with dementia. Neuropsychologia. 2010;48(13):3884–90.
81. Neary D. Dementia of frontal lobe type. J Am Geriatr Soc. 1990;38(1):71–2.
82. Rogers TT, Ivanoiu A, Patterson K, Hodges JR. Semantic memory in Alzheimer's disease and the frontotemporal dementias: a longitudinal study of 236 patients. Neuropsychology. 2006;20(3):319–35.
83. Cotelli M, Borroni B, Manenti R, Ginex V, Calabria M, Moro A, et al. Universal grammar in the frontotemporal dementia spectrum: evidence of a selective disorder in the corticobasal degeneration syndrome. Neuropsychologia. 2007;45(13):3015–23.
84. Rascovsky K, Salmon DP, Hansen LA, Thal LJ, Galasko D. Disparate letter and semantic category fluency deficits in autopsy-confirmed frontotemporal dementia and Alzheimer's disease. Neuropsychology. 2007;21(1):20–30.
85. Gasparini M, Masciarelli G, Vanacore N, Ottaviani D, Salati E, Talarico G, et al. A descriptive study on constructional impairment in frontotemporal dementia and Alzheimer's disease. Eur J Neurol. 2008;15(6):589–97.
86. Grossi D, Fragassi NA, Chiacchio L, Valoroso L, Tuccillo R, Perrotta C, et al. Do visuospatial and constructional disturbances differentiate frontal variant of frontotemporal dementia and Alzheimer's disease? An experimental study of a clinical belief. Int J Geriatr Psychiatry. 2002;17(7):641–8.
87. Diehl J, Kurz A. Frontotemporal dementia: patient characteristics, cognition, and behaviour. Int J Geriatr Psychiatry. 2002;17(10):914–8.
88. Possin KL, Laluz VR, Alcantar OZ, Miller BL, Kramer JH. Distinct neuroanatomical substrates and cognitive mechanisms of figure copy performance in Alzheimer's disease and behavioral variant frontotemporal dementia. Neuropsychologia. 2011; 49(1):43–8.
89. Rascovsky K, Salmon DP, Ho GJ, Galasko D, Peavy GM, Hansen LA, et al. Cognitive profiles differ in autopsy-confirmed frontotemporal dementia and AD. Neurology. 2002;58(12):1801–8.
90. Blair M, Kertesz A, McMonagle P, Davidson W, Bodi N. Quantitative and qualitative analyses of clock drawing in frontotemporal dementia and Alzheimer's disease. J Int Neuropsychol Soc. 2006;12(2):159–65.
91. Gregory C, Lough S, Stone V, Erzinclioglu S, Martin L, Baron-Cohen S, et al. Theory of mind in patients with frontal variant frontotemporal dementia and Alzheimer's disease: theoretical and practical implications. Brain. 2002;125(Pt 4):752–64.
92. Torralva T, Kipps CM, Hodges JR, Clark L, Bekinschtein T, Roca M, et al. The relationship between affective decision-making and theory of mind in the frontal variant of fronto-temporal dementia. Neuropsychologia. 2007;45(2):342–9.
93. Krueger CE, Bird AC, Growdon ME, Jang JY, Miller BL, Kramer JH. Conflict monitoring in early frontotemporal dementia. Neurology. 2009;73(5): 349–55.
94. Gregory CA, Orrell M, Sahakian B, Hodges JR. Can frontotemporal dementia and Alzheimer's disease be differentiated using a brief battery of tests? Int J Geriatr Psychiatry. 1997;12(3):375–83.
95. Marra C, Quaranta D, Zinno M, Misciagna S, Bizzarro A, Masullo C, et al. Clusters of cognitive and behavioral disorders clearly distinguish primary progressive aphasia from frontal lobe dementia, and Alzheimer's disease. Dement Geriatr Cogn Disord. 2007;24(5):317–26.
96. Libon DJ, Xie SX, Moore P, Farmer J, Antani S, McCawley G, et al. Patterns of neuropsychological impairment in frontotemporal dementia. Neurology. 2007;68(5):369–75.
97. Rabinovici GD, Seeley WW, Kim EJ, Gorno-Tempini ML, Rascovsky K, Pagliaro TA, et al. Distinct MRI atrophy patterns in autopsy-proven Alzheimer's disease and frontotemporal lobar degeneration. Am J Alzheimers Dis Other Demen. 2007;22(6):474–88.
98 Schroeter ML, Raczka K, Neumann J, von Cramon DY. Neural networks in frontotemporal dementia—a meta-analysis. Neurobiol Aging. 2008;29(3):418–26.
99. Rohrer JD, Geser F, Zhou J, Gennatas ED, Sidhu M, Trojanowski JQ, et al. TDP-43 subtypes are associated with distinct atrophy patterns in frontotemporal dementia. Neurology. 2010;75(24):2204–11.
100. Strauss E, Sherman EMS, Spreen O. A compendium of neuropsychological tests: administration, norms, and commentary. 3rd ed. Oxford: Oxford University Press; 2006.
101. Miyake A, Friedman NP, Emerson MJ, Witzki AH, Howerter A, Wager TD. The unity and diversity of executive functions and their contributions to

complex "frontal lobe" tasks: a latent variable analysis. Cogn Psychol. 2000;41(1):49–100.
102. Carey CL, Woods SP, Damon J, Halabi C, Dean D, Delis DC, et al. Discriminant validity and neuroanatomical correlates of rule monitoring in frontotemporal dementia and Alzheimer's disease. Neuropsychologia. 2008;46(4):1081–7.
103. O'Keeffe FM, Murray B, Coen RF, Dockree PM, Bellgrove MA, Garavan H, et al. Loss of insight in frontotemporal dementia, corticobasal degeneration and progressive supranuclear palsy. Brain. 2007;130(Pt 3):753–64.
104. Nedjam Z, Devouche E, Dalla Barba G. Confabulation, but not executive dysfunction discriminate AD from frontotemporal dementia. Eur J Neurol. 2004;11(11):728–33.
105. Beer JS, Heerey EA, Keltner D, Scabini D, Knight RT. The regulatory function of self-conscious emotion: insights from patients with orbitofrontal damage. J Pers Soc Psychol. 2003;85(4):594–604.
106. Rolls ET. The functions of the orbitofrontal cortex. Brain Cogn. 2004;55(1):11–29.
107. Hornak J, Bramham J, Rolls ET, Morris RG, O'Doherty J, Bullock PR, et al. Changes in emotion after circumscribed surgical lesions of the orbitofrontal and cingulate cortices. Brain. 2003;126 (Pt 7):1691–712.
108. Zald DH, Andreotti C. Neuropsychological assessment of the orbital and ventromedial prefrontal cortex. Neuropsychologia. 2010;48(12):3377–91.
109. Rankin KP, Santos-Modesitt W, Kramer JH, Pavlic D, Beckman V, Miller BL. Spontaneous social behaviors discriminate behavioral dementias from psychiatric disorders and other dementias. J Clin Psychiatry. 2008;69(1):60–73.
110. Eslinger PJ, Moore P, Troiani V, Antani S, Cross K, Kwok S, et al. Oops! resolving social dilemmas in frontotemporal dementia. J Neurol Neurosurg Psychiatry. 2007;78(5):457–60.
111. Rankin KP, Rosen HJ, Kramer JH, Schauer GF, Weiner MW, Schuff N, et al. Right and left medial orbitofrontal volumes show an opposite relationship to agreeableness in FTD. Dement Geriatr Cogn Disord. 2004;17(4):328–32.
112. Ruby P, Schmidt C, Hogge M, D'Argembeau A, Collette F, Salmon E. Social mind representation: where does it fail in frontotemporal dementia? J Cogn Neurosci. 2007;19(4):671–83.
113. Eslinger PJ, Dennis K, Moore P, Antani S, Hauck R, Grossman M. Metacognitive deficits in frontotemporal dementia. J Neurol Neurosurg Psychiatry. 2005;76(12):1630–5.
114. Bozeat S, Gregory CA, Ralph MA, Hodges JR. Which neuropsychiatric and behavioural features distinguish frontal and temporal variants of frontotemporal dementia from Alzheimer's disease? J Neurol Neurosurg Psychiatry. 2000;69(2):178–86.
115. Sturm VE, Rosen HJ, Allison S, Miller BL, Levenson RW. Self-conscious emotion deficits in frontotemporal lobar degeneration. Brain. 2006;129(Pt 9):2508–16.
116. Sturm VE, Ascher EA, Miller BL, Levenson RW. Diminished self-conscious emotional responding in frontotemporal lobar degeneration patients. Emotion. 2008;8(6):861–9.
117. Goodkind MS, Gyurak A, McCarthy M, Miller BL, Levenson RW. Emotion regulation deficits in frontotemporal lobar degeneration and Alzheimer's disease. Psychol Aging. 2010;25(1):30–7.
118. Werner KH, Roberts NA, Rosen HJ, Dean DL, Kramer JH, Weiner MW, et al. Emotional reactivity and emotion recognition in frontotemporal lobar degeneration. Neurology. 2007;69(2):148–55.
119. Rosen HJ, Perry RJ, Murphy J, Kramer JH, Mychack P, Schuff N, et al. Emotion comprehension in the temporal variant of frontotemporal dementia. Brain. 2002;125(Pt 10):2286–95.
120. Rosen HJ, Pace-Savitsky K, Perry RJ, Kramer JH, Miller BL, Levenson RW. Recognition of emotion in the frontal and temporal variants of frontotemporal dementia. Dement Geriatr Cogn Disord. 2004;17(4): 277–81.
121. Kipps CM, Nestor PJ, Acosta-Cabronero J, Arnold R, Hodges JR. Understanding social dysfunction in the behavioural variant of frontotemporal dementia: the role of emotion and sarcasm processing. Brain. 2009;132(Pt 3):592–603.
122. Rankin KP, Kramer JH, Miller BL. Patterns of cognitive and emotional empathy in frontotemporal lobar degeneration. Cogn Behav Neurol. 2005;18(1): 28–36.
123. Bechara A, Damasio AR, Damasio H, Anderson SW. Insensitivity to future consequences following damage to human prefrontal cortex. Cognition. 1994;50(1–3):7–15.
124. Torralva T, Roca M, Gleichgerrcht E, Bekinschtein T, Manes F. A neuropsychological battery to detect specific executive and social cognitive impairments in early frontotemporal dementia. Brain. 2009;132(Pt 5):1299–309.
125. Gleichgerrcht E, Ibanez A, Roca M, Torralva T, Manes F. Decision-making cognition in neurodegenerative diseases. Nat Rev Neurol. 2010;6(11): 611–23.
126. Rahman S, Sahakian BJ, Hodges JR, Rogers RD, Robbins TW. Specific cognitive deficits in mild frontal variant frontotemporal dementia. Brain. 1999;122(Pt 8):1469–93.
127. Folstein MF, Folstein SE, McHugh PR. "Mini-mental state". A practical method for grading the cognitive state of patients for the clinician. J Psychiatr Res. 1975;12(3):189–98.
128. Blessed G, Tomlinson BE, Roth M. Blessed-roth dementia scale (DS). Psychopharmacol Bull. 1988;24(4):705–8.
129. Nasreddine ZS, Phillips NA, Bedirian V, Charbonneau S, Whitehead V, Collin I, et al. The montreal cognitive assessment, MoCA: a brief screening tool for mild cognitive impairment. J Am Geriatr Soc. 2005;53(4):695–9.

130. Cummings JL. The neuropsychiatric inventory: assessing psychopathology in dementia patients. Neurology. 1997;48(5, Suppl 6):S10–6.
131. Srikanth S, Nagaraja AV, Ratnavalli E. Neuropsychiatric symptoms in dementia-frequency, relationship to dementia severity and comparison in Alzheimer's disease, vascular dementia and frontotemporal dementia. J Neurol Sci. 2005;236(1–2): 43–8.
132. Levy ML, Miller BL, Cummings JL, Fairbanks LA, Craig A. Alzheimer disease and frontotemporal dementias. Behavioral distinctions. Arch Neurol. 1996;53(7):687–90.
133. Blair M, Kertesz A, Davis-Faroque N, Hsiung GY, Black SE, Bouchard RW, et al. Behavioural measures in frontotemporal lobar dementia and other dementias: the utility of the frontal behavioural inventory and the neuropsychiatric inventory in a national cohort study. Dement Geriatr Cogn Disord. 2007;23(6):406–15.
134. Lennox RD, Wolfe RN. Revision of the self-monitoring scale. J Pers Soc Psychol. 1984;46(6): 1349–64.
135. Davis MH. Measuring individual differences in empathy: evidence for a multidimensional approach. J Pers Soc Psychol. 1983;44(1):113–26.

Movement Disorders with Dementia in Older Adults

22

Alexander I. Tröster and Nina Browner

Abstract

Dementias associated with movement disorders are the second most common form of dementia in old age after Alzheimer's disease. This chapter outlines the key neurological, neuropathological, neuroimaging, and neuropsychological features of two synucleinopathies (Parkinson's disease dementia and dementia with Lewy bodies) and two tauopathies (corticobasal syndrome and progressive supranuclear palsy). Neuropsychological evaluation of patients with movement disorders can be challenging, and some common pitfalls and suggestions for avoiding them are presented. Particular attention is paid to the type of information that must be elicited from medical records and the interview to plan an effective evaluation. Recommended instruments for the assessment and screening of cognition and psychiatric conditions, such as apathy and depression, are identified and some compensatory techniques are described. A case study is presented to illustrate the application of such instruments in the clinical setting.

Keywords

Dementia with Lewy bodies • Parkinson's disease • Corticobasal degeneration • Corticobasal syndrome • Basal ganglia • Progressive supranuclear palsy • Synucleinopathy • Tauopathy

A.I. Tröster, Ph.D. (✉)
Barrow Neurological Institute, 240 West Thomas Rd, Suite 301, Phoenix, Az 85013, USA
e-mail: Alexander.Troster@DignityHealth.org

N. Browner, M.D.
Department of Neurology (CB 7025), University of North Carolina School of Medicine, 170 Manning Drive, Suite 3128, Chapel Hill, NC 27599-7025, USA
e-mail: nbrowner@ad.unc.edu

L.D. Ravdin and H.L. Katzen (eds.), *Handbook on the Neuropsychology of Aging and Dementia*, Clinical Handbooks in Neuropsychology, DOI 10.1007/978-1-4614-3106-0_22,

In old age, the most common dementias associated with movement disorders are Parkinson's disease (PD) dementia (PDD), dementia with Lewy bodies (DLB), corticobasal degeneration (CBD), and progressive supranuclear palsy (PSP). These conditions can be broadly grouped according to their characteristic neuropathologic features as synucleinopathies (DLB and PDD) or tauopathies (CBD and PSP). Clinical neuropsychological test findings by themselves are not diagnostic, and differentiation between synucleinopathies and tauopathies might be easier than distinguishing among synucleinopathies or among tauopathies. Indeed, the neuropsychological features of PDD and DLB are often indistinguishable even if subtle differences occasionally emerge [1], and for this reason are considered together within this chapter. Similarly, the tauopathies have considerable symptom overlap, and CBD can present clinically resembling PSP, and vice versa (and both can present initially as a primary progressive aphasia). Despite neuropsychological overlap among dementias associated with different movement disorders, neuropsychological evaluation that carefully weighs test results, neuroimaging and neurological findings, interview information about disease course, emergence of various motor and non-motor symptoms (and their response to various treatments), and comorbidities can be helpful in supporting or ruling out a specific diagnosis. When patients with dementia and a movement disorder are referred for neuropsychological evaluation, the referral issue is often one of facilitating differential diagnosis and determining if additional factors (e.g., depression, medications, or medical conditions) are producing cognitive compromise. Other referral issues include patient selection for treatment (e.g., as in PD patients being considered for deep brain stimulation or DBS (patients with dementia are evaluated and typically excluded as candidates for DBS), documenting deficit progression with advancing disease (or improvement with treatment), and characterization of deficits to help determine potentially beneficial interventions and compensatory strategies.

Epidemiology

Parkinson's Disease Dementia and Dementia with Lewy Bodies

Prevalence estimates of PD range from 18 to 418 per 100,000 [2]. Annual incidence of PD has been estimated at 11 per 100,000, with incidence increasing from 0 per 100,000 among those 0–29 years old to 93 per 100,000 among those 70–79 years old [3]. A recent population-based study in France reported an incidence of 263 per 100,000 person-years [4]. Dementia prevalence estimates in PD vary from 8% to 93%, depending upon diagnostic criteria, sampling, and case ascertainment methods used. The most rigorous studies reveal a dementia prevalence of about 25% among patients with PD [5]. Dementia incidence is about 3% for persons with PD younger than 60 years and 15% for persons with PD older than 80 years [6–8]. Advancing age, low education, and postural instability and gait disturbance (PIGD) have been associated with increased dementia risk in PD, among other factors (see Table 22.1).

The prevalence of DLB as distinguished from PDD remains to be adequately documented, but DLB is said to be the second most common cause of dementia, accounting for up to 20% of cases

Table 22.1 Risk factors for dementia in Parkinson's disease [158]

Demographic variables	Disease variables	Neurobehavioral variables
Greater age	Later onset	Depression
Lower education	Disease duration	Poor performance on tests of
Lower socioeconomic status	Disease severity	(a) Executive/ attention
Family history of Parkinson's dementia	Susceptibility to levodopa-induced psychosis or confusion	(b) Verbal fluency
	REM sleep behavior disorder	(c) Visuoperceptual
	Akinetic-rigid symptoms	(d) List learning

coming to autopsy [9]. A review of six studies noted a DLB prevalence ranging from 0 to 5% among the general population, and from 0 to 31% among dementia cases [10]. A recent study reported an incidence of suspected DLB of 112 per 100,000 person-years [4]. A study in the USA using formal diagnostic criteria for DLB reported a similar incidence of about 0.1% in the population and 3% among dementia cases [11].

Corticobasal Degeneration

Prevalence and incidence of CBD have not been widely studied. Prevalence in Japan has been reported to be about 2 per 100,000 [12] to 9 per 100,000 [13]. A Russian study estimated age-standardized incidence at 0.02 per 100,000 person-years [14]. Dementia and neurobehavioral abnormalities were thought to be rare in CBD but are now accepted to be a common presenting problem depending perhaps on whether patients initially present to movement disorder, dementia, or psychiatry clinics. Whereas one study noted that at initial presentation, only 19% of 36 patients had "slight generalized cognitive impairment" [15], another study observed that among 13 pathologically confirmed cases, 69% had dementia at presentation [16]. The H1/H1 tau haplotype has been identified as heightening susceptibility to both CBD and PSP (with the H2 haplotype perhaps being protective) [17], but no clear genetic etiology has been identified.

Progressive Supranuclear Palsy

The population prevalence of PSP is about 5 per 100,000 [18], but these estimates may be conservative due to diagnostic inaccuracy or uncertainty and range from about 3 to 6 per 100,000. Annual incidence of PSP is estimated at 5 per 100,000 [19] in persons older than 50 years though a recent Russian study reported an age-standardized incidence of 0.14 per 100,000 person-years [14]. Neither incidence nor prevalence of PSP is strongly associated with any demographic or genetic risk factors, except older age [20]. No adequate epidemiologic studies of neuropsychological impairments in PSP have been conducted, and dementia prevalence estimates in PSP of 50–80% might be overestimates due to common visual disturbances and information processing speed abnormalities. A recent study with a sample of over 300 patients observed impairments on the Dementia Rating Scale in 57% of patients, and on the Frontal Assessment Battery in 62% of cases [21].

Clinical and Neurological Presentation

Parkinson's Disease Dementia and Dementia with Lewy Bodies

Separate criteria have been proposed for PDD [22] and DLB [23] (see Tables 22.2 and 22.3). An essential feature differentiating PDD and DLB is the time of onset of dementia in relation to onset of motor signs. When neurobehavioral symptoms precede or occur within the first 12 months of the motor signs, then a diagnosis of DLB is made. By contrast, when cognitive symptoms have their onset more than 12 months after the onset of parkinsonism, then PDD is diagnosed.

Parkinson's disease dementia requires that a prior diagnosis of Parkinson's disease has been made. Several criteria for PD diagnosis have been proposed, but the most widely accepted are those of the UK Parkinson's Disease Society Brain Bank (or Queen Square) criteria [24]. Diagnosis of PD requires the presence of a parkinsonian syndrome evidenced by bradykinesia and at least one of muscular rigidity, 4–6 Hz resting tremor, and postural instability not related to proprioceptive, vestibular, visual, or cerebellar dysfunction. The diagnosis of definite PD requires at least three supportive features: unilateral onset, persistence of symptom asymmetry, progression of symptoms, excellent response to levodopa, levodopa response sustained for 5 years, levodopa-induced dyskinesias, or a clinical course over 10 years. Exclusion of various conditions capable of producing parkinsonism is required. PD most often becomes symptomatic

Table 22.2 Clinical diagnostic criteria for PDD (based on Emre et al. [22])

Core features: (both required for probable or possible PDD)
1. Diagnosis of Parkinson's disease per UK Parkinson's Disease Society Brain Bank criteria
2. Dementia of insidious onset and slow progression in the presence of PD, defined by: (a) Impairment of more than one domain of cognition (b) Impairment represents a decline from premorbid functioning (c) Impairment in day-to-day functioning not ascribable to motor or autonomic dysfunction
Associated features: (typical cognitive profile as outlined below in at least 2 of the 4 domains, and at least one of the behavioral symptoms required for diagnosis of probable PDD; atypical cognitive profile in one or more domains allows for diagnosis of possible PDD, in which behavioral disturbance may or may not be present)
1. Cognition (a) Impaired attention which may fluctuate within or across days (b) Impaired executive functions, e.g., planning, conceptualization, initiation, rule finding, set maintenance or shifting, bradyphrenia (c) Preserved language, though word-finding and complex sentence comprehension deficits may be present (d) Impaired memory, usually with benefit from cuing and better recognition than recall
2. Behavior (a) Apathy (b) Changes in mood and personality, including features of depression and anxiety (c) Delusions; commonly of the paranoid type (d) Hallucinations; usually visual, complex, and well formed (e) Excessive daytime sleepiness/somnolence
Features making the diagnosis of PDD uncertain: (none of these features can be present when diagnosing probable PDD; one or both of these features can be present when diagnosing possible PDD)
1. Another abnormality capable of impairing cognition, but judged not to be the cause of the dementia (e.g., vascular disease on neuroimaging) 2. Time interval between onset of motor and cognitive symptoms is unknown
Features suggesting another condition as causing the mental impairment: (if present, PDD cannot be diagnosed)
1. Cognitive and behavioral abnormality occurs solely in the context of other conditions, such as confusional state due to systemic disease or intoxication, or major depressive disorder 2. Features consistent with probable vascular dementia per NINDS-AIREN criteria

during the sixth decade of life, but juvenile and young-onset forms occur. The most common initial cognitive complaint in both patients with PDD and those with DLB may involve memory. One study reported that 67% of PDD and 94% of DLB patients initially complained of memory problems [25]. However, patients may also initially complain of word-finding problems, difficulty keeping up with conversations due to slowness of thought, inefficiency with work, domestic chores and financial management, as well as problems with concentration, indecisiveness, and apathy [26]. In our experience, patients and/or their care partners may also report fairly early in PDD that the patient has problems with day-to-day and repair tasks with which they were previously facile (e.g., sequencing of recipes, trouble reassembling disassembled objects such as lawn mowers). In the case of DLB, cognitive changes are also likely to be accompanied by complaints of visual distortions and hallucinations and signs of possible rapid eye movement (REM) sleep behavior disorder (RBD) (e.g., acting out dreams while asleep).

Corticobasal Degeneration

Because the clinical features of CBD can be produced by conditions other than CBD, and pathologically confirmed CBD can have heterogeneous clinical presentations, it has been proposed that *corticobasal syndrome* (CBS) be the preferred term for conditions characterized by the core motor and cortical features of CBD regardless of etiology. In contrast, CBD has been proposed to

Table 22.3 Revised clinical diagnostic criteria for DLB (based on McKeith et al. [23])

Central feature: progressive cognitive decline that interferes with social and occupational function
Core features: (any 2 = Probable DLB; any 1 = Possible DLB)
1. Fluctuating cognition
2. Recurrent visual hallucinations
3. Spontaneous motor parkinsonism
**Suggestive features*: (1 or more + a core feature = Probable DLB, any 1 alone = Possible DLB)
1. REM sleep behavior disorder
2. Severe neuroleptic sensitivity
3. Decreased tracer uptake in striatum on SPECT dopamine transporter imaging or on MIBG myocardial scintigraphy
Supportive features: (common but lacking diagnostic specificity)
1. Repeated falls and syncope
2. Transient, unexplained loss of consciousness
3. Systematized delusions
4. Hallucinations in other modalities
5. Relative preservation of medial temporal lobe on CT or MRI scan
6. Decreased tracer uptake on SPECT or PET imaging in occipital regions
7. Prominent slow waves on EEG with temporal lobe transient sharp waves

be reserved for neuropathologically distinct CBD regardless of clinical presentation [27].

CBD onset is usually in the sixth decade of life, and mean time to death from diagnosis is about 7 years. CBD can present with either predominantly motor or cognitive dysfunction. Typical initial complaints include clumsiness, stiffness, or jerkiness of an arm and less frequently, clumsiness of a leg (stubbing one's toes when walking). The most striking motor features of CBD include markedly asymmetric, progressive, akinetic-rigid parkinsonism of gradual onset that responds minimally to levodopa, associated with focal dystonia with or without contractures, and hand, limb, gait, and speech apraxia. CBD is sometimes accompanied by focal stimulus–sensitive myoclonus, usually involving the most affected limb and jerky action-induced tremor. Common cortical signs in CBD include asymmetric ideational and ideomotor apraxia, cortical sensory deficits (e.g., astereognosis, agraphesthesia), and alien hand syndrome. The latter may involve a sense of lack of ownership in the absence of visual cues of the limb, involuntary purposeful movements, or frank interference of one limb with the other's execution of purposeful movement. Patients often complain of clumsiness with fine finger movements and abnormal reaching movements.

Progressive Supranuclear Palsy

PSP shares some pathological and clinical features with CBD and frontotemporal dementia (e.g., primary progressive aphasia). Although signs of PSP may be evident as early as age 40, formal diagnosis typically occurs after age 60, with particularly high incidence rates after age 80 [19]. Only about 5% of cases have symptom onset before age 50. At the present time, there are no effective pharmacological or neurosurgical treatments available for patients with PSP and survival rates range from approximately 5 to 10 years after diagnosis [28]. Research diagnostic criteria have been proposed wherein possible PSP criteria have better sensitivity than specificity, and probable PSP criteria have better specificity than sensitivity [29]. The diagnosis of possible PSP requires a gradually progressive disorder beginning at age 40 or later, either vertical supranuclear gaze palsy *or both* slowing of vertical saccades and prominent postural instability in the first year of disease; other diseases that could explain these features need to be excluded. Probable PSP requires vertical supranuclear gaze palsy, prominent postural instability, *and* falls in the first year of onset, and other features of possible PSP. Definite PSP requires neuropathologic confirmation after criteria for possible or probable PSP are met.

The earliest symptoms in PSP are often imbalance evident in falls, accompanied by greater axial than appendicular rigidity, impoverished postural reflexes, and dysarthria (commonly a hypophonic monotone). Other common findings are sloppy eating habits due to poor eye-hand coordination, nonspecific visual difficulties, loss of eye contact, and slowness of thought [30]. Resting tremor is unusual in PSP. Gait in individuals with PSP tends to be wide based and unstable. Symmetric bradykinesia and a masked face with a seemingly perpetually startled expression (raised brow) are common. The earliest oculomotor problem is typically a slowing of vertical saccades and fast phases with the classic vertical gaze palsy (usually affecting downgaze before upgaze) occurring later. In terms of cognitive changes, when present, patients may complain early on of visual, concentration, or executive problems.

No universally accepted clinical subtypes or categories of PSP exist. A review of 103 autopsy-proven cases of PSP revealed that all but about 15% of cases could be categorized as belonging to one of two clinical phenotypes: half the cases had the traditional PSP syndrome (with gaze palsy and early postural instability) and one-third of cases had symptoms readily confused with Parkinson's disease (PD) (asymmetric motor symptom onset, predominance of tremor among motor signs, and moderate response to levodopa therapy) [31]. The prototypical cognitive impairment was common in the traditional syndrome but rare in the parkinsonian subtype. Although disease onset for both variants is in the sixth to seventh decade of life, traditional PSP syndrome has a disease duration of approximately 6 years, whereas PSP associated with more PD-like symptoms has a duration of almost 12 years and, therefore, has a slower, less severe progression [32]. Recognizing these different clinical subtypes is not only important when considering PSP in the differential diagnosis but also for patient counseling with regard to potential medication response and prognosis.

Neuropathology

Parkinson's Disease Dementia and Dementia with Lewy Bodies

The pathological feature of PDD and DLB is the presence of aggregates of alpha-synuclein, in the form of Lewy bodies (LB; neuronal cytoplasmic inclusions) and Lewy neurites (LN; axonal and dendritic inclusions). Traditionally, PD has been defined by neuronal loss and LB in the substantia nigra. However, LB and LN are also found outside the substantia nigra. Braak et al. developed a 6-stage system [33] outlining the systematic progression of LB pathology from preclinical PD through advanced PD. In the first two stages (preclinical), olfactory and brain stem regions show LB and LN, and by the time of clinical diagnosis (usually at stage III or IV), the LB and LN extend to midbrain, including the substantia nigra, basal forebrain, transentorhinal cortex, and the hippocampal CA2 cell field. In the final two stages (V and VI), LB and LN become evident in cortical association areas and eventually in much or all of neocortex.

An instructive study evaluating the Braak staging system is the prospective Sydney Multicenter Study of PD [34]. These researchers found three phenotypes of patients: (1) a group with early, prominent dementia and akinetic-rigid PD (corresponding clinically to DLB), (2) a group of older PD patients (onset after 70 years) developing dementia in 3–10 years (corresponding clinically to PDD) who have widespread alpha-synuclein pathology, and (3) a younger PD group (onset before 70 years) in which dementia occurs late in the disease (after 10–15 years) and there is cell-loss dominant pathology with lesser alpha-synuclein deposition. Another study similarly found that PD patients developing dementia late in the disease had less cortical alpha-synuclein pathology but greater cholinergic abnormalities than those developing dementia early on, whose pathology resembles more strongly that of DLB [35].

A significant number of persons with DLB are also found to have amyloid plaques at autopsy, although amyloid pathology is likely to be less implicated in PDD. One possibility for the somewhat divergent findings obtained from studies of cerebrospinal fluid (CSF) beta-amyloid markers and functional amyloid imaging in PDD is that CSF biomarker levels may reflect biologic processes other than amyloid deposition in the brain. Although PD is initially primarily associated with dopaminergic pathophysiology, other neurotransmitter systems become involved with disease progression, and both DLB and PDD involve significant dysfunction of the dopaminergic and cholinergic systems.

Corticobasal Degeneration

The pathological hallmarks of CBD include ballooned neurons which are most numerous in frontoparietal cortex, but are also seen in the anterior cingulate, amygdala, and insular cortex. Tau-containing neuronal inclusions are evident in cortex and striatum. The frontal and frontoparietal cortices typically show asymmetric atrophy. The pons, medulla, and dentate are also atrophied, and the caudate may appear flattened. The substantia nigra shows decreased pigmentation and cell loss. Neuronal loss and gliosis, in addition to being evident in frontoparietal cortex, are seen in basal ganglia, thalamus, subthalamic nucleus, dentate, and red nucleus. Ballooned and achromatic neurons are most numerous in frontoparietal cortex but are also seen in the anterior cingulate, amygdala, and insular cortex.

Progressive Supranuclear Palsy

PSP, unlike PD, compromises the entire substantia nigra, and dopaminergic depletion is comparable in caudate and putamen. Neuronal loss and gliosis are evident in the globus pallidus, subthalamic nuclei, red nuclei, dentate, superior colliculi, and periaqueductal gray matter. Neurofibrillary tangles (different from those seen in AD), and neuropil threads, are observed in the basal ganglia, brain stem, dentate, and the nucleus basalis of Meynert, which is a major cortical cholinergic output structure.

Structural and Functional Neuroimaging Findings

Parkinson's Disease Dementia and Dementia with Lewy Bodies

Advances in structural and functional neuroimaging using radioactive tracers are beginning to confirm and clarify the role of various pathologies in the neurobehavioral features of PDD. Studies have shown an association between dementia and neocortical, medial temporal, and amygdala atrophy [36]. Findings of possibly greater temporal, parietal, and occipital [37] or frontotemporal neocortical atrophy in DLB than PDD [38], and more marked posterior reductions in fractional anisotropy on diffusion tensor imaging in DLB than PDD [39], are limited by potentially confounding group differences in duration or severity of dementia or parkinsonism.

[11C]PIB PET imaging provides an estimate of the brain's beta-amyloid load. One study reported increased PIB uptake (greater amyloid deposition) in DLB but not PDD, and in a majority of DLB but few PDD patients [40], but another study found increased PIB uptake in similar, small proportions of DLB and PDD patients. PIB uptake was associated with higher ApoE4 prevalence, dementia severity, and CSF Abeta 42 levels [41]. Cortical acetylcholinesterase (AChE) activity has been imaged in vivo using [11C] methyl-4-piperidinyl propionate (PMP) or [11C] methyl-4-piperidyl acetate (MP4A). Decreased AChE activity was associated with depression in PD/PDD [42] and with working memory and executive deficits in PDD [43]. Small sample studies concur that MP4A binding is reduced especially in posterior brain regions in PD and PDD, but the extent of the deficit in PD vs. PDD remains unclear [44, 45]. Dopaminergic imaging using PET and SPECT reveals reduced dopamine transporter binding and fluorodopa uptake in the striatum. Posterior (especially occipital) cerebral blood flow and glucose metabolism is especially reduced in DLB and PDD [46, 47].

Corticobasal Degeneration

MRI typically reveals cortical atrophy, especially frontoparietal (see Fig. 22.1), and occasionally hypointense putaminal and hyperintense subcortical white matter signals on T2-weighted images [48]. Volumetric MRI has shown parietal and callosal atrophy in CBD [49]. PET and SPECT findings are consistent with presynaptic dopaminergic abnormalities in CBD, thus revealing asymmetric decrease in fluorodopa uptake and

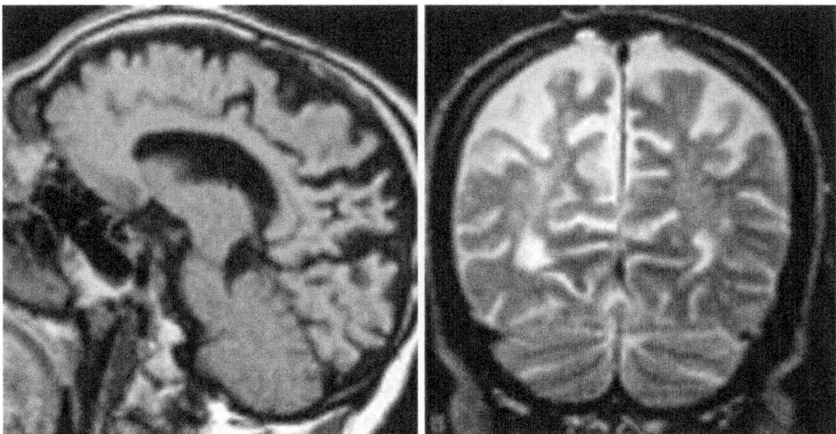

Fig. 22.1 MRI scan in corticobasal degeneration (note asymmetric atrophy, especially frontoparietal)

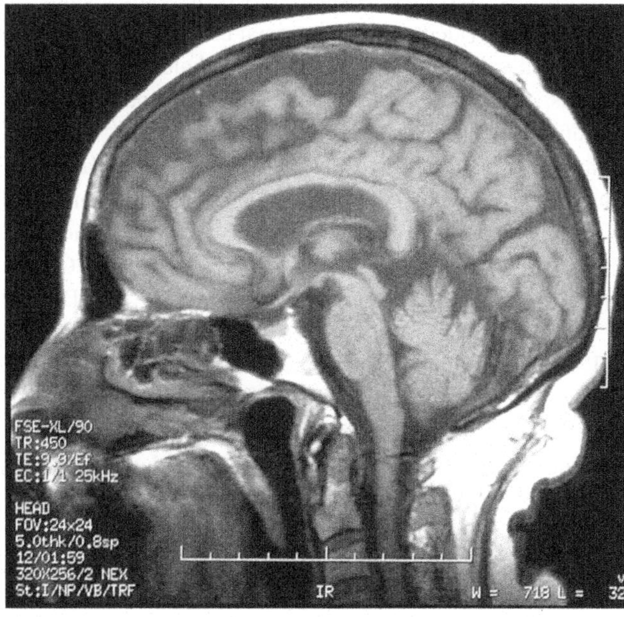

Fig. 22.2 Sagittal T1-weighted MRI in progressive supranuclear palsy: note thinning of the midbrain tegmentum and tectum and frontal atrophy

dopamine transporter binding in caudate and putamen, with the side contralateral to the hemibody most affected showing the greater reduction [50]. Mild reductions in acetylcholinesterase activity have been observed with PET imaging, especially in frontal, parietal, and occipital cortex [51].

Progressive Supranuclear Palsy

Structural MRI findings supportive of a diagnosis of PSP include midbrain atrophy correlated with oculomotor signs (see Fig. 22.2) and superior cerebellar peduncle atrophy, though putaminal atrophy which is also seen in other forms of parkinsonism may be evident [48]. Cortical (especially frontotemporal) atrophy also occurs, and frontal atrophy has been linked to scores on the Frontal Behavior Inventory [52] and executive dysfunction [53]. Reduced glucose metabolism on FDG PET is seen especially in the midbrain and mesial frontal cortex [54]. Imaging of pre- and postsynaptic dopaminergic abnormalities does not differentiate PSP from other forms of parkinsonism such as multiple system atrophy, but imaging of postsynaptic dopaminergic abnormalities can be helpful in differentiating PSP from PD [50]. Recently, PET imaging has revealed paracentral and thalamic reductions in acetylcholinesterase activity [51].

Neuropsychological Hallmarks

Parkinson's Disease Dementia and Dementia with Lewy Bodies

Recent reviews comparing cognitive performance in PDD and DLB [1, 55] can be consulted for further detail and additional references.

Attention and Working Memory

Performance on simple attention tasks, such as span tasks, is preserved in PD, but as the disease progresses, impairments may be observed even on cued attention tasks. Working memory-demanding tasks reveal impairments early in PD [56], and these deficits progress in PDD. Complex (sustained, divided) attention tasks, such as Stroop and visual cancellation tasks, are more likely than simple tasks to elicit attention impairment in DLB or PDD [25]. In comparison to PDD, DLB may involve greater impairments on tasks such as WAIS-R Arithmetic, Stroop, and Trail Making tests [57].

Executive Functions

Executive deficits may have particular importance as harbingers of PDD. Planning, often assessed with Tower tasks, can be slowed or inaccurate in PD, or even stimulus bound in PDD [58]. Card sorting tests evaluating conceptualization and maintenance and switching of set may show patients with PD to (a) be slow to conceptualize, (b) have difficulty shifting set, and (c) lose set. Set-shifting deficits are more apparent in patients with declining mental status and evident especially when extra- rather than intra-dimensional shifts are required.

DLB and PDD patients perform poorly on card sorting tasks. PDD and DLB group performance on card sorting and tower tests have not been compared, but no differences were found between these groups on the Identities and Oddities task [25].

Language

Patients with PDD have more impaired verbal fluency than PD patients, but verbal fluency may be similarly impaired in PDD and DLB [25]. Visual confrontation naming is preserved in PD. While some found naming to be comparably impaired in PDD and DLB [25], the relative preservation of naming in DLB compared to AD may have diagnostic significance [59]. Occasionally observed mild impairments in sentence comprehension or repetition have been ascribed to attention/executive limitations in PD [60], but performance in PDD is typically not impaired on comprehension and repetition tasks.

Learning and Memory

The relative integrity of recognition relative to free recall has been interpreted as indicative of a retrieval deficit in PD. It must be emphasized that recognition is not necessarily intact in PD [61, 62]. Furthermore, memory profiles in PD are heterogeneous [63], and semantic encoding may be deficient [64, 65], perhaps reflecting executive deficits or problems in the use of self-initiated rather than externally imposed learning strategies. PDD and DLB memory impairments are similarly severe (but less severe than in AD) [25]. Nonetheless, qualitative aspects of memory impairment may clinically distinguish DLB and PDD [66]. Whereas DLB manifests poorer recall and more rapid rates of forgetting, PDD makes more perseverative errors during list learning [66]. Remote memory may be impaired in PDD, but the temporal gradient of the loss is equally severe across all past decades implicating a retrieval deficit [67, 68].

Visuoperceptual and Spatial Functions

Comparably severe deficits in PDD and DLB have been observed on numerous visuospatial and constructional tasks, including pentagon copying, BVRT stimulus matching, visual cancellation, visual discrimination, and space and object perception [25, 69, 70]. Profound difficulties with

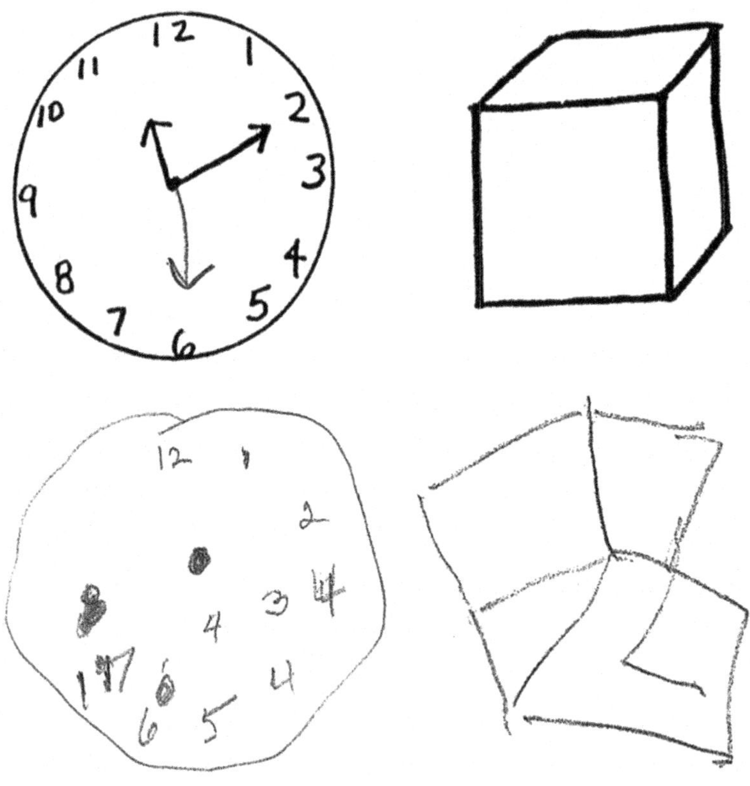

Fig. 22.3 Copies of a clock and cube by a 78-year-old patient with dementia with Lewy bodies (DLB) (Mattis Dementia Rating Scale Total Score 113/144)

visuospatial and constructional tasks, e.g., drawing and copying of figures, are often evident even in mild to moderate DLB (see Fig. 22.3).

Neuropsychiatric Features

The most recent version of the Diagnostic and Statistical Manual of Mental Disorders (DSM) [71] contains separate categories and criteria for mood and anxiety disorders due to medical conditions (including PD). The PDD criteria [22], however, do not require a separate diagnosis of a mood disorder because the criteria recognize the common coexistence of neuropsychiatric symptoms. Nonetheless, the presence of any neuropsychiatric feature is probably best documented explicitly in the medical record and neuropsychological evaluation report so that adequate treatment is undertaken. That depression is undertreated in PD is evidenced by the finding that only one-third of depressed PD patients were receiving antidepressant treatment and that, among those with persistent depression, only 11% had been tried at antidepressant dosages within the highest recommended range [72]. Similarly, it appears that anxiety and depression frequently go unrecognized by clinicians treating PD [73]. Screening for neuropsychiatric conditions is important, and recommendations for use of specific scales in various neuropsychiatric conditions by Movement Disorder Society task forces are provided in Table 22.4.

Depression is common in PD, occurring in about half of all patients, but reliable comparisons of depression prevalence estimates for PDD and DLB are not available. One study reported major depression to occur in about 13% of patients with PDD and in about 19% of patients with DLB (29% of PDD and 34% of DLB had less severe forms of depression) [74]. One meta-analysis reported a prevalence of 42% in PD studies using DSM criteria [75], but incidence and prevalence rates are higher in research than community samples (about 50% vs. 10%) [76].

Table 22.4 Recommended and suggested rating scales for the assessment of neuropsychiatric features in Parkinson's disease

Feature	Recommended scales (stronger evidence)	Suggested scales (weaker evidence)
Depression [159]	Screening (and recommended cutoff in PD): Hamilton Depression Rating Scale (HAM-D, 9/10), Beck Depression Inventory (BDI, 13/14), Hospital Anxiety and Depression Scale (HADS, 10/11), Montgomery-Åsberg Depression Rating Scale (MADRS,14/15), Geriatric Depression Scale (GDS-30, 9/10; GDS-15, 4/5)	For patients with dementia (though insufficient evidence): MADRS, GDS; Cornell Scale for Depression in Dementia (CSDD, 5/6)
Anxiety [160]	None	Beck Anxiety Inventory (BAI), HADS, Zung SAS, Zung ASI, STAI, HARS, Neuropsychiatric Inventory (NPI) anxiety section
Apathy and anhedonia [161]	Apathy Scale (Starkstein et al.); Unified Parkinson's Disease Rating Scale (UPDRS) item 4 (motivation/initiative)	Apathy Evaluation Scale (AES; Marin); Lille Apathy Rating Scale (LARS); Neuropsychiatric Inventory (NPI) item 7; Snaith-Hamilton Pleasure Scale (SHAPS)
Psychosis [162]	Neuropsychiatric Inventory (NPI); Brief Psychiatric Rating Scale (BPRS); Positive and Negative Syndrome Scale (PANSS); Schedule for Assessment of Positive Symptoms (SAPS)	Parkinson Psychosis Rating Scale (PPRS); Parkinson Psychosis Questionnaire (PPQ); Behavioral Pathology in Alzheimer's Disease Rating Scale (Behave-AD); Clinical Global Impression Scale (CGIS)
Sleep disturbances [163]	*Daytime sleepiness*: Epworth Sleepiness Scale (ESS) *Overall sleep impairment*: Parkinson's Disease Sleep Scale (PDSS); Pittsburgh Sleep Quality Index (PSQI); Scales for Outcomes in Parkinson's Disease (SCOPA-Sleep)	*Daytime sleepiness*: Inappropriate Sleep Composite Score (ISCS); Stanford Sleepiness Scale (SSS)

About 50% of patients with PD have significant symptoms of anxiety, and as many as 75% of those patients with PD *and* depression may have a comorbid anxiety disorder [77]. However, the reported prevalence of actual anxiety disorders (vs. symptoms) in PD ranges from 5% to 40% [78]. Almost 20% of PD patients had generalized anxiety, 20% had a social phobia (with another 20% experiencing significant social anxiety) [79], and recurrent panic attacks may occur in up to 24% of levodopa-treated patients [80]. Although patients with PD rarely meet the full DSM criteria for obsessive-compulsive disorder (OCD), a considerable number have symptoms of OCD. Anxiety disorders occur with comparable prevalence in PDD and DLB [74], and one study reported that anxiety may occur in about two-thirds of patients with DLB [81].

Psychosis is common in PDD and DLB (but more common than in PD) [74]. Although occurring more often in DLB than PDD, hallucinations (76% of DLB, 54% of PDD) and delusions (57% of DLB, 29% of PDD) are of a similar quality in both patient groups, with paranoid and phantom boarder delusions and well-formed visual hallucinations being among the most prominent features [74]. Apathy is another behavioral syndrome that has been observed in both PDD and DLB.

Corticobasal Degeneration

Attention and Working Memory

Impairments in digit span are not uniformly observed [82]. Autopsy-confirmed CBD patients have been shown to have mild impairments in digit span backward (but not forward span) at initial neuropsychological evaluation about 3 years after symptom onset, and more marked impairments (on average, more than 2 standard deviations below normative means) by follow-up about 2 years later [83]. In the same sample, profound impairments were noted on the Stroop interference task at both evaluations.

Executive Functions

Executive dysfunction, as indicated by poor performance on tasks such as the WCST [84–87] and Trail Making test [82, 88], is common in CBD. Performance on executive tasks such as "20 Questions" is more compromised in frontotemporal dementia (FTD) than in CBD, and therefore may be especially helpful in differentiating FTD from CBD [89].

Language

Primary progressive aphasia can be a presentation of CBD [90]. The aphasia in CBD is most commonly nonfluent (about 56% of cases), followed in frequency by anomic aphasia (30%) [91]. Fluent and mixed cases were quite rare: each about 5–7% of cases. Performance on language tests in patients with the traditional CBD presentation is somewhat inconsistent, but a key feature of the language problems in CBD is phonologic [92]. Verbal fluency is impaired [84], probably in large part due to the executive demands of those tasks [93]. Performance on semantic memory tasks such as conceptual matching and visual confrontation naming [92] and expressive vocabulary is relatively preserved and impaired in only a minority of patients [82, 94]. When naming is impaired, disproportionate benefit is derived from cuing, suggesting a retrieval rather than semantic memory deficit [88, 94].

The apraxia in CBD is most often ideomotor, but ideational and limb kinetic apraxias do occur occasionally [84, 95–97]. Patients most often have difficulty demonstrating the use of tools or utensils.

Learning and Memory

Memory impairments in CBD involve both encoding and retrieval deficits [84, 94] but may be rarer and milder than the apraxia and impairments in executive functions [83]. Remote memory impairment has been interpreted to be related to retrieval deficits given poor recall but intact recognition has been observed on remote memory tasks [88].

Visuoperceptual and Spatial Functions

Poor drawing (constructional apraxia) is commonly observed in CBD. Visuospatial impairments have also been observed [86, 91].

Neuropsychiatric Features

With respect to emotional and neuropsychiatric issues, the Neuropsychiatric Inventory (NPI) disclosed depression in 73% of CBD patients, but apathy (40%), irritability (20%), and agitation (20%) also occur at considerable rates [98]. In comparison to PSP patients, CBD patients have apathy less frequently, but depression and irritability are more frequently reported.

Progressive Supranuclear Palsy

Cognitive deficits are more likely to be evident in the classical version of PSP (Richardson syndrome) than in the parkinsonian subtype [31, 99].

Attention and Working Memory

Verbal attention is often normal on elementary tests, but deficits in visual attention are common in PSP [100]. Bradyphrenia is very common and often severe in PSP [101] and should be considered when interpreting deficits in higher-level cognitive functions.

Executive Functions

Executive dysfunction occurs early in PSP and is hypothesized to arise from a deafferentiation of the basal ganglia and prefrontal cortex [102] though imaging also reveals correlations between frontal atrophy and executive deficits and frontal behaviors [52, 103]. The executive deficits are readily observed on brief bedside and cognitive screening measures, such as the Frontal Assessment Battery and the Mattis Dementia Rating Scale (especially on the initiation/perseveration subtest) [21]. Deficits observed in CBD include compromised planning, problem solving [104], and cognitive flexibility [105]. Progression of deficits in problem solving and cognitive flexibility may be especially rapid in PSP in comparison to other frontostriatal disorders [106]. Various frontal release signs can also be observed in patients with PSP; for example, the "applause sign" (i.e., perseveration of clapping to command) may be evident in as many as three-quarters of PSP patients [107] and reliably differentiates PSP from PD and FTD [108].

Language

Speech problems like dysarthria and hypophonia occur earlier [109] and are more common in PSP as compared to other movement disorders [110]. Impairment in verbal fluency follows the classic "subcortical" pattern of letter fluency being more affected than category fluency [111], although the effects of PSP on action (verb) fluency [112] will be important to determine since PSP is associated with greater deficits in naming verbs than nouns [113]. When present, deficits in confrontation naming of nouns may be attributable to visual misperceptions, rather than semantic memory deficits [114]. Patients with PSP may also display ideomotor apraxia (associated with left posterior frontal and subcortical volume loss) [115], although it is less pronounced than in CBD [97]. Patients with PSP may present initially with primary progressive aphasia or nonfluent aphasia [116–118].

Learning and Memory

Episodic memory deficits are present in PSP, but the severity of these deficits is considerably less when compared to PDD, DLB, and AD [119]. Tests of episodic memory reveal a mixed encoding/retrieval profile whereby free recall is impaired, but recognition discrimination is generally within normal limits [85]. Remote memory is largely unaffected [120], though a mild deficit in remote autobiographical memories (without a temporal gradient) has been observed and attributed to retrieval deficits [121]. Non-declarative learning and memory deficits are observed on measures of procedural learning but not perceptual priming [101].

Visuoperceptual and Spatial Functions

Oculomotor deficits are a hallmark of PSP, with impairment in voluntary vertical eye movements considered a primary diagnostic feature. Other neuro-ophthalmologic abnormalities occasionally observed include blepharospasm and reduced blinking frequency, all of which may interfere withhigher-levelspatialcognition. Visuoperceptual abilities are also affected in PSP, including visual search and scanning [106], orienting [100], tracking, and attention, which may be correlated with more severe oculomotor deficits [122]. Even early in PSP, subtle abnormalities may be observed in clock drawing (see Fig. 22.4).

Neuropsychiatric Features

Apathy is the most common neuropsychiatric symptom in patients with PSP, perhaps reflecting pathology within medial pre-frontostriatal loops (see [123]). Apathy prevalence in PSP may be as

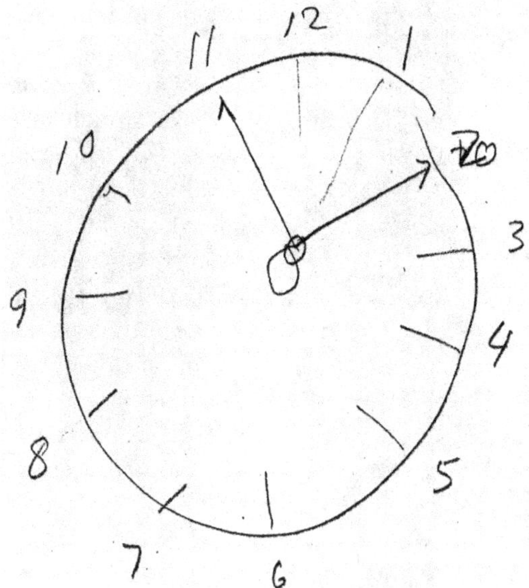

Fig. 22.4 Clock drawn to command by a patient with progressive supranuclear palsy. Note the similarly sized clock hands, indecisiveness in placing the hand origin, and double perseveration (of 1 and 2) at the number "2." The heart-shaped figure next to "2" appears to be a perseveration of the circles indicating the origin of the hands. Also, the numbers are placed outside the clockface. The difficulties seem most consistent with executive rather than visuospatial dysfunction

high as about 90% [124] and is far more common and severe in PSP as compared to PD, which is more likely to present with depression, hallucinations, and delusions [125]. Although apathy is sometimes misdiagnosed as depression, the latter does not present as a prominent neuropsychiatric feature of PSP [124]. Persons with PSP also exhibit behavioral signs of disinhibition [125]. As many as three-quarters of patients with PSP may evidence changes in "personality" [107], which can include increased irritability [125]. Given patients' possibly limited insight into their cognitive and behavioral deficits [126], neuropsychiatric symptoms often exacerbate caregiver stress and burden. A summary of the neurological, radiological, and neuropsychological features of PDD, DLB, CBD, and PSP is provided in Table 22.5.

Other Movement Disorders with Dementia

Several other movement disorders are associated with dementia. Huntington's disease is an autosomal dominant disorder associated with choreiform movements, dementia, and neuropsychiatric disturbances. The disorder is not covered in detail here since patients are typically younger. The dementia, however, is considered a prototypical "subcortical" dementia. Similarly, Sydenham's chorea (St. Vitus' dance), associated with group A beta-hemolytic streptococcal infection, is not covered here as it usually presents in childhood.

A form of parkinsonism, multiple system atrophy (MSA), not responsive to levodopa treatment, is associated with cognitive impairments, but rarely dementia, and reviews of this condition's neuropsychology have been offered elsewhere [127]. Wilson's disease, a genetic disorder of copper metabolism, can be associated with dementia, but presentation is usually in childhood or young adulthood. It is of note that cerebrovascular disease can produce parkinsonism but vascular parkinsonism accounts for a small fraction of cases with parkinsonism coming to autopsy [81]. Most cases are accounted for by Parkinson's disease, multiple system atrophy, corticobasal degeneration, and progressive supranuclear palsy. Vascular dementia and some other conditions that can be associated with parkinsonian features (e.g., normal pressure hydrocephalus, Alzheimer's disease) are discussed in separate chapters in this volume.

Neuropsychological Assessment: Practical Issues and Pointers

Review of the Medical Record

Medical records should be reviewed as in any other neuropsychological evaluation. In the case of movement disorders, especially those presenting with dementias, this review is particularly important as it allows one to plan for an adequate examination and to anticipate factors that might interfere with standardized test administration. In addition to the usual information gleaned from medical records, record reviewing for patients with movement disorders should address the following:

- Age and age at onset of movement disorder symptoms.
- Age at onset of cognitive changes, since this information may facilitate determination of PDD vs. DLB, and estimation of the rate of cognitive decline (e.g., PSP is associated with especially rapid progression of executive deficits).
- Side of onset of movement disorder symptoms such as tremor, rigidity, and bradykinesia and perceived asymmetry (PD and CBD often have asymmetric profiles, whereas DLB and PSP have more symmetric presentations, especially axial motor symptoms).
- Nature of parkinsonian symptoms (e.g., tremor, rigidity, bradykinesia, postural instability, and gait disturbance) and presence of non-parkinsonian motor features (e.g., dystonia, myoclonus, which may suggest a tauopathy).
- Timing of antiparkinsonian and other medications and when the patient is likely to be in the best motor "ON" state.
- Presence of motor fluctuations and their timing. Knowledge of fluctuations (e.g., wearing off, freezing) and involuntary movements

Table 22.5 Summary of neurological, radiological, and neuropsychological characteristics of Parkinson's disease dementia (PDD), dementia with Lewy bodies (DLB), corticobasal degeneration (CBD), and progressive supranuclear palsy (PSP)

Feature	PDD	DLB	CBD	PSP
Clinical features	Asymmetric onset of rigidity, bradykinesia or tremor; initially levodopa responsive but slow loss of levodopa responsiveness; dementia onset associated with postural instability and gait disturbance	Tremor less common than in PDD and more postural than at rest; signs less asymmetric than in PD/PDD	Markedly asymmetric rigidity; parkinsonism is minimally levodopa responsive. Other signs: apraxia, alien limb, dystonia, myoclonus, jerky tremor; cortical sensory deficits	Axial rigidity disproportionate to appendicular rigidity; "en bloc" movement; other: vertical gaze abnormality; a small subset of PSP patient's parkinsonism may be initially responsive to levodopa, but mostly unresponsive to treatment
MRI scan atrophy	Little cortical atrophy; hippocampal atrophy variable	Little cortical atrophy; hippocampal atrophy variable	Posterior frontal and parietal cortex atrophy is pronounced	Frontal and midbrain atrophy
SPECT and PET hypoperfusion	Mostly frontoparietal and occipital	Posterior: occipital-parietal	Asymmetric frontoparietal and thalamic	Frontal-subcortical
Attention/working memory/processing speed	Moderate impairment	Moderate to severe impairment; evident early	Mild to moderate impairment	Mild to moderate impairment
Executive functions	Moderate to severe impairment	Mild to moderate impairment	Normal to moderate impairment	Moderate to severe impairment; evident early and typically rapidly progressive
Language	Normal to moderately impaired; fluency impairment seen early, but visual confrontation naming and repetition relatively intact until late in disease	Normal to moderately impaired; fluency impairment is most common, but some patients may have marked naming impairment like Alzheimer's	Apraxia disproportionate to expressive and receptive language impairment	Normal to moderately impaired; verbal fluency impairment seen early
Visuospatial/perceptual and constructional	Mild to severe impairment	Moderate to severe impairment; typically seen early	Normal to moderate impairment	Mild to severe impairment, perhaps secondary to gaze abnormalities; executive dysfunction may impact
Learning and memory	Mild to severe; affects mainly encoding and retrieval, storage only later in disease; less pronounced than in Alzheimer's; remote memory impairment variable, but typically no temporal gradient and retrieval problems evident	Mild to severe; less pronounced than in Alzheimer's early on; storage (forgetting rates) variable; remote memory impairment variable but typically no temporal gradient	Mild to moderate; mainly retrieval deficits, some encoding problems; retrograde is not temporally graded	Normal to moderate; often secondary to executive deficits impacting encoding and/or retrieval strategies
Neuropsychiatric	Depression and Anxiety prominent; hallucinations (esp. visual); paranoid (esp. Othello) and phantom boarder delusions	Depression and anxiety prominent; hallucinations (esp. visual); paranoid (esp. Othello) and phantom boarder delusions	Depression with lesser apathy	Frequent apathy; disinhibition and personality changes; depression less common

(e.g., dyskinesia or dystonia) allows for planning and timing of the evaluation.

- Existence of pathological daytime sleepiness or somnolence and time of occurrence (and REM sleep behavior disorder), and if available, review of polysomnography studies. Such knowledge allows one to establish at what time of day the patient is likely best tested and how much testing might reasonably be undertaken in one appointment.
- Presence of marked tremor or apraxia that might interfere with tests with strong motor demands.
- Presence of visual problems (e.g., double vision) or gaze abnormalities (especially in PSP) that might interfere with standard test administration.
- Presence of marked attention fluctuations (especially in DLB) that might yield spurious patterns of strengths and weaknesses across cognitive tests.
- Existence of hallucinations (especially in DLB) or affective disturbance that might compromise patient effort on testing or ability to respond meaningfully.
- Comorbid medical conditions, especially endocrine conditions such as thyroid dysfunction or diabetes (patients may need snack breaks to maintain adequate blood sugar levels).
- Utilization of medications with anticholinergic effects that might impact concentration and memory (including not only agents used to treat tremor but also conditions such as urinary incontinence).
- History of prior neurosurgical intervention for movement disorder (e.g., pallidotomy, deep brain stimulation, fetal tissue transplantation). If stimulators are present, determine current setting and known side effects (e.g., dysarthria).

Interview

All information obtained from medical record review should be verified during interview along with the regularly obtained medical and psychosocial information. In addition, it should be established whether there is a family history specifically of dementias or movement disorders.

A question that arises in interview is whether patients and care partners are accurate in reporting cognitive and other behavioral and functional changes. In the case of PD, accuracy of report may vary with respect to the function being reported upon. It has been found that patients are accurate reporters of disability, even in the presence of cognitive compromise and depression [128]. In contrast, in the case of memory impairment, whereas the patient's and care partner's report is typically concordant and related to patient scores on objective cognitive measures, patient-care partner report discrepancies increase as a function of patient cognitive impairment and depression [129]. One study reported that care partners may focus on select aspects of cognitive deficit such as verbal recall [129], but another study found good concordance between caregiver report and patient's objective performance on a range of cognitive tasks, including those measuring memory, executive function, language, and psychomotor speed [130]. A useful observation to keep in mind is that patients, including those with PDD and DLB, may frequently complain of memory disorders initially [25], but what patients describe as memory disorders may actually represent other deficits. For example, reported trouble remembering names or words may refer to dysnomia, and a reported inability to recall how to operate equipment or machinery (e.g., sewing machines, lawn mowers) may refer to executive dysfunction.

During the interview, it is important to prepare the patient for evaluation. The patient's anxiety about evaluation should be allayed as far as possible, and patients should be informed that they will probably find some tasks easier than others and that variations in performance and skills are the norm rather than the exception. The patient should be encouraged to report when they feel onset of dyskinesias or dystonias, or fluctuations in motor functions. Even if it is not possible to discontinue or take a break in evaluation, the presence of these features should be noted to facilitate later interpretation of test results. Similarly, patients should be monitored for fatigue and especially in DLB, and some cases of PDD, the examiner should be alert to fluctuations in attention.

Screening Instruments

Frequently physicians and neuropsychologists need to screen for cognitive impairment in persons with movement disorders. While the use of screening instruments has been the subject of empirical investigation in PD and PDD, less attention has been paid to screening in PSP, CBD, and DLB. Thus, an important issue is how well screening instruments perform in detecting cognitive impairments in movement disorders.

In comparison to full neuropsychological evaluations, the advantages of cognitive screening instruments include their brevity, relatively simple administration and scoring, patient acceptability, and limited expense. Cognitive screening can be helpful in deciding whether a patient might require full neuropsychological evaluation. Possible disadvantages of screening instruments include the limited information obtained, the use of cutoff scores that may not be adequately corrected for demographics and base rates, and limited sensitivity and specificity for use across a broad range of disorders. Another issue is that relatively few screening instruments have been developed for movement disorders, and the application of instruments primarily developed for Alzheimer's disease may have limited applicability given such instruments emphasis on memory and relative neglect of executive functions and working memory. Recently, more emphasis has been placed on developing instruments specifically for use with PD and PDD (and presumably such instruments might have utility in other movement disorders), but no instruments have been developed specifically for PSP, CBD, and DLB. Recent studies of PSP and CBD have utilized generic screening instruments such as the Dementia Rating Scale (DRS), Addenbrooke Cognitive Examination (ACE), and Frontal Assessment Battery (FAB) for screening [21, 131].

Several overviews of screening instruments commonly used with or designed for PD have recently been published [132, 133]. It should also be borne in mind that recommendations made for cognitive assessment in PD by an American Academy of Neurology committee [134] are based on a now outdated literature review and have limited relevance.

Two commonly used screening instruments not specifically designed for PDD and DLB are the Mini-Mental State Exam (MMSE) [135, 136] and the Dementia Rating Scale (DRS and DRS-2) [137, 138]. More recently, the Montreal Cognitive Assessment (MoCA) has been used in PD [139]. Patients with PD and other dementias make qualitatively different errors on the MMSE [140]. These qualitative differences aside, the MMSE de-emphasizes working memory and executive functions and might lack sensitivity to cognitive changes associated with subcortical-frontal dysfunction. This suspicion was confirmed by a study comparing PD patients with and without mild cognitive impairment (defined by a neuropsychological test battery). The mean MMSE score of the mildly impaired group was only 1.5 points lower than that of the intact group, and in the normal range (mean 28.0, standard deviation 2.1) [141]. The MMSE also appears to be less sensitive than the DRS to cognitive deficits in atypical parkinsonian syndromes (Bak et al., 2005), and the Montreal Cognitive Assessment (MoCA) [139] in PD [142]. Nonetheless, the MMSE probably has adequate sensitivity and specificity in detecting impairment among unequivocally demented patients with PD (in whom screening may not be needed). Using DSM-IV dementia criteria as the "gold standard," a study of 126 PD patients found a MMSE cutoff of 23(dementia)/24(no dementia) to have 98% sensitivity and 77% specificity [143]. Mean annual rate of change in the MMSE score is about 1 point for persons with PD without dementia, but about 2–2.5 points for those with dementia [144].

The DRS's sensitivity and specificity in detecting cognitive impairment in PD and related disorders has not been adequately addressed, but several studies show different score profiles in PD, PDD, DLB, and AD. One study reported that whereas an AD group earned lower Memory subtest scores than a PD group with comparable severity of cognitive impairment, the PD group attained lower Construction subtest scores. Discriminant function analyses using Memory, Initiation/Perseveration, and Construction subtest scores correctly classified 75% of the sample [145]. The Construction and Initiation/Perseveration subtest scores of the DRS are the most helpful in distinguishing PD patients from healthy controls [146]. Though PDD and DLB may differ minimally in their DRS profiles (with perhaps lower Conceptualization scores in DLB early on), Memory, Construction and Initiation/Perseveration scores best distinguish between PDD/DLB and AD [119].

Another generic dementia screening instrument with potential utility in PD is the cognitive section of the Cambridge Examination for Mental Disorders (CAMCOG). Using a cutoff score of 80 points and below to identify dementia in PD, one study reported the instrument to show 95% sensitivity and 94% specificity [143]. Cognitively intact patients with PD (MMSE>25) demonstrate an average annual rate of change of about 4 points on the revised version of the instrument (CAMCOG-R) [147].

Two screening batteries for persons with frontal and subcortical dysfunction have been published, including the Frontal/Subcortical Assessment Battery (FSAB) [148] and the Frontal Assessment Battery (FAB) [149]. The latter has been used in studies of PD, but its psychometric properties still require further exploration.

Several instruments specifically for use with PD have been developed, including the Mini-Mental Parkinson (MMP) [150], the Scales for Outcomes of Parkinson's disease – Cognition (SCOPA-Cog) [151], the Parkinson Neuropsychometric Dementia Assessment (PANDA) [152], and the Parkinson's Disease Cognitive Rating Scale (PD-CRS) [153]. These instruments show promise but remain to be validated in large, independent studies. No disease-specific cognitive screening instruments have been developed for use with DLB, PSP, or CBD, though instruments developed for PD should also have utility with other movement disorders that can present with mild cognitive compromise or dementia.

Selecting Neuropsychological Test Batteries for Movement Disorders and Possible Test Modifications

As is the case for any neuropsychological evaluation, test selection should consider the patient's condition or the differential diagnosis, the referral question(s), patient and caregiver concerns, the normative and psychometric properties of the tests (e.g., availability of alternate forms, test-retest reliability, validity for use in movement disorders and dementia), and the patient's ability to tolerate and cooperate with the tests. When evaluating patients with movement disorders, awareness of the potential impact of various features of movement disorders (e.g., motor fluctuations, sleep disturbance and fatigability, choreiform and dystonic dyskinesias, gaze palsy, apraxia, dysarthria, and hypersalivation) on test performance needs to be considered (Table 22.6).

Standard test administration methods may need to be modified when working with patients with movement disorders. Downward gaze palsy, as seen in PSP, makes it difficult for patients to voluntarily look down at test forms. In such cases, stimuli may be held up for the patient to see at eye level, about 18" from the patient's face. When impediments such as slurred speech are evident, patients may be asked to repeat responses although this is frustrating to some patients, perhaps necessitating testing over multiple brief sessions. Hypophonia may be compensated for by an amplification device. Tests requiring pointing rather than oral responses may be more appropriate for patients with speech impairment.

A patient with tremor, dyskinesia, dystonia, or apraxia may require help from the examiner when completing tests or questionnaires requiring writing, circling of alternatives, or filling in of multiple choice blanks. Thus, such scales might be administered orally, with the examiner making the necessary written notation. On some tasks, such as card sorting or tower tests, the examiner may need

Table 22.6 Neuropsychological tests commonly used in movement disorders with and without dementia

Cognitive domain	Test
Premorbid estimates	North American Adult Reading Test (NAART); Wechsler Test of Adult Reading (WTAR); Wide Range Achievement Test (WRAT); Advanced Clinical Solutions Test of Premorbid Functioning (TOPF)
Neuropsychological screening	Mattis Dementia Rating Scale (DRS); Mini-Mental Status Examination; Repeatable Battery for the Assessment of Neuropsychological Status (RBANS); Montreal Cognitive Assessment (MoCA); Parkinson's Disease Cognitive Rating Scale (PD-CRS); Parkinson Neuropsychometric Dementia Assessment (PANDA); Scales for Outcomes of Parkinson's Disease – Cognition (SCOPA-Cog); Cambridge Examination for Mental Disorders (Cognitive section) (CAMCOG); Addenbrooke Cognitive Examination (ACE)
Intelligence	Raven's Progressive Matrices; Wechsler Abbreviated Scale of Intelligence (WASI); Wechsler Adult Intelligence Scale (WAIS) (recent editions)
Attention and working memory	Brief Test of Attention (BTA); Digit and Visual Span; Stroop Test[a]; Digit Ordering Test; Letter Number Sequencing; Digit Symbol or Symbol Digit test
Executive function	Delis-Kaplan Executive Function Scale (DKEFS); Booklet Category Test; Trail Making Test (TMT)[a]; Wisconsin Card Sorting Test (WCST); Tower of London (and various modifications); Cambridge Neuropsychological Test Automated Battery; Verbal fluency tests (phonemic, semantic, action)
Memory	Benton Visual Retention Test - recognition (BVRT-R); California Verbal Learning Test (CVLT/CVLT-II); Rey Auditory Verbal Learning Test (RAVLT); Selective Reminding Test; Rey Complex Figure Test (RCFT)[a]; Wechsler Memory Scale (WMS) (recent editions)[a]; Brief Visuospatial Memory Test (BVMT-R); Hopkins Verbal Learning Test (HVLT-R)
Language and praxis	Boston Naming Test (BNT); Controlled Oral Word Association Test (COWAT); Sentence Repetition; Token Test; Complex Ideational Material; Western Aphasia Battery subtests (including Apraxia)
Visual and spatial perception and construction	Benton Facial Recognition Test; Benton Judgment of Line Orientation (JLO); Hooper Visual Organization Test (VOT); Clock Drawing
Motor/fine motor	Finger Tapping[a]; Grooved Pegboard[a]
Mood state	Beck Anxiety Inventory (BAI); Beck Depression Inventory (BDI); Hamilton Depression Scale (HDS) or Inventory (HDI); The Neuropsychiatric Inventory (NPI); Profile of Mood States (POMS); State-Trait Anxiety Inventory (STAI); Maudsley Obsessional-Compulsive Inventory; Yale-Brown Obsessive Compulsive Scale (YBOCS); Hospital Anxiety and Depression Scale (HADS), Montgomery-Åsberg Depression Rating Scale (MADRS); Cornell Scales for Depression in Dementia (CSDD)
Quality of life, coping and stressors	Parkinson's Disease Questionnaire (PDQ); Medical Outcomes Study 36-item short form (SF-36); Sickness Impact Profile (SIP); Coping Responses Inventory (CRI); Ways of Coping Questionnaire; Life Stressors and Social Resources Inventory (LISRES)

[a]Note: Test may not be appropriate for patients with marked motor impairment

to hold and move the cards or blocks/beads as instructed by the patient (standard timing cannot be used in such cases). In general, tests with significant motor demands are better avoided with patients who have movement disorders. Though non-motor tasks might be administered when patients have dyskinesias, the patient may still be distracted by these movements, and this needs to be considered in interpreting the test results.

In parkinsonian patients and patients with dementia who have sleepiness or somnolence, fatigue, severe motor "OFF" periods, or frequent fluctuations, breaks will need to be taken. Although there may occasionally be a need to compare performances "ON" and "OFF" medications, it is recommended that patients be tested while on their antiparkinsonian medications (though anticholinergics are best discontinued and tapered prior to evaluation). In patients with advanced movement disorders, testing during the off state is unnecessarily challenging to patient and examiner, and the patient may also experience increased dysphoria and anxiety during off state, further complicating test interpretation.

Assessment of Neuropsychiatric Symptoms

Given the frequency with which affective and other neuropsychiatric symptoms occur in movement disorders such as PDD, DLB, PSP, and CBD, information on these conditions should be obtained during medical record review and interview. In addition, it is often helpful to quantify the severity of symptomatology to document existence and severity of a condition, and consequently, completion of various observer rating and self-report scales is recommended. The various scales recommended by the Movement Disorder Society (MDS) are listed in Table 22.4.

One particular issue in PD, PDD, and other movement disorders is that symptoms of depression and anxiety may overlap with those of the movement disorder. For example, sleep disturbance, psychomotor retardation, lack of energy, stooped posture, masked facial expression, dry mouth, and sexual dysfunction can be observed in PDD, DLB, PSP, and depression. Consequently, to improve diagnosis, it has been suggested that early morning awakening, anergia, and psychomotor slowing not be considered when diagnosing depression in PD. Due to symptoms overlap, rating scales might overestimate depression in PD/PDD/DLB, and in the case of PDD, empirically derived alternate cutoffs have been provided for several depression scales [127].

Diagnosis of an anxiety disorder in PD is also hindered by symptom overlap. Unfortunately, the validity and reliability of anxiety rating scales has not been widely studied. Elimination of anxiety inventory items reflecting autonomic and neurophysiologic dysfunction is, however, not advised, as this might lead to underestimation of anxiety [154]. PSP often features apathy, and this should be assessed carefully. CBD, though also associated with a notable frequency of apathy, more often has depression. Although the questionnaires and scales recommended for PD neuropsychiatric evaluation have not been evaluated for the most part in other movement disorders, they seem reasonable choices in the absence of other evidence.

A Case of Possible Corticobasal Degeneration (Corticobasal Syndrome)

The case described was selected because it illustrates the difficulty one may have in clinically differentiating CBD and PSP, both tauopathies. A 66-year-old, right-handed, white man with 16 years of education was seen in consultation at the request of a neurologist to facilitate differential diagnosis and treatment decision making. The patient had initially been diagnosed as having Parkinson's disease by a neurologist at an outside facility, based on left-sided cogwheel rigidity and the presence of a very slight tremor.

The patient stated at evaluation that he had experienced some cognitive changes initially about 4–5 years prior to evaluation, more specifically noticing slowness of thought and difficulty speaking at work (he had had a management position overseeing data processing). Though the patient had initiated a change in his own job duties about 1.5 years prior to the evaluation, by the time of evaluation, he had retired due to his cognitive problems. His wife had only noticed some cognitive changes in her husband for the past year or so. He seemed to be reluctant to make decisions (although the quality of his decisions seemed adequate to the wife), and she had noticed that her husband had become avoidant of chores and had begun to have difficulty with certain chores. For example, when looking at tools to fix something, or at the lawn mower, he seemed uncertain what to do with the implements and machines. He occasionally had trouble buttering his toast, but otherwise was able to cut food and use utensils.

In addition, the patient about a year before evaluation had become more hesitant to drive, had struck a mailbox, and consequently stopped driving. At evaluation, he reported that he had ceased driving due to what he described as difficulties with distance judgment and perspective.

The patient had been treated for depression with SSRIs for 6 months by his primary care physician about 2 years prior to this evaluation. His wife observed that her husband had been more easily frustrated and irritable than in the past, but the patient perceived that his depression had been a reaction to perceived cognitive and motor changes, and the loss of a close friend. Recent mood was euthymic.

Regarding motor signs, the patient had had a mild, non-bothersome tremor for 12–15 years prior to evaluation (and there was a family history of this), but in the year before evaluation developed balance problems that he sometimes referred to as "dizziness." He had had 4 or 5 falls without head injury.

At the neurological evaluation, his score on the MoCA was 17/30, and declines were noticed in memory, verbal fluency, and executive and visuospatial functions. On his movement disorders exam, resting tremor was absent, though mild postural tremor was observed in the right arm. On finger-to-nose, he had mild intention tremor on the right compared to the left. Mild rigidity in the neck and mild-to-moderate rigidity in both upper and lower extremities were noted, greater on the left. Dysdiadochokinesis and mild bradykinesia was evident bilaterally, more so on the left, and the patient had difficulty with reciprocal hand movements. Ideomotor apraxia was greater on the left. He had no difficulty arising from a chair with his hands folded across his chest. Posture was slightly stooped. Observation of gait revealed good stride length but slightly reduced arm swing. On the retropulsion test, he recovered unaided after a few steps. Strength was 5/5 throughout. His cranial nerve exam was largely unremarkable. His extraocular movements were intact, but he had mild difficulty with smooth pursuits. Facial sensation and strength was intact and symmetric. His sensory exam was intact to light touch, temperature, and vibration in all four extremities. Reflexes were 2+ and symmetric throughout. Toes were downgoing bilaterally.

The patient had had limited benefit from antiparkinsonian medications (rasagiline and ropinirole) in the year before his evaluation. A CT scan of the head done at an outside institution about 2 years prior to this evaluation was interpreted as revealing of mild cerebral atrophy given age. An MRI done about 10 months prior to evaluation was interpreted as revealing of diffuse atrophy, greater on the right than left, and especially prominent in the frontal-parietal lobes.

Neuropsychological test results are presented in Table 22.7. Particularly evident were difficulties with memory (recognition appeared relatively preserved in comparison to free recall), fine visual motor coordination, dexterity and speed, verbal fluency, apraxia, processing speed, and to lesser extent working memory. Oral language comprehension was relatively intact, and executive dysfunction was mild. Significant affective distress was denied, and the patient only reported mild symptoms of depression. Overall, the neuropsychological profile of strengths and weaknesses in the context of progressive parkinsonism fairly unresponsive to medication suggested a likely tauopathy (note CBD was more strongly suggested than PSP, but the patient developed a gaze abnormality less than 1 year after evaluation). He also began to complain of clumsiness of the legs, and stubbing his toes especially when climbing a curb.

Interested readers are referred to a recently published neuropsychology casebook for detailed case descriptions of other movement disorders with dementia, including PSP [155], CBD [156], and DLB [157].

Table 22.7 Neuropsychological test scores of a 66-year-old man with suspected corticobasal degeneration

Test	Raw score	Standard score (index (I) or T-score) or percentile*
Intelligence estimate		
Wechsler Test of Adult Reading (WTAR): Full Scale IQ estimate	48	121 (I)
Cognitive screening		
Mattis Dementia Rating Scale (DRS-2): Total score (/144)	110	23
Attention/working memory/processing speed		
Wechsler Adult Intelligence Scale (WAIS-IV): Working Memory Index		83 (I)
Wechsler Adult Intelligence Scale (WAIS-IV): Processing Speed Index		50 (I)
Digit Span maxima	5 forward, 3 backward	
Spatial Span maxima	3 forward, 3 backward	
Trail Making Parts A and B (sec)	209, 300+	15, 13
Stroop (SNST) Color and Color/Word (/112)	69, 29	<2*
Executive function		
Wisconsin Card Sorting Test (WCST-64): Categories	1	6–10*
(WCST-64): Trials to First Category	12	>16*
(WCST-64): Perseverative Errors	12	41
Language	10	19
Letter Fluency (FAS) (words/180 s)		
Category Fluency(Animals) (words/60 s)	4	7
MAE Sentence Repetition (/14)	9	7*
MAE Token Test (/44)	43	67*
Motor speed/dexterity	48.1, 34.7	46, 30
Finger Tapping (dominant/nondominant hand) (average taps/10 s)		
Grooved Pegboard (dominant/nondominant hand) (sec)	243 (all pegs placed), 300+ (only 21 pegs placed)	18, 19
Apraxia	41	
WAB Apraxia Exam (/60)		
Visuospatial/perceptual		
Benton Facial Recognition (/54)	32 (severe impairment)	
Judgment of Line Orientation (/30)	23	40*
Clock Drawing	2/3	
Verbal learning/memory		
Hopkins Verbal Learning Test-Revised (HVLT-R): Total Immediate Recall (/36)	14	22
Hopkins Verbal Learning Test-Revised (HVLT-R): Delayed (/12)	6	32
Hopkins Verbal Learning Test-Revised (HVLT-R): Recognition Discrimination Index (recognition hits—false positives) (0–12)	11–0	47
Brief Visuospatial Memory Test—Revised (BVMT-R): Total Immediate recall (/36)	10	29
Brief Visuospatial Memory Test—Revised (BVMT-R): Delayed (/12)	4	31
Brief Visuospatial Memory Test—Revised (BVMT-R): Recognition Discrimination Index (recognition hits—false positives) (0-6)	4–1	3–5*
Brief Visuospatial Memory Test—Revised (BVMT-R): Copy (/12)	12	
Mood state		
Profile of Mood States (POMS): Tension-Anxiety		50
Profile of Mood States (POMS): Depression		64
Profile of Mood States (POMS): Anger-Hostility		43
Profile of Mood States (POMS): Vigor-Activity		<30
Profile of Mood States (POMS): Fatigue-Inertia		39
Profile of Mood States (POMS): Confusion-Bewilderment		66

Clinical Pearls

- When attempting to differentiate movement disorders with dementia, consider carefully not only test scores but also qualitative features of test performance as well as the onset, evolution, and nature of motor symptoms. Also, keep in mind the base rate of disorders, their epidemiology, and typical age at onset and duration. Be familiar with the most typical neuroimaging findings.
- Bear in mind that patient terminology may not correspond to reality when making complaints of cognitive deficit. Thus, patients may complain of memory problems but in fact refer to aphasia or anomia (trouble recalling or producing words) or executive dysfunction (an inability to recall how to operate equipment and machinery such as stoves, sewing machines, and mowers).
- The best way to ensure a smooth and efficient evaluation is to be prepared for patient fatigue, fluctuations in attention and motor function, and medication effects. These should be explored carefully in the medical record or when calling the patient to schedule an appointment.
- Patients often complain of trouble recalling people's names, regardless of condition. We recommend that patients use a cellular telephone or computer to append photos of acquaintances to contact information in the computer or telephone. This information, including picture-name, can be reviewed prior to social encounters. Many of our patients have found this very helpful. Alternatively, they might review photo albums, although in our experience these contain too much information and may include too few of the persons commonly encountered.
- Patients with movement disorders, with or without dementia, often have bradyphrenia and trouble keeping up with social discourse. We encourage them to engage in conversation in small groups. One way to control the speed of the flow of conversation is by questioning. Regular questioning, without being annoying to other participants in the conversation, allows processing of information, relevant responses, and pauses that allow better encoding of information.
- In patients with movement disorders, it is critical to enquire about vision. Abnormalities of gaze and eye movements may be present and patients may have double vision and difficulty focusing or seeing test materials.

References

1. Tröster AI. Neuropsychological characteristics of dementia with Lewy bodies and Parkinson's disease with dementia: differentiation, early detection, and implications for "mild cognitive impairment" and biomarkers. Neuropsychol Rev. 2008;18(1):103–19.
2. Zhang ZX, Roman GC. Worldwide occurrence of Parkinson's disease: an updated review. Neuroepidemiology. 1993;12(4):195–208.
3. Bower JH, Maraganore DM, McDonnell SK, Rocca WA. Incidence and distribution of parkinsonism in Olmsted County, Minnesota, 1976–1990. Neurology. 1999;52(6):1214–20.
4. Perez F, Helmer C, Dartigues JF, Auriacombe S, Tison F. A 15-year population-based cohort study of the incidence of Parkinson's disease and dementia with Lewy bodies in an elderly French cohort. J Neurol Neurosurg Psychiatry. 2010;81(7): 742–6.
5. Aarsland D, Zaccai J, Brayne C. A systematic review of prevalence studies of dementia in Parkinson's disease. Mov Disord. 2005;20(10):1255–63.
6. Biggins CA, Boyd JL, Harrop FM, Madeley P, Mindham RH, Randall JI, et al. A controlled, longitudinal study of dementia in Parkinson's disease. J Neurol Neurosurg Psychiatry. 1992;55(7):566–71.
7. Marder K, Tang MX, Cote L, Stern Y, Mayeux R. The frequency and associated risk factors for dementia in patients with Parkinson's disease. Arch Neurol. 1995;52(7):695–701.
8. Mayeux R, Chen J, Mirabello E, Marder K, Bell K, Dooneief G, et al. An estimate of the incidence of dementia in idiopathic Parkinson's disease. Neurology. 1990;40(10):1513–7.
9. McKeith IG. Dementia with Lewy bodies. Br J Psychiatry. 2002;180:144–7.
10. Zaccai J, McCracken C, Brayne C. A systematic review of prevalence and incidence studies of dementia with Lewy bodies. Age Ageing. 2005;34(6):561–6.
11. Miech RA, Breitner JC, Zandi PP, Khachaturian AS, Anthony JC, Mayer L. Incidence of AD may decline in the early 90s for men, later for women: The Cache County study. Neurology. 2002;58(2):209–18.
12. Morimatsu M. Diseases other than Parkinson's disease presenting with parkinsonism. Nippon Ronen Igakkai Zasshi. 2004;41(6):589–93.

13. Osaki Y, Morita Y, Kuwahara T, Miyano I, Doi Y. Prevalence of Parkinson's disease and atypical parkinsonian syndromes in a rural Japanese district. Acta Neurol Scand. 2010;124:182–7.
14. Winter Y, Bezdolnyy Y, Katunina E, Avakjan G, Reese JP, Klotsche J, et al. Incidence of Parkinson's disease and atypical parkinsonism: Russian population-based study. Mov disord. 2010;25(3):349–56.
15. Rinne JO, Lee MS, Thompson PD, Marsden CD. Corticobasal degeneration. A clinical study of 36 cases. Brain. 1994;117(Pt 5):1183–96.
16. Grimes DA, Lang AE, Bergeron CB. Dementia as the most common presentation of cortical-basal ganglionic degeneration. Neurology. 1999;53(9):1969–74.
17. Ludolph AC, Kassubek J, Landwehrmeyer BG, Mandelkow E, Mandelkow EM, Burn DJ, et al. Tauopathies with parkinsonism: clinical spectrum, neuropathologic basis, biological markers, and treatment options. Eur J Neurol. 2009;16(3):297–309.
18. Nath U, Ben-Shlomo Y, Thomson RG, Morris HR, Wood NW, Lees AJ, et al. The prevalence of progressive supranuclear palsy (Steele-Richardson-Olszewski syndrome) in the UK. Brain. 2001;124 (Pt 7):1438–49.
19. Bower JH, Maraganore DM, McDonnell SK, Rocca WA. Incidence of progressive supranuclear palsy and multiple system atrophy in Olmsted County, Minnesota, 1976 to 1990. Neurology. 1997;49(5):1284–8.
20. Nath U, Ben-Shlomo Y, Thomson RG, Morris HR, Wood NW, Lees AJ, et al. The prevalence of progressive supranuclear palsy (Steele-Richardson-Olszewski syndrome) in the UK. Brain. 2001; 124(Pt 7):1438–49.
21. Brown RG, Lacomblez L, Landwehrmeyer BG, Bak T, Uttner I, Dubois B, et al. Cognitive impairment in patients with multiple system atrophy and progressive supranuclear palsy. Brain. 2010;133(Pt 8):2382–93.
22. Emre M, Aarsland D, Brown R, Burn DJ, Duyckaerts C, Mizuno Y, et al. Clinical diagnostic criteria for dementia associated with Parkinson's disease. Mov Disord. 2007;22(12):1689–707.
23. McKeith IG, Dickson DW, Lowe J, Emre M, O'Brien JT, Feldman H, et al. Diagnosis and management of dementia with Lewy bodies: third report of the DLB Consortium. Neurology. 2005;65(12):1863–72.
24. Hughes AJ, Ben-Shlomo Y, Daniel SE, Lees AJ. What features improve the accuracy of clinical diagnosis in Parkinson's disease: a clinicopathologic study. Neurology. 1992;42(6):1142–6.
25. Noe E, Marder K, Bell KL, Jacobs DM, Manly JJ, Stern Y. Comparison of dementia with Lewy bodies to Alzheimer's disease and Parkinson's disease with dementia. Mov Disord. 2004;19(1):60–7.
26. Caballol N, Marti MJ, Tolosa E. Cognitive dysfunction and dementia in Parkinson disease. Mov Disord. 2007;22 Suppl 17:S358–66.
27. Lang AE. Corticobasal degeneration: selected developments. Mov Disord. 2003;18 Suppl 6:S51–6.
28. Burn DJ, Lees AJ. Progressive supranuclear palsy: where are we now? Lancet Neurol. 2002;1(6):359–69.
29. Litvan I, Agid Y, Calne D, Campbell G, Dubois B, Duvoisin RC, et al. Clinical research criteria for the diagnosis of progressive supranuclear palsy (Steele-Richardson-Olszewski syndrome): report of the NINDS-SPSP international workshop. Neurology. 1996;47(1):1–9.
30. Jankovic J, Friedman DI, Pirozzolo FJ, McCrary JA. Progressive supranuclear palsy: motor, neurobehavioral, and neuro-ophthalmic findings. Adv Neurol. 1990;53:293–304.
31. Williams DR, de Silva R, Paviour DC, Pittman A, Watt HC, Kilford L, et al. Characteristics of two distinct clinical phenotypes in pathologically proven progressive supranuclear palsy: Richardson's syndrome and PSP-parkinsonism. Brain. 2005;128(Pt 6):1247–58.
32. O'Sullivan SS, Massey LA, Williams DR, Silveira-Moriyama L, Kempster PA, Holton JL, et al. Clinical outcomes of progressive supranuclear palsy and multiple system atrophy. Brain. 2008;131(Pt 5): 1362–72.
33. Braak H, Tredici KD, Rüb U, de Vos RA, Jansen Steur EN, Braak E. Staging of brain pathology related to sporadic Parkinson's disease. Neurobiol Aging. 2003;24(2):197–211.
34. Halliday GM, McCann H. The progression of pathology in Parkinson's disease. Ann N Y Acad Sci. 2010;1184:188–95.
35. Ballard C, Ziabreva I, Perry R, Larsen JP, O'Brien J, McKeith I, et al. Differences in neuropathologic characteristics across the Lewy body dementia spectrum. Neurology. 2006;67(11):1931–4.
36. Ibarretxe-Bilbao N, Tolosa E, Junque C, Marti MJ. MRI and cognitive impairment in Parkinson's disease. Mov Disord. 2009;24 Suppl 2:S748–53.
37. Beyer MK, Larsen JP, Aarsland D. Gray matter atrophy in Parkinson disease with dementia and dementia with Lewy bodies. Neurology. 2007;69(8): 747–54.
38. Sanchez-Castaneda C, Rene R, Ramirez-Ruiz B, Campdelacreu J, Gascon J, Falcon C, et al. Correlations between gray matter reductions and cognitive deficits in dementia with Lewy Bodies and Parkinson's disease with dementia. Mov Disord. 2009;24(12):1740–6.
39. Lee JE, Park HJ, Park B, Song SK, Sohn YH, Lee JD, et al. A comparative analysis of cognitive profiles and white-matter alterations using voxel-based diffusion tensor imaging between patients with Parkinson's disease dementia and dementia with Lewy bodies. J Neurol Neurosurg Psychiatry. 2010; 81(3):320–6.
40. Edison P, Rowe CC, Rinne JO, Ng S, Ahmed I, Kemppainen N, et al. Amyloid load in Parkinson's disease dementia and Lewy body dementia measured with [11C]PIB positron emission tomography. J Neurol Neurosurg Psychiatry. 2008;79(12):1331–8.
41. Maetzler W, Liepelt I, Reimold M, Reischl G, Solbach C, Becker C, et al. Cortical PIB binding in Lewy body disease is associated with Alzheimer-

like characteristics. Neurobiol Dis. 2009;34(1): 107–12.
42. Bohnen NI, Kaufer DI, Hendrickson R, Constantine GM, Mathis CA, Moore RY. Cortical cholinergic denervation is associated with depressive symptoms in Parkinson's disease and parkinsonian dementia. J Neurol Neurosurg Psychiatry. 2007;78(6):641–3.
43. Bohnen NI, Kaufer DI, Hendrickson R, Ivanco LS, Lopresti BJ, Constantine GM, et al. Cognitive correlates of cortical cholinergic denervation in Parkinson's disease and parkinsonian dementia. J Neurol. 2006;253(2):242–7.
44. Klein JC, Eggers C, Kalbe E, Weisenbach S, Hohmann C, Vollmar S, et al. Neurotransmitter changes in dementia with Lewy bodies and Parkinson disease dementia in vivo. Neurology. 2010;74(11): 885–92.
45. Shimada H, Hirano S, Shinotoh H, Aotsuka A, Sato K, Tanaka N, et al. Mapping of brain acetylcholinesterase alterations in Lewy body disease by PET. Neurology. 2009;73(4):273–8.
46. Vernon AC, Ballard C, Modo M. Neuroimaging for Lewy body disease: is the in vivo molecular imaging of alpha-synuclein neuropathology required and feasible? Brain Res Rev. 2010;65(1):28–55.
47. Teune LK, Bartels AL, de Jong BM, Willemsen AT, Eshuis SA, de Vries JJ, et al. Typical cerebral metabolic patterns in neurodegenerative brain diseases. Mov Disord. 2010;25(14):2395–404.
48. Seppi K, Poewe W. Brain magnetic resonance imaging techniques in the diagnosis of parkinsonian syndromes. Neuroimaging Clin N Am. 2010;20(1): 29–55.
49. Groschel K, Hauser TK, Luft A, Patronas N, Dichgans J, Litvan I, et al. Magnetic resonance imaging-based volumetry differentiates progressive supranuclear palsy from corticobasal degeneration. Neuroimage. 2004;21(2):714–24.
50. Tatsch K. Extrapyramidal syndromes: PET and SPECT. Neuroimaging Clin N Am. 2010;20(1):57–68.
51. Hirano S, Shinotoh H, Shimada H, Aotsuka A, Tanaka N, Ota T, et al. Cholinergic imaging in corticobasal syndrome, progressive supranuclear palsy and frontotemporal dementia. Brain. 2010;133(Pt 7):2058–68.
52. Cordato NJ, Pantelis C, Halliday GM, Velakoulis D, Wood SJ, Stuart GW, et al. Frontal atrophy correlates with behavioural changes in progressive supranuclear palsy. Brain. 2002;125(Pt 4):789–800.
53. Paviour DC, Price SL, Jahanshahi M, Lees AJ, Fox NC. Longitudinal MRI in progressive supranuclear palsy and multiple system atrophy: rates and regions of atrophy. Brain. 2006;129(Pt 4):1040–9.
54. Eckert T, Barnes A, Dhawan V, Frucht S, Gordon MF, Feigin AS, et al. FDG PET in the differential diagnosis of parkinsonian disorders. Neuroimage. 2005;26(3):912–21.
55. Metzler-Baddeley C. A review of cognitive impairments in dementia with Lewy bodies relative to Alzheimer's disease and Parkinson's disease with dementia. Cortex. 2007;43(5):583–600.
56. Possin KL, Filoteo JV, Song DD, Salmon DP. Spatial and object working memory deficits in Parkinson's disease are due to impairment in different underlying processes. Neuropsychology. 2008;22(5):585–95.
57. Mondon K, Gochard A, Marque A, Armand A, Beauchamp D, Prunier C, et al. Visual recognition memory differentiates dementia with Lewy bodies and Parkinson's disease dementia. J Neurol Neurosurg Psychiatry. 2007;78(7):738–41.
58. Culbertson WC, Moberg PJ, Duda JE, Stern MB, Weintraub D. Assessing the executive function deficits of patients with Parkinson's disease: utility of the Tower of London-Drexel. Assessment. 2004;11(1):27–39.
59. Ferman TJ, Smith GE, Boeve BF, Graff-Radford NR, Lucas JA, Knopman DS, et al. Neuropsychological differentiation of dementia with Lewy bodies from normal aging and Alzheimer's disease. Clin Neuropsychol. 2006;20(4):623–36.
60. Grossman M, Carvell S, Stern MB, Gollomp S, Hurtig HI. Sentence comprehension in Parkinson's disease: the role of attention and memory. Brain Lang. 1992;42(4):347–84.
61. Breen EK. Recall and recognition memory in Parkinson's disease. Cortex. 1993;29(1):91–102.
62. Bronnick K, Alves G, Aarsland D, Tysnes OB, Larsen JP. Verbal memory in drug-naive, newly diagnosed Parkinson's disease. The retrieval deficit hypothesis revisited. Neuropsychology. 2011;25(1): 114–24.
63. Filoteo JV, Rilling LM, Cole B, Williams BJ, Davis JD, Roberts JW. Variable memory profiles in Parkinson's disease. J Clin Exp Neuropsychol. 1997;19(6):878–88.
64. Berger HJ, van Es NJ, van Spaendonck KP, Teunisse JP, Horstink MW, van 't Hof MA, et al. Relationship between memory strategies and motor symptoms in Parkinson's disease. J Clin Exp Neuropsychol. 1999;21(5):677–84.
65. Massman PJ, Delis DC, Butters N, Levin BE, Salmon DP. Are all subcortical dementias alike? Verbal learning and memory in Parkinson's and Huntington's disease patients. J Clin Exp Neuropsychol. 1990;12(5):729–44.
66. Filoteo JV, Salmon DP, Schiehser DM, Kane AE, Hamilton JM, Rilling LM, et al. Verbal learning and memory in patients with dementia with Lewy bodies or Parkinson's disease with dementia. J Clin Exp Neuropsychol. 2009;31(7):823–34.
67. Huber SJ, Shuttleworth EC, Paulson GW. Dementia in Parkinson's disease. Arch Neurol. 1986;43(10): 987–90.
68. Leplow B, Dierks C, Herrmann P, Pieper N, Annecke R, Ulm G. Remote memory in Parkinson's disease and senile dementia. Neuropsychologia. 1997;35(4): 547–57.
69. Cormack F, Aarsland D, Ballard C, Tovee MJ. Pentagon drawing and neuropsychological performance in Dementia with Lewy Bodies, Alzheimer's disease, Parkinson's disease and Parkinson's disease

with dementia. Int J Geriatr Psychiatry. 2004;19(4): 371–7.
70. Mosimann UP, Mather G, Wesnes KA, O'Brien JT, Burn DJ, McKeith IG. Visual perception in Parkinson disease dementia and dementia with Lewy bodies. Neurology. 2004;63(11):2091–6.
71. American Psychiatric Association. Diagnostic and Statistical Manual of Mental Disorders, Fourth Edition, Text Revision: DSM-IV-TR. Washington, DC: American Psychiatric Association; 2000.
72. Weintraub D, Moberg PJ, Duda JE, Katz IR, Stern MB. Recognition and treatment of depression in Parkinson's disease. J Geriatr Psychiatry Neurol. 2003;16(3):178–83.
73. Shulman LM, Taback RL, Rabinstein AA, Weiner WJ. Non-recognition of depression and other non-motor symptoms in Parkinson's disease. Parkinsonism Relat Disord. 2002;8:193–7.
74. Aarsland D, Ballard C, Larsen JP, McKeith I. A comparative study of psychiatric symptoms in dementia with Lewy bodies and Parkinson's disease with and without dementia. Int J Geriatr Psychiatry. 2001;16(5):528–36.
75. Slaughter JR, Slaughter KA, Nichols D, Holmes SE, Martens MP. Prevalence, clinical manifestations, etiology, and treatment of depression in Parkinson's disease. J Neuropsychiatry Clin Neurosci. 2001; 13(2):187–96.
76. McDonald WM, Richard IH, DeLong MR. Prevalence, etiology, and treatment of depression in Parkinson's disease. Biol Psychiatry. 2003;54(3): 363–75.
77. Schiffer RB, Kurlan R, Rubin A, Boer S. Evidence for atypical depression in Parkinson's disease. A J Psychiatry. 1988;145(8):1020–2.
78. Walsh K, Bennett G. Parkinson's disease and anxiety. Postgrad Med J. 2001;77(904):89–93.
79. Stein MB, Heuser IJ, Juncos JL, Uhde TW. Anxiety disorders in patients with Parkinson's disease. A J Psychiatry. 1990;147(2):217–20.
80. Vazquez A, Jimenez-Jimenez FJ, Garcia-Ruiz P, Garcia-Urra D. "Panic attacks" in Parkinson's disease. A long-term complication of levodopa therapy. Acta Neurologica Scandanavica. 1993; 87(1):14–8.
81. Borroni B, Agosti C, Padovani A. Behavioral and psychological symptoms in dementia with Lewy-bodies (DLB): frequency and relationship with disease severity and motor impairment. Arch Gerontol Geriatr. 2008;46(1):101–6.
82. Mimura M, White RF, Albert ML. Corticobasal degeneration: neuropsychological and clinical correlates. J Neuropsychiatry Clin Neurosci. 1997;9(1): 94–8.
83. Murray R, Neumann M, Forman MS, Farmer J, Massimo L, Rice A, et al. Cognitive and motor assessment in autopsy-proven corticobasal degeneration. Neurology. 2007;68(16):1274–83.
84. Pillon B, Blin J, Vidailhet M, Deweer B, Sirigu A, Dubois B, et al. The neuropsychological pattern of corticobasal degeneration: comparison with progressive supranuclear palsy and Alzheimer's disease. Neurology. 1995;45(8):1477–83.
85. Pillon B, Gouider-Khouja N, Deweer B, Vidailhet M, Malapani C, Dubois B, et al. Neuropsychological pattern of striatonigral degeneration: comparison with Parkinson's disease and progressive supranuclear palsy. J Neurol Neurosurg Psychiatry. 1995; 58(2):174–9.
86. Soliveri P, Monza D, Paridi D, Radice D, Grisoli M, Testa D, et al. Cognitive and magnetic resonance imaging aspects of corticobasal degeneration and progressive supranuclear palsy. Neurology. 1999; 53(3):502–7.
87. Frasson E, Moretto G, Beltramello A, Smania N, Pampanin M, Stegagno C, et al. Neuropsychological and neuroimaging correlates in corticobasal degeneration. Ital J Neurol Sci. 1998;19(5):321–8.
88. Beatty WW, Scott JG, Wilson DA, Prince JR, Williamson DJ. Memory deficits in a demented patient with probable corticobasal degeneration. J Geriatr Psychiatry Neurol. 1995;8(2):132–6.
89. Huey ED, Goveia EN, Paviol S, Pardini M, Krueger F, Zamboni G, et al. Executive dysfunction in frontotemporal dementia and corticobasal syndrome. Neurology. 2009;72(5):453–9.
90. Kertesz A, McMonagle P. Behavior and cognition in corticobasal degeneration and progressive supranuclear palsy. J Neurol Sci. 2010;289(1–2):138–43.
91. Graham NL, Bak TH, Hodges JR. Corticobasal degeneration as a cognitive disorder. Mov Disord. 2003;18(11):1224–32.
92. Graham NL, Bak T, Patterson K, Hodges JR. Language function and dysfunction in corticobasal degeneration. Neurology. 2003;61(4):493–9.
93. Hohler AD, Ransom BR, Chun MR, Tröster AI, Samii A. The youngest reported case of corticobasal degeneration. Parkinsonism Relat Disord. 2003; 10:47–50.
94. Massman PJ, Kreiter KT, Jankovic J, Doody RS. Neuropsychological functioning in cortical-basal ganglionic degeneration: Differentiation from Alzheimer's disease. Neurology. 1996;46(3):720–6.
95. Leiguarda R, Lees AJ, Merello M, Starkstein S, Marsden CD. The nature of apraxia in corticobasal degeneration. J Neurol Neurosurg Psychiatry. 1994; 57(4):455–9.
96. Pharr V, Uttl B, Stark M, Litvan I, Fantie B, Grafman J. Comparison of apraxia in corticobasal degeneration and progressive supranuclear palsy. Neurology. 2001;56(7):957–63.
97. Soliveri P, Piacentini S, Girotti F. Limb apraxia in corticobasal degeneration and progressive supranuclear palsy. Neurology. 2005;64(3):448–53.
98. Litvan I, Cummings JL, Mega M. Neuropsychiatric features of corticobasal degeneration. J Neurol Neurosurg Psychiatry. 1998;65(5):717–21.
99. Srulijes K, Mallien G, Bauer S, Dietzel E, Groger A, Ebersbach G, et al. In vivo comparison of Richardson's syndrome and progressive supranuclear

palsy-parkinsonism. J Neural Transm. 2011;118: 1191–7.

100. Rafal RD, Posner MI, Friedman JH, Inhoff AW, Bernstein E. Orienting of visual attention in progressive supranuclear palsy. Brain. 1988;111(Pt 2): 267–80.
101. Grafman J, Litvan I, Stark M. Neuropsychological features of progressive supranuclear palsy. Brain Cogn. 1995;28(3):311–20.
102. Albert ML, Feldman RG, Willis AL. The 'subcortical dementia' of progressive supranuclear palsy. J Neurol Neurosurg Psychiatry. 1974;37(2):121–30.
103. Josephs KA, Whitwell JL, Eggers SD, Senjem ML, Jack CR, Jr. Gray matter correlates of behavioral severity in progressive supranuclear palsy. Mov Disord. 2011;26:493–8.
104. Monza D, Soliveri P, Radice D, Fetoni V, Testa D, Caffarra P, et al. Cognitive dysfunction and impaired organization of complex motility in degenerative parkinsonian syndromes. Arch Neurol. 1998;55(3): 372–8.
105. Millar D, Griffiths P, Zermansky AJ, Burn DJ. Characterizing behavioral and cognitive dysexecutive changes in progressive supranuclear palsy. Mov Disord. 2006;21(2):199–207.
106. Soliveri P, Monza D, Paridi D, Carella F, Genitrini S, Testa D, et al. Neuropsychological follow up in patients with Parkinson's disease, striatonigral degeneration-type multisystem atrophy, and progressive supranuclear palsy. J Neurol Neurosurg Psychiatry. 2000;69(3):313–8.
107. Kaat LD, Boon AJ, Kamphorst W, Ravid R, Duivenvoorden HJ, van Swieten JC. Frontal presentation in progressive supranuclear palsy. Neurology. 2007;69(8):723–9.
108. Dubois B, Slachevsky A, Pillon B, Beato R, Villalponda JM, Litvan I. "Applause sign" helps to discriminate PSP from FTD and PD. Neurology. 2005;64(12):2132–3.
109. O'Sullivan SS, Massey LA, Williams DR, Silveira-Moriyama L, Kempster PA, Holton JL, et al. Clinical outcomes of progressive supranuclear palsy and multiple system atrophy. Brain. 2008;131(Pt 5):1362–72.
110. Cordato NJ, Halliday GM, Caine D, Morris JG. Comparison of motor, cognitive, and behavioral features in progressive supranuclear palsy and Parkinson's disease. Mov Disord. 2006;21(5):632–8.
111. Rosser A, Hodges JR. Initial letter and semantic category fluency in Alzheimer's disease, Huntington's disease, and progressive supranuclear palsy. J Neurol Neurosurg Psychiatry. 1994;57(11): 1389–94.
112. Piatt AL, Fields JA, Paolo AM, Koller WC, Tröster AI. Lexical, semantic, and action verbal fluency in Parkinson's disease with and without dementia. J Clin Exp Neuropsychol. 1999;21(4):435–43.
113. Cotelli M, Borroni B, Manenti R, Alberici A, Calabria M, Agosti C, et al. Action and object naming in frontotemporal dementia, progressive supranuclear palsy, and corticobasal degeneration. Neuropsychology. 2006;20(5):558–65.
114. Podoll K, Schwarz M, Noth J. Language functions in progressive supranuclear palsy. Brain. 1991;114(Pt 3):1457–72.
115. Huey ED, Pardini M, Cavanagh A, Wassermann EM, Kapogiannis D, Spina S, et al. Association of ideomotor apraxia with frontal gray matter volume loss in corticobasal syndrome. Arch Neurol. 2009;66(10):1274–80.
116. Rohrer JD, Paviour D, Bronstein AM, O'Sullivan SS, Lees A, Warren JD. Progressive supranuclear palsy syndrome presenting as progressive nonfluent aphasia: a neuropsychological and neuroimaging analysis. Mov Disord. 2010;25(2):179–88.
117. Boeve B, Dickson D, Duffy J, Bartleson J, Trenerry M, Petersen R. Progressive nonfluent aphasia and subsequent aphasic dementia associated with atypical progressive supranuclear palsy pathology. Eur Neurol. 2003;49(2):72–8.
118. Mochizuki A, Ueda Y, Komatsuzaki Y, Tsuchiya K, Arai T, Shoji S. Progressive supranuclear palsy presenting with primary progressive aphasia–clinicopathological report of an autopsy case. Acta Neuropathologica (Berlin). 2003;105(6):610–4.
119. Aarsland D, Litvan I, Salmon D, Galasko D, Wentzel-Larsen T, Larsen JP. Performance on the Dementia Rating Scale in Parkinson's disease with dementia and dementia with Lewy bodies: comparison with progressive supranuclear palsy and Alzheimer's disease. J Neurol Neurosurg Psychiatry. 2003;74:1215–20.
120. Pillon B, Dubois B, Ploska A, Agid Y. Severity and specificity of cognitive impairment in Alzheimer's, Huntington's, and Parkinson's diseases and progressive supranuclear palsy. Neurology. 1991;41(5):634–43.
121. Zarei M, Pouretemad HR, Bak T, Hodges JR. Autobiographical memory in progressive supranuclear palsy. Eur J Neurol. 2010;17(2):238–41.
122. Bak TH, Caine D, Hearn VC, Hodges JR. Visuospatial functions in atypical parkinsonian syndromes. J Neurol Neurosurg Psychiatry. 2006;77(4):454–6.
123. Joel D. Open interconnected model of basal ganglia-thalamocortical circuitry and its relevance to the clinical syndrome of Huntington's disease. Mov Disord. 2001;16(3):407–23.
124. Litvan I, Mega MS, Cummings JL, Fairbanks L. Neuropsychiatric aspects of progressive supranuclear palsy. Neurology. 1996;47(5):1184–9.
125. Aarsland D, Litvan I, Larsen JP. Neuropsychiatric symptoms of patients with progressive supranuclear palsy and Parkinson's disease. J Neuropsychiatry Clin Neurosci. 2001;13(1):42–9.
126. O'Keeffe FM, Murray B, Coen RF, Dockree PM, Bellgrove MA, Garavan H, et al. Loss of insight in frontotemporal dementia, corticobasal degeneration and progressive supranuclear palsy. Brain. 2007;130(Pt 3):753–64.
127. Tröster AI, Fields JA. Parkinson's disease, progressive supranuclear palsy, corticobasal degeneration, and related disorders of the frontostriatal system. In:

Morgan JE, Ricker JH, editors. Textbook of clinical neuropsychology. New York: Psychology; 2008. p. 536–77.
128. Brown RG, MacCarthy B, Jahanshahi M, Marsden CD. Accuracy of self-reported disability in patients with parkinsonism. Arch Neurol. 1989;46(9): 955–9.
129. Sitek EJ, Soltan W, Wieczorek D, Robowski P, Slawek J. Self-awareness of memory function in Parkinson's disease in relation to mood and symptom severity. Aging Ment Health. 2011;15:150–6.
130. Naismith SL, Pereira M, Shine JM, Lewis SJ. How well do caregivers detect mild cognitive change in Parkinson's disease? Mov Disord. 2011;26(1):161–4.
131. Bak TH, Rogers TT, Crawford LM, Hearn VC, Mathuranath PS, Hodges JR. Cognitive bedside assessment in atypical parkinsonian syndromes. J Neurol Neurosurg Psychiatry. 2005;76(3):420–2.
132. Kulisevsky J, Pagonabarraga J. Cognitive impairment in Parkinson's disease: tools for diagnosis and assessment. Mov Disord. 2009;24(8):1103–10.
133. Chou KL, Amick MM, Brandt J, Camicioli R, Frei K, Gitelman D, et al. A recommended scale for cognitive screening in clinical trials of Parkinson's disease. Mov Disord. 2010;25(15):2501–7.
134. Miyasaki JM, Shannon K, Voon V, Ravina B, Kleiner-Fisman G, Anderson K, et al. Practice Parameter: evaluation and treatment of depression, psychosis, and dementia in Parkinson disease (an evidence-based review): report of the Quality Standards Subcommittee of the American Academy of Neurology. Neurology. 2006;66(7):996–1002.
135. Folstein MF, Folstein SE, McHugh PR. Mini-mental state. A practical method for grading the cognitive state of patients for the clinician. J Psychiatr Res. 1975;12(3):189–98.
136. Folstein MF, Folstein SE, Fanjiang G. Mini-Mental State Examination clinical guide. Lutz, FL: Psychological Assessment Resources; 2001.
137. Mattis S. Dementia Rating Scale-2. Lutz, FL: Psychological Assessment Resources, Inc.; 2001.
138. Mattis S. Dementia Rating Scale. Odessa, FL: Psychological Assessment Resources; 1988.
139. Nasreddine ZS, Phillips NA, Bedirian V, Charbonneau S, Whitehead V, Collin I, et al. The Montreal Cognitive Assessment, MoCA: a brief screening tool for mild cognitive impairment. J Am Geriatr Soc. 2005;53(4):695–9.
140. Jefferson AL, Cosentino SA, Ball SK, Bogdanoff B, Leopold N, Kaplan E, et al. Errors produced on the Mini-Mental State Examination and neuropsychological test performance in Alzheimer's disease, ischemic vascular dementia, and Parkinson's disease. J Neuropsychiatry Clin Neurosci. 2002;14(3):311–20.
141. Janvin C, Aarsland D, Larsen JP, Hugdahl K. Neuropsychological profile of patients with Parkinson's disease without dementia. Dement Geriatr Cogn Disord. 2003;15(3):126–31.
142. Hoops S, Nazem S, Siderowf AD, Duda JE, Xie SX, Stern MB, et al. Validity of the MoCA and MMSE in the detection of MCI and dementia in Parkinson disease. Neurology. 2009;73(21):1738–45.
143. Hobson P, Meara J. The detection of dementia and cognitive impairment in a community population of elderly people with Parkinson's disease by use of the CAMCOG neuropsychological test. Age Ageing. 1999;28(1):39–43.
144. Aarsland D, Andersen K, Larsen JP, Perry R, Wentzel-Larsen T, Lolk A, et al. The rate of cognitive decline in Parkinson disease. Arch Neurol. 2004;61(12):1906–11.
145. Paolo AM, Tröster AI, Glatt SL, Hubble JP, Koller WC. Differentiation of the dementias of Alzheimer's and Parkinson's disease with the Dementia Rating Scale. J Geriatr Psychiatry Neurol. 1995;8(3):184–8.
146. Brown GG, Rahill AA, Gorell JM, McDonald C, Brown SJ, Sillanpaa M, et al. Validity of the Dementia Rating Scale in assessing cognitive function in Parkinson's disease. J Geriatr Psychiatry Neurol. 1999;12(4):180–8.
147. Athey RJ, Porter RW, Walker RW. Cognitive assessment of a representative community population with Parkinson's disease (PD) using the Cambridge Cognitive Assessment-Revised (CAMCOG-R). Age Ageing. 2005;34(3):268–73.
148. Rothlind JC, Brandt J. A brief assessment of frontal and subcortical functions in dementia. J Neuropsychiatry Clin Neurosci. 1993;5(1):73–7.
149. Dubois B, Slachevsky A, Litvan I, Pillon B. The FAB: a Frontal Assessment Battery at bedside. Neurology. 2000;55(11):1621–6.
150. Mahieux F, Michelet D, Manifacier M-J, Boller F, Fermanian J, Guillard A. Mini-Mental Parkinson: first validation study of a new bedside test constructed for Parkinson's disease. Behav Neurol. 1995;8:15–22.
151. Marinus J, Visser M, Verwey NA, Verhey FR, Middelkoop HA, Stiggelbout AM, et al. Assessment of cognition in Parkinson's disease. Neurology. 2003;61(9):1222–8.
152. Kalbe E, Calabrese P, Kohn N, Hilker R, Riedel O, Wittchen HU, et al. Screening for cognitive deficits in Parkinson's disease with the Parkinson neuropsychometric dementia assessment (PANDA) instrument. Parkinsonism Relat Disord. 2008;14(2):93–101.
153. Pagonabarraga J, Kulisevsky J, Llebaria G, Garcia-Sanchez C, Pascual-Sedano B, Gironell A. Parkinson's disease-cognitive rating scale: a new cognitive scale specific for Parkinson's disease. Mov Disord. 2008;23(7):998–1005.
154. Higginson CI, Fields JA, Koller WC, Tröster AI. Questionnaire assessment potentially overestimates anxiety in Parkinson's disease. J Clin Psychol Med Settings. 2001;8(2):95–9.
155. Tröster AI, Williams RC. Progressive supranuclear palsy. In: Morgan JE, Baron IS, Ricker JH, editors. Casebook of clinical neuropsychology. New York: Oxford University; 2011. p. 596–605.
156. Lucas JA. A case of corticobasal syndrome. In: Morgan JE, Baron IS, Ricker JH, editors. Casebook

of clinical neuropsychology. New York: Oxford University; 2011. p. 559–66.
157. Ferman TJ. Clinical and neuropathologic presentation of dementia with Lewy bodies. In: Morgan JE, Baron IS, Ricker JH, editors. Casebook of clinical neuropsychology. New York: Oxford University; 2011. p. 550–8.
158. Tröster AI, Woods SP. Neuropsychological aspects. In: Pahwa R, Lyons KE, editors. Handbook of Parkinson's disease. 4th ed. New York: Informa; 2007. p. 109–31.
159. Schrag A, Barone P, Brown RG, Leentjens AF, McDonald WM, Starkstein S, et al. Depression rating scales in Parkinson's disease: critique and recommendations. Mov Disord. 2007;22(8):1077–92.
160. Leentjens AF, Dujardin K, Marsh L, Martinez-Martin P, Richard IH, Starkstein SE, et al. Anxiety rating scales in Parkinson's disease: critique and recommendations. Mov Disord. 2008;23(14): 2015–25.
161. Leentjens AF, Dujardin K, Marsh L, Martinez-Martin P, Richard IH, Starkstein SE, et al. Apathy and anhedonia rating scales in Parkinson's disease: critique and recommendations. Mov Disord. 2008;23(14):2004–14.
162. Fernandez HH, Aarsland D, Fenelon G, Friedman JH, Marsh L, Troster AI, et al. Scales to assess psychosis in Parkinson's disease: Critique and recommendations. Mov Disord. 2008;23(4): 484–500.
163. Hogl B, Arnulf I, Comella C, Ferreira J, Iranzo A, Tilley B, et al. Scales to assess sleep impairment in Parkinson's disease: critique and recommendations. Mov Disord. 2010;25(16):2704–16.

Neuropsychological Considerations for Parkinson's Disease Patients Being Considered for Surgical Intervention with Deep Brain Stimulation

23

Paul J. Mattis, Chaya B. Gopin, and Kathryn Lombardi Mirra

Abstract

In addition to their motor symptoms, patients diagnosed with idiopathic Parkinson's disease (PD) often exhibit a subcortical pattern of cognitive impairment. Deep brain stimulation (DBS) is one of the treatments used to improve motor functioning in PD patients; however, studies focusing on the effects of DBS on cognition, mood, and behavior have produced mixed findings. This chapter reviews the history of various treatments for PD, the recent literature regarding DBS, and the neuropsychological outcomes in patients who undergo such surgery for the treatment of parkinsonian motor symptoms. DBS as a treatment for several other neurologic and psychiatric disorders is also discussed. In addition, case examples and recommendations for the neuropsychologist are presented.

Keywords

Parkinson's disease • Surgery • Ablative • Deep brain stimulation • Fetal transplantation • Gene therapy • Subcortical • Subthalamic nucleus • Globus pallidus

Introduction to Parkinson's Disease

Idiopathic Parkinson's disease (PD) is a neurodegenerative disorder that is characterized by motor symptoms, including resting tremor, bradykinesia, muscle rigidity, and postural instability. Cognitive and behavioral disturbances are also common to this disease and contribute to its functional disability [1–3]. Onset is typically around age 65 years, although approximately 8% of individuals develop the illness "early," between 21 and 40 years of age [3].

P.J. Mattis (✉)
Center for Neurosciences, The Feinstein Institute for Medical Research, Manhasset, NY, 11030, USA

Department of Neurology, North Shore University Hospital, Manhasset, NY, 11030, USA
e-mail: pmattis@nshs.edu

C.B. Gopin, Ph.D. • K.L. Mirra, Ph.D.
Department of Neurology, North Shore University Hospital, Manhasset, NY, 11030, USA

Department of Psychiatry, The Zucker Hillside Hospital, 75-59 263 rd Street, Glen Oaks, NY, 11004, USA
e-mail: cgopin@nshs.edu; klombardi@nshs.edu

L.D. Ravdin and H.L. Katzen (eds.), *Handbook on the Neuropsychology of Aging and Dementia*, Clinical Handbooks in Neuropsychology, DOI 10.1007/978-1-4614-3106-0_23,

The relationship between the development of PD and the gradual death of dopamine neurons, specifically in the substantia nigra pars compacta (SNc), has been recognized since the 1950s [4–6]. It is now known that symptoms of PD manifest once a significant portion (approximately 60–70%) [7] of SNc dopaminergic cells die, resulting in increased activity within the motor circuitry (See [8] for a review). Specifically, the diminished dopamine level in the SNc reduces the inhibitory influence on the subthalamic nucleus (STN), which then exerts excessive excitatory influence on the globus pallidus pars interna (GPi). This, in turn, contributes to increased inhibition of thalamocortical neurons, which are responsible, in part, for the rhythmic tremors at rest, inability to initiate/complete voluntary movements, and cogwheel rigidity associated with PD [9].

Given the neural circuitry that has been implicated in PD, it is not surprising that patients often exhibit a subcortical pattern of cognitive impairment. The neuropsychological profile of patients with PD tends to reveal mild deficits in aspects of executive functioning, memory, and visuospatial functioning. Additionally, symptoms of depression are frequently reported [10]. Language abilities generally remain intact, although language deficits are occasionally reported and, in these instances, are largely secondary to executive dysfunction and/or motor impairment. The reader is referred to Chap. 22 for a more comprehensive discussion of the neurocognitive impairment associated with PD.

Treatment for PD

Overview

Treatments for PD attempt to restore the motor circuit's delicate balance, either through introducing dopaminergic medications that increase the output of the substantia nigra or through surgical techniques that reduce the activity of the STN or GPi [11–13]. Levodopa, a dopamine supplement, is currently the gold standard of treatment for PD [14]. Levodopa replaces dopamine in the forebrain that is lost due to the illness, consistently reversing many of the key motor symptoms: akinesia, bradykinesia, and rigidity. However, it does not prevent the progression of the disease, and for most patients, the efficacy of the medication declines after 5 years of daily treatment [14]. Long-term use of Levodopa is also hampered by treatment-induced motor complications, such as dyskinesias and motor fluctuations [15]. Furthermore, nondopaminergic symptoms (e.g., choking, drooling, sleep disturbances, mood disorders, dementia) ultimately start to emerge, contributing to the disability of late-stage PD [16]. As such, alternate treatments have been sought, including new surgical interventions.

History of Surgical Treatments for PD

The use of surgical treatment to obtain symptom relief in PD dates back over a century (for detailed review see [11] and [17]). In the early 1900s, Victor Horsley and Henry Clark introduced basic stereotactic neurosurgery techniques. After creating small openings in the skull, the researchers were able to target specific brain structures that they had previously identified using a three-dimensional Cartesian coordinate system. In 1909, Horsley began to use ablative surgery through lesioning certain areas of the sensorimotor cortex [11]. Although this technique successfully reduced the severity of resting tremors, additional impairment was evident in the performance of voluntary movements. The use of ablative surgery was further popularized in 1939 when Bucy and colleagues implemented the technique to lesion the corticospinal tracts. Also in 1939, Russell Meyers was the first to operate on the basal ganglia through an open craniotomy procedure. Although effective in alleviating some of the motor symptoms, there was a high mortality rate associated with the procedure, prompting explorations for safer treatments [11]. In the late 1940s, Spiegal and colleagues and Leskell furthered the use of stereotaxic techniques, resulting in the implementation of relatively less invasive approaches (for review, see [17]).

In 1952, while conducting a pedunculotomy of a patient with PD, Irving Cooper accidentally interrupted flow in the anterior choroidal artery. To his surprise, the patient's tremor and rigidity vastly improved postoperatively [18]. This accidental finding prompted Cooper to deliberately use this procedure over the next several years to alleviate PD motor symptoms [17].

Throughout the 1950s and 1960s, spurred by advancements in the understanding of PD neuropathology, ablative surgeries were also widely used. Destructive agents, such as alcohol, heat, or cold, were introduced to a specified location to lesion the site [11]. Targeting specific areas of the basal ganglia proved to be a relatively effective and safe approach, leading to positive outcomes and reduction of certain motor symptoms.

Levodopa was first introduced for the treatment of PD in 1968. The outcome was so promising that the use of surgical techniques decreased dramatically over the next several years [11, 17–19]; however, in the late 1970s, it became evident that some patients became refractory to levodopa treatment over time. In other patients, treatment-induced motor complications and dyskinesias were observed. These findings, in conjunction with advancements in neuroimaging techniques and neurophysiological brain mapping, resulted in the reemergence of surgical intervention [11, 20].

Ablative techniques targeting the GPi and ventral intermediate nucleus of the thalamus (Vim) were frequently employed. Then, in the early 1990s, deep brain stimulation (DBS) became an accepted and effective method of treatment [18]. Like ablative techniques, DBS treatment was aimed at the above-mentioned targets (i.e., GPi, Vim) as well as the STN. Rather than destroying the targeted tissue through lesioning [17], DBS introduced a reversible electrical impulse to the surrounding neuronal tissues near the target [18]. This technique will be discussed in detail below.

Fetal Transplantation

More recently, researchers began implanting fetal-stage neurons into the caudate-putamen or substantia nigra of PD patients. It was hypothesized that the transplanted neurons would grow, connect, and release DA, and thus, transplantation would enable the maintenance of a relatively steady supply of dopamine to remain in the synaptic clefts [21, 22]. However, double-blind clinical trials produced mixed results [23], and several transplantations resulted in the development of unforeseen, severe, off-medication dyskinesias that warranted DBS intervention [24]. Nevertheless, clinical improvement was noted for patients who were 60 years of age or younger [23], and the grafts were later found to remain viable 4 years postsurgery [25]. Further, there were no indications of cognitive decline following fetal tissue implantation [26]. At the time of this chapter, a large-scale multicenter clinical trial in Europe is being undertaken (Principal Investigator: Roger Barker, M.D. from the University of Cambridge); however, to date, the use of fetal nigral tissue transplantation for the alleviation of PD symptoms remains exclusively an experimental treatment.

Gene Therapy

Gene therapy has become the focus of a few PD treatment studies in recent years. Using modified viruses (vectors), genetic material is introduced into the neurons within the motor circuit in the hopes of reestablishing normal brain activity. Recently, researchers have demonstrated that an AAV vector can be used safely to deliver the glutamic acid decarboxylase (GAD) gene directly into STN neurons [27]. There was no evidence of cognitive decline in these patients [28]. Given that reduced GABAergic input from the GP increases the activity of the STN in PD patients [29–31], Kaplitt and colleagues [27] hypothesized that the introduction of GAD, which catalyzes the synthesis of GABA, would restore the delicate balance of neurotransmitters within the motor circuit. Indeed, prior studies conducted in animals indicated that AAV-GAD improved brain function and PD-like symptoms without causing toxic side effects [32–35]. Although this single study was not designed to assess the effectiveness of the intervention, clinical outcomes were encouraging. Substantial improvements in both the "OFF" and "ON" states were observed, beginning at 3 months after surgery and continuing until the end of the trial (i.e., 1 year postsurgery). Randomized and placebo-controlled studies are under way, and the data should be released in the coming year. This promising mode of treatment may prove to be the intervention of choice in the future, as it does not require indwelling hardware or frequent readjustments and may restore the motor network function to baseline through activity-dependent release of GABA [27].

Deep Brain Stimulation (DBS)

DBS involves the application of high-frequency electrical stimulation directly into the neurons of the motor circuit. A burr hole is performed under local anesthesia. Then, using stereotactic guidance, stimulating quadripolar electrodes are implanted using both direct MRI and CT targeting, as well as "indirect targeting" based on the known locations of these targets relative to fixed midline structures (anterior and posterior commissure). Ventriculography, involving injection of contrast into the ventricular system, was routinely used prior to the CT and MRI era and is now used by only a few centers given the invasiveness of the procedure [36]. Thin wire electrodes are aimed at the target, and intraoperative stimulation is used to predict the effects of chronic stimulation, which assists in determining the final site of electrode implantation [37]. Once the signal strength and final contact position have been verified, which typically occurs 1–2 days after surgery, one or two internal pulse generators are implanted under the skin in the subclavicular region near the collar bone [1]. These generators create an open loop system in which electrical stimulation is delivered on a set, constant, preprogrammed schedule. Finally, three-dimensional computer tomography or MRI scans are performed a few days later to confirm the position of the electrodes [9].

Risks associated with DBS surgery include air embolus, stroke, seizures, hemorrhage, hydrocephalus, infections, and lead fractures [38]. Nevertheless, the infrequent occurrence of such complications, coupled with the fact that the benefits of the surgery greatly outweigh the costs, ultimately led the FDA to approve DBS for the treatment of medically intractable symptoms of movement disorders in 2002 [9]. Since that time, thousands of patients have undergone the procedure [37].

Investigators are still not entirely certain how the treatment works at the cellular level (for review of the functional mechanism, see [39]). Micro-lesions from the procedure itself do produce motor network changes [40], but these changes dissipate over time. It is also clear that the changes in motor circuitry with STN-DBS and those with levodopa administration have much in common but are not identical [41]. It has been suggested that STN-DBS affects neuronal membrane potentials and voltage-dependent calcium channels surrounding the pathologic circuitry [9]. In doing so, DBS may be altering the firing pattern of STN neurons to immediately produce a therapeutic effect at the electrode's tip [42, 43]. It is also possible that the stimulation is not affecting the cell bodies; rather, the axons carrying signals into the STN from other areas may be the target of the stimulation's effects [9]. Support for this notion has been generated through studies of animal models of PD, in which optically stimulated cortical neurons, whose axons reach down to the STN, also diminish PD-like signs [44].

Although the STN is currently the most sought out target for DBS, stimulation of other aspects of motor network, including the GPi [45] and Vim of the thalamus [46], is also common. As the scientific community learns more about the subcortical pathophysiology of PD, target selection can be based more on the patient's most disabling symptoms, medication response (including side effects), and therapy goals [37]. Currently, DBS targeting the Vim is generally utilized to treat only the contralateral tremor, without having impact on rigidity or bradykinesia [18]. As such, the Vim is not targeted as often as other structures during DBS procedures. GPi DBS greatly reduces dyskinesias during the "ON" state, while STN-DBS helps to alleviate some of the motor impairments during the "OFF" state [18]. Further, DBS placement in the pedunculopontine nucleus has been shown to be effective in reducing freezing of gait [47].

Neuropsychological Outcome in Patients Undergoing DBS

The improvement in motor functioning following DBS has been well documented [48]. In contrast, studies focusing on the effects of DBS on cognition, mood, and behavior have yielded mixed findings. It is possible that the variation in findings is due to differences in the treatment protocols used at various centers. Other differences may include the comparison groups used and the characteristics of the patient populations, as well as small sample sizes and variable amounts of time that elapsed until follow-up. An overview of these findings are presented below.

Motor Outcome

STN-DBS and GPi DBS have both been reported to improve the cardinal motor features of PD, including tremor, bradykinesia, rigidity, akinesia, gait speed, stride length, lower limb joint movements, postural instability, and levodopa-induced dyskinesia [37, 48, 49]. Further, DBS can reduce levodopa-induced motor complications, such as prolonged "OFF" periods and dyskinesias [50]. Although the long-term implications of these treatments are not fully appreciated, multiple studies of patients who are approximately 5 years posttreatment have suggested sustained efficacy [51, 52].

Cognitive Changes

Findings regarding the cognitive changes associated with DBS vary widely (for review, see [37]), with some studies reporting cognitive improvement, others revealing cognitive decline, and still others showing no alterations in neurocognitive functioning. However, the most consistent finding is a mild decline in verbal fluency, both phonemic and semantic [53], which cannot be accounted for by changes in psychomotor speed since performance on psychomotor tasks tends to remain stable or to improve [54]. Several different explanations have been posited to explain this post-DBS cognitive weakness. Based on the activation of the left inferior frontal gyrus that was observed during neuroimaging studies of patients who underwent STN-DBS, Saint-Cyr and colleagues [55] hypothesized that stimulating the STN may impact the striato-thalamo-cortical circuit. This would then affect word generation, an ability that has been localized to the left inferior frontal gyrus. Alternatively, it is plausible that the current used to stimulate the STN may spread to adjacent cognitive circuits [54, 56], thereby disrupting the pathway associated with verbal fluency.

Decline in learning and memory has also been a consistent finding in DBS outcome studies; however, the clinical significance of these findings is questionable because the degree of decline may be limited [1]. Additionally, there is evidence to suggest that these abilities return to their pre-DBS state as time elapses [50, 57, 58]. It is possible, therefore, that the reported declines in learning and memory are due to secondary factors (e.g., edema, stimulator setting) and are not indicative of true impairment in these cognitive abilities.

Results of studies assessing the cognitive effects of STN-DBS in PD patients seem to suggest that the likelihood of decline is more frequently observed in older patients, who have a greater tendency to have presurgical cognitive impairments than younger patients [59]. However, Perriol and colleagues [60] found that neither age at time of surgery, disease duration, or performance on a cognitive screen (Dementia Rating Scale (DRS) total score), prior to surgery impacted outcome. Overall, preoperative cognitive deficits, confusion, and history of psychosis (induced by dopaminergic medication) were the factors that predicted cognitive outcome 12 months after surgery [48, 61–63].

Psychosocial Changes and Quality of Life

The findings regarding psychiatric changes following surgery have also been mixed. Reductions in symptoms of depression and anxiety are commonly described by patients [1]; however, investigations that have focused on behavioral outcome have reported either no change in mood symptoms [48, 59, 60] or significant psychological disturbances and behavioral changes following DBS. Reported increases in mood symptoms were generally associated with dysthymia or emotional lability [60, 64]. Yet, there are preliminary reports documenting that patients have experienced periods of mania/hypomania [65, 66], mirthful laughter [67], and visual hallucinations [68] after undergoing DBS surgery. York and colleagues [59] reported that patients experienced slightly elevated levels of anxiety after undergoing DBS surgery, and this was observed to be highly correlated with disease duration [59]. All other investigations conducted to date have found that anxiety symptoms remain stable [69] or improve after the surgery is performed [70, 71]. Mild improvements in obsessive-compulsive symptoms and paranoid thoughts have also been documented [69].

The factors associated with poor emotional outcome are believed to be mediated by psychiatric state prior to the surgery. It has been reported that symptoms of depression that were present one year postsurgery were associated with preexisting psychiatric disorders [60]. Additionally, advanced age seems to be associated with increased risk for postoperative mood disturbance [60]. York and colleagues [59] point out that such findings may not be truly representative of the entire sample, as the individuals who experience psychological distress may also be those who refuse to return for their follow-up evaluations.

Just as postsurgical depression appears to be associated with the presence of depressive symptoms prior to surgery, patients who present with a long-standing history of impulsivity (i.e., gambling behaviors) may be poor surgical candidates, as there has been some evidence to suggest that these individuals are at increased risk for postoperative suicide attempts [72]. In contrast, symptoms of impulsivity that have been induced by dopaminergic medications can be mitigated with STN-DBS [73].

With respect to other psychiatric symptoms, treatment with dopaminergic agents is a primary cause of hallucinations in PD [74]. Since treatment with DBS may lead to a decrease in pharmacological treatment, a reduction in these psychiatric symptoms can occur as a result. Interestingly, the existence of hallucinations presurgically does not appear to be a risk factor for the presence of these psychotic symptoms posttreatment [75, 76].

Improvements in quality of life have been reported for patients who underwent treatment with DBS [77] as well as for their families [78]. Although reduced reliance on medications has been cited as the most common reason for these improvements [79], advances in the ability to perform activities of daily living (ADLs) have also been reported [60, 70]. Further, improvement in ADLs may be present even five years posttreatment [79]. Nevertheless, the recovery of such abilities may not affect change in social adjustment. In fact, increased difficulty in interpersonal relationships has been reported in some patients postoperatively [52].

Several studies have demonstrated improvements in health status following DBS [80–82]. Improvement has reportedly been noted in sleep architecture, sleep efficiency, and nocturnal mobility; total sleep time and a reduction of sleep fragmentation and wakefulness after onset have also been demonstrated [83, 84].

Published Recommendations for Neuropsychologists

Given the varying cognitive, affective, and behavioral profiles of people diagnosed with PD, as well as the neurocognitive changes that have been reported in patients who have undergone DBS surgery, neuropsychological assessments have become an essential component of pre-DBS screening protocols at many medical centers [85]. The goal of such an evaluation is to aid in excluding patients who have Parkinson's plus syndromes (e.g., multiple systems atrophy, progressive supranuclear palsy, corticobasal degeneration) and are therefore not expected to benefit from surgery [86], as well as patients with preexisting cognitive deterioration or behavioral disorders that place them at increased risk for the exacerbation of their cognitive difficulties if they were to undergo DBS surgery [20, 55]. Additionally, neuropsychologists have historically played a role in the evaluation of cognitive outcome postsurgery [38].

In an effort to design a short (90 min) battery that could be used to exclude atypical PD candidates from undergoing DBS, Pillon [85] suggested that neuropsychologists administer the Mattis Dementia Rating Scale [87] as an estimate of global cognitive functioning, the Grober and Buschke test [88] to investigate verbal memory, the Boston Naming Test (BNT; [89]), an apraxia examination [90], and the Rey-Osterrieth Complex Figure Copying (RCFT; [91]) to assess "instrumental functions." The author also recommends conducting a neuropsychiatric interview and administering the Montgomery and Asberg Depression Rating Scale (MADRS; [92]); the latter was specifically selected because it is sensitive to changes in depressive symptoms over time [85].

Others investigators have argued that the pre-DBS battery must be more comprehensive. For example, Okun and colleagues [38] report that in addition to the Dementia Rating Scale-Second Edition (DRS-II; [93]) and the Mini-Mental State Exam (MMSE; [94]), neuropsychologists should use the Wechsler Abbreviated Scales of Intelligence (WASI; [95]) to obtain an estimate of premorbid functioning. Okun's treatment team also recommends administering a digit span subtest, as well as the Paced Auditory Serial Addition Test (PASAT; [96]), emphasizing the need to more directly assess basic attention, working memory, and auditory information processing speed, respectively. Although their battery includes the Hopkins Verbal Learning Test-Revised (HVLT-R; [97]), Okun and colleagues [38] reportedly observed that many PD patients perform poorly on such word list learning tasks. As such, they also recommend administering the Logical Memory and Faces subtests from the Wechsler Memory Scale-Third Edition (WMS-III; [98]) to glean a better understanding of whether or not the patient is amnesic. The group further states that measures of language should include the Boston Naming Test [89], Controlled Oral Word Association Test (COWAT; [99]), and a measure of category fluency. Benton's Judgment of Line Orientation (JLO) and Facial Recognition [100] are suggested as appropriate visuospatial tasks, and the Stroop is used as a measure of executive functioning [101].

Practice at North Shore: Long Island Jewish Health System

The Team and Their Roles

PD patients who are considering DBS surgery at our center, North Shore-Long Island Jewish Health System (NSLIJ), undergo a comprehensive evaluation consisting of consultations with a neurologist who specializes in movement disorders, a neurosurgeon who specializes in stereotactic surgery, and a neuropsychologist. The goal is to ensure that other treatments have been exhausted and to identify candidates who will benefit from the treatment and are physically, cognitively, and emotionally able to tolerate all aspects of surgery and postoperative care.

In general, candidates are first seen by the program's neurologist, and appointments with the neurosurgeon and neuropsychologist follow soon thereafter; however, this sequence often varies. For example, a neurologist outside of the movement disorder specialty may refer directly to neurosurgery since this is the discipline through which they would like their patients to receive treatment. In addition, sometimes movement disorder specialists refer directly to neuropsychology because they would like to understand the patient's risk for cognitive decline, and the patient's capacity to understand and tolerate the psychologically demanding procedure and follow-up, prior to referring the patient to the DBS program.

During the preoperative evaluation, a patient's levodopa response is carefully assessed using the levodopa challenge test. Although DBS has been shown to improve the motor complications of levodopa (e.g., reduce the amount of off-period time, improve dyskinesias), levodopa-resistant features tend to persist despite treatment with DBS. Therefore, a levodopa challenge test provides information regarding the potential benefits that the patient may obtain from DBS surgery. Those who respond well to the levodopa challenge are predicted to have a better prognosis (e.g., fewer levodopa-resistant features) postsurgery than those who respond poorly.

Assessment Measures Utilized

Prior to the evaluation, the neuropsychologist reviews the patient's medical record, including the neurologist and neurosurgeon's consult notes and the relevant brain scans when available (i.e., CT, MRI, FDG-PET). Patients also complete a form prior to the assessment that documents details of their developmental, educational, vocational, medical, and psychiatric history. At the outset of each neuropsychological assessment, the patient and an informant (e.g., significant other, adult child) participate in a comprehensive clinical interview lasting approximately 30 min, conducted to gather background information, gain a thorough understanding of current symptomatology, and collect additional information that may assist in making a differential diagnosis. During the course of the interview, the neuropsychologist discusses the patient's reasons for considering DBS at this time, understanding of the surgical procedure and risks associated with the treatment and expected outcome of the surgery. Information regarding any potential social stressors that may impact the patient's postoperative outcome is also discussed in detail. Conveying an understanding of treatment expectations is a key element of the neuropsychological evaluation because unreasonable expectations can result in a negative emotional response, regardless of the degree of motor improvement. Although all patients are informed about the likelihood of improvement and the types of symptoms that do and do not respond to treatment, some patients continue to believe that the surgery is a panacea. Therefore, although such patients may indeed experience an improvement in movement symptoms, their inability to fulfill an unreasonable belief (e.g., return to tennis) increases the risk that they will have a "catastrophic reaction." When there is an incongruity between patient and doctor expectations, additional patient education is required so that the discrepancies can be addressed directly.

A comprehensive neuropsychological battery is then administered in a single, extended session. Given that one of the main reasons for conducting a neuropsychological evaluation is to rule out the presence of a primary progressive dementia, it is imperative that the assessment battery adequately evaluates a range of cognitive domains including general cognition, attention/executive functioning, learning, memory, language, visuospatial functioning, sensorimotor, and mood/personality. The Dementia Rating Scale-Second Edition [93] is used to assist in distinguishing patients with dementia from those without. Because it includes measures of attention and executive functioning, it is more sensitive than the Mini-Mental State Exam [94] in assessing various subcortical degenerative diseases [85]. Additionally, the WAIS-III [102] Block Design and Similarities subtests are administered to measure current conceptual reasoning abilities.

Other subtests used at NSLIJ to assess attention and executive functioning include the Repeating Numbers subtest from the Randt Memory Test (RMT; [103]) as a measure of basic attention and working memory, the Symbol Digit Modalities Test (SDMT; written and oral; [104]) as a measure of processing speed, and the Wisconsin Card Sorting Test-64 (WCST-64; [105]) as a measure of feedback utilization and perseveration. Motor disinhibition is assessed using a motor Go/No-Go task; bimanual and unimanual tasks of motor sequencing [106] are also administered. In addition, both the patient and a family member complete the respective Frontal Systems Behavior Scale (FrSBe; [107]) to provide greater insight into the executive dysfunction that the patient is displaying in his or her everyday life.

Learning and memory are assessed for both verbal and visual information. Immediate verbal recall, learning over repeated presentations, and recall over a brief and extended delay period are assessed using the California Verbal Learning Test-Second Edition (CVLT-II; [108]). The Brief Visuospatial Memory Test-Revised (BVMT-R; [109]) is used to provide comparable information regarding the patient's visual learning and memory abilities.

For the assessment of language skills, naming is evaluated using the BNT [89], and phonemic and semantic fluencies are appraised through the COWAT (FAS; [100]) and animal naming, respectively. Auditory comprehension is assessed using the Commands subtest of the Boston Diagnostic Aphasia Examination (BDAE; [110]).

An understanding of the patient's visual perception/construction abilities is assessed using the Hooper Visual Organization Test (HVOT; [111]), Judgment of Line Orientation, and Facial Recognition [100]. Because praxis is only mildly impaired in the non-demented PD patient, the addition of an apraxia examination to the battery assists in making a differential diagnosis [85]. Finally, the severity of affective symptoms must be assessed because the presence of depressive symptoms has been shown to negatively impact recovery after DBS surgery [60]. In our center, the Beck Depression Inventory-Second Edition (BDI-II; [112]) and the Beck Anxiety Inventory (BAI; [113]) are both administered. A list of the measures administered at our center is summarized in Table 23.1.

Case Examples

Case A: Brief Presenting Information

Case A is a 71-year-old woman who was first diagnosed with Parkinson's disease approximately 10 years prior to the pre-DBS assessment. She is interested in undergoing DBS surgery as she believes it may help make her ON/OFF cycles more predictable, which will help improve her quality of life by making it possible for her to participate in enjoyable activities more often and by enabling her to decrease some of her medications. Case A feels her medication is no longer as effective as it used to be because her ON states occur less frequently and are weaker than they were several years ago. She reports physical symptoms, including balance difficulties leading to falls (none have been serious to this point), tremor, and dystonia/dyskinesias, as well as increased difficulty performing her activities of daily living independently.

Case A reports that she is having occasional difficulty with her short-term memory, mainly recalling the temporal details of events, and some word-finding difficulty. She explained that she feels "sharp" at times and "dull" at other times. According to her husband, Case A may take longer to recall details; however, he does not feel that she ever forgets information completely. Medical history is otherwise significant for hypertension, cardiac arrhythmias, and arthritis. Case A reports experiencing some depression and anxiety symptoms over the past few years, but on exam, she endorsed only mild symptoms that were not considered to be clinically significant. Case A's performance on the neuropsychological assessment battery is presented in Table 23.2.

Case B: Brief Presenting Information

Case B is a 50-year-old man diagnosed with Parkinson's disease approximately 3 years prior to the pre-DBS assessment, who mainly experiences a unilateral hand tremor that causes him distress and prevents him from performing tasks, such as driving and working in construction. In response to questions about the surgical procedure, Case B is unable to clearly state how the treatment will help him or articulate the possible risks associated with the surgery. Further, his expectations appear to be unrealistic, indicating that he will be "back to normal" and able to work and drive again. With respect to neuropsychological symptoms, he denies any cognitive difficulties but indicates a history of depressive and anxious symptoms, with recent anxiety regarding his health and inability to work. He is divorced and currently lives alone. Case B has a long history of heavy alcohol abuse; he reports

Table 23.1 Measures used for pre-DBS assessment at North Shore-Long Island Jewish Health System

Domain	Measures administered
General cognition	Dementia Rating Scale-2 (DRS-2) National Adult Reading Test (NART) WAIS-III Block Design WAIS-III Similarities
Attention/executive functioning	Repeating Numbers (Randt Memory Test) Symbol Digit Modality Test Trail-Making Test Golden Stroop Wisconsin Card Sorting Test (WCST-64) Luria Motor Sequencing Tasks Motor Go/No-Go Frontal Systems Behavior Scale (FrSBe; self and family rating)
Learning/memory	California Verbal Learning Test-2 (CVLT-II) Brief Visuospatial Memory Test-Revised (BVMT-R)
Language	Boston Naming Test (BNT) Verbal Fluency Boston Diagnostic Aphasia Examination (BDAE)-Commands
Visual perception/construction	Benton Judgment of Line Orientation Benton Facial Recognition Hooper Visual Organization Test
Sensorimotor	Praxis
Mood/personality	Beck Depression Inventory-II (BDI-II) Beck Anxiety Inventory (BAI)

Table 23.2 Examination results for Case A, Case B, and Case C

DBS candidate	**Case A**		**Case B**		**Case C**	
	Approved for DBS		**Failed prescreening**		**Approved for DBS**	
Domain	**Raw score**	**Percentile**	**Raw score**	**Percentile**	**Raw score**	**Percentile**
General cognition						
DRS-2 total	139	41–59	122	3–5	134	19–28
Attention	36	60–71	33	11–18	35	41–59
Initiation/perseveration	37	60–71	31	6–10	36	41–59
Construction	6	41–59	6	41–59	6	41–59
Conceptualization	35	29–40	31	6–10	33	11–18
Memory	23	82–89	21	6–10	24	41–59
NART	FSIQ = 126		FSIQ = 112		FSIQ = 122	
WAIS-III						
Block design	28	50	29	25	29	37
Similarities	24	75	22	37	24	63
Attention/executive functioning						
Randt Memory Test—LSF; LSB	8; 7	91; 99	6; 4	34; 30	7; 5	37; 37
SDMT—Written; Oral	39; 50	53; 63	31; 38	3; 4	35; 44	21; 30
Trail-Making Test—A and B	33; 83	73; 68	46; 199	16; 4	73; 126	<1; 2
Golden Stroop						
Word	109	50	78	7	98	30
Color	79	50	42	1	57	7
Color/Word	58	91	23	1	25	3
Interference	12	88	−4.3	34	−11.04	14

(continued)

Table 23.2 (continued)

DBS candidate	**Case A**		**Case B**		**Case C**	
	Approved for DBS		**Failed prescreening**		**Approved for DBS**	
Domain	**Raw score**	**Percentile**	**Raw score**	**Percentile**	**Raw score**	**Percentile**
WCST-64						
Categories	4	>16	3	>16	2	11–16
Perseverative errors	4	>99	12	25	19	8
Failure to maintain set	1	–	0	–	1	–
Luria motor sequencing tasks	Within normal limits		Within normal limits		Within normal limits	
Motor Go/No-Go	Within normal limits		Within normal limits		Within normal limits	
FrSBe	Raw score	T = score	Raw score	T = score	Raw score	T = score
Self—total (before; after)	97; 142	124; 146	113; 136	87; 111	65	41
Apathy	22; 53	99; >160	33; 52	74; 120	16	37
Disinhibition	34; 39	146; >160	28; 27	56; 54	16	30
Executive dysfunction	41; 50	128: 152	52; 57	100; 111	33	55
Family—total (before; after)	73; 86	114; 130			81	52
Apathy	24; 38	112; 156			27	54
Disinhibition	15; 16	84; 88			20	40
Executive dysfunction	34; 32	124; 120			34	57
Learning/memory	Raw score	Percentile	Raw score	Percentile	Raw score	Percentile
CVLT-II total	41 (3, 7, 8, 11, 12)	46	29 (3, 4, 6, 8, 8)	7	29 (4,6,5,7,7)	7
List B	6	70	3	7	4	30
Immediate recall (cued)	8 (9)	50 (30)	8 (7)	30 (16)	5 (5)	16 (2)
Delayed recall (cued)	7 (8)	30 (16)	8 (7)	30 (16)	6 (7)	16 (16)
Hits (false positives)	13 (5)	16 (3)	14 (10)	50 (2)	12 (2)	16 (50)
Forced choice	16/16	–	16/16	–	16/16	–
BVMT-R total	14 (3,5,6)	12	20 (6,7,7,)	21	15 (3,5,7,)	5
Learning	3	34	1	7	4	58
Delayed recall	7	34	7	14	5	4
Percent retention	117%	>16	100%	>16	71%	3–5
Hits (false positives)	5 (0)	>16 (>16)	5 (0)	11–16 (>16)	6 (0)	>16 (>16)
Recognition discrimination	5	>16	5	11–16	6	>16
Copy	12/12	–	11/12	–	11/12	–
Language						
BNT—correct (phonemic cues)	60 (N/A)	84	51 (3 of 9)	18	53 (5 of 7)	24
Verbal fluency—phonemic; semantic	54; 29	98; 25	47; 17	84; 1	32; 20	14; 34
BDAE Commands	15	58	14	1	15	58
Visual perception/construction						
Judgment of line orientation	30	>86	21	22	21	22
Facial recognition	49	72–85	52	88–97	41	16–21
Hooper	20	12	25.5	53	21	16
Motor						
Apraxia exam	Within normal limits		Within normal limits		Within normal limits	
Mood/personality						
BDI-II	5	Minimal	17	Mild	22	Moderate
BAI	2	Normal	17	Moderate	17	Moderate

drinking as many as 24 beers per night and notes that he has at least one blackout per week. He indicates that he has not had alcohol in 2 months as part of his preparation for surgery but reports a desire to resume his regular consumption of alcohol after undergoing DBS surgery. Table 23.2 details the results of Case B's neuropsychological assessment.

Case C: Brief Presenting Information

Case C is a 57-year-old man diagnosed with Parkinson's disease approximately 8 years prior to the pre-DBS assessment, whose presenting physical symptoms include excessive dyskinesias, "very brief" ON time, poor posture, and balance difficulties. Case C was previously considered for DBS surgery 4 years prior; however, it was determined that his psychiatric risk was too great, and his physical symptoms (just posture and balance complaints at that time) are not considered to be universally improved with the procedure. It was determined that Case C had an adverse medication response to Mirapex, and he was depressed, hypersexual, engaging in excessive gambling, performing self-mutilation, and had passive suicidal ideation. When the medication was discontinued, he responded well, and the psychiatric symptoms subsided. In response to questions about the surgical procedure, Case C is hoping to increase his ON time and decrease the severity of his dyskinesias. He was able to appropriately articulate the possible risks associated with the surgery, and he seemingly realistic expectations regarding treatment outcome.

With respect to neuropsychological symptoms, Case C reported that he has experienced a cognitive decline over the past 5–10 years, with a more significant drop over the past 6 months. Symptoms include word-finding difficulty and confusion during his OFF state, including comprehension and memory problems. While he denied any changes in mood, he reported that he has always been an anxious person, with some depression since his divorce several years ago. Although he is not receiving psychotherapy or psychopharmacologic treatment at the present time, he has in the past. Case C currently lives in residential housing, due to his psychiatric history, and he works part time in security. Table 23.2 outlines the results of Case C's neuropsychological assessment.

Case A: Summary and Conclusions

Case A has identified a realistic treatment outcome that matches her neurological state and has associated this outcome with a plausible change in her life circumstances. There is little concern regarding Case A's cognitive functioning. Attention, executive, learning, memory, and visuospatial functions are all generally intact. Her performance does reveal a mild weakness in initial encoding, and she reports difficulties with executive functions. However, she does not exhibit rapid forgetting, and there is no evidence of a significant anomia. This pattern is typical of cognition in Parkinson's disease.

In sum, the patient is entering into the process fully informed and fully aware of the surgical procedure, as well as its risks and possible benefits. Her cognitive difficulties are relatively mild and in a pattern typical of Parkinson's disease. Therefore, there is no evidence of a secondary neurodegenerative disorder, and she is not at risk for greater than typical cognitive side effects. Finally, although she exhibits some mood issues, she does not have a clinically significant psychiatric disorder that would interfere with postsurgical quality of life or put her at risk for greater mood difficulties. In such a case, participation in a series of psychotherapy sessions before and after surgical intervention could be considered.

Case B: Summary and Conclusions

Case B is experiencing significant difficulties across multiple cognitive domains, with his greatest impairment in complex attention and memory functions. This pattern of dysfunction is consistent with the frontosubcortical dysfunction associated with Parkinson's disease; however, the degree of impairment is somewhat greater than expected in an individual his age, especially considering that the time since diagnosis is only 3 years. It is very likely that his difficulties are compounded by more diffuse brain dysfunction associated with long-term alcohol abuse. Further, Case B exhibits mild to moderate mood difficulties, with greater anxiety than depressive symptoms.

Several issues should be considered in reference to his possible participation in surgical intervention. First, Case B does not appear to fully understand the procedure itself and the associated risk, but more importantly, his expectation for the treatment appears to be unrealistic. Second, he exhibits significant cognitive and mood difficulties. Finally, and most concerning, is his history of alcohol abuse. Given the patient's history and report during the exam, the prognosis for successful cessation is poor. If he is to be further considered for surgical treatment, enrollment in a formal substance abuse treatment program would be recommended, with the period of abstinence set by the surgical risk.

Case C: Summary and Conclusions

Case C is experiencing some difficulties across multiple cognitive domains, with the area of greatest concern being executive functioning. He is experiencing slowed processing speed, cognitive inflexibility, and perseveration. More mild difficulties are apparent in memory and visuospatial functioning, but performance in these domains is in part implicated by his executive dysfunction. His memory difficulties are characterized by poor learning and retrieval, but he has intact retention over time for information previously encoded. He has intact basic perceptual and construction abilities, with difficulties in spatial processing and integration. Language functions are largely intact with some retrieval difficulties apparent. In addition, Case C is endorsing significant emotional symptoms.

Overall, Case C's pattern of cognitive difficulties is fully consistent with what is seen in Parkinson's disease. Despite the severity of deficits, there is no indication of a secondary neurological illness that would put him at risk for greater than typical cognitive side effects from the DBS procedure. He exhibits realistic expectations for the procedure, has a strong support network, including living in a supported environment, and has close relationships with his siblings who live locally and see him regularly. Case C is reporting significant, albeit mitigated, symptoms of depression and anxiety that are currently not being treated directly and present some concern for the procedure. Therefore, it is strongly recommended that Case C participates in individual psychotherapy, as well as have a psychopharmacological consultation, prior to moving forward with the DBS procedure. These treatments will not only help address his long-standing affective symptoms but will also provide him with an additional support system while he engages in the process of considering the procedure, undergoing the surgery, and recovering thereafter. Although Case C is experiencing significant cognitive deficits and emotional symptoms, it was determined that he would be considered a viable surgical candidate with appropriate supports in place to monitor his psychiatric state. His medical risk for surgery is low, given his age and health, and a clinical judgment was made in this case that the potential benefit to his quality of life postoperatively is greater than his risk factors, considering that his symptoms are fully consistent with the disease.

Other Patient Populations Treated with DBS and Clinical Considerations

DBS has proven to be an effective method of treatment for several other disorders, as well. In fact, the FDA approved of this surgery for the amelioration of symptoms associated with essential tremor (ET) 5 years before it was approved for use in PD patients. Since that time, DBS surgery has been used to mitigate the symptoms of numerous movement and affective disorders. Neuropsychologists continue to be an integral part of the treatment team for these surgical indications; however, there is less evidence on which to base clinical practice. In general, the role of the neuropsychologist remains the same, assessing the patients' understanding of the procedure and quantifying the patients' cognitive, behavioral, and emotional status to aid in the prediction of outcome. However, the focus of course is different, especially in psychiatric indications.

DBS and Essential Tremor

ET is a slowly progressive disease that is usually characterized by postural tremor; intention tremor is seen in approximately half of ET patients, as well [114, 115]. These patients also have a disorder of tandem gait, which is usually mild. Propranolol and primidone tend to be the first-line treatments, and in most cases, the symptoms of ET can be treated solely with one or both of these medications [116]. As the illness progresses, the frequency of the tremors tend to decrease; however, their amplitude increases, exacerbating the resultant disability and significantly impacting daily activities and quality of life. When the disease progression has reached such a point, or when symptoms are not properly managed with pharmacotherapy, DBS of the ventralis intermedius nucleus (Vim) of the thalamus is often considered [37]. Outcome studies have revealed that it is very likely that the pure postural tremor of the upper extremities will improve after DBS of the ventralis intermedius/zona incerta (for review, see [116]). The success rate is slightly decreased if the patient presents with an intention tremor or a more proximal tremor predominates. In fact, only 50% of patients with intention tremors experience long-term improvement [117]. Results of outcome studies further suggest that bilateral DBS may be considered if head, voice, or trunk tremors are the main reason for surgery [118], yet bilateral thalamotomy is associated with high risks of complications and should not be conducted [119].

Tourette's Syndrome

According to the DSM-IV-TR [120], Tourette's syndrome (TS) is a chronic, neurobehavioral disorder that is characterized by motor and phonic tics that persist for a minimum of 12 months. Patients who have been diagnosed with TS and who experience functional impairment in their ability to socialize are usually treated with neuroleptics, adrenergic agonists, and dopamine agonists [121]. Pharmacotherapy is often accompanied with behavioral treatment in which techniques such as habit reversal training are implemented. Because symptoms are often refractory to these various treatments and are frequently reported to cause significant distress, various neurosurgical procedures have been attempted to mitigate both motor and phonic tics [122]. Among these procedures, DBS is considered to be an appropriate technique to use when TS symptoms are refractory to medications [121], yet it has not yet been FDA approved. Part of the intralaminar nucleus of the thalamus, known as the centromedian-parafascicular complex (CM-PF), is considered to be the preferred target for DBS treatment of TS symptoms [123], as stimulation in this area has effectively allayed tics and improved the behavioral aspects of TS [124]. However, it has been suggested that stimulating the GPi or the anterior limb of the internal capsule may prove to be even more advantageous than DBS of the CM-PF for other behavioral features of the disorder [121]. Future studies are necessary to ascertain which site should be targeted for which patients.

Major Depressive Disorder

More recently, DBS has been used to treat endogenous depression [42]. Like PD, major depressive disorder (MDD) was initially treated using ablative surgeries until monoamine oxidase inhibitors and tricyclic antidepressants were found to effectively improve depressive symptoms [125]. Nevertheless, a large number of patients diagnosed with depression remain refractory to these classes of medications and to the selective serotonin reuptake inhibitors (SSRIs). Although electroconvulsive therapy (ECT) can be used to treat medically resistant depression, many patients are hesitant to undergo such a procedure due to the stigma associated with it [126] or because they are apprehensive that the ECT may result in long-standing neurocognitive side effects [125]. This has spurred investigations into the effectiveness of other nonpharmacologic therapies, including vagus nerve stimulation, transcranial magnetic stimulation, ketamine infusion therapy, and DBS (for review, see

[125, 127–129], respectively). Investigators who have studied the safety and efficacy of DBS for the treatment of MDD symptoms have targeted a wide array of areas, including the orbitofrontal cortex, anterior cingulate gyrus, corpus striatum, GP, subgenual cingulate, ventral capsule/ventral striatum, ventral capsule/ventral commissure, nucleus accumbens, and inferior thalamic peduncle [129]. The various outcome studies that have been conducted to date have been fairly compelling [130–135]. Across investigations, treatment resulted in sustained effects in most patients, and thus far, only minor complications from the surgery have been reported [125].

Obsessive-Compulsive Disorder

DBS has also been used in the treatment of symptoms associated with obsessive-compulsive disorder (OCD). An estimated 30–40% of patients diagnosed with OCD do not respond to medications, which frequently prompts off-label use of alternative treatments [136], including DBS. To date, the thalamic/capsular area seems to be the target of choice in the preliminary studies that have been conducted. Over a decade ago, Nuttin and colleagues [137] used DBS to treat six patients with severe OCD through implanting quadripolar electrodes into the anterior limb of the internal capsule. Of the four people who continued in the study, three were reportedly "much improved" and one remained "unchanged"; a follow-up study conducted 21 months postsurgery indicated that individuals who had improved did not remit [138]. Further, the stimulation resulted in changes in regional activity, particularly in the pons, as measured by fMRI, and lower frontal metabolism as seen on PET imaging, 3 months after surgery [139]. Other investigators who implanted the same location also reported that most patients were improved post-DBS [140, 141]. The right nucleus accumbens has also been the target of DBS surgery for the treatment of OCD [142]; stimulation resulted in complete symptom remission 24–30 months after surgery in three of the four patients. Single case studies have suggested that stimulation of the caudate [143] or the inferior thalamic peduncle [144] can also be effective in reducing or eliminating OCD symptoms.

Conclusions

Over the past decade, DBS has proven to be an effective treatment for several medically refractory movement disorders and appears to have promising palliative effects for a variety of psychiatric disorders. Although a number of investigators have studied the neuropsychological implications of DBS surgery in an effort to identify inclusionary and exclusionary criteria for the procedure, no consensus has been reached regarding the degree of neurocognitive or psychiatric dysfunction that would render a patient to be an inappropriate candidate [38]. Therefore, neuropsychologists must keep abreast of the ever increasing literature on this topic and create and explicitly state the criterion to be used within their program.

Clinical Pearls

- Take the time to learn about PD, parkinsonian disorders, and the disorders that can interfere with treatment success. Without a clear understanding of the natural history of cognitive and emotional symptoms in PD and other movement disorders, it is difficult to interpret the exam findings.
- Antiparkinson medication may need to be withheld for the purposes of other assessments, and this can potentially confound the neuropsychological evaluation. Try to coordinate the neuropsychological exam at a time when patients have taken their medications, and they will be in the "ON" state.
- Do not restrict your differential diagnosis to those disorders common to PD. PD is a disorder of mid- to late-adulthood, and each individual has many risk factors that are related to his or her genetic, environmental, emotional, and medical status, which are not necessarily a

result of the patient's PD or common concerns such as Alzheimer's disease.

- Remember that the role of the neuropsychologist includes being a psychologist. Depression and anxiety are symptoms of PD, not just a reaction to a disabling disease, and these difficulties affect quality of life.
- Although mood symptoms can potentially be treated with DBS in other brain regions, they are not treated by DBS in the STN, GPi, or Vim. Mood symptoms can persist even after successful DBS for motor aspects of PD, resulting in threats to quality of life.
- Expectations are everything. Just as mood disturbances limit treatment success, so do unrealistic expectations. The neuropsychologist plays a key role in assessing the patient's understanding of the anticipated postsurgical outcome. Presurgical counseling and additional education about treatment expectations may be needed.
- Although the treatment team will take the patient's level of motoric disability into account in their final decision, care must be taken to not let this factor bias your interpretation of the neuropsychological data.
- There are no pathognomonic signs for exclusion and risk. However, the following are often considered as negative findings:
  - Generalized cognitive decline at a level that is suggestive of dementia, for example, a Dementia Rating Scale less than 123.
  - Pattern of cognitive deficits associated with focal cortical dysfunction.
  - Memory performance suggesting greater deficits in the retention of learned information than in learning and retrieval.
  - Language difficulties out of proportion to executive deficits.
  - History of impulsive/obsessive behaviors associated with disease onset and treatment, such as pathological gambling.
  - History of suicidal ideation/attempts.
  - Major depressive disorder, or other axis I psychiatric disorder, that has gone unrecognized or intractable to treatment.
  - Specific phobias related to medical procedures.
  - A hyperfocus on a single outcome specific to their environment. For example, a patient may have a restriction in a hobby in which he or she needs to use a particular tool.
  - Expectations that include environmental changes, such as having better access to job opportunities.

References

1. Woods SP, Fields JA, Troster AI. Neuropsychological sequelae of subthalamic nucleus deep brain stimulation in Parkinson's disease: a critical review. Neuropsychol Rev. 2002;12:111–26.
2. Emre M, Aarsland D, Brown R, Burn DJ, Duyckaerts C, Mizuno Y, et al. Clinical diagnostic criteria for dementia associated with Parkinson's disease. Mov Disord. 2007;22:1689–707.
3. Pallone JA. Introduction to Parkinson's disease. Disease-A-Month. 2007;53:195–9.
4. Olanow CW, Stern MB. Parkinson's disease: unresolved issues. Ann Neurol. 2008;64:S1–2.
5. Rosenthal A. Auto transplants for Parkinson's disease? Neuron. 1998;20:169–72.
6. Rothstein TL, Olanow CW. The neglected side of Parkinson's disease. Am Sci. 2008;96:218–25.
7. Youdim MB, Riederer P. Understanding Parkinson's disease. Sci Am. 1997;1:52–9.
8. DeLong M, Wichmann T. Update on models of basal ganglia function and dysfunction. Parkinsonism Relat Disord. 2009;15:S239–40.
9. Torres G, Fraley GS, Hallas BH, Leheste JR, Phillippens I. New frontiers in Parkinson's disease therapy: deep brain stimulation. Kopf Carrier. 2010; 69:1–8. Retrieved from http://www.kopfinstruments.com/Carrier/downlaod/carrier 69.pdf.
10. Fernandez HH, See RH, Gary MF, Bowers D, Rodriguez RL, Jacobson C, Okun MS. Depressive symptoms in Parkinson disease correlate with impaired global and specific cognitive performance. J Geriatr Psychiatry Neurol. 2009;22:223–7.
11. Cozzens JW. Surgery for Parkinson's disease. Disease-A-Month. 2007;53:227–42.
12. Henderson JM, Dunnett SB. Targeting the subthalamic nucleus in the treatment of Parkinson's disease. Brain Res Bull. 1998;46:467–74.
13. Pollak P, Benabid AL, Gross C, Gao DM, Laurent A, Benazzouz A, Hoffmann D, Gentil M, Perret J. Effects of the stimulation of the subthalamic nucleus in Parkinson's disease. Rev Neurol. 1993;149:175–6.
14. Fahn S. How do you treat motor complications in Parkinson's disease: Medicine, surgery, or both? Ann Neurol. 2008;64:S56–64.
15. Schrag A, Quinn N. Dyskinesias and motor fluctuations in Parkinson's disease. A community-based study. Brain. 2000;123:2297–305.

16. Fox SH, Brotchie JM, Lang AE. Non-dopaminergic treatments in development for Parkinson's disease. Lancet Neurol. 2008;7:927–38.
17. Rezai AR, Machado AG, Deogaonkar M, Azmi H, Kubu C, Boulis NM, et al. Surgery for movement disorders. Neurosurgery. 2008;62:S809–39.
18. Espay AJ, Mandybur GT, Revilla FJ. Surgical treatment of movement disorders. Clin Geriatr Med. 2006;22:813–25.
19. Gildernberg PL. Management of movement disorders. An overview. Neurosurg Clin N Am. 1995;6:43–53.
20. Fields JA, Troster A. Cognitive outcomes after deep brain stimulation for Parkinson's disease: a review of initial studies and recommendations for future research. Brain Cogn. 2000;42:268–93.
21. Cooper O, Astradsson A, Hallett P, Robertson H, Mendez I, Isacson O. Lack of functional relevance of isolated cell damage in transplants of Parkinson's disease patients. J Neurol. 2009;256:S310–316.
22. Olanow CW, Kordower JH, Freeman TB. Fetal nigral transplantation as a therapy for Parkinson's disease. Trends Neurosci. 1996;19:102–9.
23. Spencer DD, Robbins RJ, Naftolin F, Marek KL, Vollmer T, Leranth C, Roth RH, Price LH, Gjedde A, Bunney BS, Sass KJ, Elsworth JD, Kier L, Majuch R, Hoffer PB, Redmond DE. Unilateral transplantation of human fetal mesencephalic tissue into the caudate nucleus of patients with Parkinson's disease. N Engl J Med. 1992;327:1541–8.
24. Olanow CW, Fahn S. Fetal nigral transplantation as a therapy for Parkinson's disease. In: Brundin P, Olanow CW, editors. Restorative therapist in Parkinson's disease. New York, NY: Springer Science+Business Media, LLC; 2006. p. 93–118.
25. Ma Y, Tang C, Chaly T, Greene P, Breeze R, Fahn S, Freed C, Dhawan V, Eidelberg D. Dopamine cell implantation in Parkinson's disease: Long-term clinical and ^{18}F-FDOPA PET outcomes. J Nucl Med. 2010;51:7–15.
26. Trott CT, Fahn S, Greene P, Dillon S, Winfield H, Winfield L, Kao R, Eidelberg D, Freed CR, Breeze RE, Stern Y. Cognition following bilateral implants of embryonic dopamine neurons in PD: a double blind study. Neurology. 2003;60(12):1938–43.
27. Kaplitt MG, Feigin A, Tang C, Fitzsimons H, Mattis P, Lawlor PA, Bland RJ, Young B, Strybing K, Eidelberg D, During MJ. Safety and tolerability of gene therapy with an adeno-associated virus (AAV) borne GAD gene for Parkinson's disease: an open label, phase I trial. Lancet. 2007;369:2097–105.
28. Mattis P, Zgaljardic D, Feigin A. Neuropsychological functioning in pre-symptomatic but gene positive patients with Huntington's disease. J Int Neuropsychol Soc. 2002;8:276.
29. Obeso JA, Rodriguez-Oroz MC, Rodriguez M, Marcias R, Alvarez L, Guridi J, Vitek J, Delong MR. Pathophysiologic basis of surgery for Parkinson's disease. Neurology. 2000;55:S7–S12.
30. Wichmann T, DeLong MR. Pathophysiology of Parkinson's disease: the MPTP primate model of the human disorder. Ann N Y Acad Sci. 2003; 991:199–213.
31. Erlander MG, Tillakaratne NJ, Feldblum S, Patel N, Tobin AJ. Two genes encode distinct glutamate decarboxylases. Neuron. 1991;7:91–100.
32. Emborg ME, Carbon M, Holdern JE, During MJ, Ma Y, Tang C, Moirano J, Fitzsimons J, Roitberg BZ, Tuccar E, Roberts A, Kaplitt MG, Eidelberg D. Subthalamic glutamic acid decarboxylase gene therapy: changes in motor function and cortical metabolism. J Cereb Blood Flow Metab. 2007;27:501–9.
33. Kaplitt MG, Leone P, Samulski RJ, Xiao X, Pfaff DW, O'Malley KL, During MJ. Long-term gene expression and phenotypic correction using adeno-associated virus vectors in the mammalian brain. Nat Genet. 1994;8:148–54.
34. Lee B, Lee H, Nam YR, Oh JH, Cho YH, Chang JW. Enhanced expression of glutamate decarboxylase 65 improves symptoms of rat parkinsonian models. Gene Ther. 2005;12:1215–22.
35. Luo J, Kaplitt MG, Fitzsimons HL, Zuzga DS, Liu Y, Oshinsky ML, During MJ. Subthalamic GAD gene therapy in a Parkinson's disease rat model. Science. 2002;298:425–9.
36. Dormont D, Seidenwurm D, Galanaud D, Cornu P, Yelnik J, Bardinet E. Neuroimaging and deep brain stimulation. Am J Neuroradiol, 2010; 15–23.
37. Benabid AL, Chabardes S, Seigneuret E. Deep-brain stimulation in Parkinson's disease: long-term efficacy and safety—What happened this year? Curr Opin Neurol. 2005;18:623–30.
38. Okun MS, Rodriguez RL, Miller AMK, Kellison I, Kirsch-Darrow L, Wint DP, Springer U, Fernandez HH, Foote KD, Crucian G, Bowers D. Deep brain stimulation and the role of the neuropsychologist. Clin Neuropsychol. 2007;21:162–89.
39. Vitek JL. Deep brain stimulation: how does it work? Cleveland Clinical J Med. 2008;75:S59–65.
40. Pourfar M, Tang C, Lin T, Dhawan V, Kaplitt MG, Eidelberg D. Assessing the microlesion effect of subthalamic deep brain stimulation surgery with FDG PET. J Neurosurg. 2009;110:1278–82.
41. Asanuma K, Tang C, Ma Y, Dhawan V, Mattis P, Edwards C, Kaplitt MG, Feigin A, Eidelberg D. Network modulation in the treatment of Parkinson's disease. Brain. 2006;129:2667–78.
42. Chang J. Brain Stimulation for neurological and psychiatric disorders, current status and future direction. J Pharmacol Exp Ther. 2004;309:1–7.
43. Chan CS, Guzman JN, Ilijic E, Mercer JN, Rick C, Tkatch T, Meredith GE, Surmeier DJ. "Rejuvenation" projects neurons in mouse models of Parkinson's disease. Nature. 2007;447:1081–5.
44. Histed MH, Bonin V, Reid RC. Direct activation of sparse, distributed populations of cortical neurons by electrical micro-stimulation. Neuron. 2009;63:508–22.
45. Volkmann J, Allert N, Voges J, Sturn V, Schnitzler A, Freund H. Long term results of bilateral pallidal stimulation in Parkinson's disease. Ann Neurol. 2004;55:871–5.

46. Machado A, Rezai AR, Kopell BH, Gross RE, Sharan AD, Benabid A. Deep brain stimulation for Parkinson's disease: surgical technique and perioperative management. Mov Disord. 2006;21:S247–58.
47. Schweder PM, Hansen PC, Green AL, Quaghebeur G, Stein J, Aziz TZ. Connectivity of the pedunculopontine nucleus in parkinsonian freezing of gait. NeuroReport: For Rapid Communication of Neuroscience Research. 2010;21:914–6.
48. Morrison CE, Borod JC, Perrine K, Beric A, Brin MF, Rezai A, Kelly P, Sterio D, Germano I, Weisz D, Olanow CW. Neuropsychological functioning following bilateral subthalamic nucleus stimulation in Parkinson's disease. Arch Clin Neuropsychol. 2002;19:165–81.
49. St George RJ, Nutt JG, Burchiel KJ, Horak FB. A meta-regression of the long-term effects of deep brain stimulation on balance and gait in PD. Neurology. 2010;75:1292–9.
50. Moro E, Scerrati M, Romito LMA, Roselli R, Tonali P, Albanese A. Chronic subthalamic nucleus stimulation reduces medication requirements in Parkinson's disease. Neurology. 1999;53:85–90.
51. Moro E, Hamani C, Poon Y, Al-Khairallah T, Dostrovsky JO, Hutchinson WD, Lozano AM. Unilateral pedunculopontine stimulation improves falls in Parkinson's disease. Brain. 2010;133:215–24.
52. Schupbach WMM, Chastan N, Welter ML, Houeto JL, Mesnage V, Bonnet AM, Czernecki V, Maltete D, Hartmann A, Mallet L, Pidoux B, Dormont D, Navarro S, Cornu P, Mallet A, Agid Y. Stimulation of the subthalamic nucleus in Parkinson's disease: a 5 year follow up. J Neurol Neurosurg Psychiatry. 2005;76: 1650–44.
53. Parsons TD, Rogers SA, Broaten AJ, Woods SP, Troster AI. Cognitive sequelae of subthalamic nucleus deep brain stimulation in Parkinson's disease: a meta-analysis. Lancet Neurol. 2006;5:578–88.
54. Jahanshahi M, Ardouin CMA, Brown RG, Rothwell JC, Obeso J, Albanese A, Rodriguez-Oroz MC, Moro E, Benabid AL, Pollak P, Lomousin-Dowsey P. The impact of deep brain stimulation on executive function in Parkinson's disease. Brain. 2000;123: 1142–54.
55. Saint-Cyr JA, Trepanier LL, Kumar R, Lozano AM, Lang AE. Neuropsychological consequences of chronic bilateral stimulation of the subthalamic nucleus in Parkinson's disease. Brain. 2000;123:2091–108.
56. Ashby P, Kim YJ, Kumar R, Lang AE, Lozano AM. Neurophysiological effects of stimulation through electrodes in the human subthalamic nucleus. Brain. 1999;122:1919–31.
57. Dujardin K, Defebvre L, Krystkowiak P, Blond S, Destee A. Influence of chronic bilateral stimulation of the subthalamic nucleus on cognitive function in Parkinson's disease. J Neurol. 2001;248: 603–11.
58. Pillon B, Ardouin C, Damier P, Krack P, Houeto JL, Klinger H, Bonnet AM, Pollak P, Benabid AL, Agid Y. Neuropsychological changes between "off" and "on" STN or GPi stimulation in Parkinson's disease. Neurology. 2000;55:411–8.
59. York MK, Dulay M, Macias A, Levin HS, Grossman R, Simpson R, Jankovic J. Cognitive declines following bilateral subthalamic nucleus deep brain stimulation for the treatment of Parkinson's disease. J Neurol Neurosurg Psychiatry. 2008;79:789–95.
60. Perriol MP, Krystkowiak P, Defebvre L, Blond S, Destee A, Dujardin K. Stimulation of the subthalamic nucleus in Parkinson's disease: Cognitive and affective changes are not linked to the motor outcome. Parkinsoniam Relat Disord. 2006;12:205–10.
61. Hariz MI, Johansson F, Shamsgovara P, Johansson E, Hariz GM, Fagerlund M. Bilateral subthalamic nucleus stimulation in parkinsonian patient with preoperative deficits in speech and cognition: Persistent improvement in mobility but increased dependency: A case study. Movement Disoders. 2000;15:136–9.
62. Trepanier LL, Kumar R, Lozano AM, Lang AE, Saint-Cyr JA. Neuropsychological outcome of GPi pallidotomy and GPi or STN deep brain stimulation in Parkinson's disease. Brain Cogn. 2000;42:324–47.
63. Perozzo P, Rizzone M, Bergamasco B, Castelli L, Lanotte M, Tavella A, Torre E, Lopiano L. Deep brain stimulation of the subthalamic nucleus in Parkinson's disease: comparison of pre- and postoperative neuropsychological evaluation. J Neurol Sci. 2001; 192:9–15.
64. Smeding HMM, Speelman JD, Koning-Haanstra M, Schuurman PR, Nijssen P, Van Laar T, Schmand B. Neuropsychological effects of bilateral STN stimulation in Parkinson's disease: a controlled study. Neurology. 2006;66:1830–6.
65. Funkiewiez A, Ardouin C, Caputo E, Krack P, Fraix V, Klinger H, Chabardes S, Foote K, Benabid AL, Pollak P. Long term effects of bilateral subthalamic nucleus stimulation on cognitive function, mood, and behaviour in Parkinson's disease. J Neurol Neurosurg Psychiatry. 2004;75:834–9.
66. Kulisevsky J, Berthier ML, Gironell A, Gironell A, Pascual-Sedano B, Molet J, Pares P. Secondary mania following subthalamic nucleus deep brain stimulation for the treatment of Parkinson's disease [abstract]. Neurology. 2001;56:S49.
67. Krack P, Kumar R, Ardouin C, Limousin-Dowsey P, McVicker JM, Benabid AL, Pollak P. Mirthful laughter induced by subthalamic nucleus stimulation. Mov Disord. 2001;16:867–75.
68. Diederich NJ, Alesch F, Goetz CG. Visual hallucinations induced by deep brain stimulation in Parkinson's disease. Clin Neuropharmacol. 2000;23:287–9.
69. Castelli L, Perozzo P, Zibetti M, Crivelli B, Morabito U, Lanotte M, Cossa F, Bergamasco B, Lopiano L. Chronic deep brain stimulation of the subthalamic nucleus for Parkinson's disease: Effects on cognition, mood, anxiety and personality traits. Eur Neurol. 2006;55:136–44.
70. Daniele A, Albanese A, Contarino MF, Zinzi P, Barbier A, Gasparini F, Romito LMA, Bentivoglio AR, Scerrati M. Cognitive and behavioural effects of

chronic stimulation of the subthalamic nucleus in patients with Parkinson's disease. J Neurol Neurosurg Psychiatry. 2003;74:175–82.
71. Witt K, Daniels C, Reiff J, Krack P, Volkmann J, Pinsker MO, Krause M, Tronnier V, Kloss M, Schnitzler A, Wojtecki L, Botzel K, Danek A, Hilker R, Sturm V, Kupsch A, Karner E, Deuschl G. Neuropsychological and psychiatric changes after deep brain stimulation for Parkinson's disease: a randomized, multicentre study. Lancet Neurol. 2008;7:605–14.
72. Voon V, Krack P, Lang AE, Lozano AM, Dujardin K, Schupbach M, et al. A multicentre study on suicide outcome following subthalamic stimulation for Parkinson's disease. Brain. 2008;131:2720–8.
73. Ardouin C, Voon V, Worbe Y, Abouazar N, Czernecki V, Hosseini H, et al. Pathological gambling in parkinon's disease improves on chronic subthalamic nucleus stimulation. Mov Disord. 2006;21:1941–6.
74. Brun DJ, Troster AI. Neuropsychiatric complications of medical and surgical therapies for Parkinson's disease. J Geriatr Psychiatry Neurol. 2004;17:172–80.
75. Papapetropoulos S, Katzen H, Schrag A, Singer C, Scanlon BK, Nation D, Guevara A, Levin B. A questionnaire-based (UM-PDHQ) study of hallucinations in Parkinson's disease. BMC Neurol. 2008;8:21.
76. Yoshida F, Miyagi Y, Kishimoto J, Morioka T, Murakami N, Hashiguchi K, Samura K, et al. Subthalamic nucleus stimulation does not cause deterioration of preexisting hallucinations in Parkinson's disease patients. Sterotact Funct Neurosurg. 2009;87:45–9.
77. Siderowf A, Jaggi JL, Xie SX, Loveland-Jones C, Leng L, Hurtig H, Colcher A, Stern M, Chou KL, Liang G, Maccarone H, Simuni T, Baltuch G. Long-term effects of bilateral subthalamic nucleus stimulation on health-related quality of life in advanced Parkinson's disease. Mov Disord. 2006;21:746–53.
78. Lezcano E, Gomez-Esteban JC, Zarranz JJ, Lambarri I, Madoz P, Bilbao G, Pomposo I, Garibi J. Improvement in quality of life in patients with advanced Parkinson's disease following bilateral deep-brain stimulation in subthalamic nucleus. Eur J Neurol. 2004;11:451–4.
79. Krack P, Batir A, Van Blercom N, Chabardes S, Fraix V, Ardouin C, Koudsie A, Limousin PD, Benazzouz A, LeBas JF, Benabid AL, Pollak P. Five-year follow-up of bilateral stimulation of the subthalamic nucleus in advanced Parkinson's disease. N Engl J Med. 2003;349:1925–34.
80. Den Oudsten BL, Van Heck GL, De Vries J. Quality of life and related concepts in Parkinson's disease: a systemic review. Mov Disord. 2007;22:1528–37.
81. Diamond A, Jankovic J. The effect of deep brain stimulation on quality of life in movement disorders. J Neurol Neurosurg Psychiatry. 2005;76:188–1193.
82. Martinez-Martin P, Deuschl G. Effect of medical and surgical interventions on health-related quality of life in Parkinson's disease. Mov Disord. 2007;22:757–65.
83. Antonini A, Landi A, Mariani C, DeNotaris R, Pezzoli G. Deep brain stimulation and its effect on sleep in Parkinson's disease. Sleep Med. 2004;5:211–4.
84. Cicolin A, Lopiano L, Zibetti M, Torre E, Tavella A, Guastamacchia G, Terreni A, Makrydakis G, Fattori E, Lanotte MM, Bergamasco B, Mutani R. Effects of deep brain stimulation on the subthalamic nucleus on sleep architecture in parkinsonian patients. Sleep Med. 2004;5:207–10.
85. Pillon B. Neuropsychological assessment for management of patients with deep brain stimulation. Mov Disord. 2002;17:S116–22.
86. Pillon B, Dubois B, Agid Y. Testing cognition may contribute to the diagnosis of movement disorders. Neurology. 1996;46:329–33.
87. Mattis S. Dementia rating scale. Odessa, FL: Psychological Assessment Resources; 1988.
88. Grober E, Buschke H. Genuine memory deficits in dementia. Dev Neuropsychol. 1987;3:13–36.
89. Kaplan EF, Goodglass H, Weintraub S. The Boston Naming Test. 2nd ed. Philadelphia, PA: Lea and Febiger; 1983.
90. Heilman KM, Gonzalez Rothi LJ. Apraxia. In: Heilman KM, Valenstein E, editors. Clinical Neuropsychology. 2nd ed. Oxford, England: Oxford University; 2003. p. 215–35.
91. Meyers J, Meyers K. The Meyers scoring system for the Rey Complex Figure and the Recognition Trial: professional manual. Odessa, FL: Psychological Assessment Resources; 1995.
92. Montgomery SA, Asberg MA. A new depression scale designed to be sensitive to change. Br J Psychiatry. 1979;134:382–9.
93. Jurica PJ, Leitten CL, Mattis S. Dementia Rating Scale-2: professional manual. Lutz: Psychological Assessment Resources; 2001.
94. Folstein MF, Folstein SE, McHugh PR. Mini-mental state: a practical method for grading the cognitive state of patients for the clinician. J Psychiatr Res. 1975;12:189–98.
95. Wechsler D. Wechsler Abbreviated Scales of Intelligence. San Antonio, TX: Psychological Corporation; 1999.
96. Gronwall DM. Paced Auditory Serial Addition Task: a measure of recovery from concussion. Percept Mot Skills. 1977;44:363–73.
97. Brandt J, Benedict RHB. The Hopkins Verbal Learning Test Revised: professional manual. Odessa, FL: Psychological Assessment Resources; 2002.
98. Wechsler D. Wechsler Memory Scale: manual. 3rd ed. San Antonio, TX: Psychological Corporation; 1997.
99. Benton AL, Hamsher K, Sivan AB. Multilingual Aphasia Examination—Third Edition. 3rd ed. Iowa City, IA: AJA Associates; 1983.
100. Benton AL, Hamsher K, Varney NR, Spreen O. Contributions to Neuropsychological Assessment. A clinical manual. New York, NY: Oxford University; 1983.
101. Golden CJ. Stroop Color and Word Test: a manual for clinical and experimental uses. Cleveland, OH: Stoelting Co; 1978.

102. Wechsler D. Wechsler Adult Intelligence Scale. 3rd ed. San Antonio, TX: Psychological Corporation; 1997.
103. Randt CT, Brown ER. Administration Manual: Randt Memory Test. Bayport, NY: Life Science Associates; 1983.
104. Smith A. Symbol Digit Modalities Test: manual. Los Angeles, CA: Western Psychological Services; 1982.
105. Kongs SK, Thompson LL, Iverson GL, Heaton RK. Wisconsin Card Sorting Test-64 Card Version. Lutz, FL: Psychological Assessment Resources; 2000.
106. Luria AR. Higher Cortical Functions in Man. New York, NY: Basic Books; 1980.
107. Grace J, Malloy P. Frontal Systems Behavior Scale (FrSBe): professional manual. Lutz, FL: Psychological Assessment Resources; 2001.
108. Delis DC, Kramer JH, Kaplan E, Ober BA. California Verbal Learning Test-Second Edition, Adult Version manual. San Antonio, TX: The Psychological Corporation; 2000.
109. Benedict RHB. Brief Visuospatial Memory Test-Revised: manual. Odessa, FL: Psychological Assessment Resources; 1997.
110. Goodglass H, Kaplan E. Boston diagnostic aphasia examination. Philadelphia, PA: Lea and Febiger; 1983.
111. Hooper H. Hooper Visual Organization Test (HVOT). Los Angeles: Western Psychological Services; 1983.
112. Beck AT, Steer RA, Brown GK. BDI-II, Beck depression inventory: manual. 2nd ed. Boston, MA: Harcourt Brace; 1996.
113. Beck AT, Steer RA. Beck anxiety inventory: manual. San Antonio, TX: Psychological Corporation; 1990.
114. Deuschel G, Wenzelburger R, Loffler K, Raethjen J, Stolze H. Essential tremor and cerebellar dysfunction clinical and kinematic analysis of intention tremor. Brain. 2000;123:1568–80.
115. Louis ED, Ford B, Wendt KJ, Cameron G. Clinical characteristics of essential tremor: data from a community-based study. Mov Disord.1998;13:803–8.
116. Deuschl G, Bain P. Deep brain stimulation for trauma: patient selection and evaluation. Mov Disord. 2002;17:S102–11.
117. Pollak P, Benabid AL, Krack P, Lomousin P, Benazzouz A. Deep brain stimulation. In: Jankovic J, Tolosa E, editors. Parkinson's disease and movement disorders. Baltimore, MD: Williams and Wilkoins; 1998. p. 1085–102.
118. Pahwa R, Lyons KL, Wilkonson SB, Carpenter MA, Troster AI, Searl JO, Overman J, Pickering S, Koller WC. Bilateral thalamic stimulation for the treatment of essential tremor. Neurology. 1999;53:1447–50.
119. Schuurman PR, Bosch DA, Bossuyt PM, Bonsel GJ, van Someren EJ, de Bie RM, Merkus MO, Speelman JD. A comparison of continuous thalamic stimulation and thalamotomy for suppression of severe tremor. N Engl J Med. 2000;342:461–8.
120. American Psychiatric Association. Diagnostic and statistical manual of mental disorders. 4th ed. Washington, DC: American Psychiatric Association; 2000. p. 111–4.
121. Serrvello D, Sassi M, Porta M. Deep brain stimulation in Tourette syndrome. Clin Neuropsychiatry. 2009;6:266–73.
122. Temel Y, Visser-Vandewalle V. Surgery in Tourette syndrome. Mov Disord. 2004;19:3–14.
123. Houeto JL, Karachi C, Mallet L, Pillon B, Yelnik J, Mesnage V, Welter ML, Navarro S, Pelissolo A, Damier P, Pidoux B, Dormont D, Cornu P, Agid Y. Tourette's syndrome and deep brain stimulation. J Neurol Neurosurg Psychiatry. 2005;76: 992–5.
124. Servello D, Porta M, Sassi M, Brambilla A, Robertson MM. Deep brain stimulation in 18 patients with severe Gilles de la Tourette syndrome refractory to treatment: the surgery and stimulation. J Neurol Neurosurg Psychiatry. 2008;79:136–42.
125. Alterman RL, Dumitriu D, Mathew S. Deep brain stimulation for major depressive disorder. Clin Neuropsychiatry. 2009;6:259–65.
126. Dowman J, Patel A, Rajput K. Electroconvulsive therapy: attitudes and misconceptions. J Electroconvulsive Therapy. 2005;21:84–7.
127. Daban C, Martinez-Aran A, Cruz N, Vieta E. Safety and efficacy of Vagus Nerve Stimulation in treatment-resistant depression. A systematic review. J Affect Disord. 2008;110:1–15.
128. Loo CK, MaFarquhar TF, Mitchell PB. A review of the safety of repetitive transcranial magnetic stimulation as a clinical treatment for depression. Int J Neuropsychopharmacol. 2008;11:131–47.
129. Price RB, Nock MK, Charney DS, Mathew SJ. Effects of intravenous ketamine on explicit and implicit measures of suicidality in treatment-resistant depression. Biol Psychiatry. 2009;66:522–6.
130. Jimenez F, Velasco F, Salin-Pascual R, Hernandez JA, Velasco M, Criales JL, Nicolini H. A patient with a resistant major depression disorder treated with deep brain stimulation in the inferior thalamic peduncle. Neurosurgery. 2005;57:585–93.
131. Mayberg HS, Lozano AM, Voon V, McNeely HE, Seminowicz D, Hamani C, Schwalb JM, Kennedy SH. Deep brain stimulation for treatment-resistant depression. Neuron. 2005;45:651–60.
132. Schlaepfer TE, Lieb K. Deep brain stimulation for treatment of refractory depression. Lancet. 2005; 366:1420–2.
133. Lozano AM, Maybery HS, Giacobbe O, Hamani C, Craddock RC, Kennedy SH. Subcallosal cingulated gyrus deep brain stimulation for treatment-resistant depression. Biol Psychiatry. 2008;64:461–7.
134. Malone Jr DA, Doughtery DD, Rezai AR, Carpenter LL, Friehs GM, Eskandar EN, Rauch SL, Rasmussen SA, Machado AG, Jubu CS, et al. Deep brain stimulation of the ventral capsule/ventral striatum for treatment-resistant depression. Biol Psychiatry. 2009;65:267–75.
135. Wang X, Chang C, Geng N, Li N, Wang J, Ma J, Xue W, Zhao W, Wu H, Wang P, Gao G. Long-term effects of bilateral deep brain stimulation of the subthalamic nucleus on depression in patients with Parkinson's disease. Parkinsonism Relat Disord. 2009;15:587–91.
136. Lakhan SE, Callaway E. Deep brain stimulation for obsessive-compulsive disorder and treatment-resistant

depression: systematic review. BMC Research Notes. 2010;3:60.

137. Nuttin B, Cosyns P, Demeulemeester H, Gybels J, Meyerson B. Electrical stimulation in anterior limbs of internal capsules in patients with obsessive-compulsive disorder. Lancet. 1999;354:1526.
138. Nuttin BJ, Gabriels LA, Cosyns PR, Meyerson BA, Andreewitch S, Sunaert SG, Maes AF, Dupont PJ, Gybels JM, Gilen F, Demeulemeester HG. Long-term electrical capsular simulation in patients with obsessive-compulsive disorder. Neurosurgery. 2003;52:1263–72.
139. Nuttin BJ, Gabriels LA, Cosyns PR, Meyerson BA, Andreewitch S, Sunaert SG, Maes AF, Dupont PJ, Gybels JM, Gielen F, Demeulemeester HG. Long-term electrical capsular stimulation in patients with obsessive-compulsive disorder. Neurosurgery. 2008;62:966–77.
140. Gabriels L, Cosyns P, Nuttin B, Demeulemeester H, Gybels J. Deep brain stimulation for treatment-refractory obsessive-compulsive disorder: psychopathological and neuropsychological outcome in three cases. Acta Psychiatr Scand. 2003;107:275–82.
141. Abelson JL, Curtis GC, Sagher O, Albucher RC, Harrigan M, Taylor SF, Martis B, Giordani B. Deep brain stimulation for refractory obsessive-compulsive disorder. Biol Psychiatry. 2005;57:510–6.
142. Sturm V, Lenartz D, Koulousakis A, Treuer H, Herholz K, Klein JC, Klosterkotter J. The nucleus accumbens: a target for deep brain stimulation in obsessive-compulsive- and anxiety-disorder. J Chem Neuroanat. 2003;26:293–9.
143. Aouizerate B, Cuny E, Bardinet E, Yelnik J, Martin-Guehl C, Rotge JY, Rougier A, Bioulac B, Tignol J, Mallet L, et al. Distinct striatal targets in treating obsessive-compulsive disorder and major depression. J Neurosurg. 2009;111:775–9.
144. Jimenez F, Velasco F, Salin-Pascual R, Velasco M, Nicolini H, Velasco AL, Castro G. Neuromodulation of the inferior thalamic peduncle for major depression and obsessive compulsive disorder. Acta Neurochir. 2007;97:S393–8.

Idiopathic Normal Pressure Hydrocephalus

24

Lisa D. Ravdin and Heather L. Katzen

Abstract

Idiopathic normal pressure hydrocephalus (INPH) is characterized by the clinical triad of gait disturbance, cognitive dysfunction, and urinary symptoms, observed in the context of enlargement of the cerebral ventricular system. Mean age of onset is approximately 60 years, which complicates the diagnosis since there is the potential for multiple age-related comorbidities in this population. Typically, gait disturbance is the presenting symptom that brings an individual to medical attention, but cognitive decline can be the initial symptom in some cases. NPH is an important diagnostic entity for the neuropsychologist working with older adults to be familiar with, since it is one of the few progressive cognitive disturbances that can be effectively treated. The current standard of care treatment is placement of a ventriculoperitoneal shunt, which can lead to reversal of symptoms, but shunt surgery is not without complications and careful patient selection is prudent. The neuropsychologist can be a key contributor in clinical settings for diagnostic considerations and in the evaluation of treatment response. In this chapter, we present a discussion of the clinical presentation and characteristic features of INPH, explore recent evidence-based diagnostic criteria, and provide guidelines for neuropsychological evaluation of INPH. A case example documenting post-shunt recovery of function is presented.

Keywords

Normal pressure hydrocephalus • Gait disorders • Urinary symptoms • Executive dysfunction

L.D. Ravdin, Ph.D. (✉)
Department of Neurology & Neuroscience,
Weill Cornell Neuropsychology Service,
Weill Medical College of Cornell University,
New York Presbyterian Hospital, 428 East 72nd Street,
Suite 500, New York, NY 10021, USA
e-mail: ldravdin@med.cornell.edu

H.L. Katzen, Ph.D.
Division of Neuropsychology, Department of Neurology,
University of Miami Miller School of Medicine,
1120 NW 14th Street, Room 1337, Miami,
FL 33136, USA
e-mail: hkatzen@med.miami.edu

L.D. Ravdin and H.L. Katzen (eds.), *Handbook on the Neuropsychology of Aging and Dementia*,
Clinical Handbooks in Neuropsychology, DOI 10.1007/978-1-4614-3106-0_24,

Clinical Presentation

The clinical symptom triad of cognitive impairment, gait disorder, and incontinence is considered the classic presentation of INPH, hence the well-known mnemonic "wacky, wobbly, and wet." However, contrary to clinical lore, it is now widely recognized that all three symptoms are not required for diagnosis. Most commonly, disturbed gait is the presenting symptom which brings the individual to medical attention, followed in frequency by cognitive impairment and urinary symptoms [2, 3]. In rare instances, cognitive dysfunction can predate the onset of gait abnormalities in INPH [4]. Nevertheless, variations in symptom presentation, with cognitive symptoms greater in severity than the disturbance in gait, should always raise the suspicion of comorbid disease (e.g., diagnosis of both Alzheimer's disease and INPH).

Gait

As described above, gait abnormalities are typically the first symptoms to become apparent and are the most readily recognized feature of INPH. The gait dysfunction in INPH has been described as "magnetic," "glue-footed," "short-stepped," or "shuffling." While the term "gait apraxia" has also been used, this may not be accurate given the observation that many patients can execute correct walking movements in a recumbent or supine position [5]. This clinical observation has been qualitatively described in the literature and may differentiate INPH from other movement disorders, yet it has never been carefully studied. INPH patients typically present with complaints of fatigue brought on by walking, difficulty with chair and bed transfers, halting ambulation down a sloping surface, and inability to walk at an expected pace [6]. Abnormal turning ("en bloc" turning) is also a characteristic feature of the gait abnormality, with multiple steps being needed to turn in place. It is notable that many standardized gait scales employ a cutoff of greater than two steps to indicate abnormal turning; however, we have found that many healthy older adults tend to take multiple steps to make a 180° turn on command. In our experience, up to four steps is within the normal range and should not be considered an indication of en bloc turning. INPH patients often require 5 or 6 steps and in some cases as many as 10–12 steps. In severe cases, patients with INPH may be unable to turn at all without someone to hold their hands and guiding them around. It is important to note that in the very early stages of the disease, individuals may present with relatively normal turning but may go on to develop worsening gait and en bloc turning if left untreated.

Urinary Symptoms

Urinary incontinence has not been well characterized in INPH and is the least common symptom to be reported at the time of diagnosis. While frank incontinence is present in about half the cases, particularly in advanced stages, increased frequency and urinary urgency are far more common in the early stages of the disease. This is very important to note, as questions about urinary symptoms need to extend beyond asking about the presence or absence of frank incontinence. Specific follow-up questions regarding frequency of urination and a sense of urgency should be included and may reveal subtle bladder symptoms that would otherwise go unreported. It is also not uncommon for patients to develop a "functional incontinence," where the gait disturbance may interfere with successful toileting. Since they may attribute occasional episodes of incontinence to their inability to walk fast enough to get to the bathroom, they may not report these as bladder symptoms unless specifically asked. Bowel incontinence can also occur in the late stages of INPH.

Cognitive Dysfunction

Cognitive deficits in INPH range from subtle cognitive dysfunction to a frank dementia [7]. It is estimated that INPH may be a contributing factor in to up to 6% of dementia cases [8], yet that figure is likely an underestimate given the challenge of parceling out INPH in the context of other dementing disorders. Early cognitive symptoms can readily go undetected or can falsely be attributed to normal aging. In our experience, many high functioning patients do not report subjective cognitive changes early in the disease course and perform well on global measures that are typically employed in neurology and neurosurgery clinics (e.g., MMSE, 3MS). However, detailed neuropsychological assessment frequently reveals more subtle executive deficits and psychomotor slowing, even when cognitive symptoms are denied by the patient.

In its purest form, the cognitive profile associated with INPH reflects frontal systems dysfunction and can include reduced psychomotor and information processing speed, executive deficits, as well as compromised complex attention and memory. [7, 9–12] Deficits in memory are characterized predominantly by difficulty acquiring new information and retrieval. This is typically secondary to deficits in the organization and efficient processing of information. Delayed recall is impaired but can often be prompted by cueing. Early cognitive compromise attributable to INPH presents as mild frontal systems dysfunction. If unrecognized and left untreated, cognitive symptoms may progress to a more severe frontal dysexecutive syndrome. Lack of treatment for a prolonged period may lead to the development of profile that appears to be consistent with a more generalized dementia. As true with other progressive dementing disorders, advanced untreated cases result in cognitive compromise indistinguishable from other forms of dementia. The presence of cortical deficits such as aphasia, agnosia, and alexia can be seen in the more advanced stages of INPH but likely signal comorbid disease or alternate diagnoses if present early on. As always, onset and duration of symptoms are critical factors to be considered in the differential diagnosis.

With regard to the cognitive profile, there are many occasions in which the neuropsychological test results suggest involvement of not only frontal systems but a more widespread cognitive decline that may indicate comorbid Alzheimer's disease (AD), vascular cognitive impairment, or another neurodegenerative process. However, the presence of another disorder does not negate the fact that INPH may contribute to the presentation, and even more importantly, is not necessarily a contraindication for treatment. In our experience, many patients with comorbid neurodegenerative conditions have been successfully treated for INPH. While the cognitive symptoms typically do not show substantial improvements post-shunt in patients with significant comorbid disease, improvements in gait can be associated with increased independence in activities of daily living and can significantly improve the patient's quality of life as well as make physical management easier for the caregiver.

Behavioral/Psychiatric Symptoms

Several case reports of psychiatric disturbances in association with INPH have appeared in the literature, including depression [13, 14], bipolar mania [15], psychosis [16, 17], aggressivity [18, 19], and obsessive–compulsive disorder [20]. Although atypical, psychiatric symptoms can emerge as a presenting feature and may complicate the diagnostic process [17]. The pathogenesis of psychiatric presentations in INPH is not well understood. Symptoms may develop due to neurochemical changes associated with the underlying brain disorder. In some cases, behavioral symptoms, such as depression, may be "reactive" or arise secondary to the physical and mental disability. Nevertheless, it is important to recognize the behavioral disturbances associated with INPH since they may be refractory to conventional pharmacological treatment and may, in some cases, be responsive to shunt placement. Case reports have suggested an improvement in specific psychiatric symptoms with shunt placement; however, this has not been systematically studied [16, 17].

Demographics

Symptoms of INPH typically develop with an insidious onset in the sixth and seventh decade of life. [2, 21] It has been estimated that approximately one half of a percent of the population over

65 suffers from NPH-related symptoms; however, few definitive incidence or prevalence studies of INPH have been conducted. [22, 23] Many NPH experts feel that this is an underestimate of the true prevalence of this condition. A recent review of five population-based studies from three countries revealed estimates ranging from 0.4% to 3.0%, concluding that approximately 1% of the population will develop NPH by the age of 80 [24]. Although no large-scale epidemiological studies have been conducted, there does not appear to be a gender or racial predilection [25]. The vast majority of INPH cases are sporadic, yet detailed linkage studies have not been performed.

Pathophysiology

The cause of ventricular enlargement in INPH is poorly understood. A CSF absorption deficit in or an imbalance between CSF production and absorption has been postulated; the exact pathophysiologic mechanism and specific neuroanatomic substrates underlying the symptoms in INPH remain unknown. Ventricular dilatation may cause disruption of descending periventricular fibers from the supplementary motor areas or compression of deeper subcortical circuits involving the globus pallidus. It has been proposed that ventricular enlargement may lead to increased vascular stretching, thereby decreasing compliance and decreasing capacitance of the system [26, 27]. It has also been suggested that infarction in the deep white matter fibers leading to decreased periventricular tensile strength could be a mechanism underlying INPH [28, 29].

Differential Diagnosis

The differential diagnosis of INPH often includes primary neurodegenerative disorders such as Parkinson's disease (PD) and Alzheimer's disease (AD).

Like PD, INPH presents with gait changes, motor slowing, and a profile of frontal systems dysfunction on cognitive testing. In particularly challenging cases when it is difficult to differentiate the two conditions, the treating physician may sometimes consider a trial of Levodopa (L-dopa) to see if there is a clinical response. While there are some reports of INPH showing brief or partial response to L-dopa, this is atypical and may be indicative of comorbid disease (i.e., PD). L-dopa treatment failures would rule out idiopathic PD, and these cases may then be directed to a tap test to prognosticate about shunt responsiveness. Other Parkinsonian syndromes may also be nonresponsive to L-dopa and tap test.

INPH patients can also be misdiagnosed with AD. Historically, gait disorder is more prominent and noted to be the initial presenting feature in the majority of INPH cases, whereas cognitive decline is the predominant presenting feature in AD. However, this notion may be in part due to the fact that objective cognitive testing was not historically part of the diagnostic workup of INPH. Rather, basic mental status screening instruments such as the MMSE were most frequently used. The MMSE is not sensitive to frontal subcortical dysfunction, the pattern of impairment most associated with INPH, and reports of normal mental status based on these screening measure do necessarily negate the presence of cognitive deficits.

Neuroimaging can be helpful in terms of the differential diagnosis of AD versus INPH. The degree and pattern of ventricular enlargement is key, but the differences are often subtle and are not always interpreted accurately to an untrained eye. Scans revealing ventricular enlargement with cerebral atrophy greater than expected for age are typically interpreted as consistent with AD. In these cases, the ventricular changes are attributed to a secondary consequence of cerebral atrophy. When close inspection of the pattern of ventricular enlargement reveals rounded frontal horns and marked enlargement of the temporal horns and third ventricle, this would suggest the changes are not simply a consequence of atrophy but rather that they are consistent with INPH. In these cases, the degree of ventricular enlargement is out of proportion to the cerebral atrophy. The term *hydrocephalus ex vacuo* is sometimes used to describe ventricular enlargement in association with brain atrophy and can

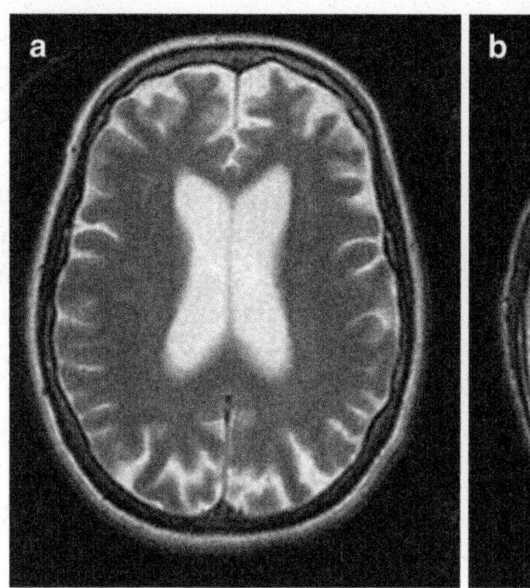

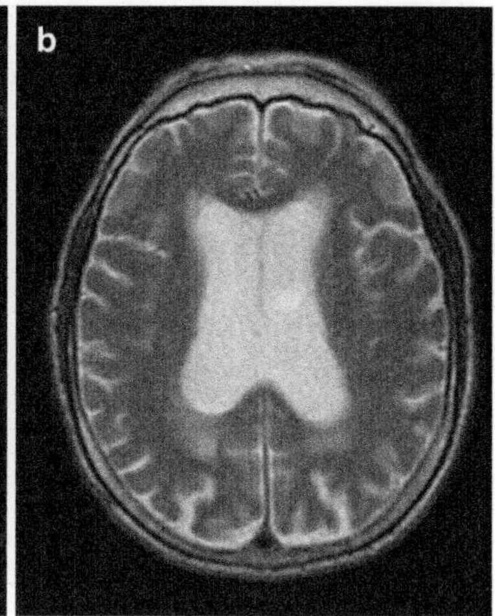

Fig. 24.1 Imaging characteristics in INPH versus AD. Comparison of AD and INPH on brain MRI. Axial images show (**a**) ventriculomegaly with significant cortical atrophy in AD and (**b**) ventriculomegaly without significant cortical atrophy in INPH

be differentiated from INPH. Neuroimaging will often be repeated over time to aid in diagnosis and to track disease progression or response to treatment; however, the presence or absence of ventricular changes does not always directly correspond to changes in clinical symptoms or deficits on formal testing. Axial MRI images of an INPH and AD brain are shown in Fig. 24.1.

There are several other conditions with varying etiologies that are common in aging populations that can produce gait changes, bladder symptoms, and cognitive dysfunction. Gait signs and symptoms can be associated with joint disorders such as hip, groin, or knee pain and other neurologic disorders (peripheral neuropathy and spinal stenosis), as well as slowing and other gait changes that can be attributable to normal aging. There are a host of etiologies underlying cognitive disorders in the elderly. A frontal systems disturbance can be observed secondary to other neurologic disorders (FTD and vascular disease), psychiatric disorders (depression, bipolar), and a multitude of other causes. Urinary symptoms are also common in older adults and can present with urinary tract infections, diabetes, a variety of bladder conditions, prostate problems in men, and gynecological abnormalities in women. Table 24.1 shows a list of neurologic diagnoses that are often considered in the differential diagnosis of INPH.

Table 24.1 INPH differential diagnosis

Neurodegenerative disorders	Other conditions
Alzheimer's disease	Spinal stenosis
Parkinson's disease	Noncommunicating hydrocephalus
Vascular dementia	HIV
Dementia with Lewy bodies	Lyme disease
Frontotemporal dementia	B_{12} deficiency
Spongiform encephalopathy	Collagen vascular disorders
Corticobasal degeneration	Neurosyphilis
Multisystem atrophy	Bladder spasticity
Progressive supranuclear palsy	Osteoarthritis

Evidence-Based Diagnostic Criteria

In 2005, a set of evidence-based guidelines were published to aid in the diagnosis and management of INPH [30]. These guidelines recommend the classification of INPH into "probable," "possible," and "unlikely" cases based on data gathered from clinical history, neuroimaging, physical exam, and physiological criteria (see Table 24.2).

Probable INPH

A diagnosis of "probable" INPH requires a history of gait disturbance and at least one of the other symptoms in the classic triad (cognitive or urinary). Also required is an insidious onset after the age of 40 years, a suggestion of progression over time, a minimum duration of 3–6 months, no antecedent event, and no evidence of another medical, neurologic, or psychiatric condition that could fully explain the symptoms.

There must also be brain imaging (CT or MRI) performed after the onset of symptoms that indicates ventricular enlargement not entirely explained by cerebral atrophy or congenital enlargement. This can be quantified by an Evan's index of 0.3 or greater [31, 32] or some other equivalent measurement of the ratio of ventricular size to cranial diameter. No evidence of macroscopic obstruction to CSF flow should be observed. In addition, either enlargement of the temporal horns of the lateral ventricles not fully accounted for by hippocampal atrophy, callosal angle of 40° or more, evidence of altered brain water content not attributable to microvascular ischemia or demyelination, or an aqueductal or fourth ventricular flow void on MRI must be observable on brain imaging.

The clinical examination must confirm the history criteria above including the presence of gait/balance disturbance as well as impairment in either cognition or urinary function. Gait and balance disturbance requires the presence of at least two of nine possible characteristics, including (1) decreased step height, (2) decreased step length, (3) decreased walking speed, (4) increased trunk sway during walking, (5) widened standing base, (6) toes turned outward on walking, (7) retropulsion, (8) turning requiring three or more steps for 180°, and (9) impaired walking balance. If cognitive symptoms are present, they must not be attributed to another condition. The criteria specifically state that there must be a documented impairment in performance on a cognitive screening instrument or evidence of deficits in at least two cognitive domains (e.g., psychomotor functioning, fine motor speed, fine motor accuracy, attention, memory, executive functions, or behavioral/personality). To document symptoms in the domain of urinary continence, patients must have either (1) episodic or persistent urinary incontinence not attributable to primary urological disorders, (2) persistent urinary incontinence or urinary and fecal incontinence, or (3) two of the following: urinary urgency (frequent perception of a pressing need to void), urinary frequency (more than six voiding episodes in an average 12-h period despite normal fluid intake), or nocturia (the need to urinate more than two times in an average night).

In addition to the above requirements, a diagnosis of "probable" INPH requires a CSF opening pressure in the range of 5–18 mm Hg (or 70–245 mm H_2O) as determined by a lumbar puncture or a comparable procedure. Pressures that are significantly higher or lower than this range are not consistent with a "probable" INPH diagnosis.

Possible INPH

The criteria required for a diagnosis of "possible" INPH are somewhat less rigorous. The history may indicate a subacute or indeterminate mode of onset, symptoms may be nonprogressive, duration may be less than 3 months, and symptoms may begin at any age after childhood. Also, as long as an antecedent event is not judged by the clinician to be causally related to the onset, mild head trauma, remote history of intracerebral hemorrhage, childhood and adolescent meningitis, or other condition may be present. Further, a comorbid neurologic, psychiatric, or medical condition does not prohibit the INPH "possible" diagnosis, as long as it is not thought to entirely explain the presentation. The brain imaging must demonstrate ventricular enlargement consistent with hydrocephalus but can show evidence of cerebral atrophy or structural lesions that may influence ventricular size. Clinical findings may include gait disturbance or dementia alone, or incontinence and cognitive impairment without gait disturbance. CSF opening pressure may be unavailable or can be outside the defined range (5–18 mm Hg or 70–245 mm H_2O).

Table 24.2 Idiopathic normal pressure hydrocephalus classification: probable, possible, and unlikely categories

Probable INPH	Possible INPH	Unlikely INPH
I. *Clinical findings must include*:	I. *Clinical findings include*:	
a. Gait/balance disturbance consistent with NPH b. Symptoms in at least one other domain (cognition, control of urination) c. Insidious onset (versus acute) after 40 years of age d. Minimum symptom duration of 3–6 months e. Evidence suggesting progression of symptoms over time f. No antecedent neurologic, psychiatric, or general medical conditions sufficient to explain in the presentation	a. Symptoms of either: 1. Incontinence and/or cognitive impairment in the absence of an observable gait/balance disturbance 2. Gait disturbance or dementia alone b. Reported symptoms may: 1. Have subacute or indeterminate mode of onset 2. Be nonprogressive or not clearly progressive 3. Begin at any age after childhood 4. Have <3 months or unknown duration 5. Follow *remote* events that in the judgment of the clinician are not likely to be causally related (e.g., mild head trauma, history of intracerebral hemorrhage, childhood/adolescent meningitis, or other conditions) 6. Coexist with other neurologic, psychiatric, or general medical disorders but in the judgment of the clinician not entirely explained by these conditions	1. No evidence of ventriculomegaly 2. Signs of increased intracranial pressure such as papilledema 3. No component of the clinical triad of INPH is present 4. Symptoms fully explained by other causes (e.g., spinal stenosis)
II. *Brain imaging* (*CT or MRI*) *must show*:	II. *Brain imaging* (*CT or MRI*) must show ventricular enlargement consistent with hydrocephalus but can be associated with:	
a. Enlargement of the ventricular system not entirely attributable to cerebral atrophy or congenital enlargement b. No macroscopic obstruction to CSF flow c. At least one of the following supportive features 1. Enlargement of the temporal horns of the lateral ventricles not entirely attributable to hippocampal a trophy 2. Callosal angle >40° 3. Evidence of altered brain water content, including periventricular signal changes (CT/MRI) not attributable to microvascular ischemic changes or demyelination 4. An aqueductal or fourth ventricular flow void on MRI	a. Evidence of cerebral atrophy sufficient to potentially explain ventricular size b. Structural lesions that may influence ventricular size	
III. *Physiological*: CSF opening pressure in the range of 5–18 mm Hg (or 70–245 mm H_2O)	III. *Physiological*: Opening pressure measurement not available or pressure outside range required for probable INPH	

Details regarding specific gait, cognitive, and urinary symptoms necessary for diagnosis are reviewed elsewhere [30]
INPH idiopathic normal pressure hydrocephalus, *CT* computed tomography, *MRI* magnetic resonance imaging, *CSF* cerebrospinal fluid, *SPECT* single-photon emission computed tomography

Unlikely INPH

An improbable or "unlikely" INPH diagnosis is simply defined by a presentation in which there is (1) no evidence of ventriculomegaly, (2) no signs of increased intracranial pressure such as papilledema, (3) no component of the clinical triad, and (4) symptoms explained by other causes (e.g., spinal stenosis).

Clinical Evaluation

Routine clinical evaluation for INPH includes clinical history and neurologic examination, bedside assessment of mental status, gait evaluation, and structural brain imaging. Without additional procedures, research indicates a 46–61% response rate to surgical treatment [33]. Consensus guidelines [30] also recommend lumbar puncture, CSF drainage, and outflow resistance studies, as well as neuropsychological testing. While functional brain imaging, urodynamic studies, video or computerized gait evaluation, and other laboratory investigations may provide additional information in some case, these were deemed as lacking sufficient evidence to include as part of the INPH consensus criteria [30].

Interestingly, CSF tap test is not required according to the consensus criteria, but it is the most widely used diagnostic test performed to prognosticate shunt responsiveness. The procedure, also called a large volume lumbar puncture, involves removal of approximately 50 cc of CSF. Improvement in clinical symptoms following a tap test is associated with an increased likelihood of a positive surgical outcome; however, this technique has also been found to have a high false-negative rate [34–36]. While the standard of care has typically been for the clinician to make subjective observations of the patient's gait and mental function following tap test, these methods have inherent bias. More objective detailed clinical assessment should be performed both before tap test and about 2–4 h after CSF removal to evaluate change. The pre- and posttap assessment should include standardized gait and cognitive assessment. In the event of equivocal results, a repeat test or referral for another type of CSF drainage procedure may be helpful. Given the high false-negative rate, lack of tap test response does not completely rule out a diagnosis of INPH nor does it preclude shunt responsiveness [30].

External lumbar drainage (ELD) is a more prolonged CSF drainage procedure in which larger volumes of fluid are removed, typically over several days. CSF is typically drained at a rate of 10 cc/h through a catheter placed temporarily in the lumbar region. ELD has been shown to have good prognostic value with a sensitivity of 50–100%, specificity of 60–100%, and positive predictive value of 80–100% [33]. If there is a strong suspicion of INPH and the tap test is negative or equivocal, the ELD procedure may be considered. Until recently, ELD had only been performed at a limited number of sites in the USA, yet, a growing number of clinical research settings have implemented it as part of the standard presurgical workup. It is important to note that this procedure requires hospitalization and can be associated with complications such as infection or nerve root irritation, and the clinical decision of whether or not to conduct ELD should be considered on case-by-case basis. As with a tap test, detailed assessment of gait, cognition, and urinary symptoms should be performed to objectively assess response. The postdrainage neuropsychological evaluation and standardized gait assessment are key factors in determining response. The neuropsychologist plays an integral role in these evaluations by providing objective data regarding changes in performance.

Treatment Response

Response following shunt placement for INPH varies dramatically, with reported improvement rates ranging from 30% to 96% [37]. While treatment response rates for INPH are traditionally thought to be lower than in secondary forms of hydrocephalus, a recent study found that this can be explained primarily by the fact that INPH patients frequently have comorbid disease. With favorable preconditions (e.g., low comorbidity), INPH patients were shown to have an approximately 80% chance of good outcome, even among patients with advanced age [38].

While the insertion of a shunt is a relatively minor neurosurgical procedure, morbidity rates have been reported to be approximately 30% [39]. Major complications have been reported to occur in about 10%, and minor complications occur in approximately 14% of patients [40]. Common complications include intracerebral hemorrhage, subdural effusions, subdural hematomas, infection, shunt malfunction, over drainage, and hypotensive headaches.

Although all three symptoms in the clinical triad can show dramatic improvement following treatment, a substantial number of patients show incomplete resolution of one or more of the symptoms. In general, gait is reported to be the earliest and most frequent symptom to improve. Research has suggested that both a greater duration of symptoms prior to intervention and the existence of comorbid disease are factors associated with poorer outcome. Also, there is agreement that if left untreated or inadequately managed, INPH often progresses to a severe state of impairment and dependency, resulting in markedly compromised mobility as well as a full-blown dementia. While all three symptoms in the clinical triad are not required for a diagnosis, several studies have shown that the presence of the complete triad is associated with better outcome following treatment [41, 42].

There has been great variability in the literature regarding recovery of cognitive functions. Some studies report no change in mental status, while others suggest improvement in up to 90% of patients. Conflicting findings may be explained by variations in the depth of cognitive examination and the way in which cognitive improvement is defined, as well as length of study follow-up intervals. Several studies have documented improvement in overall mental status using screening measures, but there is less agreement about whether specific cognitive deficits may respond differentially to treatment [2, 7, 43]. It has been shown that patients with overt dementia exhibit clear gains in mental status following surgery, whereas patients with more subtle impairment in executive skills tend to show less striking improvement [7, 12]. Others have suggested that the more severe impairments may be more likely to be refractory to treatment, but this has not been empirically studied. In our experience, even patients with subtle cognitive compromise show objective improvement in cognitive functioning and report an overall sense of improved cognitive efficiency. In severely impaired patients that are basically untestable before surgery, there are sometimes changes in affect and in the ability to participate in basic aspects of the evaluation that provide qualitative evidence of improvement.

Another methodological issue that contributes to our limited understanding about the recovery of specific cognitive functions in INPH is that most investigations lack a control group, making it difficult to disentangle practice effects from a true treatment effect. One recent study used comparison data from a control sample and found post-shunt improvement on most tasks; however, effects of prior exposure to test material could not be examined since the controls were only tested at one time point [44]. We recently evaluated 12 INPH patients and nine controls with comprehensive neuropsychological testing at baseline and at 6-month follow-up [45]. The INPH group showed greater improvement than controls on a timed test of mental tracking and sequencing (Trail Making B). INPH caregivers also reported improved activities of daily living (ADLs) and reduced caregiver distress, suggesting functional and quality of life improvements for both the shunt responder and their caregiver.

Neuropsychological Assessment

A neuropsychologist may encounter INPH in the context of a diagnostic evaluation, follow-up assessment to track changes over time, an examination to help establish response to intervention (tap test, ELD, shunt), or for research purposes. Detailed cognitive testing is recommended, particularly in patients with more subtle abnormalities, since screening measures and bedside testing may not pick up these mild deficits. Mental status screening tests have poor sensitivity to the subcortical pattern of cognitive dysfunction typically observed in INPH [46]. Repeat neuropsychological assessment is useful in monitoring disease progression and response to treatment or may be used to help identify shunt malfunction. Fatigue, both physical and mental, can contribute to reduced performance, and we have found that obtaining the patient's best performance is most readily accomplished when conducting the exam in two sessions.

Taking the Clinical History

Cognitive difficulties, including deficits in insight and/or memory, may interfere with a patient's ability to provide a complete and accurate history. It is therefore critical for the clinician to gather history and background information from a collateral source. A well-informed caregiver or third party who is knowledgeable about the patient's premorbid and current level of functioning should be interviewed.

In order to understand the disease presentation and course, one should ascertain whether the onset of symptoms was acute or insidious, whether the symptoms have been static or progressive, and the severity of deficits and degree with which they impact everyday functioning. Since INPH does not have a known antecedent cause by definition, inquiries regarding potential precipitating factors should be made to rule out SNPH. Although familial occurrence of INPH is rare, other heritable conditions should be ruled out. Family history questions should focus on neurodegenerative disorders such as PD, AD, Huntington's disease, and other neurologic conditions that are often considered in the differential diagnosis. Falls are common, and questions about gait changes should also inquire about head injuries or loss of consciousness that may have occurred during those events. Detailed questions about subtle bladder symptoms need to be addressed with particular attention to frequency and urgency as well as frank incontinence. Personal and family psychiatric histories should also be reviewed since behavioral symptoms can sometimes appear or be exacerbated in INPH. As always, a standard review of past medical and surgical history is also an important part of the evaluation.

Selection of Neuropsychological Measures

As always, selection of tests will vary based on the nature of the referral and the patient's presentation. Most initial referrals are for diagnostic purposes or for characterization of the extent of cognitive impairment. In these cases, a relatively comprehensive battery should be employed that mirrors that of a typical memory disorders evaluation, especially since comorbid conditions may need to be ruled out. When more specific referral questions, such as assessing potential response to intervention (tap test, ELD, shunt), are at hand, a more selective battery can be implemented. A sample neuropsychological battery for use in NPH is listed in Table 24.3. This is a core group of tests that we have found to be sensitive to changes in NPH and that we use in our NPH research program.

Not surprisingly, many of the traditional neuropsychological measures of higher cortical functions are unchanged in the posttap session or immediately following surgery, but measures of processing and motor speed often show improvements. We have found that measures of upper extremity motor speed can be helpful in determining response to tap test [47], particularly since there are many cases where lower extremity motor functioning is severely compromised and cannot be formally assessed with standard gait scales (i.e., the patient is unable to ambulate without assistance). The recommended battery for assessing change pre- to post-CSF drainage (tap test or ELD) is heavily weighted toward motor and psychomotor tests in order to maximize the ability to realize small gains over the short term. Many of these tests are standardized measures that are regularly used in neuropsychological clinics. Two less well-known measures that we have incorporated into our battery that have not been well standardized, but provide excellent qualitative data, are the Line Tracing

Test and the Serial Dotting Test [48]. These two psychomotor speed and precision tests shown in Fig. 24.2 have been demonstrated to be sensitive to change in NPH [47].

We have found that to minimize fatigue and to optimize performance, the pretap evaluation should be done on a day prior to the day of the spinal tap, preferably 1 or 2 days before and always within 1 week if possible. The posttap assessment should always be done on the same day as the spinal tap. Although there is limited data regarding the optimal time for measuring posttap performance, and there are likely great individual differences in the response peak, the majority of experts suggest conducting the post-tap assessment between 2 and 4 h after the removal of spinal fluid [49]. Not uncommonly, family members report improved gait and sometimes improved attentiveness within 24 h after the tap test. We recommend routinely contacting patients the day after the tap to obtain this type of qualitative data. Post-shunt evaluations can also be useful to evaluate response to treatment and in some cases help determine whether there may be a shunt malfunction. For example, if a patient that initially demonstrated a clear response post-shunt developed a reemergence of symptoms, neuropsychological assessment may be helpful in documenting the nature and severity of the change to provide evidence of a possible shunt obstruction or other type of shunt malfunction. Repeated assessments post-shunt can be useful in documenting recovery of function, as illustrated in the case example provided below.

Table 24.3 Core neuropsychological battery for repeat assessment in INPH

Global cognitive measures (i.e., Dementia Rating Scale [50] or 3MS [1])
Boston Naming Test [51]
Controlled Oral Word Association [52]
Hopkins Verbal Learning Test—Revised [53]
Wechsler Adult Intelligence Scale IV [54] (Digit Span)
Trail Making Test A and B [55]
Symbol Digit Modalities Test [56]
Grooved Pegboard Test [55]
Finger Tapping Test [55]
Line Tracing Test [57]
Serial Dotting Test [57]
Gait scale [2] (videotaping of gait is helpful)

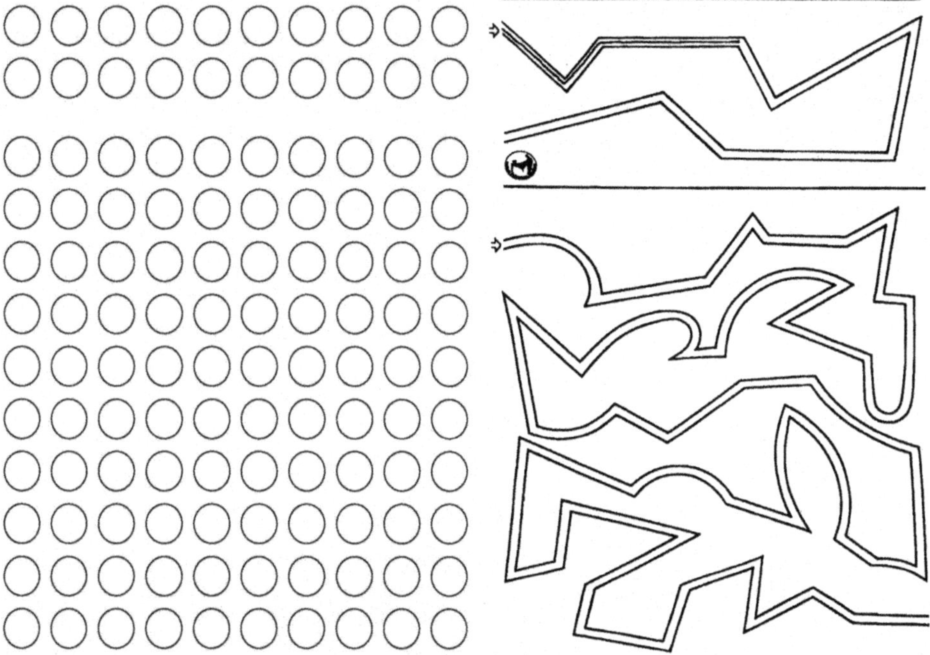

Fig. 24.2 Line tracing and serial dotting

Management of NPH is accomplished with a multidisciplinary approach to patient care. The neuropsychologist is a key member of the team and can play an important role in the diagnostic process, prognosticating about candidacy for treatment and monitoring recovery of function. A case example that demonstrates neuropsychological assessment of recovery of function post-shunt is presented below.

Case Example: Recovery of Function Following Shunt

A brief summary is provided for Mr. X, an 82-year-old right-handed gentleman who underwent of a series of neuropsychological assessments before and after shunt placement (baseline and follow-up post-shunt exams at 2, 5, and 8 months). The patient initially presented with severe gait disturbance, moderate cognitive decline, and mild urinary symptoms of approximately 1 year's duration with a reportedly progressive course. Neuroimaging reportedly revealed prominent ventriculomegaly out of proportion to cerebral atrophy. The patient was diagnosed with INPH and underwent shunt placement.

At the time of diagnosis, Mr. X enrolled in a clinical research protocol, which included baseline and post-shunt neuropsychological and gait evaluations. A brief summary of his performance on select measures administered as part of the research protocol is provided below.

Baseline Results

The pattern of baseline cognitive test scores reflected significant decline from premorbid functioning, which was estimated to be in the high average range. Mr. X demonstrated borderline to impaired performance on two global cognitive screening measures (3MS = 82/100; DRS total = 118/144). Detailed neuropsychological testing revealed impairments in memory, semantic fluency, executive functions, visuospatial abilities, processing speed, and motor skills (dominant > nondominant). Attention, confrontation naming, and phonemic fluency were intact. Overall, the observed pattern of performance revealed moderate frontal subcortical dysfunction, and this was interpreted as consistent with INPH.

Follow-Up Results

Comparison of baseline and post-shunt evaluations suggested considerable improvement in cognition as evidenced by significant gains on a global scale of cognitive functioning (see Fig. 24.3). Several measures of motor speed and dexterity, rapid motor processing, and mental tracking demonstrated moderate improvement

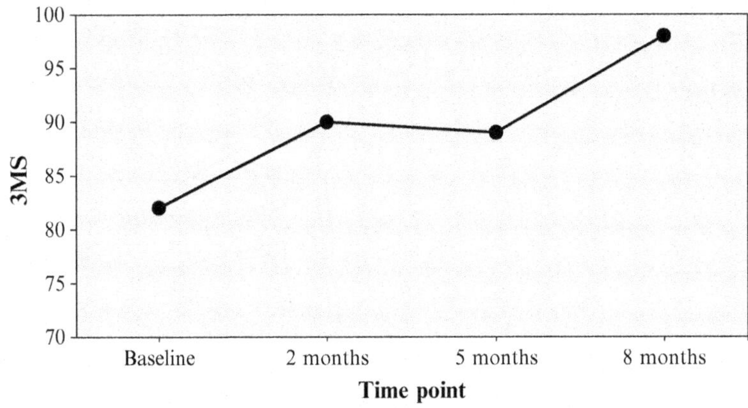

Fig. 24.3 Case example of post-shunt change in Modified Mini-Mental Exam (3MS)

over time (see Fig. 24.4). Moderate improvement was also observed on verbal fluency and memory by the 8-month follow-up exam (see Fig. 24.5). Dramatic improvement in gait was observed clinically as well as documented on a standardized gait scale (see Fig. 24.6). At baseline, Mr. X walked 10 m in 20.5 s and 23 steps. At the final follow-up visit 8 months postsurgery, Mr. X walked 10 m in 10 s and 9 steps, a clinically significant improvement. Not all cognitive measures reflected improvement; deficits persisted on some tasks of psychomotor speed, and relative

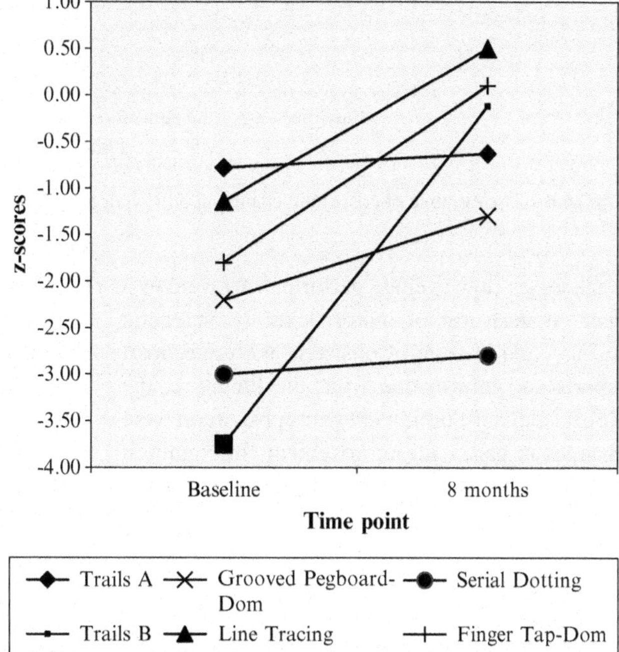

Fig. 24.4 Case example of post-shunt change in motor and psychomotor tests

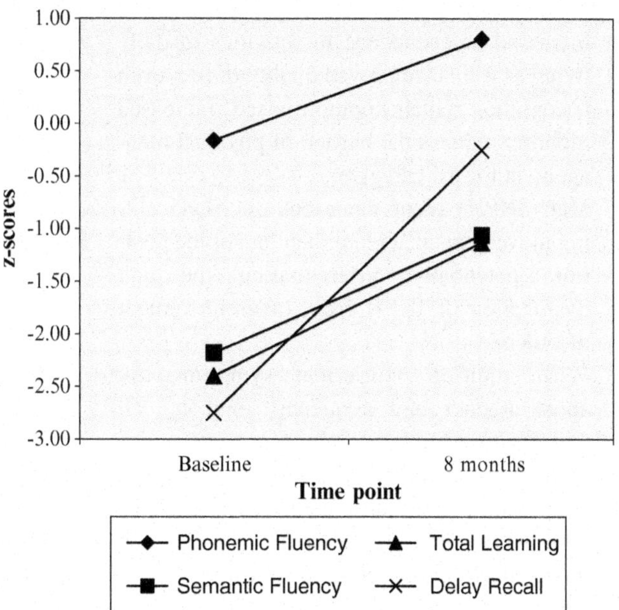

Fig. 24.5 Case example of post-shunt change in fluency and memory tests

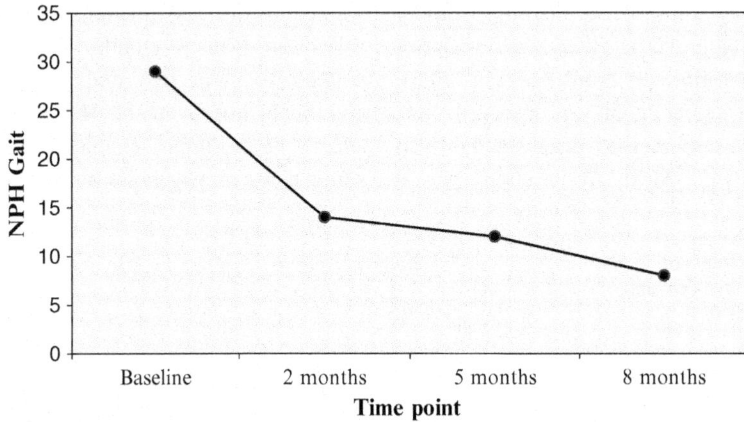

Fig. 24.6 Case example of post-shunt change in NPH Gait Scale. *Note*: Higher scores indicate greater impairment

weaknesses (low average performance) were evident on measures of motor dexterity, semantic fluency, and learning. Consistent with anecdotal reports and information from the literature, the earliest and most prominent gains post-shunt were changes in gait, with improvements in cognition evolving over the extended recovery period.

Clinical Pearls

- Comorbidity is common in INPH but does not preclude shunt candidacy or response.
- Post-shunt improvements in gait can lead to increased independence in activities of daily living as well as improved quality of life, even if cognition remains compromised. Increased mobility reduces the burden of physical management for the caregiver.
- Many INPH patients can execute correct walking movements in a recumbent or supine position, potentially differentiating the gait dysfunction of INPH from other movement disorders.
- When inquiring about urinary symptoms, ask about urgency and frequency, since not all patients have frank incontinence.
- Despite reports of intact cognition as assessed by bedside mental status testing, many patients with INPH exhibit frontal systems dysfunction on detailed neuropsychological testing.
- The gold standard for gait assessment in INPH is typically a neurologist's subjective assessment of gait; the neuropsychologist can bring a unique set of skills that provide objective measures of response.
- In cases where gait is severely compromised or postdrainage changes are subtle, tests which rely on the integrity of upper extremity motor functioning can provide additional data to inform management.
- Consistent with the literature demonstrating a high false-negative rate for tap tests, we have seen INPH patients with negative tap test respond to shunt.
- ELD can be superior to tap test for prognosticating about shunt responsiveness, but it may not be appropriate for all patients and it is only performed at specialty centers.

References

1. Teng EL, Chui HC. The Modified Mini-Mental State (3MS) examination. J Clin Psychiatry. 1987;48:314–8.
2. Boon AJ, Tans JT, Delwel EJ, et al. Dutch normal-pressure hydrocephalus study: prediction of outcome after shunting by resistance to outflow of cerebrospinal fluid. J Neurosurg. 1997;87:687–93.
3. Boon AJ, Tans JT, Delwel EJ, et al. Dutch Normal-Pressure Hydrocephalus Study: the role of cerebrovascular disease. J Neurosurg. 1999;90:221–6.
4. Ravdin LD, Katzen HL. Idiopathic normal pressure hydrocephalus. In: Morgan JE, Baron IS, Ricker JH,

editors. Casebook of clinical neuropsychology. Oxford University Press: New York; 2010.
5. Fisher CM. Hydrocephalus as a cause of disturbances of gait in the elderly. Neurology. 1982;32:1358–63.
6. Knutsson E, Lying-Tunell U. Gait apraxia in normal-pressure hydrocephalus: patterns of movement and muscle activation. Neurology. 1985;35:155–60.
7. Iddon JL, Pickard JD, Cross JJ, Griffiths PD, Czosnyka M, Sahakian BJ. Specific patterns of cognitive impairment in patients with idiopathic normal pressure hydrocephalus and Alzheimer's disease: a pilot study. J Neurol Neurosurg Psychiatry. 1999;67:723–32.
8. Casmiro M, D'Alessandro R, Cacciatore FM, Daidone R, Calbucci F, Lugaresi E. Risk factors for the syndrome of ventricular enlargement with gait apraxia (idiopathic normal pressure hydrocephalus): a case-control study. J Neurol Neurosurg Psychiatry. 1989;52:847–52.
9. Caltagirone C, Gainotti G, Masullo C, Villa G. Neurophysiological study of normal pressure hydrocephalus. Acta Psychiatr Scand. 1982;65:93–100.
10. Klinge P, Berding G, Brinker T, Schuhmann M, Knapp WH, Samii M. PET-studies in idiopathic chronic hydrocephalus before and after shunt-treatment: the role of risk factors for cerebrovascular disease (CVD) on cerebral hemodynamics. Acta Neurochir Suppl. 2002;81:43–5.
11. Merten T. Neuropsychology of normal pressure hydrocephalus. Nervenarzt. 1999;70:496–503.
12. Thomsen AM, Borgesen SE, Bruhn P, Gjerris F. Prognosis of dementia in normal-pressure hydrocephalus after a shunt operation. Ann Neurol. 1986;20:304–10.
13. Price TR, Tucker GJ. Psychiatric and behavioral manifestations of normal pressure hydrocephalus. A case report and brief review. J Nerv Ment Dis. 1977;164:51–5.
14. Rosen H, Swigar ME. Depression and normal pressure hydrocephalus. A dilemma in neuropsychiatric differential diagnosis. J Nerv Ment Dis. 1976;163:35–40.
15. Schneider U, Malmadier A, Dengler R, Sollmann WP, Emrich HM. Mood cycles associated with normal pressure hydrocephalus. Am J Psychiatry. 1996;153:1366–7.
16. Lying-Tunell U. Psychotic symptoms in normal-pressure hydrocephalus. Acta Psychiatr Scand. 1979;59:415–9.
17. Pinner G, Johnson H, Bouman WP, Isaacs J. Psychiatric manifestations of normal-pressure hydrocephalus: a short review and unusual case. Int Psychogeriatr. 1997;9:465–70.
18. Crowell RM, Tew Jr JM, Mark VH. Aggressive dementia associated with normal pressure hydrocephalus. Report of two unusual cases. Neurology. 1973;23:461–4.
19. McIntyre AW, Emsley RA. Shoplifting associated with normal-pressure hydrocephalus: report of a case. J Geriatr Psychiatry Neurol. 1990;3:229–30.
20. Abbruzzese M, Scarone S, Colombo C. Obsessive-compulsive symptomatology in normal pressure hydrocephalus: a case report. J Psychiatry Neurosci. 1994;19:378–80.
21. Mori K. Management of idiopathic normal-pressure hydrocephalus: a multiinstitutional study conducted in Japan. J Neurosurg. 2001;95:970–3.
22. Casmiro M, Benassi G, Cacciatore FM, D'Alessandro R. Frequency of idiopathic normal pressure hydrocephalus. Arch Neurol. 1989;46:608.
23. Trenkwalder C, Schwarz J, Gebhard J, et al. Starnberg trial on epidemiology of Parkinsonism and hypertension in the elderly. Prevalence of Parkinson's disease and related disorders assessed by a door-to-door survey of inhabitants older than 65 years. Arch Neurol. 1995;52:1017–22.
24. Conn H. Normal pressure hydrocephalus (NPH): more about NPH by a physcian who is the patient. Clin Med. 2010;10:1–4.
25. Marmarou A, Bergsneider M, Relkin N, Klinge P, Black PM. Development of guidelines for idiopathic normal-pressure hydrocephalus: introduction. Neurosurgery. 2005;57:S1–3. discussion ii-v.
26. Greitz D, Hannerz J, Rahn T, Bolander H, Ericsson A. MR imaging of cerebrospinal fluid dynamics in health and disease. On the vascular pathogenesis of communicating hydrocephalus and benign intracranial hypertension. Acta Radiol. 1994;35:204–11.
27. Sklar FH, Diehl JT, Beyer Jr CW, Clark WK. Brain elasticity changes with ventriculomegaly. J Neurosurg. 1980;53:173–9.
28. Bradley Jr WG, Whittemore AR, Watanabe AS, Davis SJ, Teresi LM, Homyak M. Association of deep white matter infarction with chronic communicating hydrocephalus: implications regarding the possible origin of normal-pressure hydrocephalus. AJNR Am J Neuroradiol. 1991;12:31–9.
29. Tullberg M, Hultin L, Ekholm S, Mansson JE, Fredman P, Wikkelso C. White matter changes in normal pressure hydrocephalus and Binswanger disease: specificity, predictive value and correlations to axonal degeneration and demyelination. Acta Neurol Scand. 2002;105:417–26.
30. Relkin N, Marmarou A, Klinge P, Bergsneider M, Black PM. Diagnosing idiopathic normal-pressure hydrocephalus. Neurosurgery. 2005;57:S4–16. discussion ii-v.
31. Evans WA. An encephalographic ratio for estimating ventricular enlargement and cerebral atrophy. Arch Neurol Psychiatry. 1937;93:1–7.
32. Williams MA, Razumovsky AY, Hanley DF. Evaluation of shunt function in patients who are never better, or better than worse after shunt surgery for NPH. Acta Neurochir Suppl. 1998;71:368–70.
33. Marmarou A, Bergsneider M, Klinge P, Relkin N, Black PM. The value of supplemental prognostic tests for the preoperative assessment of idiopathic normal-pressure hydrocephalus. Neurosurgery. 2005;57:S17–28. discussion ii-v.
34. Vanneste JA. Three decades of normal pressure hydrocephalus: are we wiser now? J Neurol Neurosurg Psychiatry. 1994;57:1021–5.
35. Malm J, Kristensen B, Karlsson T, Fagerlund M, Elfverson J, Ekstedt J. The predictive value of cere-

brospinal fluid dynamic tests in patients with th idiopathic adult hydrocephalus syndrome. Arch Neurol. 1995;52:783–9.
36. Bret P, Chazal J, Janny P, et al. Chronic hydrocephalus in adults. Neurochirurgie. 1990;36 Suppl 1:1–159.
37. Klinge P, Marmarou A, Bergsneider M, Relkin N, Black PM. Outcome of shunting in idiopathic normal-pressure hydrocephalus and the value of outcome assessment in shunted patients. Neurosurgery. 2005;57:S40–52. discussion ii-v.
38. Kiefer M, Meier U, Eymann R. Does idiopathic normal pressure hydrocephalus always mean a poor prognosis? Acta Neurochir Suppl. 2010;106:101–6.
39. Vanneste J, Augustijn P, Dirven C, Tan WF, Goedhart ZD. Shunting normal-pressure hydrocephalus: do the benefits outweigh the risks? A multicenter study and literature review. Neurology. 1992;42:54–9.
40. Wilson RK, Williams MA. The role of the neurologist in the longitudinal management of normal pressure hydrocephalus. Neurologist. 2010;16:238–48.
41. Black PM. Idiopathic normal-pressure hydrocephalus. Results of shunting in 62 patients. J Neurosurg. 1980; 52:371–7.
42. Hebb AO, Cusimano MD. Idiopathic normal pressure hydrocephalus: a systematic review of diagnosis and outcome. Neurosurgery. 2001;49:1166–84. discussion 84–6.
43. Raftopoulos C, Deleval J, Chaskis C, et al. Cognitive recovery in idiopathic normal pressure hydrocephalus: a prospective study. Neurosurgery. 1994;35:397–404. discussion -5.
44. Hellstrom P, Edsbagge M, Blomsterwall E, et al. Neuropsychological effects of shunt treatment in idiopathic normal pressure hydrocephalus. Neurosurgery. 2008;63:527–35. discussion 35-6.
45. Katzen H, Ravdin LD, Assuras S, Heros R, Kaplitt M, Schwartz TH, Fink M, Levin BE, Relkin NR. Post-shunt cognitive and functional improvement in idiopathic Normal Pressure Hydrocephalus (iNPH). Neurosurgery. 2011;68(2):416–9.
46. Tombaugh TN, McIntyre NJ. The mini-mental state examination: a comprehensive review. J Am Geriatr Soc. 1992;40:922–35.
47. Tsakanikas D, Katzen H, Ravdin LD, Relkin NR. Upper extremity motor measures of Tap Test response in normal pressure hydrocephalus. Clin Neurol Neurosurg. 2009;111:752–7.
48. Klinge P, Ruckert N, Schuhmann M, Dorner L, Brinker T, Samii M. Neuropsychological testing to improve surgical management of patients with chronic hydrocephalus after shunt treatment. Acta Neurochir Suppl. 2002;81:51–3.
49. Katzen H, Relkin N. Normal pressure hydrocephalus: a review. In: Geldmacher D, editor. Other dementias. Delray Beach: Carma Publishing; 2008.
50. Mattis S. Dementia Rating Scale: professional manual. Odessa: Psychological Assessment Resources; 1988.
51. Goodglass H, Kaplan E. The assessment of aphasia and related disorders. 2nd ed. Philadelphia: Lea and Febiger; 1987.
52. Spreen O, Benton AL. Neurosensory Centory Comprehension Examination for Aphasia (NCCEA). Victoria: University of Victoria; 1969.
53. Benedict RHB, Schretlen D, Groninger L, Brandt J. Hopkins verbal learning test-revised: normative data and analysis of inter-form and test-retest reliability. Clin Neuropsychol. 1998;12:43–55.
54. Wechsler D. WAIS-IV manual. New York: The Psychological Corporation; 2008.
55. Reitan RM, Wolfson D. The Halstead-Reitan neuropsychological test battery. Tucson: Neuropsychological Press; 1985.
56. Smith A. Symbol digit modalities test manual. Los Angeles: Western Psychological Services; 1973.
57. Klinge P, Rückert N, Weißenborn K, Dörner L, Samii M, Brinker T, A practical neuropsychological test battery for measurement of cognitive and motor function in patients with Normal-pressure hydrocephalus (NPH). Poster at the 3rd International Hydrocephalus Workshop. Kos: Greece; May 17–20, 2001.

Episodic and Semantic Memory Disorders

25

Taylor Kuhn and Russell M. Bauer

Abstract

In its most pure form, the human amnesic syndrome involves a disabling impairment in new learning accompanied by some degree of impairment in aspects of remote memory in the context of relatively normal intellectual ability, language, and attention span. Neuropsychological research has clearly shown that lesions within the brain's extended memory system (medial temporal lobe, diencephalon, and basal forebrain) produce anterograde amnesia while leaving other aspects of memory (retrieval of general knowledge, vocabulary, names) relatively intact. The episodic–semantic distinction has been useful in explaining key characteristics of the human amnesic syndrome. This chapter provides a framework for characterizing the distinction between "episodic" and "semantic" memory, and discusses the clinical features and assessment of disordered function in each of these two domains.

Keywords

Episodic memory • Semantic memory • Amnesia • Memory systems • Neurobehavioral assessment

It has been nearly five decades since the famous patient H.M., who represents a paradigmatic case of the human amnesic syndrome, was first described in the literature. In its most pure form, the human amnesic syndrome involves a disabling impairment in new learning accompanied by some degree of impairment in aspects of remote memory in the context of relatively normal intellectual ability, language, and attention span. The hallmark feature, *anterograde amnesia*, involves "recent" memory; the essential feature of the deficit is that the patient is impaired in the conscious, deliberate recall of information initially learned after illness onset. In cases where remote memory is impaired (*retrograde amnesia*), the deficit is often temporally graded or time-limited and is generally worse for memories acquired in

T. Kuhn, M.S. • R.M. Bauer, Ph.D., ABPP (✉)
Department of Clinical and Health Psychology, University of Florida, PO Box 100165 HSC, Gainesville, FL 32610-1065, USA
e-mail: tkuhn@phhp.ufl.edu; rbauer@phhp.ufl.edu

L.D. Ravdin and H.L. Katzen (eds.), *Handbook on the Neuropsychology of Aging and Dementia*, Clinical Handbooks in Neuropsychology, DOI 10.1007/978-1-4614-3106-0_25,

Table 25.1 Diseases and problems producing disorders of episodic and semantic memory

Disorders of episodic memory	Disorders of semantic memory
Alzheimer's disease (early)	Alzheimer's disease (mid/late)
Amnesic mild cognitive impairment	Semantic dementia
Stroke (PCA, thalamic perforators)	Herpes simplex encephalitis
Aneurysm rupture/repair (ACoA)	Neurosyphilis
Cerebral anoxia	Stroke (MCA, PCA, cortical)
Wernicke–Korsakoff syndrome	Focal retrograde amnesia
Herpes simplex and HSV-6 encephalitis	Dissociative (psychogenic) amnesia
Autoimmune limbic encephalitis	
Traumatic brain injury	
Transient global amnesia (TGA)	
Electroconvulsive therapy (ECT)	
Dissociative (psychogenic) amnesia	

recent time periods than it is for memories acquired in the very remote past.

Neuropsychological research has clearly shown that lesions within the brain's extended memory system (medial temporal lobe, diencephalon, and basal forebrain) produce anterograde amnesia while leaving other aspects of memory (retrieval of general knowledge, vocabulary, names) relatively intact. This chapter focuses on one way of characterizing this difference, the distinction between "episodic" and "semantic" memory, and discusses the clinical features and assessment of disordered function in each of these two domains. A list of disorders producing primary impairments in episodic or semantic memory is provided in Table 25.1.

The Episodic–Semantic Distinction

The episodic–semantic distinction has historical roots dating back to William James [1]. Hebb's [2] proposed distinction between short-term and long-term memory, along with ubiquitous evidence from neuropsychological investigations of brain-damaged patients, gave rise to a variety of two-component models of memory, each attempting to characterize spared versus impaired memory function in amnesia. In 1972, Tulving [3] first distinguished between two memory systems ("episodic" and "semantic" memory). Although these two systems differ in content (episodic memory has come to be synonymous with memory for specific events and their context, while semantic memory involves general knowledge), the core difference involves the subjective experience of remembering associated with each system. Episodic memories are accompanied by an experience of autobiographical remembering (in Tulving's terms, self-knowing or "autonoetic"), while semantic memories lack this quality and are accompanied by a feeling of "knowing" rather than "remembering." Over time, the episodic–semantic distinction has been useful in explaining key characteristics of the human amnesic syndrome.

Spared Function in Amnesia

Many authors have argued that selective impairment of episodic, but not semantic, memory accounts for the finding that amnesic patients retain substantial intellectual, linguistic, and social skill despite profound impairments in the ability to recall specific information encountered in prior learning episodes [4–6].

Retrograde Amnesia

The episodic–semantic distinction may explain temporally graded retrograde amnesia [4]. Cermak suggested that, as biographical material ages, it becomes progressively more semantic. Through retelling, it becomes less tied to specific recollective episodes and increasingly incorporated into one's personal/family history or "folklore." More recent memories are less likely to have been retold or elaborated beyond their original form and thus may retain more of a distinct episodic quality.

If amnesia reflects a selective impairment in episodic memory, then memories from more remote time periods would be relatively more semantic and relatively spared as a result of this process.

Anatomy of Memory

The episodic–semantic distinction is broadly consistent with anatomic facts. Lesions to the brain's extended memory system (hippocampus/medial temporal lobe, diencephalon, and basal forebrain) predominantly produce episodic memory impairment, while cortical lesions to anterior temporal and parietal cortices tend to produce semantic memory impairments [7]. This distinction is further elucidated within a contemporary clinico-anatomic model of human memory called "Multiple Trace Theory" (MTT; [8]) that is reminiscent of Cermak's [4] ideas. MTT posits that as long as memories retain their episodic quality (e.g., autobiographical mode of recollection, context dependency, sensory-perceptual vividness), they remain hippocampus dependent. Each time an episodic memory is retrieved, it is subsequently re-encoded within the hippocampus and by dynamic networks of activation between the hippocampus and cortical processing areas. Activation of these networks leads to formation of multiple traces in a network that becomes increasingly distributed with each recollective episode. As a result, older episodic memories (i.e., those that have been retrieved numerous times in different contexts) are more widely distributed within the MTL than are recent ones, and different structures/regions within the MTL come to make their own contribution. Moreover, as the distributed network widens via multiple encodings, it eventually can become independent of the hippocampus and supported solely by neocortex. These memories lose their context dependency or autobiographic quality over time to the extent to which they have been retrieved in multiple contexts. By this process, some episodic memory can gradually become "semantic" in quality. Thus, semantic memory results at least in part from gradual transfer of memory from hippocampus-dependent networks to cortical ones.

Although it is tempting to regard anterograde amnesia as "episodic" and retrograde amnesia/remote memory disturbance as "semantic," evidence supports the view that both episodic and semantic memories can exist within each of these compartments. With respect to amnesia, MTT predicts that MTL damage will result in impairment of both recent and remote episodic memories, with more extensive damage leading to more extensive impairment. Although early studies with amnesic patients such as H.M. reportedly found largely intact remote memory, recent reevaluations support the existence of more extensive retrograde amnesia than previously thought (e.g., [9].).

Double Dissociation Between Episodic and Semantic Memory

If the episodic–semantic distinction reflects a general principle of brain organization, then these domains of memory should show double dissociation in cases of focal brain disease. While data described above provide ample evidence that episodic memory can be impaired in the absence of a deficit in semantic memory [3], what about the opposite? There have been several case reports demonstrating impaired semantic retrieval in the absence of a deficit in episodic/autobiographical retrieval [10–12]]. Several well-described cases of focal retrograde amnesia (i.e., disproportionately impaired retrograde memory with relatively spared anterograde memory) have also contributed to our understanding of the relationship between episodic and semantic memory [13–19]. In some cases [18], a distinction within remote memory has been found in which the patient is impaired in retrieval of general knowledge but unimpaired in retrieval of remote autobiographical events. Damage to the anterior temporal cortex is involved in most cases of focal retrograde amnesia, and damage to limbic-diencephalic structures contributes to impairment in remote "autobiographical" memory. However, not all cases of focal retrograde amnesia are clearly suggestive of an episodic–semantic distinction, since careful analysis of the memory loss in some cases reveals equivalent impairments in remote autobiographical memory and factual knowledge [20]. Finally, there is also ample evidence that a developmental impairment in episodic memory does not preclude the acquisition of factual knowledge or language competence during development [21]. The acquisition of semantic knowledge is largely independent from episodic memory processes and takes place through spared cortical regions subjacent to the hippocampi [21].

Although dissociations have been reported, amnesics can have both episodic and semantic impairments [22–26]. For example, Cermak et al. [23] found that Korsakoff patients had difficulty generating words from "conceptual" semantic memory ("name a fruit that is red"). Butters and colleagues [22] similarly found Korsakoff amnesics to be deficient on a verbal fluency task.

A fundamental problem is that episodic and semantic memories are not easily dissociable behaviorally [24] and may in some circumstances involve activation of the same or similar structures in functional imaging studies [27]. One confound is that they interact in complex ways (e.g., episodic learning can have a stimulating effect on semantic search rate; [28]).

As indicated earlier, multiple trace theory provides a contemporary reformulation of the episodic–semantic memory distinction within a functional-anatomic account of the activity of the hippocampal system. From the perspective of multiple memory systems accounts of spared and impaired function, MTT offers a promising way to conceptualize episodic and semantic memory as points on a processing continuum. Of equal importance, it provides a neurobiologically realistic model of memory dissociations that accounts for a large amount of clinical and research data.

Disorders of Episodic Memory

Clinical Features

The primary clinical features of episodic memory disorders have already been described and involve impairment in new learning (anterograde amnesia) and at least some degree of remote memory loss (retrograde amnesia). Depending upon etiology, remote memory loss can be worse for more recent time periods, confined to a specific time period or nonspecific [7]. As mentioned earlier, the classic amnesic syndrome is most commonly accompanied by relative sparing of intellectual and attentional ability, language, and other performance domains that rely on established knowledge. Memory function that is not dependent on conscious, explicit recollection (i.e., implicit memory) is also relatively spared.

Etiology

Serious episodic memory loss is a common problem in clinical neuropsychological evaluations and has considerable localizing significance. It is also a helpful diagnostic finding since it is a distinguishing feature of several neurological disorders. Episodic memory disorders impair functional capacity along a spectrum of severity, with only the most severe types qualifying as "amnesic." Below, we review some of the more important disorders.

Mild Cognitive Impairment

Recently, the concept of *mild cognitive impairment* (MCI) was introduced to describe older adults with a memory complaint in the context of normatively impaired memory, intact activities of daily living, generally intact cognitive function, and no dementia [29, 30]. At least three subtypes of MCI are widely recognized, including amnesic, multi-domain (encompassing more than one cognitive area), and single-domain nonamnesic, forms [30]. The primary importance of the MCI concept relates to its role as a possible prodromal stage of dementia. Longitudinal studies indicate that approximately 10–15% of patients with MCI convert to Alzheimer's disease each year, compared to overall conversion rates of 1–2% in cognitively normal elders [31]. Behavioral markers and concurrent presence of entorhinal and hippocampal atrophy appear to most strongly predict eventual conversion [32]. It is important to note that MCI encompasses both objective evidence and subjective report (often including an informant) of age-related memory impairment. Many objectively normal adults may complain of memory loss, particularly if they are in intellectually demanding positions. The isolated presence of a memory complaint without objective evidence may indicate the presence of depression or adjustment difficulties that are themselves worthy of independent clinical attention. By the same token, depression, anxiety, and other neuropsychiatric symptoms that may give rise to a subjective memory complaint are quite common in MCI [33].

Degenerative Disorders

Many degenerative dementias such as Pick's, Huntington's, and Parkinson's disease eventually affect memory, but Alzheimer's disease (AD) initially manifests with an episodic memory impairment [34]. Nearly all of the neural systems thought to be important in memory are affected by AD, including the medial temporal lobe [35–37], basal forebrain [38], thalamus [39], and neocortex. Memory impairment in Alzheimer's disease primarily affects episodic memory first but may also affect some aspects of semantic memory such as verbal fluency [40]. Eventually, semantic memory is more severely affected, as are other cognitive domains including language, visuoperceptual ability, and executive function. While the memory deficit seen in AD and other cortical dementias primarily involves episodic memory, significant loss of semantic memory can be seen in a variant of frontotemporal dementia, so-called semantic dementia [41, 42]. Thus, the memory loss found in AD and frontotemporal dementia is not as "pure" as in other forms of amnesia and takes place in the context of broader cognitive decline. Semantic dementia is discussed more fully below.

Effects of Anticholinergic Medication

Many commonly used medications have significant central anticholinergic actions, including antihistamines commonly used in nonprescription sleep and allergy medications, some antidepressants, and medications used to manage urinary frequency and incontinence. Anticholinergic drugs can impair memory [43], and withdrawal of these medications in patients with memory deficits may result in dramatic improvement in memory [44].

Vascular Disease

Stroke can produce amnesia when critical areas are infarcted. Strokes affecting the posterior cerebral artery territory (posterior medial temporal lobe and retrosplenial cortex; [45]) and the thalamic penetrating arteries [46] have been implicated, as has basal forebrain amnesia from anterior communicating artery aneurysm hemorrhage or surgery [47]. Infarction of the fornix with or without basal forebrain lesions can also present with isolated amnesia [48, 49]. In vascular cases, the onset of amnesia is abrupt. Improvement is variable, and patients may be left with serious permanent deficits, even following small infarctions.

Cerebral Anoxia

Depending upon the degree and duration of ischemia and/or hypoxia, neuronal loss may be widespread or very focal. Amnesia has been reported following cardiac arrest in which the only pathological feature identified was loss of neurons in field CA1 of the hippocampus [50]. Issues related to characterizing the extent of damage from anoxic or ischemic insults have been reviewed [51].

Wernicke–Korsakoff Syndrome

Alcoholic Korsakoff syndrome most frequently develops after years of alcohol abuse and nutritional deficiency [52–54] but can also result from chronic avitaminosis secondary to malabsorption syndromes [55] or in patients who refuse to eat in the context of a psychiatric disorder [56]. Patients first undergo an acute stage of the illness, Wernicke's encephalopathy, in which symptoms of confusion, disorientation, oculomotor dysfunction, and ataxia are present. After this resolves, amnesia can persist as a permanent symptom. Severe anterograde amnesia and an extensive, temporally graded retrograde amnesia are characteristic features. Substantial deficits in memory encoding, coupled with signs of frontal executive and visuospatial dysfunction are common.

Herpes Simplex and HSV-6 Encephalitis

Herpes simplex causes inflammation and necrosis, particularly in the orbitofrontal and inferior temporal regions. It thus involves limbic structures, including the hippocampus, parahippocampal gyrus, amygdala and overlying cortex, the polar limbic cortex, cingulate gyrus, and the orbitofrontal cortex [34]. Patients may present with personality change, confusion, headache, fever, and seizures and are often amnesic. Prompt treatment with antiviral agents can control the illness, and full recovery is possible. However, damage to the aforementioned structures often leaves the patient with severe anterograde and retrograde amnesia. The amnesic syndromes in patient D.R.B. (also known as Boswell; [57]) and patient S.S. [58, 59] have been particularly well characterized. Recent reports indicate that herpes simplex infection can occasionally lead to a syndrome of focal retrograde amnesia that is described more completely below [13, 60, 61]. Human herpes virus-6 (HHV-6) also can target the limbic system and present with amnesic syndromes, confusion, sleep disorders, and seizures [62]. Hokkanen and Launes [63] review other infectious agents that can leave residual neuropsychological sequelae, including memory loss.

Autoimmune Limbic Encephalitis

This condition usually presents with personality change, agitation, and amnesic symptoms. It was first described as a paraneoplastic syndrome [64–67], but it can also occur in patients without neoplasm [68]. Over the past decade, several autoantibodies have been associated with different forms of limbic encephalitis (see [69, 70]). Neuronal antibodies (Hu, Ma2, CV2/CRMP5, amphiphysin, and atypical intracellular antibodies) in patients with various neoplasms (small cell and non-small cell lung cancer, testicular tumors, thymomas, and others) have been associated with an inflammatory disorder affecting neurons throughout the neuraxis but often with particular intensity in limbic structures including the hippocampus. Although the pathogenesis is autoimmune, response to immunotherapy is usually poor. However, patients with Ma-2 antibodies in association with testicular cancers often improve after surgery. Patients with antibodies to voltage-gated potassium channels (VGKC), sometimes associated with thymoma or small cell lung cancer, but more often without known neoplasm, can have a more selective limbic encephalitis that often responds to immunotherapy with steroids, IVIG, or plasma exchange [68]. A syndrome of amnesia, psychosis, seizures, and central hypoventilation progressing to coma has been attributed to antibodies that react with NMDA receptors [71], and this syndrome may respond dramatically to immunotherapy. Although first described in association with neoplasms, only 60% of a large series had cancer [72], and the same syndrome has now been reported in children, many without neoplasms [73]. Similar autoantibodies have been identified in patients with epilepsy and systemic lupus [74].

Trauma

Following closed head injury, patients may have an acute anterograde and retrograde amnesia, the duration of which correlates with the severity of the injury as measured by the Glasgow Coma Scale or the duration of unconsciousness [75]. The duration of posttraumatic amnesia (memory for ongoing events after trauma) is a good predictor of long-term functional outcome [76–78]. The retrograde amnesia typically improves along with improvement in anterograde amnesia, providing evidence that a retrieval deficit is responsible for the portion of the retrograde memory loss that recovers. Residual memory impairment is usually a feature of broader cognitive and attentional impairment, but it can be prominent with severe injuries [79, 80]. Pathological changes are variable and widespread. Memory dysfunction may be caused by anterior temporal lobe contusions, temporal lobe white matter necrosis, or diffuse axonal disruption [75, 81]. Cases of focal retrograde amnesia in the relative absence of a new learning defect have been reported after closed head trauma [15, 16].

Transient Global Amnesia

This distinctive form of amnesia begins suddenly and typically resolves within a day [82–85]. A severe impairment in new learning and patchy loss of information learned prior to onset is seen.

The patient often asks repetitive questions and may be aware of the memory deficit. After resolution, neuropsychological testing is usually normal except for amnesia for the episode [84]. Although the etiology of transient global amnesia (TGA) is unclear, epilepsy [86–88], emotional stress [89], occlusive cerebrovascular disease [90, 91], migrainous vasospasm [83, 92, 94] head trauma [95], vertebrobasilar dyscontrol [82], and venous insufficiency [96] have all been mentioned as possibilities. There are now many reports of small diffusion-weighted imaging (DWI) abnormalities in CA1 of the hippocampus in patients with TGA within the first 48 h [97–100]; these lesions typically are transient [101, 102] and are more likely to be evident after 24–48 h of symptom onset (and hence, after resolution in the majority of patients). The striking predilection of these punctate lesions for the lateral hippocampus leaves little doubt as to their relevance to the clinical findings; however, their pathogenesis remains enigmatic. Although the DWI characteristics are suggestive of ischemia, patients with TGA do not appear to be at greater risk for cerebrovascular disease than controls [83, 103]. Epileptic TGA [104, 105] usually has a shorter duration, is more likely to recur, and may be associated with EEG abnormalities.

Electroconvulsive Therapy

Used for relief of depression, electroconvulsive therapy (ECT) can produce rapidly recovering anterograde and temporally limited retrograde amnesia [106–108]. More severe impairment is seen after bilateral versus unilateral application. The anterograde defect is related in severity to the number of treatments and is characterized by rapid forgetting and poor delayed recall [109]. Substantial, often complete, recovery takes place in the few months after treatment ends [107, 110, 111]. The retrograde amnesia appears to be temporally limited, involving only the few years prior to treatment onset. It, too, recovers almost completely in the months after treatment [112, 113]. Though the data is by no means clear, some authors have suggested that ECT-induced memory loss models bilateral temporal lobe disease [109].

Dissociative (Psychogenic) Amnesias

Psychologically induced loss of memory may be normal, as in amnesia for events of childhood [114–116] or for events during sleep [117]. Alternatively, they may be pathological, as in the amnesias associated with dissociative states, multiple personality, or with simulated amnesia [118–120]. A striking loss of personal autobiographical memory is a hallmark of functional amnesia, and amnesia for one's own name (in the absence of aphasia or severe cognitive dysfunction in other spheres) is seen exclusively in this form of memory loss. Retrograde loss is often disproportionate to anterograde amnesia, and some patients will demonstrate loss of skills or other procedural memories typically retained by organic amnesic patients. Some studies have reported disproportionate loss of "personal" as opposed to "public" information in the retrograde compartment [121], a fact that is discussed in terms of the episodic–semantic distinction by Reinhold and Markowitsch [122]. A good general review is provided by Kihlstrom and Schacter [123].

Disorders of Semantic Memory

Clinical Features

In contrast to the patient with episodic memory impairment, the patient with semantic memory loss finds it difficult to retrieve and use previously stored factual, linguistic, or perceptual knowledge. The impairment may affect the comprehension or production of words, concepts, facts, semantic relationships, and general knowledge. Episodic memory, though not entirely normal, is relatively spared, and the patient typically has no great disability in learning and retrieving knowledge of ongoing day-to-day events. A closer look at the pattern of disruption over time reveals that the loss of semantic knowledge initially affects the ability to retrieve specific exemplars within broad categories and the patient may be capable eventually of identifying only typical items that show high family resemblance of their parent category. The disorder affects naming, language comprehension, expressive and receptive vocabulary, and fact retrieval. Behavioral changes coincident with semantic loss may occur and may include withdrawal, a reduction in interests, or the development of new preferences for food or activity [124], but these are not typically predominant features or reasons for referral.

Although disorders of semantic memory are typically nonspecific (i.e., do not differentially affect specific semantic categories), several well-described cases of category-specific semantic deficits have left little doubt that selective loss of semantic memory exists. Warrington and Shallice [125] reported four cases of category-specific semantic loss for living versus nonliving things after partial recovery from herpes simplex encephalitis. Since Warrington and Shallice's initial demonstration, a large literature has accumulated showing that *selective impairment of living things* is most common [126]. Substantial literature has examined the implications of category specificity for understanding the organization of semantic memory. While these cases are most consistent with a categorical, meaning-based organization of the memory store, other data either indicate that category specificity can be accommodated within a modality-specific semantic network affecting visually based category distinctions [127] or which outright favor a more interactive, modality-specific view [128]. Category specificity is relatively rare (fewer than 150 reported cases exist) and is most common after herpes simplex encephalitis. It is not commonly seen in degenerative conditions that produce semantic memory impairments, including Alzheimer's disease [129] and semantic dementia [130].

Etiology

Semantic memory impairments are seen in a variety of disease states, with the most common causes being degenerative disease (semantic dementia variant of frontotemporal dementia, mid-stage Alzheimer's disease) or a post-acute outcome of CNS infection (herpes simplex encephalitis; HSVE). These diseases affect semantic memory differently and each presents with a unique neuropsychological profile and associated comorbidities. However, all of these diseases are associated with relatively intact somatosensory and motor abilities, procedural memory, verbal abilities, and visuospatial skills. As such, knowledge of the disease course, outcome, neurologic and neuropsychological profile, and treatment are all necessary in order to successfully complete a differential diagnosis and provide effective medical care to affected patients. All three of these diseases affect the neural substrates that mediate semantic memory, primarily the temporal cortex. Both lateral and medial structures of the temporal lobe that are involved in the encoding, consolidation, and retrieval of semantic information can be affected. The semantic memory impairment seen in these conditions is briefly reviewed below.

Semantic Dementia

Semantic dementia (SD) is one of three prominent subtypes of frontotemporal dementia (progressive nonfluent aphasia and behavioral variant are the others), which results from frontotemporal lobar degeneration. Patients with SD may present with word-finding difficulties, aphasia, anomia, visual associative agnosia, or impaired understanding of semantic words and images. Pathologically, most patients have ubiquitin-positive, tau-negative inclusion bodies, though some may have pathology consistent with Pick's disease or Alzheimer's disease [124, 131].

The most prominent early feature in semantic dementia is the reduction of expressive vocabulary, commonly described as a "loss of memory for words" [132, 133]. Episodic memory problems may also be present but are typically mild in comparison [134]. Receptive vocabulary also deteriorates, though changes may be subtle initially. As the disease progresses, spontaneous speech becomes increasingly anomic, with word-finding pauses and substitution of more generic words (e.g., "thing") for specific lexical items [124]. Many patients with SD also have defective *person knowledge*, manifested in impairments in naming people, generating information about them from their names or faces, and, in severe cases, recognizing the identity of faces or determining whether they are familiar [124].

Alzheimer's Disease (Later Stages)

AD begins focally in the transentorhinal cortex of the temporal lobe, affecting the hippocampus early in the disease. As the disease progresses, pathological features move in a posterior and lateral fashion to affect the lateral temporal lobe, basal forebrain, thalamus, and neocortex of the parietal and frontal lobes, ultimately affecting virtually all areas thought to be important for memory. Because of increasing cortical involvement later in the disease, a broad spectrum of neuropsychological deficits may eventually emerge. In the later stages of the disease, executive function, language, and even postural stability and gait may be affected.

Semantic memory impairment in AD may be reflected in reduced receptive vocabulary and reduced ability to retrieve and understand words [135]. The impairment is greater for more recently acquired words than for words learned earlier in life [136], which has been postulated to result from the richer semantic embeddedness of earlier-acquired words [137, 138]. A recent study suggested that this effect was related to the degree of involvement in left anterior temporal neocortex as measured by voxel-based morphometry [139].

How does the semantic impairment in AD compare to that of SD? A recent longitudinal study by Xie et al. [140] showed that, while SD and AD patients were not different early in the disease, the semantic impairment in SD eventually outstripped that seen in AD later on. In this study, the SD patients performed more poorly than AD on semantic memory at all time points, whereas measures of episodic memory, initially worse in AD, eventually converged as the diseases progressed. A recent study suggested that SD patients performed more poorly than AD patients on word sorting and naming tests from the Cambridge Semantic Memory Test (CMST), though the overall test was not able to differentiate the groups [40]. Particularly, in early stages of the disease, substantial overlap in deficits might exist. However, it is reasonable to postulate that episodic memory impairments typically exceed semantic memory impairments in early AD, while the reverse is true of SD. Tests of other functions (e.g., visuospatial function) differentially affected in AD versus SD might prove useful in differential diagnosis. The Adlam et al. [40] study suggests that, despite some semantic memory impairment in AD [141, 142] and episodic memory difficulties in SD [143], the two groups can be differentiated when measures of the two types of memory are combined with measures of visuospatial ability.

Herpes Simplex Encephalitis

HSE is an acute inflammation and necrosis of the brain resulting from a herpes simplex virus-1 strain infection of the limbic structures, including the hippocampus, parahippocampal gyrus amygdala and overlying cortex, polar limbic cortex, cingulate gyrus, and the orbitofrontal cortex. HSE often presents acutely with fever, personality changes, confusion, seizures, hemiparesis, and headaches. In the post-acute period, HSE is associated with a range of neuropsychological impairments owing to the typically bilateral, though sometimes asymmetrical, medial, and lateral temporal lobe involvement. Remote memory is typically impaired with a "flat" temporal gradient [144]. Episodic and semantic memory can both be profoundly impaired, including the ability to retrieve remote autobiographical information [61]. Classic amnesic syndromes after HSE have been reported by McCarthy and Warrington [145] and Cermak [58, 59].

Some HSE cases suffer a more restricted impairment of semantic memory, often in the form of a category-specific deficit. Most commonly reported are patients who have selective impairment in accessing information pertaining to "living things" [146], though the opposite has been found and methodological issues in defining "category specificity" may be useful for the clinician to consider [147]. The fact that category specificity is seen more commonly after HSE (which predominantly affects anteromedial temporal cortex) than it is in SD (which involves more anterolateral temporal cortex) is intriguing. Noppeney et al. [148] suggest that the medial temporal cortex may represent semantic categories that are more interrelated (in their words, "tightly packed") in semantic space, while the lateral temporal cortex might play a more general semantic role.

Other Etiologies

Other forms of brain disease can produce semantic memory deficits (e.g., neurosyphilis, stroke), usually in the context of other impairments that correlate with the site of damage. Capitani et al. [149] found that 12 of 18 patients with left posterior cerebral artery stroke involving the fusiform gyrus displayed semantically based naming deficits and 5 showed distinct category specificity. Half of the left PCA patients showed additional deficits in verbal semantic knowledge. Unlike the majority of HSE cases, who showed differential impairments for animals, some of the left PCA patients showed distinct impairments in naming plants, with relative sparing of animals. Other cases are the result of trauma affecting orbitofrontal and anterolateral temporal regions or reflect comorbid symptoms of serious neurologic disturbances (e.g., brain tumor). In general, the clinician should be aware of the fact that most patients with significant semantic memory impairments have (typically bilateral) damage to the lateral anterior temporal lobe or parietotemporal association cortex, and should clinically evaluate semantic memory with appropriate tests in any patient who has damage within these regions.

Clinical Examination

Pre-examination interview of the patient suspected of having semantic memory impairment is critical and offers insight into the broad cognitive domain in which impairment is suspected. Critical data include age, mode of onset (acute vs. insidious), progression of cognitive decline, duration, and degree of impairment in activities of daily living. The onset of the impairment should be clearly determined along with its course (remitting, stable, or progressive). An insidious onset suggests a dementia such as AD or SD-FTD. An acute onset suggests an infectious, vascular, or traumatic origin. HSE can occur at any time point across the adult lifespan whereas dementia typically begins primarily after the age of 40. Within the degenerative disorders, a younger age of onset has been associated with SD which has a mean age of onset of 59 or FTD which has a mean age of onset of 63 [150]. Although there are exceptions, AD tends to onset later. The mean age of onset of AD is 68, with early onset defined as that which begins prior to the age of 60 and late onset that which begins after 65 years of age [151]. Acute onset of febrile illness followed by more chronic semantic memory impairment should suggest an infectious process such as HSE. Conversely, gradual, progressive impairment of semantic memory most likely signals a neurodegenerative process. HSE can remit and often does so in a pattern of alternative remission and relapse. HSE can be effectively treated, and when treated, survival is assured in the significant majority of cases. However, survivors can be left with a range of impairments from complete recovery to mild impairment from restricted impairment of language or memory to severe dementia [152]. In terms of independent activities of daily living (IADLs), patients with AD will be initially impaired by episodic memory failure, while those with SD or HSE may lose the ability to follow customary routines or to understand key concepts such as finances. The pattern of loss should be ascertained during the clinical interview and should inform test selection during the neuropsychological examination.

While a fixed battery of tests is attractive due to broad applicability to research databases and to ease of comparison with existing norms and already evaluated patient populations, it is not common to include comprehensive tests of semantic memory in standard neuropsychological batteries. In the patient suspected of semantic memory impairment, a well-validated battery of tests, the Cambridge Semantic Memory Test (CSMT) Battery, can be used to parse semantic from autobiographical memory impairment and can determine whether the impairment is modality or category specific. Good normative data exists. However, while the CSMT is useful for evaluation of the type and nature of semantic memory deficits, it is not sufficiently sensitive to differentiate advanced AD from SD [40]. Additionally, research has shown that the Four Mountains Test, a compilation of a topographical perception task with a topographical short-term memory task and a nonspatial perception and related short-term memory task, is a sensitive measure than can be used to distinguish AD from FTD [153]. These authors showed that patients with AD and amnesic MCI were impaired on the topographical short-term memory task but not on perception when compared to the FTD participants. While the non-topographical task revealed no group differences, this task suggests that short-term memory for topographical information can be impaired in AD, regardless of stage of disease, and is therefore a useful diagnostic measure [153].

The neuropsychologist should be aware that differential diagnosis depends critically on the relative patterning of semantic memory deficits compared to other aspects of the performance profile. SD will tend to exhibit semantic language impairments and executive dysfunction early in the disease in the context of intact visuospatial skills and relatively intact episodic memory. By the time AD patients exhibit disabling semantic memory impairments, their episodic memory problems will be quite significant, but they may show relatively preserved language and visuospatial skills and varying executive function that declines as a function of disease progression. HSE-related semantic memory deficits more commonly are category specific, such that selection of standard neuropsychological tests may be insufficient to disclose their deficit. Standardized tests of semantic memory are critical in evaluating these patients. HSE affects executive functioning while leaving language and visuospatial skills primarily intact.

Regardless of the preferred type of battery, special considerations and techniques should be employed when assessing potential semantic memory deficits. "Testing the limits" should be employed when working with patients who do not perform the tasks in the allotted time but who are capable of completing the tasks given enough time. Since speed of memory retrieval is often a sign of a degraded semantic memory system, relaxing time constraints allows the clinician to investigate the boundaries of a patient's capability. Although many other factors are involved, improvement with relaxation of time constraints suggests some deficit in semantic access, while lack of improvement may indicate a loss of semantic representations.

SD is the primary cause of semantic language impairment in FTD. Language should be fully assessed to rule out other forms of FTD (e.g., behavioral variant, progressive nonfluent aphasia). The concomitant, equal impairment of production *and* comprehension may distinguish SD from progressive nonfluent aphasia. Standardized aphasia batteries (Western Aphasia Battery, Boston Diagnostic Aphasia Examination) provide an overview of performance that can be supplemented by individual tests of naming (Boston Naming Test), auditory comprehension (Token Test), semantic processing (Pyramids and Palm Trees, a subtest of the Cambridge Semantic Memory Test), grammar and syntax (Test for Recognition of Grammar), repetition (Western Aphasia Battery), fluency (Controlled Oral Word Association, DKEFS Fluency), and tests of writing and reading. SD patients have been shown to exhibit more significant impairment on the Boston Naming Test than either FTD or AD patients [154]. The COWA is particularly useful, as research suggests that temporal lobe-damaged patients and AD patients perform worse on semantic fluency measures (e.g., fruits/vegetables) than on letter fluency (e.g., S). Patients with frontal lobe disease tend to perform worse on letter fluency than on semantic fluency, due to the increased demand on strategic retrieval processes [155]. However, this discrepancy was observed only when fruits and the letter S were used. No group differences were observed when animals and the letter F were compared. This finding illustrates the necessity of a broad assessment of language so that such potential confounds may be more fully understood.

In cases where remote memory/knowledge is affected, the assessment should be sufficiently thorough to enable an understanding of the type of memory impaired (autobiographical vs. semantic), time of memory impaired (remote vs. retrograde vs. anterograde amnesia), and whether or not the memory deficit is context specific. First, it must be established that the memory impairment is one of semantic memory rather than autobiographical memory. This can be achieved by using such batteries as the Wechsler Memory Scale (WMS-IV), which are composed of measures designed to assess the full range of memory domains. Additional standardized measures of episodic memory include the Hopkins Verbal Learning Test, the California Verbal Learning Test—II, the Rey Complex Figure, the Continuous Visual Memory Test, and the Brief Visual Memory Test—Revised. Focused measures which assess either autobiographical or semantic memory are available as well. For remote autobiographical memory, the Crovitz task ("describe an event from your past that involved a 'flag'"), the Autobiographical Memory Interview [156], or Squire's TV Test [157] may be useful, though clinicians are cautioned about the lack of precise normative data. General tests of vocabulary (WAIS-IV) are useful, as are tests of factual event knowledge that require patients to identify famous faces (Famous Faces Task; Presidents Test) or to show knowledge of well-known public events from different decades that were not part of their personal life experience (Boston Remote Memory Battery). By assessing the patient's ability to recognize and recall information that is not bound to their own life-event memory, these tasks measure deficits in semantic memory. While semantic memory can be impaired in AD and SD, episodic, autobiographical knowledge is an early sign of AD. Both episodic and semantic memory can be impaired in varying extents in HSE. Semantic memory impairments that are not language bound in terms of either perception or production and are also not context specific are more likely the result of AD. Both FTD and AD have been shown to be impaired on verbal memory tasks; AD may be more likely to display visual memory deficits [154]. HSE and focal stroke are the most likely disorders to produce a category-specific semantic memory impairment, and the clinician should, if necessary, develop in-house tests to informally assess for this possibility if more extensive, standardized tests of semantic memory are unavailable

Assessing executive function can be useful for further differentiating SD-FTD from AD. Common measures include Wisconsin Card Sort Test (WCST), The Delis–Kaplan Executive Functioning Scales, the Category Test, the Stroop Color Word Test, and measures of motor organization and inhibition (Luria's contrasting programs, Go–No Go, recursive figures and serial hand sequences). Ideally, executive functioning should be assessed as part of any neuropsychological evaluation and is important in the investigation of semantic memory impairment. As executive function is primarily mediated by frontal lobe structures, and SD is a subset of frontal lobar degeneration, executive dysfunction is common in SD patients. However, this does not necessarily distinguish SD from AD or HSE, since some executive dysfunction should be expected in association with all etiologies we have discussed, particularly in later disease stages. HSE often presents with comorbid personality changes and alterations in consciousness, and later-stage AD frequently involves personality changes, disinhibition, emotional lability, and apathy.

Other Neurodiagnostic Considerations

In most cases, neuropsychologists who are asked to evaluate patients with episodic and semantic memory disorders will function within an interdisciplinary team that includes specialty physicians (neurologists, psychiatrists, neurosurgeons). It is obvious that the neurobehavioral workup of these patients should supplement available neurodiagnostic information from the neurologic and physical exam, laboratory studies, and neuroradiologic investigations. Neuroimaging data suggest that both SD and HSE involve pathological changes in similar, though not identical regions. HSE often results in bilateral anterior temporal damage extending into the amygdala and may include gray matter atrophy in the medial structures of the anterior temporal lobe and the insula. These medial structures are relatively spared in SD; atrophy is more commonly observed in the lateral temporal cortex, either unilaterally or bilaterally. The hallmark of early onset AD is focal hippocampal atrophy that is often readily apparent on MRI. Finally, genetic testing can add informative but not definitive data to a diagnostic profile. Carriers of the apolipoprotein E ε4 allele (*APOE* ε4) have been found to be at increased risk for developing AD; the *APOE* ε2 allele has been suggested to serve a protective effect against the development of AD. Simply having an *APOE* ε4 allele does not denote future development of AD, but this information can be added to a preponderance of evidence during a dementia consensus debate. Parallel developments in the genetics and neurohistochemistry of frontotemporal dementia are beginning to elucidate specific genetic and immunohistochemical markers that might be useful in the differential diagnosis of SD and other FTD variants [158].

As has been demonstrated, there are numerous etiologies of acquired and degenerative semantic memory impairment, each with a unique disease onset, course and neuropsychological profile, and numerous tools to measure and evaluate these deficits. Thorough understanding and implementation of appropriate measures, as well as educated

Table 25.2 Evaluation of episodic and semantic memory disorders

Domain	Test	Norms	AFP[a]?	Reference
Episodic/recent memory				
Verbal memory	WMS-IV Logical Memory	√	√	Wechsler et al. [159]
	Hopkins Verbal Learning Test-Revised	√	√	Benedict et al. [160]
	California Verbal Learning Test—II	√	√	Delis et al. [161]
	Rey Auditory Verbal Learning Test	√	√	Schmidt [162]
Nonverbal memory	WMS-IV Visual Reproduction	√	√	Wechsler et al. [159]
	Rey Complex Figure	√	√	Meyers and Meyers [163]
	Brief Visual Memory Test	√	√	Benedict [164]
	Continuous Visual Memory Test	√	√	Trahan and Larrabee [165]
Prospective memory	Cambridge Test of Prospective Memory	√	√	Wilson et al. [166]
Episodic/remote memory	Crovitz Paradigm			Crovitz and Schiffman [167]
	Autobiographical Memory Interview	+/−	√	Kopelman et al. [156]
	TV Test, Remote events test			Squire and Slater [157]
Semantic memory	Cambridge Semantic Memory Test	√	PPT[b]	Adlam et al. [40]
	WAIS-IV Vocabulary, Information	√	√	Wechsler et al. [168]
Language/semantic processing	Western Aphasia Battery—Revised	√	√	Kertesz [169]
	Boston Diagnostic Aphasia Examination	√	√	Goodglass et al. [170]
	Boston Naming Test	√	√	Goodglass et al. [170]
	Controlled Oral Word Association	√	√	Benton et al. [171]
	DKEFS Fluency	√	√	Delis et al. [172]
	Test for Reception of Grammar	√	√	Bishop [173]
	Reading, Writing Tests			Various available
Executive functioning	Wisconsin Card Sorting Test	√	√	Grant and Berg [174]
	Booklet Category Test	√	√	DeFilippis and McCampbell [175]
	Delis–Kaplan Executive Functioning Scales	√	√	Delis et al. [172]
	Stroop Test	√	√	Stroop [176]
	Luria Motor Programming			Luria [177]

[a]Denotes whether test is available for purchase on the commercial market
[b]The Pyramid and Palm Trees Test (a subtest of the CSMT) is commercially available

and concise interaction between health care providers, is essential for the proper evaluation, diagnosis, and treatment of amnesic syndromes.

Clinical Pearls

- Evaluation of patients with suspected episodic or semantic memory disorders should always include the participation of a collateral informant who can verify the patient's report, which may appear accurate to the naïve examiner.
- Examination of the patient with episodic memory impairment should be capable of separating encoding, retention, and retrieval processes through the use of multiple tests.
- Virtually any neurologic disorder above the cervical vertebrae can affect episodic memory function; diagnosis typically relies on interdisciplinary evaluation.
- Although the commonly used neuropsychological tests are capable of screening for aspects of semantic memory dysfunction (e.g., vocabulary, fluency measures), systematic evaluation of semantic memory disorders will typically require the use of instruments specifically designed for this purpose (see text).
- Episodic memory is most affected by disease processes affecting the medial temporal lobe, diencephalon, and basal forebrain, while semantic memory is most affected by cortical dysfunction.
- Episodic and semantic memories are distinguished primarily as different modes of retrieval; episodic memory has an autobiographical character, while semantic memory does not.
- The clinician should keep in mind that the episodic–semantic memory distinction is not the same as the recent–remote memory distinction. Episodic memories can be quite old and retrieved from the remote compartment, just as new semantic memories are acquired all of the time (Table 25.2).

References

1. James W. The principles of psychology. New York: Dover; 1890.
2. Hebb DO. The organization of behavior: a neuropsychological theory. New York: Wiley; 1949.
3. Tulving E. Episodic and semantic memory. In: Tulving E, Donaldson W, editors. Organization of memory. New York: Academic; 1972. p. 381–403.
4. Cermak LS. The episodic-semantic distinction in amnesia. In: Squire L, Butters N, editors. Neuropsychology of memory. New York: Guilford Press; 1984. p. 55–62.
5. Kinsbourne M, Wood F. Short-term memory processes and the amnesic syndrome. In: Deutsch D, Deutsch JA, editors. Short-term memory. New York: Academic; 1975. p. 258–91.
6. Weingartner H, Grafman J, Boutelle W, Kaye W, Martin P. Forms of cognitive failure. Science. 1983;221:380–2.
7. Bauer R, Reckess G, Kumar A, Valenstein E. Amnesic disorders. In: Heilman KM, Valenstein E, editors. Clinical neuropsychology. 5th ed. New York: Oxford University Press; 2011.
8. Moscotitch M, Rosenbaum RS, Gilboa A, Addis DR, Westmacott R, Grady CL, et al. Functional neuroanatomy of remote episodic, semantic, and spatial memory: A unified account based on multiple trace theory. Journal of Anatomy. 2005;207:35–66.
9. Steinvorth S, Levine B, Corkin S. Medial temporal lobe structures are needed to re-experience remote autobiographical memories: Evidence from H.M. & W.R. Neuropsychologia. 2005;43:479–96.
10. De Renzi E, Liotti M, Nichelli P. Semantic amnesia with preservation of autobiographic memory. A case report. Cortex. 1987;23(4):575–97.
11. Grossi D, Trojano L, Grasso A, Orsini A. Selective "semantic amnesia" after closed-head injury. A case report. Cortex. 1988;24(3):457–64.
12. Yasuda K, Watanabe O, Ono Y. Dissociation between semantic and autobiographic memory: a case report. Cortex. 1997;33(4):623–38.
13. Carlesimo GA, Sabbadini M, Loasses A, Caltagirone C. Analysis of the memory impairment in a post-encephalitic patient with focal retrograde amnesia. Cortex. 1998;34(3):449–60.
14. Hodges JR, McCarthy RA. Loss of remote memory: a cognitive neuropsychological perspective. Curr Opin Neurobiol. 1995;5(2):178–83.
15. Hunkin NM, Parkin AJ, Bradley VA, Burrows EH, Aldrich FK, Jansari A, Burdon-Cooper C. Focal retrograde amnesia following closed head injury: a case study and theoretical account. Neuropsychologia. 1995;33(4):509–23.
16. Kapur N, Ellison D, Smith MP, McLellan DL, Burrows EH. Focal retrograde amnesia following bilateral temporal lobe pathology. A neuropsycho-

logical and magnetic resonance study. Brain. 1992;115(Pt 1):73–85.
17. Kapur N, Young A, Bateman D, Kennedy P. Focal retrograde amnesia: a long term clinical and neuropsychological follow-up. Cortex. 1989;25(3): 387–402.
18. Markowitsch HJ, Calabrese P, Neufeld H, Gehlen W, Durwen HF. Retrograde amnesia for world knowledge and preserved memory for autobiographic events. A case report. Cortex. 1999;35(2):243–52.
19. O'Connor M, Butters N, Miliotis P, Eslinger P, Cermak LS. The dissociation of anterograde and retrograde amnesia in a patient with herpes encephalitis. J Clin Exp Neuropsychol. 1992;14(2):159–78.
20. Kapur N. Syndromes of retrograde amnesia: a conceptual and empirical synthesis. Psychol Bull. 1999;125(6):800–25.
21. Vargha-Khadem F, Gadian DG, Watkins KE, Connelly A, Van Paesschen W, Mishkin M. Differential effects of early hippocampal pathology on episodic and semantic memory. Science. 1997;277(5324):376–80.
22 Butters N, Granholm E, Salmon E, Grant I, Wolfe J. Episodic and semantic memory: a comparison of amnesic and demented patients. J Exp Clin Neuropsychol. 1987;9:479–97.
23 Cermak LS, Reale L, Baker E. Alcoholic Korsakoff patients' retrieval from semantic memory. Brain Lang. 1978;5:215–26.
24. Squire LR, Zola SM. Episodic memory, semantic memory, and amnesia. Hippocampus. 1998;8(3):205–11.
25. Verfaellie M, Cermak LS. Acquisition of generic memory in amnesia. Cortex. 1994;30(2):293–303.
26. Zola-Morgan S, Cohen NJ, Squire LR. Recall of remote episodic memory in amnesia. Neuropsychologia. 1983;21:487–500.
27. Schacter DL, Wagner AD, Buckner RL. Memory systems of 1999. In: Tulving E, Craik FIM, editors. The Oxford handbook of memory. New York: Oxford University Press; 2000. p. 627–43.
28. Loftus EF, Cole W. Retrieving attribute and name information from semantic memory. J Exp Psychol. 1974;102:1116–22.
29. Petersen RC, Stevens J, Ganguli M, Tangalos EG, Cummings JL, DeKosky ST. Practice parameter: early detection of dementia: mild cognitive impairment (an evidence-based review): report of the Quality Standards Subcommittee of the American Academy of Neurology. Neurology. 2001;56:1133–42.
30. Petersen RC. Mild cognitive impairment: aging to Alzheimer's disease. New York: Oxford University Press; 2004.
31. Petersen RC. Mild cognitive impairment: transition between aging and Alzheimer's disease. Neurologia. 2000;15:93–101.
32. Devanand DP, Liu X, Tabert MH, Pradhaban G, Cuasay K, Bell K, et al. Combining early markers strongly predicts conversion from mild cognitive impairment to Alzheimer's disease. Biol Psychiatry. 2008;64:871–79.
33. Monastero R, Mangialasche F, Camarda C, Ercolani S, Camarda R. A systematic review of neuropsychiatric symptoms in mild cognitive impairment. J Alzheimers Dis. 2009;18:11–30.
34. Damasio AR, Tranel D, Damasio H. Amnesia caused by herpes simplex encephalitis, infarctions in basal forebrain, Alzheimer's disease, and anoxia/ischemia. In: Boller F, Grafman J, editors. Handbook of neuropsychology. Amsterdam: Elsevier; 1989. p. 149–66.
35. Hyman BT, Van Hoesen GW, Damasio AR, Barnes CL. Cell specific pathology isolates the hippocampal formation in Alzheimer's disease. Science. 1984;225:1168–70.
36. Jack CR, Petersen RC, Xu Y, O'Brien PC, Smith GE, Ivnik RJ, et al. Rate of medial temporal lobe atrophy in typical aging and Alzheimer's disease. Neurology. 1998;51:993–9.
37. Scott SA, DeKosky ST, Scheff SW. Volumetric atrophy of the amygdala in Alzheimer's disease: quantitative serial reconstruction. Neurology. 1991;41:351–6.
38. Whitehouse PJ, Price DL, Clark AW, Coyle JT, DeLong MR. Alzheimer disease: evidence for selective loss of cholinergic neurons in the nucleus baslis. Ann Neurol. 1981;10:122–6.
39. Xuereb JH, Perry RH, Candy JM, Perry EK, Marshall E, Bonham JR. Nerve cell loss in the thalamus in Alzheimer's disease and Parkinson's disease. Brain. 1991;114:1363–79.
40. Adlam A-L, Patterson K, Bozeat S, Hodges JR. The Cambridge Semantic Memory Test Battery: detection of semantic deficits in semantic dementia and Alzheimer's disease. Neurocase. 2010;16:193–207.
41. Bozeat S, Lambon Ralph MA, Patterson K, Garrard P, Hodges JR. Non-verbal semantic impairment in semantic dementia. Neuropsychologia. 2000;38:1207–15.
42. Davies RR, Halliday GM, Xuereb JH, Kril JJ, Hodges JR. The neural basis of semantic memory: evidence from semantic dementia. Neurobiol Aging. 2009;30(12):2043–52.
43. Drachman DA, Leavitt J. Human memory and the cholinergic system. A relationship to aging? Arch Neurol. 1974;30:113–21.
44. Womack KB, Heilman KM. Tolterodine and memory: dry but forgetful. Arch Neurol. 2003;60:771–3.
45. Benson DF, Marsden CD, Meadows JC. The amnesic syndrome of posterior cerebral artery occlusion. Acta Neurol Scand. 1974;50:133–45.
46. Graff-Radford NR, Tranel D, Van Hoesen GW, Brandt JP. Diencephalic amnesia. Brain. 1990;113:1–25.
47. Volpe BT, Hirst W. Amnesia following the rupture and repair of an anterior communicating artery aneurysm. J Neurol Neurosurg Psychiatry. 1983;46:704–9.
48. Part SA, Hahn JH, Kim JI, Na DL, Huh K. Memory deficits after bilateral anterior fornix infarction. Neurology. 2000;54:1379–82.
49. Renou P, Ducreux D, Batouche F, Denier C. Pure and acute Korsakoff syndrome due to a bilateral anterior

fornix infarction: A diffusion tensor tractography study. Arch Neurol. 2008;65:1252–53.
50. Zola-Morgan S, Squire LR, Amaral DG. Human amnesia and the medial temporal region: enduring memory impairment following a bilateral lesion limited to field CA1 of the hippocampus. J Neurosci. 1986;6:2950–67.
51. Squire LR, Zola SM. Ischemic brain damage and memory impairment: a commentary. Hippocampus. 1996;6(5):546–52.
52. Butters N. Alcoholic Korsakoff's syndrome: an update. Semin Neurol. 1984;4:226–44.
53. Butters N, Cermak LS. Alcoholic Korsakoff's syndrome: an information processing approach to amnesia. New York: Academic; 1980.
54. Victor M, Adams RD, Collins GH. The Wernicke-Korsakoff Syndrome. Philadelphia: F.A. Davis Co.; 1971.
55. Becker JT, Furman JMR, Panisset M, Smith C. Characteristics of the memory loss of a patient with Wernicke-Korsakoff's syndrome without alcoholism. Neuropsychologia. 1990;28:171–9.
56. Newman ME, Adityanjee A, Sobolewski E, Jampala VC. Wernicke-Korsakoff amnestic syndrome secondary to malnutrition in a patient with schizoaffective disorder. Neuropsychiatry Neuropsychol Behav Neurol. 1998;11(4):241–4.
57. Damasio AR, Eslinger PJ, Damasio H, Van Hoesen GW, Cornell S. Multimodal amnesic syndrome following bilateral temporal and basal forebrain damage. Arch Neurol. 1985;42:252–9.
58. Cermak LS. The encoding capacity of a patient with amnesia due to encephalitis. Neuropsychologia. 1976;14(3):11–326.
59. Cermak LS, O'Connor M. The anterograde and retrograde retrieval ability of a patient with amnesia due to encephalitis. Neuropsychologia. 1983;21:213–34.
60. Fujii T, Yamadori A, Endo K, Suzuki K, Fukatsu R. Disproportionate retrograde amnesia in a patient with herpes simplex encephalitis. Cortex. 1999; 35(5):599–614.
61. Tanaka Y, Miyazawa Y, Hashimoto R, Nakano I, Obayashi T. Postencephalitic focal retrograde amnesia after bilateral anterior temporal lobe damage. Neurology. 1999;53(2):344–50.
62. Wainwright MS, Martin PL, Morse RP, Lacaze M, Provenzale JM, Coleman RE, Morgan MA, Hulette C, Kurtzberg J, Bushnell C, Epstein L, Lewis DV. Human herpes virus 6 limbic encephalitis after stem cell transplantation. Ann Neurol. 2001;50:612–9.
63. Hokkanen L, Launes J. Neuropsychological sequelae of acute-onset sporadic viral encephalitis. Neuropsychol Rehabil. 2008;17(4–5):450–77.
64. Corsellis JA, Goldberg GJ, Norton AR. "Limbic encephalitis" and its association with carcinoma. Brain. 1968;91:481–96.
65. Khan N, Wieser HG. Limbic encephalitis: a case report. Epilepsy Res. 1994;17(2):175–81.
66. Martin RC, Haut MW, Goeta Kreisler K, Blumenthal D. Neuropsychological functioning in a patient with paraneoplastic limbic encephalitis. J Int Neuropsychol Soc. 1996;2(5):460–6.
67. Gultekin SH, Rosenfeld MR, Voltz R, Eichen J, Posner JB, Dalmau J. Paraneoplastic limbic encephalitis: neurological symptoms, immunological findings and tumor association in 50 patients. Brain. 2000;123:1481–94.
68. Bien CG, Schulze-Bonhage A, Deckert M, Urbach H, Helmstaedter C, Grunwalt T, Schaller C, Elger CE. Limbic encephalitis not associated with neoplasm as a cause of temporal lobe epilepsy. Neurology. 2000;55:1823–8.
69. Dalmau J, Bataller L. Clinical and immunological diversity of limbic encephalitis: a model for paraneoplastic neurological disorders. Hematol Oncol Clin North Am. 2006;20:1319–35.
70. Darnell RB, Poser JB. Autoimmune encephalopathy (editorial). Ann Neurol. 2009;66:1–2.
71. Nokura K, Yamamoto H, Okawara Y, Koga H, Osawa H, Sakai K. Reversible limbic encephalitis caused by ovarian teratoma. Acta Neurol Scand. 1997;95:367–73.
72. Dalmau J, Gleichman AJ, Hughes EG, Rossi JE, Peng X, Lai M, et al. Anti-NMDA-receptor encephalitis: Case series and analysis of the effects of antibodies. Lancet Neurol. 2008;7:1091–98.
73. Florance NR, Davis RL, Lam C, Szperka C, Zhou L, Ahmad S, Campen CJ, Moss H, Peter N, Gleichman AJ, Glasere CA, Lynch DR, Rosenfeld MR, Dalmau J. Anti-N-methyl-D-aspartate receptor (NMDAR) encephalitis in children and adolescents. Ann Neurol. 2009;66:11–8.
74. Levite M, Ganor Y. Autoantibodies to glutamate receptors can damage the brain in epilepsy, systemic lupus erythematosus and encephalitis. Expert Rev Neurother. 2008;8:1141–60.
75. Levin HS. Memory deficit after closed head injury. In: Boller F, Grafman J, editors. Handbook of neuropsychology, vol. 3. Amsterdam: Elsevier; 1989. p. 183–207.
76. Ownsworth T, McKenna K. Investigation of factors related to employment outcome following traumatic brain injury: a critical review and conceptual model. Disabil Rehabil. 2004;26:765–83.
77. Ponsford J, Draper K, Schonberger M. Functional outcome 10 years after traumatic brain injury: Its relationship with demographic, injury severity, and cognitive and emotional status. J Int Neuropsychol Soc. 2008;14:233–42.
78. Ponsford JL, Olver JH, Curran C, Ng K. Prediction of employment status 2 years after traumatic brain injury. Brain Inj. 1995;9:11–20.
79. Russell WR, Nathan PW. Traumatic amnesia. Brain. 1946;69:290–300.
80. Whitty CD, Zangwill OL, editors. Amnesia. London: Butterworths; 1977.

81. Vannorsdall TD, Cascella NG, Rao V, Pearlson GD, Gordon B, Schretlen DJ. A morphometric analysis of neuroanatomic abnormalities in traumatic brain injury. J Neuropsychiatry Clin Neurosci. 2010;22: 173–81.
82. Caplan LB. Transient global amnesia. In: Frederiks JAM, editor. Handbook of clinical neurology, vol. 1. Amsterdam: Elsevier; 1985. p. 205–18.
83. Hodges JR, Warlow CP. Syndromes of transient amnesia: towards a classification. A study of 153 cases. J Neurol Neurosurg Psychiatry. 1990;53:834–43.
84. Kritchevsky M. Transient global amnesia. In: Boller F, Grafman J, editors. Handbook of neuropsychology, vol. 3. Amsterdam: Elsevier; 1989. p. 167–82.
85. Kritchevsky M, Squire LR, Zouzounis JA. Transient global amnesia: characterization of anterograde and retrograde amnesia. Neurology. 1988;38:213–9.
86. Bilo L, Meo R, Ruosi P, de Leva MF, Striano S. Transient epileptic amnesia: an emerging late-onset epileptic syndrome. Epilepsia. 2009;50 Suppl 5: 58–61.
87. Fisher CM. Transient global amnesia: precipitating activities and other observations. Arch Neurol. 1982;39:605–8.
88. Fisher CM, Adams RD. Transient global amnesia. Trans Am Neurol Assoc. 1958;83:143–5.
89. Olesen J, Jørgensen MB. Leao's spreading depression in the hippocampus explains transient global amnesia: a hypothesis. Acta Neurol Scand. 1986;73:219–20.
90. Heathfield KWG, Croft PB, Swash M. The syndrome of transient global amnesia. Brain. 1973;96:729–36.
91. Shuping JR, Rollinson RD, Toole JF. Transient global amnesia. Ann Neurol. 1980;7:281–5.
92. Caplan L, Chedru F, Lhermitte F, Mayman C. Transient global amnesia and migraine. Neurology. 1981;31:1167–70.
93. Schmidtke K, Ehmsen L. Transient global amnesia and migraine. A case control study. European Neurol. 2008;40:9--14.
94. Tosi L, Righetti CA. Transient global amnesia and migraine in young people. Clin Neurol Neurosurg. 1997;99:63–65.
95. Haas DC, Ross GS. Transient global amnesia triggered by mild head trauma. Brain. 1986;109:251–7.
96. Chung C-P, Hsu H-Y, Chao A-C, Chang F-C, Sheng W-Y, Hu H-H. Detection of intracranial venous reflux in patients of transient global amnesia. Neurology. 2006;66:1873–7.
97. Alberici E, Pichiecchio A, Caverzasi E, Farina LM, Persico A, Cavallini A, Bastianello S. Transient global amnesia: hippocampal magnetic resonance imaging abnormalities. Funct Neurol. 2008;23:149–52.
98. Ay H, Furie KL, Yamada K, Koroshetz WJ. Diffusion-weighted MRI characterizes the ischemic lesion in transient global amnesia. Neurology. 1998;51:901–3.
99. Woolfenden AR, O'Brien MW, Schwartzberg RE, Norbash AM, Tong DC. Diffusion-weighted MRI in transient global amnesia precipitated by cerebral angiography. Stroke. 1997;28:2311–4.
100. Bartsch T, Deuschl G. Transient global amnesia: functional anatomy and clinical implications. Lancet Neurol. 2010;9:205–14.
101. Sedlaczek O, Hirsch JG, Grips E, Peters CN, Gass A, Wöhrle J, Hennerici M. Detection of delayed focal MR changes in the lateral hippocampus in transient global amnesia. Neurology. 2004;62:2165–70.
102. Toledo M, Pujadas R, Grivé E, Álvarez-Sabin J, Quintana M, Rovira A. Lack of evidence for arterial ischemia in transient global amnesia. Stroke. 2008;39:476–9.
103. Miller JW, Petersen RC, Metter EJ, Millikan CH, Yanagihara T. Transient global amnesia: clinical characteristics and prognosis. Neurology. 1987;37:733–7.
104. Kapur N. Transient epileptic amnesia—a clinical update and reformulation. J Neurol Neurosurg Psychiatry. 1993;56:1184–90.
105. Butler CR, Zeman A. A case of transient epileptic amnesia with radiological localization. Nat Clin Pract Neurol. 2008;4:516–21.
106. Sackeim HA. The cognitive effects of electroconvulsive therapy. In: Moos WH, Gamzu ER, Thal LJ, editors. Cognitive disorders: pathophysiology and treatment. New York, NY: Marcel Dekker; 1992. p. 183–228.
107. Semkovska M, McLoughlin DM. Objective cognitive performance associated with electroconvulsive therapy for depression: a systematic review and meta-analysis. Biol Psychiatry. 2010;15:568–77.
108. Squire LR. A stable impairment in remote memory following electroconvulsive therapy. Neuropsychologia. 1975;13:51–8.
109. Squire LR. ECT and memory dysfunction. In: Lerer B, Weiner RD, Belmaker RH, editors. ECT: basic mechanisms. Washington, DC: American Psychiatric Press; 1984. p. 156–63.
110. Squire LR, Chace PM. Memory functions six to nine months after electroconvulsive therapy. Arch Gen Psychiatry. 1975;32:1157–64.
111. Squire LR, Slater PC. Electroconvulsive therapy and complaints of memory dysfunction: a prospective three-year follow-up study. Br J Psychiatry. 1983; 142:1–8.
112. Squire LR, Chace PM, Slater PC. Retrograde amnesia following electroconvulsive therapy. Nature. 1976;260:775–77.
113. Squire LR, Slater PC, Miller P. Retrograde amnesia following ECT: Long-term follow-up studies. Arch Gen Psychiatry. 1981;38:89–95.
114. Eacott MJ, Crawley RA. Childhood amnesia: on answering questions about very early life events. Memory. 1999;7(3):279–92.
115. Usher JA, Neisser U. Childhood amnesia and the beginnings of memory for four early life events. J Exp Psychol Gen. 1993;122(2):155–65.

116. Wetzler SE, Sweeney JA. Childhood amnesia: a conceptualization in cognitive-psychological terms. J Am Psychoanal Assoc. 1986;34(3):663–85.
117. Roth T, Roehrs T, Zwyghuizen Doorenbos A, Stepanski E, Wittig R. Sleep and memory. Psychopharmacol Ser. 1988;6:140–5.
118. Markowitsch HJ. Functional neuroimaging correlates of functional amnesia. Memory. 1999;7(5–6):561–83.
119. Kessler J, Markowitsch HJ, Huber M, Kalbe E, Weber-Luxenburger G, Kock P. Massive and persistent anterograde amnesia in the absence of detectable brain damage: anterograde psychogenic amnesia or gross reduction in sustained effort? J Clin Exp Neuropsychol. 1997;19(4):604–14.
120. Kopelman MD. Amnesia: organic and psychogenic. Br J Psychiatry. 1987;150:428–42.
121. Kapur N. Amnesia in relation to fugue states—distinguishing a neurological from a psychogenic basis. Br J Psychiatry. 1991;159:872–7.
122. Reinhold N, Markowitsch HJ. Retrograde episodic memory and emotion: a perspective from patients with dissociative amnesia. Neuropsychologia. 2009;47:2197–206.
123. Kihlstron JF, Schacter DL. Functional amnesia. In: Boller F, Grafman J, editors. Handbook of neuropsychology, vol. 2. 2nd ed. Amsterdam: Elsevier; 2000. p. 409–27.
124. Hodges JR, Patterson K. Semantic dementia: a unique clinicopathological syndrome. Lancet Neurol. 2007;6:1004–14.
125. Warrington EK, Shallice T. Category specific semantic impairments. Brain. 1984;107:829–54.
126. Capitani E, Laiacona M, Mahon B, Caramazza A. What are the facts of semantic category-specific deficits? A critical review of the clinical evidence. Cogn Neuropsychol. 2003;20:213–62.
127. Farah MJ, McClelland JI. A computational model of semantic memory impairment: modality specificity and emergent category specificity. J Exp Psychol. 1991;120:339–57.
128. Thompson-Schill SL, Aguirre GK, D'Esposito M, Farah MJ. A neural basis for category and modality specificity of semantic knowledge. Neuropsychologia. 1999;37:671–6.
129. Tippett LJ, Meier SL, Blackwood K, Diaz-Asper C. Category specific deficits in Alzheimer's disease: fact or artifact? Cortex. 2007;43:907–20.
130. Lambon Ralph MA, Lowe C, Rogers TT. Neural basis of category-specific semantic deficits: evidence from semantic dementia, HSVE, and a neural network model. Brain. 2007;130:1127–37.
131. Davies RR, Kipps CM, Mitchell J, Kril JJ, Halliday GM, Hodges JR. Progression in frontotemporal dementia: identifying a benign behavioral variant by magnetic resonance imaging. Arch Neurol. 2006;63:1627–31.
132. Pijnenburg YA, Gillissen F, Jonker C, Scheltens P. Initial complaints in frontotemporal lobar degeneration. Dement Geriatr Cogn Disord. 2004;17:302–6.
133. Thompson SA, Patterson K, Hodges JR. Left/right asymmetry of atrophy in semantic dementia: behavioural cognitive implications. Neurology. 2003;61:1196–203.
134. Hodges JR, Graham KS. Episodic memory: insights from semantic dementia. Phil Trans R Soc Lond: B Biol Sci. 2001;356:1423–34.
135. Altmann LJ, McClung JS. Effects of semantic impairment on language use in Alzheimer's disease. Semin Speech Lang. 2008;29:18–31.
136. Cuetos F, Herrera E, Ellis AW. Impaired word recognition in Alzheimer's disease: the role of age of acquisition. Neuropsychologia. 2010;48:3329–34.
137. Johnston RA, Barry C. Age of acquisition in semantic processing of pictures. Mem Cognit. 2005;33:905–12.
138. Juhasz BJ. Age of acquisition effects in word and picture identification. Psychol Bull. 2005;131:684–712.
139. Venneri A, McGeown WJ, Heitanen H, Guerrini C, Ellis AW, Shanks MF. The anatomical basis of semantic retrieval deficits in early Alzheimer's disease. Neuropsychologia. 2008;46:497–510.
140. Xie SX, Libon DJ, Wang X, Massimo L, Moore P, et al. Longitudinal patterns of semantic and episodic memory in frontotemporal lobar degeneration and Alzheimer's disease. J Int Neuropsychol Soc. 2010;16:278–86.
141. Adlam A-LR, Bozeat S, Arnold R, Watson P, Hodges JR. Semantic knowledge in mild cognitive impairment and mild Alzheimer's disease. Cortex. 2006;42:675–84.
142. Hodges JR, Patterson K. Is semantic memory consistently impaired early in the course of Alzheimer's disease? Neuroanatomical and diagnostic implications. Neuropsychologia. 1995;33:441–59.
143. Scahill VL, Hodges JR, Graham KS. Can episodic memory tasks differentiate semantic dementia from Alzheimer's disease? Neurocase. 2005;11:441–51.
144. Kopelman MD, Stanhope N, Kingsley D. Retrograde amnesia in patients with diencephalic, temporal lobe, or frontal lesions. Neuropsychologia. 1999;37:939–58.
145. McCarthy RA, Warrington EK. Actors but not scripts: the dissociation of people and events in retrograde amnesia. Neuropsychologia. 1992;30(7):633–44.
146. Gainotti G. What the locus of brain lesion tells us about the nature of the cognitive defect underlying category-specific disorders: a review. Cortex. 2000;36:539–59.
147. Laws KR, Sartori G. Category deficits and paradoxical dissociations in Alzheimer's disease and herpes simplex encephalitis. J Cogn Neurosci. 2005;17:1453–9.
148. Noppeney U, Patterson K, Tyler LK, Moss H, Stamatakis EA, Bright P, Mummery C, Price CJ. Temporal lobe lesions and semantic impairment: a comparison of herpes simplex virus encephalitis and semantic dementia. Brain. 2007;130:1138–47.
149. Capitani E, Laiacona M, Pagani R, Capasso R, Zampetti P, Miceli G. Posterior cerebral artery infarcts and semantic category dissociations: a study of 28 patients. Brain. 2009;132:965–81.

150. Johnson JK, Diehl J, Mendez MF, Neuhaus J, Shapria JS, et al. Frontotemporal lobar degeneration: demographic characteristics of 353 patients. Arch Neurol. 2005;62:925–30.
151. Saunders AM, Strittmatter WJ, Schmechel D, et al. Association of apolipoprotein E allele epsilon 4 with late-onset familial and sporadic Alzheimer's disease. Neurology. 1993;43:1467–72.
152. Pietrini V, Nertempi P, Vaglia A, Revello MG, Pinna V, Ferro-Milone F. Recovery from herpes simplex encephalitis: selective impairment of specific semantic categories with neuroradiological correlation. J Neurol Neurosurg Psychiatry. 1988;51:1284–93.
153. Bird CM, Chan D, Hartley T, Pijnenburg YA, Rossor MN, Burgess N. Topographical short-term memory differentiates Alzheimer's disease from frontotemporal lobar degeneration. Hippocampus. 2010;20: 1154–69.
154. Kramer J, Jurik J, Sha S. Distinctive neuropsychological pattern in frontotemporal dementia, semantic dementia, and Alzheimer's disease. Cogn Behav Neurol. 2003;16:211–8.
155. Hodges JR, Patterson K, Ward R, Garrard P, Bak T, Perry R, Gregory C. The differentiation of semantic dementia and frontal lobe dementia (temporal and frontal variants of frontotemporal dementia) from early Alzheimer's disease: a comparative neuropsychological study. Neuropsychol. 1999;13:31--40.
156. Kopelman MD, Wilson BA, Baddeley A. Autobiographical memory interview. Oxford: Pearson Assessments; 1990.
157. Squire LR, Slater PC. Forgetting in very long term memory as assessed by an improved questionnaire technique. J Exp Psychol. 1975;104:50–4.
158. Seelaar H, Rohrer JD, Pijnenburg YAL, Fox NC, van Swieten JC. Clinical, genetic and pathological heterogeneity of frontotemporal dementia: a review. J Neurol Neurosurg Psychiatry. 2010. doi:10.1136/jnnp.2010.212225.
159. Wechsler D, Holdnack JA, Drozdick LW. Wechsler Memory Scale, fourth edition. Technical and interpretive manual. San Antonio, TX: Pearson Assessments; 2009.
160. Benedict RHB, Schretlen D, Groninger L, Brandt J. Hopkins Verbal Learning Test-Revised: Normative data and analysis of inter-form and test-retest reliability. Clin Neuropsychol. 1998;12:43–55.
161. Delis DC, Kramer JH, Kaplan E, Ober BA. California Verbal Learning Test—second edition (CVLT-II). San Antonio, TX: Psychological Corporation; 2000.
162. Schmidt M. Rey Auditory and Verbal Learning Test: a handbook. Los Angeles: Western Psychological Services; 1996.
163. Meyers JE, Meyers KR. Rey Complex Figure Test and Recognition Trial. Odessa, FL: Psychological Assessment Resources; 1995.
164. Benedict R. Brief Visuospatial Memory Test-Revised professional manual. Odessa, FL: Psychological Assessment Resources, Inc.; 1997.
165. Trahan DE, Larrabee GJ. Continuous Visual Memory Test. Odessa, FL: Psychological Assessment Resources; 1988.
166. Wilson AB, Shiel A, Foley J, Smslie H, Groot Y, Hawkins K, Watson P. Cambridge Test of Prospective Memory (CAMPROMPT). San Antonio, TX: Pearson Assessments; 2005.
167. Crovitz HF, Schiffman H. Frequency of episodic memories as a function of their age. Bull Psychonom Soc. 1974;4:517–8.
168. Wechsler D, Coalson DL, Raiford SE. Wechsler Adult Intelligence Test: fourth edition technical and interpretive manual. San Antonio: Pearson Assessments; 2008.
169. Kertesz A. Western aphasia battery-revised. San Antonio, TX: Pearson Assessments; 2006.
170. Goodglass H, Kaplan E, Barresi B. Boston Diagnostic Aphasia Examination. 3rd ed. San Antonio, TX: Pearson Assessments; 2000.
171. Benton AL, Hamsher K deS, Sivan A. Multilingual Aphasia Examination. 3rd ed. Iowa City, IA: AJA Associates; 1994.
172. Delis DC, Kaplan E, Kramer J. Delis-Kaplan Executive Function Scale. San Antonio: Psychological Corporation; 2001.
173. Bishop D. Test for the reception of grammar—second edition (TROG-2). Sydney, AU: Pearson Assessments; 2003.
174. Grant DA, Berg EA. A behavioral analysis of the degree of reinforcement and ease of shifting to new responses in a Weigl-type card sorting problem. J Exp Psychol. 1948;38:404–11.
175. DeFilippis NA, McCampbell E. Booklet Category Test. 2nd ed. Odessa, FL: Psychological Assessment Resources; 1997.
176. Stroop JR. Studies of interference in serial verbal reactions. J Exp Psychol. 1935;18:643–62.
177. Luria AR. Higher cortical functions in Man. New York: Basic Books; 1966.

Epilepsy and Aging

26

Brian D. Bell and Anna Rita Giovagnoli

Abstract

Epilepsy is the third most common neurological disorder of old age and a substantial public health problem. As the elderly population rises, the elderly will account for a large percentage of all new-onset seizures. However, while the study of epilepsy in adults in general has led to major advances in neuropsychology, epilepsy in the aged has been one of the more neglected areas within the field. Geriatric epilepsy is now an emerging field for all health-care practitioners, including neuropsychologists. Patient management requires assessment and treatment of cognitive and functional impairment and psychological issues. A thorough assessment of cognitive function is essential in discriminating epilepsy from classic progressive dementias and for assessing functioning prior to treatments for seizures once they are diagnosed. Neuropsychological assessment plays an important role to characterize cognitive impairments, reveal preserved abilities, help monitor medication treatment, track for coexistence of MCI or dementia, and assess for emotional distress.

Keywords

Epilepsy • Aging • Memory • Executive functions • Brain plasticity • Comorbitities • Antiepileptic drugs

B.D. Bell, Ph.D. (✉)
Charles Matthews Neuropsychology Laboratory, Department of Neurology, University of Wisconsin School of Medicine and Public Health, MFCB, 1685 Highland Ave, Madison, WI 53705-2281, USA

W.S. Middleton Memorial Veterans Hospital, Madison, WI, USA
e-mail: bell@neurology.wisc.edu

A.R. Giovagnoli, M.D., Ph.D.
Department of Clinical Neurosciences, Neuropsychology Laboratory, Carlo Besta Neurological Institute, Milan, Italy
e-mail: r.giovagnoli@istituto-besta.it

L.D. Ravdin and H.L. Katzen (eds.), *Handbook on the Neuropsychology of Aging and Dementia*, Clinical Handbooks in Neuropsychology, DOI 10.1007/978-1-4614-3106-0_26,

Background

Seizures and Epilepsy Defined

A seizure is a sudden, transitory event characterized by positive or negative mental or physical symptoms associated with neuronal discharge and electroencephalographic (EEG) changes. In 1981, the International League Against Epilepsy (ILAE) classified two major categories of seizure type, characterized by either partial or generalized onset [1]. Partial (focal) seizures begin in a local area of the brain and are further subdivided into simple partial (no alteration in consciousness) and complex partial seizures (CPS) (alteration of consciousness). Generalized seizures may have partial onset with secondary generalization (there is a clinical aura or an EEG focal discharge) or generalized onset (involving the entire brain simultaneously). In some cases, seizure type may remain unclassifiable. Seizure symptoms vary across the life span, with more challenging diagnostic demands in older adults.

Epilepsy is defined by recurrent (two or more) epileptic seizures, unprovoked by any immediate identified cause [2–4]. Idiopathic epilepsies generally have a genetic basis and onset during childhood, symptomatic epilepsies are caused by brain lesion, and cryptogenic epilepsies have an unknown cause that potentially could be identified with sufficient investigation [2]. Multiple seizures occurring in a 24-h period or an episode of status epilepticus (SE) are considered a single event for diagnostic purposes. A single unprovoked seizure does not constitute epilepsy, nor do isolated febrile seizures, neonatal seizures, or acute symptomatic seizures provoked by acute systemic illness, intoxication, or substance abuse or withdrawal [5]. Seizure classifications and terminology are undergoing revision by the ILAE to incorporate advances in neuroimaging, genomics, and molecular biology [4].

Although epilepsy is the most common neurological condition overall (average prevalence 1%) [6], there are disparities in its prevalence and incidence across the world due to variations in diagnostic definition, socioeconomic status, access to health care and environmental exposures [7]. Furthermore, prevalence and incidence may be underestimated in geographic areas where the condition is greatly stigmatized. Gender-specific disparity (higher incidence in males than females) is small [8, 9]. The classic rule that epilepsy is most common in the first 10 years of life has changed. In fact, older adults now have the highest prevalence of epilepsy per decade of any age group [10].

Seizures in Older Adults: A Growing but Understudied Problem

Because the world's population is aging and the risk of acute symptomatic seizures, epilepsy, and SE is highest in older adults, the number of older adults with epilepsy is rising [11–15]. By the year 2025, greater than 30% of the population of many developed countries will be older than 60, and at that point, the aged population will account for a high percentage of all new-onset seizures [16, 17]. This is due in part to increases in long-term survival after acute neurological insults and the likelihood of correct diagnosis compared to past decades. In the USA, epilepsy affects nearly 1.5% of those ≥65 years old, and the prevalence is higher in nursing homes (exceeding 5%). Epilepsy is now the third most common neurological disorder of old age, and it is therefore not surprising that it has been described as a substantial public health problem [10, 12, 14, 18–26].

Despite the rising prevalence of epilepsy in older adults, epilepsy and aging issues have received limited attention in both human and animal research [27–29]. While the study of epilepsy in children and young adults has led to major advances in neuropsychology [30, 31], epilepsy and aging are thought to be one of the more neglected areas of research within the field of neuropsychology [32]. This may be because older patients with epilepsy have been infrequently referred to neuropsychologists. This pattern is likely to change with the advancing wave of baby boomers and increasing recognition of geriatric seizures and their morbidity.

Geriatric epilepsy is an emerging field for all health-care practitioners, including neuropsychologists, who can make a key contribution to the care of older adults with suspected epilepsy. In addition to diagnosis and use of medications, medical management requires assessment of cognitive and behavioral impairments, as well as social or psychological problems that are caused not only by epilepsy-related brain dysfunction but also by chronic pathology and aging itself [11, 18, 33–37]. Abnormalities in cognition are relatively common in patients with epilepsy, including affected older adults [38–41]. Leading epileptologists have emphasized that a thorough assessment of cognitive function is essential in discriminating epilepsy-related impairment from dementia, and should be conducted prior to the initiation of treatment for newly diagnosed seizures [22, 42].

There are two broad groups of older adults with seizures, those who come to old age having had epilepsy since earlier in life and those who experience the onset of seizures or epilepsy at an advanced age in the context of either an acute medical or neurological illness (stroke, tumor, trauma, infection, metabolic abnormality, or drug interaction) or a non-acute setting, perhaps including the aging process itself [11, 13, 14, 28, 32]. Across the full age range, the majority of seizures are cryptogenic, while 33–50% of seizures have an unknown etiology in the elderly [7, 43]. These figures may decrease as diagnostic procedures improve [12, 21, 22, 44].

Many conditions can cause seizures in older adults. Cerebrovascular disease, dementia, tumor, and head trauma are the brain disorders most often associated with new-onset epilepsy in older adults. A fundamental distinction is made between epileptic seizures and non-epileptic seizures that occur due to other neurological attacks such as migraine, sleep-related disorders, and narcolepsy or to a medical condition such as cardiac syncope, paroxysmal abdominal pain, metabolic derangement, respiratory compromise, or alcohol abuse [45].

Seizure and Epilepsy Etiologies in Older Adults

Stroke

Stroke is the most common cause of new-onset seizures and epilepsy in older adults, accounting for 30–50% of all epilepsies in this group. Stroke-related seizures can be divided into early onset and late onset, which reflect different etiopathogenesis. The 5-year risk of developing a post-stroke seizure is roughly 10%, and about one-third of those with seizures will develop epilepsy [46–49]. The risk of poststroke seizures might be higher after a longer follow-up period [14, 23]. Moreover, mild cerebrovascular disease may be the etiology of epilepsy even in some patients with cryptogenic epilepsy [11, 14, 15, 22]. In a study of US veterans, stroke and dementia had an additive effect. Older adults with a combination of stroke and dementia were four times as likely to have epilepsy as those without either condition [21].

Seizure risk is highest in severe, disabling strokes, in hemorrhagic strokes, and in those with cortical involvement [20, 26, 44, 47]. Further, the relationship between stroke and epilepsy is bidirectional, in that individuals with late-onset seizures are at higher risk of an initial stroke, owing to a coexistence of vascular risk factors such as hypertension, ischemic heart disease, diabetes, and antiepileptic drug (AED)-related alteration of folate metabolism. When a late-onset seizure occurs after a stroke, the possibility of a new cerebrovascular accident should be investigated. The possibility of a decline in cognition also should be investigated, especially in the case of late-onset recurrent seizures or SE [50]. It has been recommended that older adults with new-onset seizures undergo a thorough cerebrovascular workup [23].

TIA

Transient ischemic attacks (TIAs) are rarely associated with seizures. TIAs usually can be differentiated from seizures, because negative motor phenomena such as hemiparesis are quite uncommon in seizures. However, “inhibitory seizures" do occur, most often characterized by aphasia or dysarthria. An aphasic disturbance that has a sudden onset and then remains stable until its subsequent gradual resolution is more likely to be a TIA [15]. A normal EEG is expected in TIA, whereas the EEG is likely to be abnormal in "inhibitory seizures," showing diffuse slowing or intermittent rhythmic delta activities. In about two-thirds of inhibitory seizures patients, the negative symptoms are associated with some degree of confusion or a subsequent partial retrograde amnesia for the event, whereas focal vascular insults do not usually produce confusion [15, 50].

Alzheimer's Disease and Other Degenerative Dementias

There is no evidence that seizure risk is elevated in patients with mild cognitive impairment (MCI), which can represent prodromal Alzheimer's disease (AD) [51]. Studies of the prevalence of seizures in patients with AD have led to conflicting results. One investigation reported that from 10 to 17% of patients with autopsy-confirmed AD presented with unprovoked seizures after disease onset [52]. On the other hand, a recent multi-site study of 453 patients indicated unprovoked seizures are a "quite uncommon feature" in AD, although more common than in the general elderly population [53]. CPS, including those with secondary generalization, are the most common type of seizure in AD [51, 53]. It is possible that CPS are sometimes underdiagnosed because AD patients may be unaware of sudden changes or not able to report subjective symptoms, while caregivers may find it difficult to distinguish behavioral alterations caused by seizures and fluctuations in behavior related to dementia [53]. It should also be kept in mind that demented patients sometimes exhibit orofacial movements, outbursts of temper, wandering, fluctuating confusion, and memory lapses that may not necessarily be seizure related [15].

Seizures are most common in the advanced stages of AD, but early age of onset also is associated with greater risk of seizures, perhaps because of its association with gene mutations [20, 23, 51, 53, 54]. The frequency of seizures is high in patients with AD and Down syndrome, affecting up to 56% of cases [55]. Experimental studies have shown that high levels of β-amyloid, the main constituent of AD plaques, and the apolipoprotein ε4 allele, a genetic risk factor for AD, were associated with seizures [56], supporting the clinical evidence of association between AD and epilepsy. An additional factor is the potentially proconvulsant effect of acetylcholinesterase inhibitors, which are used in the treatment of dementia.

New-onset epilepsy in older adults sometimes may cause cognitive decline leading to an incorrect diagnosis of dementia. Further, AED treatment (e.g., valproate) may provoke reversible chronic cognitive impairment that can also be misdiagnosed as dementia [57]. Thus, if dementia and epilepsy start together, then it is probable that dementia is a consequence of epilepsy or AED treatment, rather than an expression of AD.

Dementia with Lewy bodies (DLB) can be associated with seizures. Reports on EEG in DLB have been conflicting, but recent diagnostic guidelines indicate EEG abnormalities are supportive of the diagnosis. In one study that examined EEG abnormalities, a "Grand Total EEG" index was derived from six variables: rhythmic background activity, diffuse slow-wave activity, reactivity, paroxysmal activity, focal abnormalities, and sharp-wave activity. The patients with DLB had a higher index than patients with AD, and DLB was identified with a sensitivity of 72% and a specificity of 85% using an EEG cutoff score. The association between DLB and this EEG abnormality was independent of age and MMSE score [58].

Frontotemporal lobe dementia (FTD) appears to be rarely associated with seizures [51, 54, 59]. However, a family has been reported with a novel phenotype characterized by a combination of early onset and rapidly progressive FTD, parkinsonism, and epileptic seizures [60].

Alcohol and Drugs, Brain Tumor, Head Trauma, and HIV/AIDS

The peak incidence of initial seizures related to alcohol withdrawal occurs late in life [25]. About 10% of seizures in older adults are associated with use of alcohol or prescription drugs, and seizures sometimes occur after withdrawal from certain sedative medications following chronic use [15]. Two other neurological disorders commonly seen by neuropsychologists, brain tumor and head trauma, account for some cases of epilepsy in older adults. Seizures are the first sign of a brain tumor in 50% of older patients [23]. In the case of head trauma, an age of 65 years or greater is one of the factors that increase the risk of post-traumatic epilepsy. Also, a sizable minority of individuals with HIV or AIDS is more than 50 years old, and this percentage is increasing. Seizures in this group usually occur later in the disease process, resulting from mass lesions of various etiologies, or due directly to cerebral HIV infection [15].

Clinical Issues

Diagnostic Challenges

The diagnosis of epilepsy mainly rests on the patient's history and should be considered in any patient who suffers from recurrent attacks of consistently or relatively stereotyped involuntary behavior or subjective experience. Specific diagnostic criteria depend on the seizure type, while general diagnostic points broadly support an epilepsy diagnosis. The first step is to define a critical symptom or fixed combination of symptoms (seizure diagnosis), the second is to establish the nature of the seizure (epileptic versus non-epileptic), and the third is to determine the cause of seizures or epilepsy (symptomatic, idiopathic, cryptogenic). As for EEG, no diagnostic test can absolutely confirm or exclude epilepsy unless the registration of epileptiform discharges is contemporaneous to seizure symptoms. Other contributory diagnostic techniques include neuroimaging, ambulatory electrocardiography (ECG), orthostatic blood pressure management, tilt table testing, hematological and biochemical profiles, and thyroid function testing [61].

Seizures are both underdiagnosed and overdiagnosed in specific subgroups of older adults [11, 20, 22]. Unnecessary treatment with AEDs can lead to deleterious side effects, while lack of appropriate treatment in undiagnosed geriatric epilepsy patients can have dire consequences. Many older patients' new-onset seizures are not diagnosed or there is a significant delay to diagnosis, with a mean time to correct diagnosis in one study of more than 18 months [11, 15, 19–22, 62]. In general, reasons for difficulty in securing a seizure diagnosis in older adults include (1) atypical or nonspecific presentation or semiology of partial seizures; (2) absence of classic symptoms due to relative infrequency of tonic–clonic seizures; (3) coexisting cognitive impairment that may lead to an incomplete history, underreporting of events, or failure to recognize transitory confusional states; (4) absence of witnesses due to patient living alone and/or being retired; (5) low sensitivity and/or specificity in diagnostic investigations such as interictal EEG or ECG; (6) decreased continuity of patient/physician relationships; and (7) the absence of specialists in the diagnostic process [20, 22, 26, 59, 63, 64]. Because it can be difficult for physicians to differentiate seizures from various other conditions, neuropsychologists are likely to evaluate patients who have not yet received a definitive diagnosis. It also is important to keep in mind that two different disorders may coexist in the same patient [65].

The etiology, semiology or clinical presentation, and prognosis of a seizure disorder often differ between younger and older patients. In fact, "novel diagnostic paradigms" have been recommended because of the diverse etiologies and atypical presentations of seizures in the elderly [15, 20, 22, 59] (cf. [62]). Tables 26.1 and 26.2 [59] present some common characteristics of seizures in older adults and clues to the diagnosis, respectively. Generalized tonic–clonic seizures can occur in older adults, including primary generalized seizures that reemerge in old age after initial occurrence in early life [22]. About two-thirds of geriatric seizures have a focal onset, with or without secondary generalization. Focal motor seizures are the most frequently reported type of partial seizure. However, this may reflect not only a real occurrence but also the difficulty in collecting details about the

Table 26.1 Characteristics of epilepsy in older adults

Partial epilepsy is most common
New-onset frontal lobe seizures more common than temporal lobe seizures
Motor or sensory symptoms more common than psychic symptoms
Auras less common and may present in a nonspecific way (e.g., dizziness)
Automatisms less common than in young adults
Secondary generalization less common
Prolonged postictal state can occur
Status epilepticus appears to be more common than in young adults
Focal slowing on EEG less likely to be indicative of epilepsy

Table 26.2 Clues to the possibility of epileptic seizures in older adults [59]

Confusional state with sudden onset and end
Rhythmic muscular contractions in a focal territory
Paroxysmal behavior disorder with or without a focal neurological sign
Impairment of consciousness
A prior history of epilepsy
Focal slow waves on interictal EEG

seizure semiology in older people who may fail to report psychic symptoms [66]. CPS in particular account for about 40% of all seizures in the aged population [14, 15, 19, 22, 61, 67].

CPS with a mesial temporal lobe onset are most common in young adults and often are associated with an aura, disturbance of consciousness, behavioral arrest, oral-facial and limb automatisms, and a period of post-ictal confusion of seconds to minutes. Secondary generalization also is relatively common. It also should be noted that widespread volumetric changes on imaging and cognitive deficits are common in this group [39], and older patients with long-standing temporal lobe epilepsy (TLE) also can be expected to show impairment in more domains than memory. While new-onset temporal lobe seizures can occur quite late in life [68], new-onset CPS in older adults is most likely to be extratemporal, often originating in the frontal lobe. This is at least in part due to the link between anterior frontal cortical areas and stroke.

There is often a lack of specific clinical signs of epilepsy in older adults. In a study of individuals older than 60 years who had a mean duration of partial epilepsy of 44 years, many demonstrated progressively less elaborate and briefer seizures over the course of their lives [69]. Auras are uncommon and often nonspecific when they occur, and automatisms and secondary generalization also are relatively uncommon. A disturbance of consciousness accompanied by a blank stare may be the only manifestation of a CPS in an older adult [12, 15, 22]. Postictal symptoms result from seizure-induced reversible alterations in neuronal function. Both the postictal focal motor deficits and confusional state can be prolonged in older patients, with the former lasting for hours and the latter for days. The prolonged post-ictal confusion may even be mistaken for dementia [15, 20, 22, 23, 26, 32].

Transient Epileptic Amnesia Versus Transient Global Amnesia

Transient epileptic amnesia (TEA), also called epileptic amnesic syndrome, is a specific and probably underdiagnosed type of TLE that tends to have a late onset [37, 70–72]. It usually strikes in the sixth or seventh decade of life and is associated with recurrent, abrupt, transient, and relatively severe anterograde memory disturbance (median duration = 30–60 min). Cognition is otherwise generally intact during the occurrence of the amnesic event. TEA may be associated with an abnormal EEG, especially a sleep-deprived EEG, and is almost always responsive to an AED such as carbamazepine. Before treatment is instituted, TEA tends to occur upon awakening and sometimes is associated with other temporal lobe symptomatology such as olfactory hallucinations, oral automatisms, or brief unresponsiveness. But transient amnesia may be the sole ictal symptom. Interictal memory impairment is commonly reported by TEA patients and may not resolve with treatment. Although standard memory testing might reveal only subtle difficulty, some TEA patients report considerable problems with remote memory loss and accelerated long-term forgetting (ALF).

In the latter, information tends to be recalled normally for a day or more, but then fades at an accelerated rate compared to healthy controls. The subjective report of this phenomenon by a subset of TEA patients has been confirmed by means of innovative memory assessment over long intervals [73]. ALF may reflect a problem with a late stage of memory consolidation and perhaps a disturbance restricted to the hippocampus bilaterally. Thus, epilepsy should be ruled out in patients with credible reports of intermittent and clear-cut amnesic attacks, ALF, and/or isolated retrograde amnesia [37, 70, 72, 74].

A late life onset of transient memory loss is characteristic of both TEA and transient global amnesia (TGA). TGA is not an epileptic event and so is associated with a normal EEG or slowing only, tends to last longer than TEA, and is usually a one-time event [37, 70]. Table 26.3 lists characteristics of TEA versus TGA and TIA.

Status Epilepticus

It is noteworthy that 30% of first seizures in older adults present as SE [75], defined as any seizure lasting more than 30 min or intermittent seizures lasting for more than 30 min during which the patient does not regain consciousness [76]. Stroke is the most common etiology of SE in older adults [47]. Two main types of SE are distinguished: generalized (convulsive, nonconvulsive) and partial (simple, complex). Incidence of SE is substantially higher in older adults in comparison to younger ages, and mortality is elevated in older adults, particularly in patients with brain anoxia [77, 78]. SE is often underdiagnosed. In particular, nonconvulsive and partial complex SE can present as prolonged confusion or unusual behavior such as lethargy, agitation, automatisms, or mild personality change, which may prevent a timely diagnosis in elderly patients. When nonconvulsive SE is suspected, an EEG should be performed so that, if it is confirmed, treatment can be provided quickly [75].

Non-epileptic Paroxysmal Syndromes

There is a range of disorders with symptoms that can cause or mimic a seizure, including cerebrovascular, cardiovascular, endocrine/metabolic, infectious, sleep, migraine, and psychiatric conditions. The main differential diagnosis in older adults is convulsive syncope. Syncope is loss of consciousness due to an acute decrease in cerebral blood flow, and if it is prolonged, convulsions may occur. This type of seizure may result from a cardiac cause (heart block, ventricular tachycardia, ventricular fibrillation, asymmetric septal hypertrophy, aortic stenosis), carotid sinus hypersensitivity, or vasovagal attack. Clinical observation (e.g., heart rate, blood pressure, skin vegetative signs) facilitates diagnosis. Whether or not an attack is observed, diagnosis is aided by simultaneous EEG and ECG.

Other causes of non-epileptic seizures include sleep-related disorders such as sleep attacks (irresistible episodes of sleep), cataplexy (sudden loss of postural tone sparing consciousness, often stimulated by strong emotions such as fear), sleep paralysis (lasting a few minutes on awakening or when falling to sleep), hypnagogic hallucinations, and REM behavior disorders. Diagnosis is

Table 26.3 Differential diagnosis of transient epileptic amnesia (TEA), transient global amnesia (TGA), and transient ischemic attack (TIA)

	TEA	TGA	TIA
Duration	<1 h	4–6 h	Variable
Ictal amnesia	Retro-anterograde	Dense anterograde, variable retrograde	Not well characterized
Other symptoms	Sometimes olfactory hallucinations, automatisms, brief loss of awareness	Headache, nausea	Focal neurological deficits
Recurrence	~Monthly	Rare	Not well characterized
Interictal memory	Includes accelerated long-term forgetting, remote memory loss	No permanent deficits	Risk of permanent deficits from strokes

Note: Adapted with permission from Zeman and Butler [37]

based on a characteristic history and the typical EEG pattern showing sleep-onset REM. Another differential condition is migraine which may cause sudden loss of consciousness owing to brainstem vasomotor changes. Clinical history and EEG may easily discriminate epilepsy and migraine, although patients with migraine may show EEG epileptic abnormalities and some patients can be affected of course by both disorders. When a seizure is caused by electrolyte imbalance, febrile illness, or hypoglycemia or hyperglycemia, chronic AED treatment is not required after the condition is successfully treated [20, 79].

Psychogenic Non-epileptic Seizures

Psychogenic non-epileptic seizures (PNES) are sudden involuntary attacks of sensation, movement, autonomic alteration, or complex behavior, such as anesthesia, crying, bizarre postural changes, hyperventilation, or sudden fear expression, that are not caused by cortical discharges, although they may, in some cases, perfectly mimic epileptic seizures. PNES are pseudo-neurological manifestations of psychological distress or psychiatric disorders (conversion, somatization). After Charcot's definition of hystero-epilepsy and later terms such as pseudo-seizures or hysterical seizures, the term PNES has been preferred. PNES appear to be about as common in older as in younger adults and sometimes can have an onset late in life [62, 80]. Diagnosis of PNES requires differentiation not only from epileptic seizures but also other forms of non-epileptic episodes. Video-EEG recording documenting the absence of epileptiform discharges during an event is the gold standard for diagnosis of PNES. In the absence of ictal EEG, no single symptom, clinical sign, or demographic variable allows for the diagnosis of PNES. Differential diagnosis is important to prevent unnecessary AED treatment, iatrogenic complications, and delayed referral to adequate psychiatric treatment.

Some studies suggest that PNES represents approximately one-half of the non-epileptic seizures identified during video-EEG monitoring in patients over age 60 [80, 81]. In younger adults, approximately 75% of PNES patients are women, but this ratio may decrease significantly in late-onset (>age 55) patients [82, 83]. In addition, it appears that a history of sexual abuse, which is relatively common in early-onset PNES patients, is rare in late-onset patients, who are more likely to have severe physical health problems (e.g., cardiovascular illness) and report health-related traumatic experiences. Older-onset patients also seem to be less likely to have baseline psychiatric disturbances [83].

In general, PNES may be longer than average epileptic seizures (>2 min), have motor features with a gradual onset and a fluctuating course, and be associated with thrashing, violent movements, side-to-side head movements, asynchronous movements, and closed eyes. Other possible signs of PNES include crying or speaking during seizures, noninvolvement of the face during generalized movements, no seizures during sleep, stronger seizures when the staff is present, resistance when trying to open the patient's eyes, and frequent hospitalizations. A history of multifaceted symptoms and features that are unusual for epilepsy and an absence of incontinence, tongue laceration, and self-injury support this diagnosis. PNES patients also are more likely to recall details from the unresponsive period compared to patients with epilepsy [15].

At the group level, epilepsy and PNES patients typically perform similarly on neuropsychological testing. However, symptom validity tests and personality measures can help with differential diagnosis. When present in young adult PNES patients, neuropsychological impairment is often a function of suboptimal motivation during the assessment or an emotional disturbance. For example, PNES patients tend to perform worse than those with epilepsy on the Portland Digit Recognition Test and Word Memory Test. While there is no single psychological profile that differentiates PNES from epilepsy, extreme scores on the Hs and Hy scales of the MMPI-2 are more common in PNES patients [82, 84]. Initial work with the MMPI-2-RF suggests that the RC1 (Somatic Complaints) correctly classifies about two-thirds of epilepsy and PNES patients. In addition, two newly created supplementary scales

(PNES Physical Complaints and PNES Attitudes) show promise, as they provided slightly better accuracy in correctly classifying 73% of patients [85]. Careful assessment of personality style and psychopathology, emotional–behavioral distress symptoms, pre-illness life and medical events, personal resources, and coping attitudes plays a role in determining the psychic origin of PNES, as well as in defining epilepsy-related psychological disorders which in relatively rare cases can result in coexistence of non-epileptic seizures.

EEG

Discharges on EEG are not rare in older patients without epileptic seizures, and interictal epileptiform activity is present on routine EEG only in a minority of patients with onset of seizures after age 60 [86]. Benign EEG variants that are most common in older adults include subclinical rhythmic electrical discharges of adulthood (SREDA), wicket spikes, and small sharp spikes [64, 75]. Nevertheless, EEG often can be helpful in the diagnostic process [59, 63, 68, 87], including extended/ambulatory EEG and long-term inpatient video-EEG monitoring. The latter tends to be underused in older adults, as they account for about 5% of video-EEG inpatient admissions [62, 64]. Long-term monitoring (typically lasting 3–5 days) can be cost effective and especially valuable in diagnosing recurrent spells, classifying epilepsy, and determining candidates for epilepsy surgery [22, 61, 62, 75, 80, 88, 89]. Long-term video-EEG does require precautions to be in place for prevention of falls and prompt detection and treatment of adverse events; tertiary epilepsy centers generally offer the highest level of experience and care [89].

Brain Imaging

In recent years, brain imaging of course has become more sophisticated, allowing for various structural and functional studies. For the most part, these techniques have been applied for the diagnosis of younger, drug-resistant epilepsy patients or to experimental study designs. Age-related changes on brain imaging are common and not necessarily related to onset of epilepsy. For other abnormalities, computerized tomography (CT) scans can reveal tissue contrasts such as the presence of blood, calcified lesions, and encephalomalacia, whereas magnetic resonance (MRI) is more effective in identifying subtle changes in tissue density such as glial tumors or hippocampal changes [11, 14, 19, 32, 80]. CT- and MRI-detected brain lesions are not a necessary or sufficient criterion for epilepsy. However, in older patients, the detection of a focal brain lesion represents a significant diagnostic criterion that supports diagnosis when typical clinical and EEG signs are present [59]. In particular, in older patients with SE or prolonged behavior/mental symptomatology of uncertain origin (e.g., nonconvulsive SE versus metabolic failure), CT and MRI are important emergency measures [90].

Antiepileptic Drug Treatment

AEDs are the most common treatment for epilepsy, while other approaches may be applied in patients with drug-resistant seizures. Major drug selection criteria (i.e., the seizure type to be treated and side effects) are considered in the context of individual patient characteristics in order to determine the probable relative efficacy and tolerability of a drug. This process has become more complex as many new AEDs have been introduced to clinical practice in the last few decades, requiring systematic trials to determine efficacy in the individual patient.

Epilepsy usually is diagnosed after two or more unprovoked seizures occur [14]. The question of whether a physician should begin treatment with an AED immediately after a first seizure is controversial. Studies have demonstrated that deferring treatment until more than one seizure has occurred does not adversely affect the long-term remission rate. However, it has been recommended that treatment be instituted after a single unprovoked seizure, especially in the context of a history of stroke, because of the high risk of subsequent seizures and their potential serious consequences, includ-

Table 26.4 AED use in older adults

AED selection depends on comorbid conditions, co-medications, and expected side effects
Increased vulnerability to side effects and toxicity
Increased likelihood of failing medication trials due to adverse effects
Slower, more gradual titration and lower dosage recommended
Serum drug concentrations tend to vary
AED combined with another medication may amplify adverse effects common to both

ing falls, fractures, etc. [22, 45, 47, 50]. Fortunately, up to 80% of patients who develop epilepsy in old age are rendered seizure free with AED treatment [22, 44], with better outcome when an AED is started within 2 years of the first seizure compared to after 2 years [61].

Taking into account the selection criterion of the seizure type, the narrow-spectrum AEDs (e.g., carbamazepine, gabapentin, lacosamide, oxcarbazepine, phenobarbital, phenytoin, pregabalin, primidone, tiagabine), which are typically effective in partial seizures with or without secondary generalization, are primary choices in the treatment of late-onset epilepsy in older adults. However, broad-spectrum AEDs (e.g., lamotrigine, levetiracetam, rufinamide, topiramate, valproate, zonisamide), effective both in partial and generalized seizures, are useful when diagnosis is uncertain. Older adults are more likely than younger patients to become seizure free with low AED doses [12]. Characteristics of AED use in older adults are listed in Table 26.4.

AEDs rank fifth among all drug categories in capacity to elicit adverse side effects in older adults. In a recent survey, 64% of a sample of elderly community dwelling patients with intractable partial epilepsy listed medication side effects as an illness-related concern [91]. AED adherence among elderly patients often is suboptimal, and this is associated with increases in both seizures and health-care costs [92]. It is worth keeping in mind that compliance may be affected by ability to afford an AED; elderly individuals are more likely to rely on government insurance and may have to pay out of pocket for some medications [26, 79, 91, 93]. Medication side effects may be dose dependent or drug specific, and the spectrum of side effects may differ from that seen in younger patients. The pharmacokinetics (absorption, distribution, and metabolism) and pharmacodynamics (receptor function) of AEDs generally are different in older adults, who are more susceptible to the adverse side effects of these drugs and toxicity, as well as interactions with other types of medications. Older adults are often more susceptible to AED-induced cognitive side effects, ataxia, and dizziness, with a secondary increased tendency to confusion and falls. The coexistence of various medical (e.g., cardiac, hepatic or renal failure, obesity), neurological (e.g., sleep-related disorders, migraine), or psychiatric comorbidities (e.g., depression, psychosis, anxiety) may be a factor in choosing a particular AED. For instance, valproate and pregabalin are associated with weight gain; valproate and topiramate may be effective in migraine; levetiracetam, primidone, phenobarbital, topiramate, and zonisamide may contribute to worsen depression; levetiracetam, phenobarbital, and primidone may cause behavioral reactions; carbamazepine and valproate may have positive psychotropic effects; and many AEDs (in particular phenobarbital, primidone, topiramate) may cause cognitive deficits. Detailed discussions of AED risks and benefits in older adults are provided elsewhere [14, 19, 22, 23].

Comorbidities in older adults are also related to the use of other medications that may implicate pharmacological interactions and co-toxicities. Co-medications can alter the absorption, distribution, and metabolism of AEDs, effects which increase the risk of either toxicity or therapeutic failure [79]. Common medications that interact with AEDs include warfarin, digoxin, theophylline, cyclosporine, and corticosteroids. Because depression and anxiety are common in patients with epilepsy, the proconvulsive properties of tricyclic antidepressants have to be considered. All tricyclic antidepressants can lower seizure threshold; seizures caused by these drugs typically are generalized tonic–clonic [20]. It has been estimated that 33% of the pharmaceutical expenditure by older adults is for over-the-counter products. Some over-the-counter allergy, weight loss, and memory aids may also have proconvulsive properties [14, 20].

In line with the conclusions of the ILAE [94], a low dose of lamotrigine, gabapentin, or carbamazepine has been recommended for treatment of poststroke seizures [50]. A few recent studies have described the effectiveness and tolerability of AEDs in patients with AD, suggesting no difference in clinical efficacy between phenobarbital, levetiracetam, and lamotrigine but minor side effects for levetiracetam [95]. Levetiracetam has been demonstrated to be safe in the treatment of older patients with partial or generalized SE [96]. Use of phenobarbital and phenytoin is advised against in older adults, in part due to risk of sedation and falls (for a combination of reasons, epilepsy doubles the risk of fractures), but phenytoin remains commonly prescribed in this age group, in part because it is relatively inexpensive and its properties are well known [12, 14, 18, 19, 22, 23, 32, 44, 97].

It should be noted that the cutoff of age 65 to designate older age is arbitrary, with no particular biological significance, because the gradual health changes associated with aging manifest themselves at different times in different people. Thus, older adults are "not a single cohort" [14, 45, 79]. In addition to chronological age, a patient's biological age, based on a physician's clinical judgment, is an important factor when medication choices are made [14, 19]. Attempting to minimize AED side effects while also controlling seizures is a delicate balance [22, 33, 35, 39].

Epilepsy Surgery

Surgery is a potentially curative treatment for disabling, medically refractory epilepsy, and in TLE in particular, it is the standard of care in selected patients [98, 99]. There have been few studies of epilepsy surgery in older adults, and no consensus exists on an upper age limit for epilepsy surgery candidates [100]. But the overall findings from a small series of studies of epilepsy surgery in patients more than 50 years old [101, 102] and two recent studies addressing surgery in those more than 60 years old [42, 98] suggest older patients often are viable candidates for epilepsy surgery. One study [42] described postsurgical seizure and neuropsychological outcome in TLE patients with a mean age of 56 and a mean duration of epilepsy of 33 years. Seizure outcome after temporal lobe excisions was not significantly different in patients older than 50 years compared to a sample consisting of patients younger than 50. In fact, even a subset of patients more than 60 years old ($n = 11$) had an outcome similar to the younger group. Although surgical and neurological complications were infrequent, they were significantly higher in the >50 years group. In addition, the >50 group was more likely to show significant decline when assessed about 12 months after surgery on an index of attention, and the >60 years old group was especially vulnerable to decline in verbal memory, even though 91% of them underwent a right-sided surgery. A report from Germany [42] concluded that, although there is modestly increased risk of complications and neuropsychological decline, epilepsy surgery is effective in older TLE patients. Another report that reviewed results from seven patients who underwent temporal resection after age 60 also concluded that surgery in this group generally is safe and effective [98]. Similarly, based on studies of patients with a mean age in the early to mid-50s, other authors concluded that neither chronological age nor duration of epilepsy should necessarily exclude patients from consideration for epilepsy surgery [100, 102]. While recognizing that the risk of any operative procedure is higher in elderly patients and that there may be obstacles to surgery for some, these authors emphasized the potential benefits of surgery in the context of possible medication intolerance, persisting seizures, and corresponding physical injuries, loss of independence, cognitive decline, and psychiatric disorders in the absence of surgery. More research is needed about cognitive outcome and quality of life (QOL) after epilepsy surgery in older adults.

Cognition, Behavior, and Quality of Life

Quality of Life and Mood

On generic measures of health-related QOL, scores for both physical and mental health status tend to be lower in epilepsy patients than in the general population, particularly for those with uncontrolled seizures. The few studies of elderly epilepsy patients suggest they also have significantly lower QOL compared to the general population [93, 103]. On epilepsy-specific QOL measures [35, 104], elderly patients with epilepsy generally do not experience poorer QOL compared to younger patients, but QOL can suffer in those with new-onset epilepsy, especially those diagnosed after retirement [103, 104]. As just one example of the potential long-reaching impact of the illness, veterans with epilepsy were about 1.5 times more likely than those without to report getting no regular exercise which, among other things, may lead to decreased muscle mass, falls, hip fractures, and frailty [103].

Young and old epilepsy patients share many of the same QOL concerns [91], but the impact of an epilepsy diagnosis on QOL is potentially different in older adults. For example, it may lead to premature admission to a nursing home or other long-term care facility [19, 61], and the diagnosis of epilepsy in the context of existing age-related physical and cognitive changes may lead to a debilitating sense of loss of control or a fear of losing one's mind [20, 32, 105]. Also, some senior citizens may be distressed by their own recall of a time when there were limited treatments for epilepsy, people did not understand why seizures occurred and were afraid of them, and families sometimes sent people with seizures to institutions or kept them isolated from others [106–108]. Different epilepsy-specific QOL measures have not been compared in an elderly population [29]. It may prove useful to develop a QOL instrument specifically for older adults and their caregivers [29, 93].

A few studies show that age is not always a significant predictor for QOL in patients with epilepsy [109]. The impact of epilepsy on the aged population may be more complex than on younger groups because health and perceptions of life success have different definitions that are dependent on the modified perspectives, aims, and physiological ability associated with aging. In the general population, the main determinants of successful aging include absence of disability, arthritis and diabetes, and being a nonsmoker and, to a lesser extent, social interaction, physical activity, and absence of cognitive impairment and depression [110]. The impact of epilepsy on QOL in older adults may depend on a combination of such determinants, as well as on the subjective perception of aging and personal resources. The subjective perception of epilepsy, stigma, loneliness, low self-esteem, poor mastery, and disease-related distress and, on the other side, life fulfillment and coping abilities interact in the individual patient, explaining 20–35% of the variance of QOL [111]. Spiritual aspects may also contribute to determine overall well-being, irrespective of age [109]. Improving the factors that enhance QOL in the non-epileptic elderly (e.g., physical exercise, calorie restriction, cognitive and social stimulation, and psychological support) also would be expected to combat the deleterious effects of epilepsy in older adults [112].

Depression is common in older epilepsy patients and is associated with poor subjective QOL [113]. Suicide risk is elevated in people with epilepsy and in older adults [114, 115], occurring more frequently in patients with chronic long-lasting epilepsy and medical and psychiatric comorbidities. Other disabling mental health symptoms also are common among people with epilepsy [116]. More research is needed to understand QOL issues and the causes and consequences of depression and other psychiatric disorders in geriatric epilepsy [12].

Studies of Aging and Cognitive Functioning in Epilepsy Patients

In young adults with epilepsy, memory and word-finding difficulties are predominant [117]. These complaints also are common with normal aging of course, and so they are likely to be frequent among older epilepsy patients. The latter are more likely to be concerned about the possibility that they are developing dementia compared to younger patients. At the group level, older people with partial epilepsy show a variety of cognitive impairments as compared to healthy subjects matched for gender, age, and education [38, 40, 41, 118]. For example, abstraction, divided attention, word fluency, and episodic memory were impaired in this group, although between-group differences generally were not large [40, 41]. In one study, results remained stable over a 3-year period [38], although there was failure to benefit from a test–retest effect. Early age of onset of epilepsy, a known etiology, and a high number of years with seizures, number of years taking medications, number of medications taken, and lifetime number of generalized tonic–clonic seizures are factors that have been associated with poorer neuropsychological functioning in the general population of patients with epilepsy [35]. Other factors associated with cognition are brain lesion, genetic abnormalities, seizure frequency, type of seizure, SE, and surgery [119].

Although variables such as age of onset and duration of illness are associated with manifestation of cognitive deficits [40], recent cross-sectional studies suggest that cognitive deficits characteristic of early-onset TLE are established early in life and tend to remain relatively stable with aging [120, 121]. In older patients with partial epilepsy, AED polytherapy so far appears to be the strongest determinant of cognitive performance, regardless of whether seizures are controlled or refractory [40, 41], with effects on initiation, shifting, attention, and memory. Older epilepsy patients on AED polytherapy were impaired compared to patients with amnesic MCI, whereas those on AED monotherapy showed comparable deficits to the MCI group [118]. See Table 26.5 for a summary of the results of studies of cognition in older adults with epilepsy.

Framework for Neuropsychological Assessment

The neuropsychological approach to epilepsy, often assumed as a model to test patients with focal brain lesions, aims to produce a functional map of impaired and preserved functions, highlighting the interactions between weaknesses and strengths and contributing to determination of the type and severity of brain damage. Other aims are clinical monitoring, in particular the follow-up of AED changes and surgery, and the determination of baseline cognitive and emotional status. The neuropsychological approach to presurgical assessment is evolving in the face of advances in neuroimaging [122]. Aspects of the therapeutic assessment model can be applicable in geriatric neuropsychology, including the tenets of addressing the patient's presenting concerns and the potentially threatening nature of the assessment, treating the patient as a collaborator, and providing feedback relevant to the individual's questions and everyday functioning and circumstances [123, 124].

Neuropsychological data reflect a combination of fixed factors, such as neuropathology and its localization, disease course factors, including history of recent SE or epilepsy surgery, and potentially remediable factors, such as medication effects, fatigue, and mood [122, 123]. When cognitive status is in question, neuropsychologists can help determine a patient's ability to understand the rationale for medications, written instructions about the regimen, use of dosing trays, and the potential need for close involvement of a family member and interaction with a multidisciplinary health-care team. The treatment goal for an epilepsy patient is to achieve seizure freedom with minimal AED side effects and the least possible decrease in QOL. Since no ideal AED exists [19, 26, 61], interdisciplinary efforts can strive for maximization of QOL.

Health-care professionals and epilepsy advocacy groups have worked together to publish specific recommendations concerning driving applicable to people with epilepsy [125], yet formal driving restrictions vary widely across different states and countries [126]. Neuropsychologists may play a role in advising about driving restrictions related to aging and epilepsy. In particular, neuropsychologists can provide information about a patient's awareness of cognitive impairments and risks for driving, and about the status of the main cognitive resources that are important to complex

Table 26.5 Results of neuropsychological studies of older patients with epilepsy

Study sample	Cognitive domain investigated	Neuropsychological tests	Findings	Reference
26 Epilepsy pts 26 MCI pts 26 Healthy older controls	Overall cognitive abilities Immediate and long-term memory Lexical ability	Dementia Rating Scale Wechsler Memory Scale-III Logical Memory subtest CFL Word Fluency test	Epilepsy pts impaired with respect to healthy controls. Epilepsy pts on AED polytherapy more impaired than MCI pts	Griffith et al. [118]
40 Epilepsy pts 40 Healthy older controls	Selective and divided attention Abstraction Memory, learning Language	Attentional Matrices, Trail Making Tests Raven CPM Short story, Paired words test, Rey Complex Figure Verbal Fluency test, Token test	Epilepsy pts impaired on all tests, with the worst deficits in those on AED polytherapy	Piazzini et al. [41]
25 Epilepsy pts 27 Healthy older controls	Overall cognitive functioning Immediate and long-term memory	Mattis Dementia Rating Scale Wechsler Memory Scale-III Logical Memory subtest	Epilepsy pts impaired on all tests. Pts on AED polytherapy more impaired than pts on monotherapy	Martin et al. [40]
17 Epilepsy pts 17 Older controls	Overall cognitive functioning	Dementia Rating Scale Wechsler Memory Scale-III Logical Memory subtest	Epilepsy pts impaired on all tests, with stable pattern over 3 years	Griffith et al. [38]
95 pts with epilepsy and AD treated with phenobarbital, levetiracetam or lamotrigine 68 Controls	Overall cognitive functioning	Mini-Mental State Examination Alzheimer's Disease Assessment-Cognitive	At 1-year follow-up, levetiracetam was associated with seizure decrease and improved attention, short-term memory, and verbal fluency; lamotrigine with mild cognitive decline; and phenobarbital with significant worsening	Cumbo and Ligori [95]

Pts patients

driving behavior (e.g., visuospatial functions) [127]. This baseline information may be helpful during other examinations relevant to fitness to drive, including structured assessment of driving performance (e.g., driving simulation test).

Exclusion of cognitive decline requires at least two examinations, usually separated by a minimum of 12 months. Especially at advanced ages, variability in cognitive reserve may lead to quite different individual trajectories of cognitive change. Cognitive reserve, as a product of intelligence level, education, lifestyle, social stimulation, personal experiences, and motivation, can modify or buffer the impact of aging and epilepsy on cognitive functions. It is a common experience that older patients affected by similar brain pathology may be heterogeneous at the physical, mental, and behavioral levels. Cognitive functions may reflect previous neural and functional reorganizations, resulting in selectively impaired or preserved function irrespective of epilepsy. This underlines the importance of obtaining a comprehensive neuropsychological profile in older patients with epilepsy and assessing in detail different cognitive abilities. Mental control, episodic memory, the inhibition of interference, set shifting, lexical-semantic competence, constructive praxis, and social cognition may show different trajectories. The understanding of social situations, in particular, might be relatively preserved with respect to memory and executive functions. A neuropsychological battery sensitive to epilepsy- and aging-related variables should assess multiple domains, but the battery should be cognizant of fatigability and fluctuating compliance. The tests should not be redundant or excessively time-consuming, preferably divided into 30–40 min sections. In addition to the necessary psychometric properties, the tests ideally should have alternative forms for serial assessment and be sensitive at the lowest levels of performance, allowing for detection of small changes.

Test Battery

There is no consensus neuropsychological test battery for older patients with epilepsy. However, the neuropsychology subcommittee of the NINDS Epilepsy Common Data Element (CDE) Project very recently published a recommended test battery for adult epilepsy patients that could be adopted for older adults (see Table 26.6) [128, 129]. The subcommittee recommended that when WAIS-IV or WASI short forms are used, the Vocabulary and Block Design tests should be administered, at a minimum. The entire battery, depending on whether an IQ short form or the optional tests are used, should take from 2 to 3.5 h [129]. The CDE recommendations emphasize that the tests do not have to constitute a "fixed battery." Alternative or novel measures can be included to maintain continuity within an existing program or to advance the field [129, 130]. As just a few examples, additions might include measures of planning, theory of mind, semantic knowledge, and visual perception. The battery listed here does not include psychiatric measures, but the Epilepsy CDE also does provide a list of recommended psychiatric scales [129].

Table 26.6 NINDS Epilepsy Common Data Element Project: Recommended neuropsychological test battery [128]

General IQ estimation	American National Adult Reading Test (AmNART)
Formal IQ	WAIS-IV, a WAIS-IV short form, or WASI
Verbal memory	Rey Auditory Verbal Learning Test
Naming	Boston Naming Test
Phonemic fluency	Controlled Oral Word Association (aka FAS)
Semantic fluency	Animal fluency
Set shifting	Trail Making Tests A and B
Simple attention span	WAIS-IV Digit Span
Processing speed	WAIS-IV PSI (see WAIS-IV above)
Motor speed	Grooved Pegboard
Optional or potential tests	
Hypothesis testing	Wisconsin Card Sorting Test short form (WCST-64)
Visual memory	Brief Visuospatial Memory Test-Revised (BVMT-R)

WAIS-IV Wechsler Adult Intelligence Scale-IV, *WASI* Wechsler Abbreviated Scale of Intelligence, *PSI* Processing Speed Index

Memory Self-Report

Decades ago, a review of the extant self-report memory questionnaire literature led to the conclusion that it is "prudent to employ memory questionnaires with caution" [131]. This advice continues to hold true, because there is no close correlation between self-reported memory ability and objective test results across patient groups [132]. Presurgical adult TLE patients, the most consistently studied epilepsy group, most often overestimate their degree of memory impairment [130]. Complaints of recent memory dysfunction may be associated with a number of factors, including a stable chronic deficit, increased seizure activity, medication side effects, mood, or a combination of these factors [34], with depression and anxiety playing a central role in self-perception of memory [39, 132]. Thus, it is possible that, in some older patients with epilepsy, identification of mood problems during a neuropsychological evaluation may lead to both effective psychiatric/psychological treatment and reassurance that a feared dementia is not present. With the patient's consent, information acquired from family members may help determine the severity of the problem in everyday life. When memory impairment is identified, external memory aids, such as a calendar and a personal digital assistant (PDA), can be recommended.

Information for Patients and Family

Guides that may be helpful for patients and families include those published on-line by the Epilepsy Foundation, The Epilepsy Project, and Epilepsy Action [133–135]. For additional sources of information, see Loring, Hermann, and Cohen [136]. As noted above, the term epilepsy may have unfortunate connotations and stigma associated with it for some older patients, and so it may be best to avoid the term in those cases [11]. Family members and caregivers can be taught about the signs of AED toxicity to help prevent falls and other consequences [13]. A 7-day pillbox aids adherence to AEDs and some patients may benefit from having a family member fill the pillbox once per week. A visiting nurse also may enhance AED adherence.

Case Report

A 77-year-old, right-handed, married woman (FC) with primary schooling reported long-lasting mental and physical fatigue and recurrent depression. Since age 71, FC experienced CPS that were incompletely controlled by carbamazepine. Her seizures were characterized by sudden gastric distress, nausea, and loss of consciousness in the absence of falls or motor symptoms; sometimes she appeared disoriented or mildly confused for almost 1 h. After the onset of her seizure disorder, FC also complained of naming difficulties and autobiographical, immediate, and spatial memory failures. Some of the memory failures were characterized by sudden interruption of the processing or learning of new information (e.g., taking note of a phone call). Minor problems concerned motor planning, with slowing and abnormal sequencing and execution of fine actions such as sewing. Past medical history included undefined digestive and bowel problems, anemia, chronic hypokalemia, hypothyroidism and hypocalcemia with secondary hypoparathyroidism following surgical resection of a thyroid adenoma, and beneficial treatment of some of these conditions with thyroxin, calcium, and potassium. Family history was negative.

At neurological examination, FC was oriented in time and space, depressed but cooperative; her behavior was sometimes reactive, with theatrical manifestations or repeated demands for help. Speech was fluent and communicative, and comprehension was fully preserved. Immediate memory and autobiographical memory were clinically impaired. No other cognitive, motor, sensorial, balance, or cranial nerve defects were observed. The seizures, as well as some sudden memory failures, were strongly indicative of epilepsy, while cognitive decline, in the light of medical history, suggested a vascular or secondary metabolic encephalopathy, although a degenerative disease had to be excluded. Brain CT showed cortical atrophy in the posterior parietal and occipital brain areas and small vascular lacunae in the deep white matter. Positron emission CT showed normal brain perfusion. EEG documented left temporal slow waves and spikes. Carotid Doppler sonography showed mild acceleration of the blood flow at the origin of the internal carotids.

The first neuropsychological assessment, at age 77, showed impaired working memory, verbal and visuospatial long-term memory, word fluency on phonemic and semantic cues, word-list learning, and constructive praxis, with spared short-term memory span, set shifting, and abstract reasoning. A year later, neuropsychological testing revealed a similar qualitative pattern, with worsening of visuoperceptual and praxis abilities. At this time, due to the persistence of medical symptoms, especially anemia, asthenia, and bowel problems, and drug-resistant seizures, she underwent blood testing for antigliadin antibodies that was indicative of gluten intolerance. Biopsy specimens from the small bowel showed villous atrophy and crypt hyperplasia, indicating celiac disease alterations. After a 6-month gluten-free diet, she reported weight loss and significant improvement of physical strength and mental concentration. Moreover, seizures disappeared. Neuropsychological follow-up, at age 80, showed long-term memory and word fluency deficits but improvement of visuospatial abilities, constructive praxis, and divided attention. The neurological and neuropsychological picture was unchanged at the age 82 follow-up.

This is a rare case of treatable epilepsy-related cognitive impairment in an older adult. The patient was affected by late-onset seizures and cognitive decline associated with celiac disease. Seizures were reversed after dietary restrictions. At the clinical level, it is worth noting that the seizures were characterized by longer compromise of consciousness compared to typical young-adult seizures and that sudden memory failures, quite different from the other everyday difficulties reported by the patient, may have been the result of TEA. In regard to diagnosis, this case underlines the importance of considering the medical symptoms and comorbidities that may raise the suspicion of unexpected etiologies, although many adult patients with celiac disease may be asymptomatic or have only non-intestinal symptoms. Recent reports have described different neurological complications of celiac disease, such as ataxia, peripheral neuropathy, and epilepsy. Prevalence of celiac disease is increased among patients with epilepsy of unknown etiology, and humoral immune mechanisms may explain the neurological complications [137]. This case suggests a link between gluten sensitivity and epilepsy. Thus, it is worthwhile to investigate celiac disease in any elderly patient with partial epilepsy of unknown origin, even in the absence of digestive symptoms. FC's cognitive decline was in great part reversible, with the cognitive changes identified by serial neuropsychological assessment. After specific dietary restrictions, she reached an age-appropriate level of functioning and did not lose her autonomy. The findings from the cognitive evaluations excluded degenerative or vascular dementia, supporting a diagnosis of normal cognitive aging.

Clinical Pearls

- The neuropsychologist should explain to the patient the nature of neuropsychological assessment in the context of a multidisciplinary approach.
- Older patients may be reluctant to acknowledge problems they view as "psychological" or may not be aware of seizure symptoms or their significance.
- Include spouse or other collateral source in the interview to acquire additional information about seizure type(s) and frequency, patient's level of everyday cognitive functioning, etc.
- Determine when the most recent seizure occurred and get detailed information about recent medication changes, adherence, and any known side effects.
- Take into account comorbid conditions and risks for cognitive impairment, including AEDs and other medications, head trauma, alcohol use, family history of dementia, etc.
- Administer a test battery appropriate to age and stamina; key abilities to assess include

psychomotor speed, attention, executive functions, and learning (see Table 26.6). Make sure to assess for depression, anxiety, suicidality, and quality of life.

- Remember that driving restriction is a prime quality-of-life concern.
- Both the patient and spouse may benefit from psychosocial support.

References

1. Commission on Classification and Terminology of the International League Against Epilepsy. Proposal for revised classification of epilepsies and epileptic syndromes. Epilepsia. 1981;30:389–99.
2. Commission on Classification and Terminology of the International League Against Epilepsy. Proposal for revised clinical and electroencephalographic classification of epileptic seizures. Epilepsia. 1989; 22:489–501.
3. Commission on Epidemiology and Prognosis, International League Against Epilepsy. Guidelines for epidemiological studies on epilepsy. Epilepsia. 1993;34:592–6.
4. Berg AT, Berkovic SF, Brodie MJ, et al. Revised terminology and concepts for organization of seizures and epilepsies: report of the ILAE Commission on Classification and Terminology, 2005–2009. Epilepsia. 2010;51:676–85.
5. Beghi E, Carpio A, Forsgren L, et al. Recommendation for a definition of acute symptomatic seizure. Epilepsia. 2010;51:671–5.
6. WHO. World Health Organization: epilepsy: epidemiology, aetiology, and prognosis (WHO Fact Sheet). Geneva: World Health Organization; 2001.
7. Banerjee PN, Filippi D, Hauser WA. The descriptive epidemiology of epilepsy—a review. Epilepsy Res. 2009;85:31–45.
8. Lavados J, Germain L, Morales A, Campero M, Lavados P. A descriptive study of epilepsy in the district of El Salvador, Chile, 1984–1988. Acta Neurol Scand. 1992;85:249–56.
9. Birbeck GL, Kalichi EM. Epilepsy prevalence in rural Zambia: a door-to-door survey. Trop Med Int Health. 2004;9:92–5.
10. Wallace H, Shorvon S, Tallis R. Age-specific incidence and prevalence rates of treated epilepsy in an unselected population of 2 052 922 and age-specific fertility rates of women with epilepsy. Lancet. 1998;352:1970–3.
11. Brodie MJ, Elder AT, Kwan P. Epilepsy in later life. Lancet Neurol. 2009;8:1019–30.
12. Cloyd J, Hauser W, Towne A, et al. Epidemiological and medical aspects of epilepsy in the elderly. Epilepsy Res. 2006;68:39–48.
13. Jacobson MP. Epilepsy in aging populations. Curr Treat Options Neurol. 2002;4:19–30.
14. Leppik IE, Birnbaum AK. Epilepsy in the elderly. Ann N Y Acad Sci. 2010;1184:208–24.
15. Ramsay RE, Macias FM, Rowan AJ. Diagnosing epilepsy in the elderly. In: Ramsay RE (ed. in Chief), Cloyd JC, Kelly KM, Leppik IE, Perucca E (editors). The neurobiology of epilepsy and aging. New York: Elsevier; 2007. p. 129–151.
16. Hauser WA. Epidemiology of seizures and epilepsy in the elderly. In: Rowan AJ, Ramsay RE, editors. Seizures and epilepsy in the elderly. Newton, MA: Butterworth-Heinemann; 1997. p. 7–18.
17. Leppik IE. Introduction to the International Geriatric Epilepsy Symposium (IGES). Epilepsy Res. 2006;68 Suppl 1:1–4.
18. Baker GA, Jacoby A, Buck D, Brooks J, Potts P, Chadwick DW. The quality of life of older people with epilepsy: findings from a UK community study. Seizure. 2001;10:92–9.
19. Brodie MJ, Kwan P. Epilepsy in elderly people. Br Med J. 2005;331:1317–22.
20. DeToledo JC. Changing presentation of seizures with aging: clinical and etiological factors. Gerontology. 1999;45:329–35.
21. Pugh MJ, Knoefel JE, Mortensen EM, Amuan ME, Berlowitz DR, Van Cott AC. New-onset epilepsy risk factors in older veterans. J Am Geriatr Soc. 2009;57:237–42.
22. Ramsay RE, Rowan AJ, Pryor FM. Special considerations in treating the elderly patient with epilepsy. Neurology. 2004;62 Suppl 2:24–9.
23. Sheorajpanday R, De Deyn PP. Epileptic fits and epilepsy in the elderly: general reflections, specific issues and therapeutic implications. Clin Neurol Neurosurg. 2007;109:727–43.
24. Tallis R, Hall G, Craig I, Dean A. How common are epileptic seizures in old age? Age Ageing. 1991;20:442–8.
25. Tebartz van Elst L, Baker G, Kerr M. The psychosocial impact of epilepsy in older people. Epilepsy Behav. 2009;15 Suppl 1:17–9.
26. Waterhouse E, Towne A. Seizures in the elderly: nuances in presentation and treatment. Cleve Clin J Med. 2005;72 Suppl 3:26–37.
27. Hermann BP, Seidenberg M, Sager M, Carlsson C, Gidal B, Rutecki P, Asthana S. Growing old with epilepsy: the neglected issue of cognitive and brain health in aging and elder persons with chronic epilepsy. Epilepsia. 2008;49:731–40.
28. Leppik IE, Kelly KM, deToledo-Morrell L, Patrylo PR, DeLorenzo RJ, Mathern GW, White HS. Basic research in epilepsy and aging. Epilepsy Res. 2006;68 Suppl 1:21–37.
29. Martin RC, Vogtle L, Gilliam F, Faught E. Health-related quality of life in senior adults with epilepsy: what we know from randomized clinical trials and suggestions for future research. Epilepsy Behav. 2003;4:626–34.
30. Loring DW. History of neuropsychology through epilepsy eyes. Arch Clin Neuropsychol. 2010; 25:259–73.

31. Novelly R. The debt of neuropsychology to the epilepsies. Am Psychol. 1992;47:1126–9.
32. Snyder PJ, McConnell HW. Neuropsychological aspects of epilepsy in the elderly. In: Nussbaum PD, editor. Handbook of neuropsychology and aging. New York: Plenum; 1997. p. 271–9.
33. Aldenkamp AP, Baker GA, Meador KJ. The neuropsychology of epilepsy: what are the factors involved? Epilepsy Behav. 2004;5 Suppl 1:1–2.
34. Baker GA, Goldstein LH. The dos and don'ts of neuropsychological assessment in epilepsy. Epilepsy Behav. 2004;5 Suppl 1:77–80.
35. Dodrill CB, Matthews CG. The role of neuropsychology in the assessment and treatment of persons with epilepsy. Am Psychol. 1992;47:1139–42.
36. Hayashi PJ, O'Connor M. Neuropsychological assessment and application to temporal lobe epilepsy. In: Schachter SC, Shomer DL, editors. The comprehensive evaluation and treatment of epilepsy: a practical guide. New York: Elsevier; 1997. p. 111–30.
37. Zeman A, Butler C. Transient epileptic amnesia. Curr Opin Neurol. 2010;23:610–6.
38. Griffith HR, Martin RC, Bambara JK, Faught E, Vogtle LK, Marson DC. Cognitive functioning over three years in community dwelling older adults with chronic partial epilepsy. Epilepsy Res. 2007;74:91–6.
39. Hermann BP, Meador KJ, Gaillard WD, Cramer JA. Cognition across the lifespan: antiepileptic drugs, epilepsy, or both? Epilepsy Behav. 2010;17:1–5.
40. Martin RC, Griffith HR, Faught E, Gilliam F, Mackey M, Vogtle L. Cognitive functioning in community dwelling older adults with chronic partial epilepsy. Epilepsia. 2005;46:298–303.
41. Piazzini A, Canevini MP, Turner K, Chifari R, Canger R. Elderly people and epilepsy: cognitive function. Epilepsia. 2006;47 Suppl 5:82–4.
42. Grivas A, Schramm J, Kral T, et al. Surgical treatment for refractory temporal lobe epilepsy in the elderly: seizure outcome and neuropsychological sequels compared with a younger cohort. Epilepsia. 2006;47:1364–72.
43. Scheuer ML, Cohen J. Seizures and epilepsy in the elderly. Neurol Clin. 1993;11:787–804.
44. Ruggles KH, Haessly SM, Berg RL. Prospective study of seizures in the elderly in the Marshfield Epidemiologic Study Area (MESA). Epilepsia. 2001;42:1594–9.
45. Leppik IE. Epilepsy in the elderly. Epilepsia. 2006;47 Suppl 1:65–70.
46. Burn J, Dennis M, Bamford J, et al. Epileptic seizures after a first stroke: the Oxfordshire community stroke project. Br Med J. 1997;315:1182–7.
47. Ferro JM, Pinto F. Poststroke epilepsy: epidemiology, pathophysiology, and management. Drugs Aging. 2004;21:639–53.
48. Myint PK, Staufenberg EFA, Sabanathan K. Post-stroke seizure and post-stroke epilepsy. Postgrad Med. 2006;82:568–72.
49. So EL, Annegers JF, Hauser WA, O'Brien PC, Whisnant JP. Population-based study of seizure disorders after cerebral infarction. Neurology. 1996;46: 350–5.
50. De Reuck J. Management of stroke-related seizures. Acta Neurol Belg. 2009;109:271–6.
51. Larner AJ. Epileptic seizures in AD patients. Neuromolecular Med. 2010;12:71–7.
52. Mendez MF, Catanzaro P, Doss RC, Arguello R, Frey 2nd WH. Seizures in Alzheimer's disease: clinicopathologic study. J Geriatr Psychiatry Neurol. 1994;7:230–3.
53. Scarmeas N, Honig LS, Choi H, et al. Seizures in Alzheimer's disease: Who, when, and how common? Arch Neurol. 2009;66:992–7.
54. Caramelli P, Castro LH. Dementia associated with epilepsy. Int Psychogeriatr. 2005;17 Suppl 1:195–206.
55. McCarron M, Gill M, McCallion P, Begley C. Health co-morbidities in ageing persons with Down syndrome and Alzheimer's dementia. J Intellect Disabil Res. 2005;49:560–6.
56. Palop JJ, Mucke L. Epilepsy and cognitive impairment in Alzheimer disease. Arch Neurol. 2009;66: 435–40.
57. Armon C, Shin C, Miller P, et al. Reversible parkinsonism and cognitive impairment with chronic valproate use. Neurology. 1996;47:626–35.
58. Roks G, Korf ES, van der Flier WM, Scheltens P, Stamm PJ. The use of EEG in the diagnosis of dementia with Lewy bodies. J Neurol Neurosurg Psychiatry. 2008;79:377–80.
59. Dupont S, Verny M, Harston S, et al. Seizures in the elderly: development and validation of a diagnostic algorithm. Epilepsy Res. 2010;89:339–48.
60. Sperfeld AD, Collatz MB, Baier H, et al. FTDP-17: an early-onset phenotype with parkinsonism and epileptic seizures caused by a novel mutation. Ann Neurol. 1999;46:708–15.
61. Brodie MJ, Stephen LJ. Outcomes in elderly patients with newly diagnosed and treated epilepsy. In: Ramsay RE (ed. in Chief), Cloyd JC, Kelly KM, Leppik IE, Perucca E (editors). The neurobiology of epilepsy and aging. New York: Elsevier; 2007. p. 253–263.
62. Kellinghaus C, Loddenkemper T, Dinner DS, Lachhwani D, Luders HO. Seizure semiology in the elderly: a video analysis. Epilepsia. 2004;45:263–7.
63. Ito M, Echizenya N, Nemoto D, Kase M. A case series of epilepsy-derived memory impairment resembling Alzheimer disease. Alzheimer Dis Assoc Disord. 2009;23:406–9.
64. Van Cott AC. Epilepsy and EEG in the elderly. Epilepsia. 2002;43 Suppl 3:94–102.
65. Seidenberg M, Pulsipher DT, Hermann B. Association of epilepsy and comorbid conditions. Future Neurol. 2009;4:663–8.
66. Bladin CF. Seizures in the elderly. Neurology. 1994;44: 194–5.
67. Jetter GM, Cavazos JE. Epilepsy in the elderly. Semin Neurol. 2008;28:336–41.
68. O'Donovan CA, Lancman ME, Luders HO. New-onset mesial temporal lobe epilepsy in a 90-year-old:

clinical and EEG features. Epilepsy Behav. 2004;5:1021–3.
69. Tinuper P, Provini F, Marini C, et al. Partial epilepsy of long duration: changing semiology with age. Epilepsia. 1996;37:162–4.
70. Gallassi R. Epileptic amnesic syndrome: an update and further considerations. Epilepsia. 2006;47 Suppl 2:103–5.
71. Kapur N. Transient epileptic amnesia: a clinical update and a reformulation. J Neurol Neurosurg Psychiatry. 1993;56:1184–90.
72. Mendes MHF. Transient epileptic amnesia: an underdiagnosed phenomenon? Three more cases. Seizure. 2002;11:238–42.
73. Muhlert N, Milton F, Butler CR, Kapur N, Zeman AZ. Accelerated forgetting of real-life events in Transient Epileptic Amnesia. Neuropsychologia. 2010;48:3235–44.
74. Theodore WH. The postictal state: effects of age and underlying brain dysfunction. Epilepsy Behav. 2010;19:118–20.
75. Towne AR. Epidemiology and outcomes of status epilepticus in the elderly. In: Ramsay RE (ed. in Chief), Cloyd JC, Kelly KM, Leppik IE, Perucca E (editors). The neurobiology of epilepsy and aging. New York: Elsevier; 2007. p. 111–127.
76. Gastaut H. Classification of status epilepticus. Adv Neurol. 1983;34:15–35.
77. Coeytaux A, Jallon P, Galobardes B, et al. Incidence of status epilepticus in French-speaking Switzerland: (EPISTAR). Neurology. 2000;55:693–7.
78. Logroscino G, Hesdorffer DC, Cascino G, et al. Mortality after a first episode of status epilepticus in the United States and Europe. Epilepsia. 2005;46:46–8.
79. Leppik IE. Epilepsy in the elderly: scope of the problem. In: Ramsay RE (ed. in Chief), Cloyd JC, Kelly KM, Leppik IE, Perucca E (editors). The neurobiology of epilepsy and aging. New York: Elsevier; 2007. p. 1–14.
80. McBride AE, Shih TT, Hirsch LJ. Video-EEG monitoring in the elderly: a review of 94 patients. Epilepsia. 2002;43:165–9.
81. Kawai M, Hrachovy RA, Franklin PJ, Foreman PJ. Video-EEG monitoring in a geriatric veteran population. J Clin Neurophysiol. 2007;24:429–32.
82. Drane DL, Coady EL, Williamson DJ, Miller JW, Benbadis S. Neuropsychology of psychogenic nonepileptic seizures. In: Schoenberg MR, Scott JG, editors. The little black book of neuropsychology: a syndrome-based approach. New York: Springer; 2011. p. 521–50.
83. Duncan R, Oto M, Martin E, Pelosi A. Late onset psychogenic nonepileptic attacks. Neurology. 2006;66:1644–7.
84. Binder LM, Salinsky MC. Psychogenic nonepileptic seizures. Neuropsychol Rev. 2007;17:405–12.
85. Locke DE, Thomas ML. Initial development of Minnesota Multiphasic Personality Inventory-2-Restructured Form (MMPI-2-RF) scales to identify patients with psychogenic nonepileptic seizures. J Clin Exp Neuropsychol. 2011;33:335–43.
86. Ramsay RE, Pryor F. Epilepsy in the elderly. Neurology. 2000;55 Suppl 1:9–14.
87. Hogh P, Smith SJ, Scahill RI, et al. Epilepsy presenting as AD: neuroimaging, electroclinical features, and response to treatment. Neurology. 2002;58: 298–301.
88. Drury I, Selwa LM, Schuh LA, et al. Value of inpatient diagnostic CCTV-EEG monitoring in the elderly. Epilepsia. 1999;40:1100–2.
89. Noe KH, Drazkowski JF. Safety of long-term video-electroencephalographic monitoring for evaluation of epilepsy. Mayo Clin Proc. 2009;84:495–500.
90. Veran O, Kahane P, Thomas P, Hamelin S, Sabourdy C, Vercueil L. De novo epileptic confusion in the elderly: a 1-year prospective study. Epilepsia. 2010;51: 1030–5.
91. Martin RC, Vogtle L, Gilliam F, Faught E. What are the concerns of older adults living with epilepsy? Epilepsy Behav. 2005;7:297–300.
92. Ettinger AB, Baker GA. Best clinical and research practice in epilepsy of older people: focus on antiepileptic drug adherence. Epilepsy Behav. 2009;15 Suppl 1:60–3.
93. Laccheo I, Ablah E, Heinrichs R, et al. Assessment of quality of life among the elderly with epilepsy. Epilepsy Behav. 2008;12:257–61.
94. Glauser T, Ben-Menachem E, Bourgeois B, et al. ILAE treatment guidelines: evidence-based analysis of antiepileptic drug efficacy and effectiveness as initial monotherapy for epileptic seizures and syndromes. Epilepsia. 2006;47:1094–120.
95. Cumbo E, Ligori LD. Levetiracetam, lamotrigine, and phenobarbital in patients with epileptic seizures and Alzheimer's disease. Epilepsy Behav. 2010;17: 461–6.
96. Fattouch J, Di Bonaventura C, Casciato S, et al. Intravenous levetiracetam as first-line treatment of status epilepticus in the elderly. Acta Neurol Scand. 2010;121:418–21.
97. Pugh MJ, Van Cott AC, Cramer JA, Knoefel JE, Amuan ME, Tabares J, Ramsay RE, Berlowitz DR, et al. Trends in antiepileptic drug prescribing for older patients with new-onset epilepsy: 2000–2004. Neurology. 2008;70:2171–8.
98. Acosta I, Vale F, Tatum IV WO. Epilepsy surgery after age 60. Epilepsy Behav. 2008;12:324–5.
99. Wiebe S, Blume WT, Girvin JP, Eliasziw M. Effectiveness and Efficiency of Epilepsy Surgery for Temporal Lobe Epilepsy Study Group. A randomized, controlled trial of surgery for temporal-lobe epilepsy. N Engl J Med. 2001;345:311–8.
100. Costello DJ, Shields DC, Cash SS, Eskandar EN, Cosgrove GR, Cole AJ. Consideration of epilepsy surgery in adults should be independent of age. Clin Neurol Neurosurg. 2009;111:240–5.
101. Cascino GD, Sharbrough FW, Hirschorn KA, Marsh WR. Surgery for focal epilepsy in the older patient. Neurology. 1991;41:1415–7.

102. Murphy M, Smith PD, Wood M, et al. Surgery for temporal lobe epilepsy associated with mesial temporal sclerosis in the older patient: a long-term follow-up. Epilepsia. 2010;51:1024–9.
103. Pugh MJ, Berlowitz DR, Kazis L. The impact of epilepsy on older veterans. In: Ramsay RE (ed. in Chief), Cloyd JC, Kelly KM, Leppik IE, Perucca E (editors). The neurobiology of epilepsy and aging. New York: Elsevier; 2007. p. 221–233
104. Baker GA, Smith DF, Dewey M, Jacoby A, Chadwick DW. The initial development of a health-related quality of life model as an outcome measure in epilepsy. Epilepsy Res. 1993;16:65–81.
105. Morrison JH, Hof PR. Life and death of neurons in the aging cerebral cortex. In: Ramsay RE (ed. in Chief), Cloyd JC, Kelly KM, Leppik IE, Perucca E (editors). The neurobiology of epilepsy and aging. New York: Elsevier; 2007. p. 41–57
106. de Boer HM. Epilepsy stigma: moving from a global problem to global solutions. Seizure. 2010;19: 630–6.
107. Kobau R, DiIorio CA, Anderson LA, Price PH. Further validation and reliability testing of the Attitudes and Beliefs about Living with Epilepsy (ABLE) components of the CDC Epilepsy Program Instrument on Stigma. Epilepsy Behav. 2006; 8:552–9.
108. www.epilepsyfoundation.org/living/seniors.
109. Giovagnoli AR, Meneses RF, da Silva AM. The contribution of spirituality to quality of life in focal epilepsy. Epilepsy Behav. 2006;9:133–9.
110. Depp CA, Jeste DV. Definitions and predictors of successful aging: a comprehensive review of larger quantitative studies. Am J Geriatr Psychiatry. 2006;14:6–20.
111. Suurmeijer TP, Reuvekamp MF, Aldenkamp BP. Social functioning, psychological functioning, and quality of life in epilepsy. Epilepsia. 2001;42:1160–8.
112. Vahia IV, Depp CA, Palmer BW, et al. Correlates of spirituality in older women. Aging Ment Health. 2010;4:1–6.
113. Hermann BP, Seidenberg M, Bell B. Psychiatric comorbidity in chronic epilepsy: identification, consequences, and treatment of major depression. Epilepsia. 2000;41 Suppl 2:31–41.
114. Kramer G. Broadening the perspective: treating the whole patient. Epilepsia. 2003;44 Suppl 5:16–22.
115. Jones JE, Hermann BP, Barry JJ, Gilliam FG, Kanner AM, Meador KJ. Rates and risk factors for suicide, suicidal ideation, and suicide attempts in chronic epilepsy. Epilepsy Behav. 2003;4 Suppl 3:31–8.
116. Butterbaugh G, Rose M, Thomson J, et al. Mental health symptoms in partial epilepsy. Arch Clin Neuropsychol. 2005;20:647–54.
117. Giovagnoli AR. Characteristics of verbal semantic impairment in left hemisphere epilepsy. Neuropsychology. 2005;19:501–8.
118. Griffith HR, Martin RC, Bambara JK, Marson DC, Faught E. Older adults with epilepsy demonstrate cognitive impairments compared with patients with amnestic mild cognitive impairment. Epilepsy Behav. 2006;8:161–8.
119. Meador KJ. Cognitive outcomes and predictive factors in epilepsy. Neurology. 2002;58 Suppl 5:21–6.
120. Helmstaedter C, Elger CE. Chronic temporal lobe epilepsy: a neurodevelopmental or progressively dementing disease? Brain. 2009;132:2822–30.
121. Baxendale S, Heaney D, Thompson PJ, et al. Cognitive consequences of childhood-onset temporal lobe epilepsy across the adult lifespan. Neurology. 2010;75:705–11.
122. Baxendale S, Thompson P. Beyond localization: the role of traditional neuropsychological tests in an age of imaging. Epilepsia. 2010;51:2225–30.
123. Jamora CW, Ruff RM, Connor BB. Geriatric neuropsychology: implications for front line clinicians. NeuroRehabilitation. 2008;23:381–94.
124. Potter GG, Attix DK. An integrated model for geriatric neuropsychological assessment. In: Attix DK, Welsh-Bohmer KA, editors. Geriatric neuropsychology: assessment and intervention. New York: Guilford; 2006. p. 5–26.
125. American Academy of Neurology, American Epilepsy Society and Epilepsy Society, Epilepsy Foundation of America. Consensus statement, sample statutory provisions and model regulations regarding driver licensing and epilepsy. Epilepsia. 1994;35:696–705.
126. Drazkowski J. An overview of epilepsy and driving. Epilepsia. 2007;48 Suppl 9:10–2.
127. Reger MA, Welsh RK, Watson GS, et al. The relationship between neuropsychological functioning and driving ability in dementia: a meta-analysis. Neuropsychology. 2004;18:85–93.
128. Loring DW, Lowenstein DH, Barbaro NM, et al. Common data elements in epilepsy research: development and implementation of the NINDS epilepsy CDE project. Epilepsia. 2011;52(6):1186–91.
129. http://www.commondataelements.ninds.nih.gov/Epilepsy.aspx.
130. Loring DW. Material, modality, or method? Manageable modernization of measurement. Epilepsia. 2010;51:2364–5.
131. Herrmann DJ. Know thy memory: the use of questionnaires to assess and study memory. Psychol Bull. 1982;92:434–52.
132. Hall K, Isaac CL, Harris P. Memory complaints in epilepsy: an accurate reflection of memory impairment or an indicator of poor adjustment? A review of the literature. Clin Psychol Rev. 2009;29:354–67.
133. www.epilepsyfoundation.org.
134. www.epilepsy.com.
135. www.epilepsy.org.uk.
136. Loring DW, Hermann BP, Cohen MJ. Neuropsychology advocacy and epilepsy. Clin Neuropsychol. 2010;24:417–28.
137. Peltola M, Kaukinen K, Dastidar P, et al. Hippocampal sclerosis in refractory temporal lobe epilepsy is associated with gluten sensitivity. J Neurol Neurosurg Psychiatry. 2009;80:626–30.

Neuropsychological Assessment of Older Adults with a History of Cancer

27

Mariana E. Witgert and Jeffrey S. Wefel

Abstract

Older adults are at increased risk for developing cancer. Given the aging population, the incidence of cancer is predicted to rise and, as a result, cancer is likely to become an even greater public health concern. Anticancer therapies can have potential untoward impacts on cognitive functioning, which is of particular concern for aging individuals that are already at increased risk for cognitive decline. This chapter reviews the potential cognitive side effects varies of cancer therapies and presents the most common considerations for differential diagnosis of memory complaints in this population. Instructive case examples are provided along with clinical pearls for the neuropsychologist working with older adults in an oncology setting.

Keywords

Neuropsychological assessment • Cancer • Cognition • Older adults

Adults over the age of 65 have a 9.6 times greater risk of cancer diagnosis and 17.4 times greater risk of cancer-related mortality [1]. In fact, it is estimated that 54.2% of cancer incidence and 69.5% of cancer-related mortality occur in individuals aged 65 or older. The US Census Bureau predicts a rapid rise in the number of individuals in the United States who are over the age of 65. In 2010, it was estimated that there were 40.2 million people aged 65 or older; this number is projected to rise to 88.5 million by the year 2050 [2]. As a result, cancer is likely to become an even greater public health concern. Significant advances have been made in multimodal drug therapy and have resulted in increased success in the management of many cancers. However, since many anticancer therapies are not highly specific, healthy tissues are also placed at risk. This can have potential untoward impacts on cognitive functioning, which may be of particular importance for an aging population whose

M.E. Witgert, Ph.D. (✉) • J.S. Wefel, Ph.D.
Section of Neuropsychology, Department of Neuro-Oncology, University of Texas M.D. Anderson Cancer Center, 1515 Holcombe Blvd, Unit 431, Houston, TX 77030-4009, USA
e-mail: mwitgert@mdanderson.org; jwefel@mdanderson.org

L.D. Ravdin and H.L. Katzen (eds.), *Handbook on the Neuropsychology of Aging and Dementia*, Clinical Handbooks in Neuropsychology, DOI 10.1007/978-1-4614-3106-0_27,

members are at increased risk for cognitive decline and toxicities related to cancer therapies.

Cancer-Related Cognitive Impairment

In order to determine whether or not cancer therapies impact cognitive functioning, one must first understand the presence and pattern of cognitive symptoms prior to the initiation of treatment. Patients with brain tumors may present with a variety of cognitive complaints as tumors destroy, crowd, and infiltrate brain tissue; the nature and severity of cognitive impairments vary in association with lesion location and lesion momentum, or the rate at which tumors grow. Cancer-related cognitive dysfunction is not limited to central nervous system (CNS) cancers. Several studies have demonstrated cancer-related cognitive dysfunction in non-CNS cancers as well. For example, cognitive dysfunction in at least a subgroup of women with breast cancer has been demonstrated prior to initiation of chemotherapy, with estimates ranging from 11% to 35% of patients [3–6]. The first of these studies revealed particularly frequent difficulties (18–25%) on measures assessing learning and memory [3]. Pretreatment cognitive dysfunction has also been found in other patient populations, including acute myelogenous leukemia (AML) and myelodysplastic syndrome (MDS), with pretreatment impairments in learning and memory (41–44%), cognitive processing speed (28%), aspects of executive dysfunction (29%), and upper extremity fine motor dexterity (37%) [7]. Patients with small cell lung cancer have also been shown to exhibit pretreatment cognitive impairments. Meyers et al. [8] demonstrated that 70–80% of patients with small cell lung cancer exhibited memory deficits, 38% had deficits in executive functions, and 33% showed impaired motor coordination *before* treatment was initiated. Without a clear understanding of the pretreatment cognitive status, impairments in cognition that are observed posttreatment could be erroneously attributed to a specific treatment, when in fact they might have been associated with the cancer itself.

Treatment-Related Cognitive Impairment

In addition to the potential for cognitive impairment related to cancer itself, cancer therapies, including surgery, radiation, chemotherapy, immunotherapy, and hormonal therapy, may have an untoward impact on cognitive functioning.

Surgery

Undergoing surgery and associated exposure to anesthesia may carry differential risk for older patients, who appear to be more vulnerable to developing postoperative cognitive dysfunction, or POCD, affecting memory, attention and concentration, and speed of processing [9]. We are not aware of any data to suggest that the surgical resection of non-CNS cancers carries any greater risk than other non-CNS surgeries. However, in patients with brain tumors, surgery may result in damage to normal tissue that surrounds the tumor. This can engender relatively focal cognitive impairments or more diffuse impairments secondary to the disconnection of subcortical networks.

Radiation

It is well known that radiation to the brain may be associated with the development of neuropsychological dysfunction both during and after treatment. The acute phase (during treatment) is characterized by transient symptoms of headache, fatigue, fever, and nausea, as well as exacerbation of preexisting neurologic deficits. Early delayed toxicity typically develops 2–5 months after completion of radiotherapy and has been associated with declines in information processing speed, attention, learning efficiency and memory retrieval, executive functioning, and fine motor dexterity; these symptoms may resolve spontaneously. Late-delayed toxicity can occur months to years after completion of radiation therapy and includes progressive dementia, personality changes, and leukoencephalopathy; unlike acute and early delayed effects, late-delayed toxicity tends to be irreversible [10]. Numerous risk factors for developing radiation-induced cognitive dysfunction and necrosis have been identified and include age over 60 years, greater than 2 Gy dose per fraction, higher total dose, greater total volume of brain irradiated, hyperfractionated schedules, shorter overall treatment time, concomitant or subsequent treatment with chemotherapy, and the presence of comorbid vascular risk factors [11, 12]. Current practice utilizes lower doses of radiation in an attempt to reduce exposure of the surrounding healthy brain tissue. Continued advances in treatment modalities (i.e., intensity modulated radiation therapy, whole brain radiation with hippocampal sparing, and proton therapy) should further improve the therapeutic ratio and limit incidental brain irradiation, thereby minimizing associated neurobehavioral complications. The risks and benefits of focal versus whole brain radiation are still being debated, but it has been shown that patients with 1–3 newly diagnosed brain metastases treated with stereotactic radiosurgery plus whole brain radiation were at increased risk of significant declines in learning and memory at 4 months after treatment compared to those treated with stereotactic radiosurgery alone [13]. The most profound effects of radiation treatment may not be evident for several years posttreatment. Therefore, careful monitoring of cognitive function in patients over time remains necessary.

Chemotherapy

The majority of research regarding chemotherapy-related side effects has been conducted in patients with breast cancer; cognitive dysfunction has most frequently been observed in learning and memory, attention, executive function, and processing speed, with estimates of dysfunction ranging from 13% to 70% [4, 5, 14–20]. Posttreatment follow-up has revealed that a subset of these women fails to achieve complete recovery [20]. More recent studies have also raised concern for ongoing, progressive cognitive decline after completion of chemotherapy [21], which may be of particular concern for older individuals who are already at increased risk for cognitive decline secondary to noncancer-related factors [21].

Cognitive and emotional dysfunction associated with hematopoietic stem cell transplant (HSCT) has also been reported by a number of investigators and is thought to result from the intense treatment regimen utilizing high-dose chemotherapy and total-body irradiation during pre-transplant conditioning [22, 23]. Studies in this group of patients are limited by small sample size and cross-sectional designs; however, the available prospective neuropsychological assessment data suggest a decline in executive functions [23] and memory [24] following HSCT.

Biological Response Modifiers

Biological response modifiers (BRMs; also known as immunotherapies) are aimed at modifying the immune response of cancer patients in hopes of yielding a therapeutic effect [25]. Such agents include a wide variety of treatments, including cytokines, vaccines, monoclonal antibodies, thymic factors, and colony-stimulating factors [26]. In normal, healthy controls, a single dose of only 1.5 million international units of the cytokine interferon alpha (IFN-alpha) worsened reaction time at 6 and 10 h after injection. When used as a treatment for cancers such as chronic myelogenous leukemia and melanoma, IFN-alpha is delivered at much higher doses for longer periods of time. Posttreatment cognitive impairments have been documented on measures of memory, psychomotor speed, and executive functioning, especially when used in combination with chemotherapy [27, 28]. In addition, IFN-alpha has been associated with depression [29] and the so-called dysphoric mania, characterized by extreme irritability or agitation that is often accompanied by poor insight and does not respond to treatment with antidepressants [30]. Although antidepressants may be used prophylactically for symptom prevention/reduction in some patients, pretreatment screening in combination with close serial monitoring of a patient's mood may help avoid unnecessary medications and potential side effects [30, 31].

Hormonal Therapies

Estrogen and testosterone have been found to impact cognitive functioning [32, 33], and treatments affecting these hormones are commonly used in the care of breast and prostate cancer patients. Studies in breast cancer have investigated both selective estrogen receptor modulators (SERMs) such as tamoxifen (TAM) and aromatase inhibitors such as anastrozole or exemestane. Patients receiving TAM, anastrozole, or a combination of those therapies performed more poorly than noncancer controls on measures of memory and processing speed [23]. One year of treatment with TAM was associated with declines in memory and executive functioning, whereas no such decline was observed in patients treated with exemestane [34].

In prostate cancer, LHRH agonists such as leuprolide and goserelin have been found to be associated with alterations in visuospatial processing, including visual memory, and executive functioning, with contradictory findings with regard to verbal memory performance [33]. While group analyses of mean change often fail to demonstrate a statistically significant effect, reliable change index based analyses have demonstrated cognitive decline in up to 50% of men treated with an LHRH agonist [35].

Cognitive Profile Associated with Cancer Therapy

The cognitive deficits associated with brain tumors are often specific to lesion location; however, the pattern of treatment-related cognitive decline tends to be suggestive of frontal-subcortical dysfunction. This pattern includes impairments in executive functioning, speed of processing, and speeded motor coordination, as well as inefficiencies in learning and memory retrieval in the context of relatively well-preserved memory consolidation processes [36]. These impairments typically manifest in complaints of difficulty with short term memory, such as forgetting the details of recent conversations and events as well as misplacing possessions. They also frequently describe problems with sustained attention, organization, and multitasking.

Cancer in Older Adults

Prognosis appears to worsen with age for some cancers such as acute myeloid leukemia and non-Hodgkin's lymphoma. In contrast, older age is associated with more favorable tumor biology in breast cancers. In non-small cell lung cancer (NSCLC), research has found no impact or a favorable impact of age on prognosis. It appears that overall, prognosis is impacted more by characteristics of the tumor than by age [37]. Despite this, older adults are generally less likely to be included in clinical trials, despite an equal willingness to participate in trials when offered, and this appears to potentially be due to age bias and toxicity concerns [38]. Indeed, older adults are more likely to have comorbid conditions which may make them more vulnerable to treatment-related toxicity [39]. Age is associated with reduced renal function and bone marrow reserves, as well as increased anemia, which could influence the way chemotherapies are tolerated [37] As a result of comorbid conditions and greater toxicities, older patients are less likely to receive optimal doses of chemotherapy [40, 41].

Although concerns regarding increased risk of toxicity should not be dismissed, it has been demonstrated that older adults do benefit from cancer treatment. In a recent study, patients aged 70 years or older with newly diagnosed glioblastoma and a poor performance status treated with chemotherapy (temozolomide) alone were found to have an acceptable toxicity profile and increased survival as compared to supportive care, and an improvement in functional status was observed in 30% of cases [42]. Studies using a combination of chemotherapy (temozolomide) and radiation therapy have also revealed a survival benefit and acceptable rates of toxicity in adults over the age of 65 [43, 44]. This suggests that more studies should consider inclusion of older adults.

It has been suggested that evaluation of comorbid conditions is a more appropriate surrogate for life expectancy than chronological age and should be taken into consideration over and above age when making treatment decisions for older adults [39]. The European Organization for Research and Treatment of Cancer (EORTC) elderly task force recommends design of specific trials for older patients, with separate trials for those patients considered fit, vulnerable, and frail. The task force also advocates for inclusion of geriatric assessment in clinical trials, such as the Comprehensive Geriatric Assessment (CGA), which evaluates functional, nutritional, and mental status, as well as the presence of comorbid conditions, use of associated pharmacologic interventions, and the individual's level of social support. In addition, the task force suggested consideration of "elderly-specific" outcomes, such as functional independence, time to progression, or a combination of efficacy and toxicity, as well as close monitoring and early intervention for toxicities to which older adults are more vulnerable, including myelotoxicity, anemia, mucositis, diarrhea, and dehydration [37].

Cognition in Older Adults with a History of Cancer

While the above data regarding the ability of older adults to tolerate and benefit from cancer therapies is promising, it is noted that those studies did not include formal measures of cognitive functioning. Few studies have investigated the impact of cancer and cancer therapies on cognition in older adults, despite the higher incidence of cancer diagnosis and potential increased risk of treatment-related morbidity in that population. The majority of studies investigating the impact of chemotherapy on cognition in patients with breast cancer have been performed in younger women, despite the fact that the majority of breast cancers occur in women over the age of 65 and aging is the number one risk factor for breast cancer [45]. This tendency to focus on younger adults is prevalent across cancer types; only 17% of studies investigating cognition in cancer patients that were identified in a recent literature review included patients whose mean or median age was 65 or above; of these, 27% utilized the MMSE as a measure of cognitive status [46].

Data available from the limited number of studies that have investigated the presence and pattern of cancer and cancer treatment-related cognitive symptoms in older adults suggest that, similar to younger adults, a subset of older adult cancer patients exhibits cognitive impairment prior to the initiation of treatment. For example, in older men diagnosed with prostate cancer, 45% scored ≥1.5 standard deviations below the normative mean on at least two neuropsychological tests prior to beginning androgen ablation therapy [47].

Posttreatment cognitive changes have also been documented in older adults. In one of the few prospective studies focusing on chemotherapy-related cognitive dysfunction in older adults, patients aged 65–84 with a diagnosis of breast cancer underwent neuropsychological and geriatric assessment prior to the initiation of chemotherapy and 6 months after treatment. Consistent with research performed in younger women, results revealed a subset of patients who demonstrated posttreatment cognitive decline, most often in the domains of memory, psychomotor speed, and attention [6]. A more recent study found that breast cancer patients in the older age group (60–70) performed more poorly on a measure of processing speed than younger patients or healthy controls [48].

Hormonal therapies also appear to impact older adults in a manner similar to that observed in younger adults. Older women (≥65) treated with TAM were found to perform significantly worse than healthy controls on measures of memory and information processing speed [34]. In older men treated with LHRH agonists for prostate cancer, patients who scored in the average range or above on cognitive tests at baseline displayed improvements in visuospatial planning and phonemic fluency posttreatment; those who performed below expectation at baseline displayed no significant change in cognition. It was hypothesized that this lack of improvement (presumably due to practice effects) may in and of itself be representative of impairment [47].

Cancer and Dementia

It has been suggested that there may be a link between cancer and the development of dementia, particularly Alzheimer's disease (AD). This concern was raised in a retrospective study of Swedish twin pairs discordant for cancer history, which reported that twins with a history of cancer were more likely to be classified as cognitively impaired based on a telephone mental status screening measure [49]. However, as was highlighted in an editorial response to that study, screening measures are inadequate to make such a conclusion. Further, there was no statistically significant difference in the rate of clinician-determined dementia between twins with and without a history of cancer [50]. Results of a more recent study indicate that in White older adults, AD is actually associated with a reduced risk of cancer and that a history of cancer is associated with a reduced risk of AD [51]. It was suggested by another investigator that this finding might reflect underdiagnosis of cancer in AD patients [52]; however, the same study that found a reduced risk of cancer in AD patients found no association between cancer and vascular dementia, and the authors point out that underdiagnosis, if present, would be just as likely to exist in this patient group as in AD patients [51]. A longitudinal study confirmed a slower rate of cancer development in individuals with a preexisting diagnosis of AD; the authors hypothesize that this may reflect a protective relationship between the two conditions or that they may share a common biological mechanism which affects the vulnerability of cells to apoptosis, which is excessive in AD and may be insufficient in cancer [53]. It is noted that these studies included cancers of all types; patients with cancer requiring radiation to the brain should be considered separately, as they are at an increased risk of treatment-related dementia. As noted above, in patients who have been treated with whole brain radiation (WBRT), late effects of treatment are of concern, and progressive dementia secondary to WBRT is more likely to emerge in patients who survive at least 6–12 months following radiation [54]. Severe dementia requiring full-time caregiving was documented in 10% of anaplastic glioma patients treated with accelerated radiotherapy followed by chemotherapy [55].

Neuropsychological Assessment of Older Adults with a History of Cancer

Occasionally, older adults are referred for neuropsychological evaluation prior to undergoing cancer treatment to help with decision making regarding appropriate therapies. Most commonly, patients are referred during or after their cancer treatment with complaints of memory loss. Some of the most common considerations for differential diagnosis are listed in Table 27.1; in addition to the untoward impact of cancer and cancer treatments or metastatic disease, alternative etiological considerations include those seen in older adults without a history of cancer, such as neurodegenerative dementias, potentially reversible metabolic or electrolyte imbalances, and cognitive change secondary to mood disturbance.

Baseline evaluations of neuropsychological functioning allow for the identification of even subtle treatment-related neurotoxicities; such information can prevent misclassification of patients who do experience clinically and functionally meaningful declines in cognitive function but continue to perform within normal limits

Table 27.1 Common etiologies for memory loss in older adult patients with a history of cancer

Cancer- and treatment-related toxicity
Brain metastases
Dementia including
Cerebrovascular disease
Alzheimer's disease
Lewy body dementia
Frontotemporal dementia
Potentially reversible conditions including
B12 deficiency
Thyroid abnormalities
Electrolyte abnormalities
Complications of mood disturbance and fatigue

relative to normative standards. For example, in a prospective, longitudinal study, Wefel et al. [20] found that classifying posttreatment cognitive performance as impaired using a conventional classification criterion (e.g., 1.5 SDs below the normative mean), without consideration of their pretreatment baseline level of performance, resulted in false-negative classification errors approximately 50% of the time. While baseline cognitive evaluation is critical for research, it is rarely available as a point of comparison for clinicians, who are most often asked to address referral questions in the absence of baseline data and in the aftermath of cancer and cancer treatment. Thus, as with any evaluation, one must conduct a thorough interview investigating the premorbid level of functioning, including information regarding educational and occupational attainment and any developmentally-based weaknesses, as well as the use of neuropsychological tests to estimate premorbid functioning.

Information regarding medical comorbidities and the type of cancer treatment received should also be obtained during the clinical interview, and can be of particular importance when the obtained cognitive profile and clinical correlates, such as imaging studies, may be ambiguous. For example, a patient's cognitive performance may reveal a pattern suggestive of frontal-subcortical dysfunction, and imaging studies might reveal white matter changes, which could be secondary to vascular disease or may reflect leukoencephalopathy secondary to treatment with certain cancer treatments such as methotrexate. Knowledge regarding the presence or absence of risk factors for cerebrovascular disease and the type of cancer therapy utilized may therefore elucidate the underlying etiology of observed cognitive impairments. The clinician should also determine the onset and course of cognitive symptoms, and how that timeline relates to cancer diagnosis and treatment. In the most straightforward case, patients and their family members are likely to describe cognitive difficulties that had onset during treatment or became noticeable shortly thereafter, when the patient was presented with increased cognitive challenges. These difficulties are often described as nonprogressive. Greater challenges arise when cognitive problems are perceived prior to initiation of treatment and are exacerbated during treatment.

Appropriate neuropsychological assessment of patients with cancer includes careful selection of reliable and valid measures that are sensitive to subtle changes in functioning and are robust to practice effects [36]. In this patient population, there is often a heavy emphasis on tests assessing frontal-subcortical network functioning. Additional test selection may vary in association with cancer diagnosis; for example, tests of visuospatial functioning are likely less sensitive to treatment-related cognitive decline in women with breast cancer, but may be critical in the assessment of treatment-related cognitive decline in men with prostate cancer. Similarly, test selection for patients with brain tumors may vary somewhat depending on lesion location.

In addition to the above considerations, a thorough neuropsychological examination includes an assessment of fatigue and affective distress, which can have an untoward impact on cognitive performance, particularly with regard to aspects of attention and memory. It is important to note that in cancer patients, self-report of cognitive complaints has been shown to correlate more strongly with fatigue and mood disturbance than with objective evidence of cognitive dysfunction, as assessed by standardized neuropsychological tests [56]. Thus, a thorough assessment may be needed to elucidate whether perceived difficulties are secondary to cancer- and treatment-related cognitive dysfunction and/or affective distress and fatigue.

Case Examples

Ms. A, Ms. B, and Ms. C are college-educated women in their mid-70s who have a history of breast cancer and were treated with standard dose adjuvant chemotherapy including fluorouracil, Adriamycin, and cyclophosphamide. All three women presented with similar complaints, namely problems with recent memory characterized by difficulty remembering recent conversations, forgetting to pay bills, and difficulty with medication management. Ms. C and her family members also described word-finding difficulty. As a result of these complaints, the women were referred for evaluation of their cognitive functioning in an effort to determine whether cognitive symptoms reflected the impact of cancer and associated treatment or whether there was concern for an additional neurodegenerative process.

Neuropsychological evaluation of Ms. A revealed a pattern consistent with frontal-subcortical dysfunction and characterized by mild impairments in memory retrieval (in the context of intact memory consolidation processes), working memory, and bilateral fine motor dexterity. The latter impairments were believed to reflect her peripheral neuropathy, which is commonly associated with the chemotherapies she received. The observed pattern of performance, and the fact that her reported functional difficulties had onset during her chemotherapy and developed simultaneously with her peripheral neuropathy, is consistent with the untoward impact of her breast cancer and cancer treatment.

Ms. B's cognitive profile was very similar to that of Ms. A's; however, in Ms. B's case, the etiology of her cognitive impairments is less clear, as her medical history was also notable for numerous cerebrovascular risk factors, including hypertension, hypercholesterolemia, and a previous transient ischemic attack. Thus, it is possible that the observed cognitive impairments result from cerebrovascular disease, her cancer and chemotherapy, or from a combined effect of vascular burden and treatment effect.

Finally, Ms. C's neuropsychological evaluation revealed moderate to severe impairments in learning and memory, with little to no benefit from the provision of retrieval cues. In addition, she evidenced disorientation, dysnomia, and impairments in processing speed and visuoconstruction. Basic attention span and reasoning skills remained relatively preserved. The severity and pattern of the observed difficulties exceeded that which might be expected secondary to breast cancer and associated treatment alone; in addition, it was noted that while her cancer diagnosis and treatment were quite remote, her cognitive difficulties had more recent onset and, per her family's report, had been gradually progressive. This was worrisome for a neurodegenerative process. The patient was therefore referred to neurology for a further diagnostic work-up.

Preventing Cognitive Sequelae of Cancer and Cancer Therapy

Risk factors for treatment-related cognitive dysfunction (i.e., high dose, agent, and schedule of administration) can be adjusted to reduce neurotoxicity while maintaining adequate disease control [57, 58]. Pharmacologic interventions targeted at specific underlying mechanisms of some neurotoxic side effects have also been investigated; it remains unclear whether these interventions are differentially effective for older versus younger patients. Psychostimulant medications have been shown to be effective in addressing fatigue and cognitive dysfunction in cancer patients. A commonly used psychostimulant is methylphenidate, which has been found to be beneficial in reducing fatigue in non-CNS cancer patients [59–61]. In patients with primary brain tumors, methylphenidate has been effective in combating cognitive symptoms associated with treatment-related frontal-subcortical dysfunction, such that patients demonstrated significant improvements in memory, psychomotor speed, visual-motor function, executive function, and fine motor speed [62]. Patients with cardiovascular diseases may not be ideal candidates for this medication, as stimulants have been associated with increased blood pressure and elevated heart rate. As with patients of all ages, medical comorbidities must be taken into account when considering the appropriateness of this and other pharmacological interventions. Other medications that have been used in oncology populations include modafinil to alleviate fatigue and donepezil to combat difficulties with cancer-related fatigue, attention, and memory [63]. The use of high-dose vitamin E has been shown to be beneficial in patients with nasopharyngeal carcinoma who had imaging evidence of unilateral or bilateral temporal lobe necrosis, such that patients who were treated with vitamin E demonstrated greater improvement on measures of learning, memory, and cognitive flexibility than nontreated controls [64].

Animal studies have identified additional potential pharmacologic interventions. For example, the severe memory impairment observed in rats treated with chemotherapy was fully prevented by supplementation with an antioxidant, *N*-acetyl cysteine [65]. Similarly, administration of the peroxisomal proliferator-activated receptor-γ agonist pioglitazone prevented memory disturbance associated with whole brain irradiation in rats [66]. Radiation-induced memory loss was also attenuated via transplantation of human embryonic stem cells into the rat hippocampus [67].

In addition to making adjustments to primary treatments and using pharmacological interventions to combat cognitive inefficiencies and fatigue, goal-focused compensatory interventions and behavioral strategies may be useful in minimizing the impact of neurobehavioral symptoms on daily life in patients with cancer. Physical exercise has been linked to improvements in at least some aspects of cognitive functioning in patients with mild cognitive impairment and Alzheimer's disease [68, 69] and has been associated with increased patient self-reported quality of life, including cognitive functioning, in cancer patients [70]. Animal studies provide support for exercise as a protective factor against cancer treatment-related cognitive side effects; daily running after WBRT prevented declines in spatial memory in mice [71]. Further studies are needed with regard to physical activity as an intervention against cognitive dysfunction in human cancer patients.

Knowledge gained from traditional rehabilitation disciplines treating survivors of traumatic brain injury or stroke has yielded important information regarding evidenced-based compensatory strategies that may be applicable to patients with cancer-related cognitive dysfunction. Such multidisciplinary therapeutic interventions, provided by a team of psychologists, speech/language pathologists, occupational therapists, and vocational specialists, was found to improve community independence and employment outcomes in brain tumor patients at a significantly lower cost and shorter treatment length than was typical of survivors of traumatic brain injury who took part in the same program [72]. Training in the use of compensatory strategies and attention retraining has also shown promise in addressing both cognitive complaints and mental fatigue [73]. Compensatory tools might include external memory aids such as memory notebooks, user-programmable paging systems, and medication reminder systems to assist neurologically impaired patients compensate for difficulties with forgetfulness. Older adults, particularly those with multiple comorbidities, may require adjustments to their environment and increased support to make certain that demands do not exceed capacity while maintaining safety and ensuring treatment compliance.

Summary

Older adults are at increased risk for developing cancer, thus the incidence of cancer is predicted to increase with an aging population [1, 2]. Despite the possibility of treatment-related cognitive declines for some patients, these treatments remain a critical component in the management and eradication of many cancers. Thus, the potential side effects of these therapies must be considered in the context of the overall health benefit they provide. Continued research into the mechanisms of treatment-related cognitive dysfunction may afford opportunities for the development of neuroprotective therapies, effective adjuvant supportive pharmacotherapies, or modification of primary treatments. Advances in behavioral interventions will help minimize the impact of cancer and cancer therapy on cognitive function, mood, quality of life, and functional abilities. It appears that older adults can benefit from cancer treatments; as with younger adults, medical comorbidities, cognitive status, and social support are important clinical considerations. To date, older adults have often been excluded from studies investigating the impact of cancer and cancer therapies on cognitive functioning, and more research is needed to determine whether older adults are differentially affected.

Clinical Pearls

- Cognitive changes can result from CNS and non-CNS cancers, even prior to the initiation of treatment.
- Treatment-related cognitive changes may result from surgical intervention, radiation, chemotherapy, immunotherapy, and hormonal therapy.
- Treatment-related cognitive declines most often occur during or immediately after surgery, chemotherapy, and hormonal therapy. In contrast, late-onset cognitive decline can occur, and is more likely to be progressive, after treatment with radiation.
- The neuropsychological profile of treatment-related cognitive decline often suggests frontal-subcortical dysfunction.
- Screening measures such as the MMSE are insufficient to detect the subtle cognitive changes often associated with cancer and cancer treatment.
- Neuropsychological assessment should include measures that are sensitive to frontal-subcortical network dysfunction; test selection may vary depending on cancer type and location.
- Older adults have additional risk of cognitive impairment, as age independently increases risk and they are also more likely to have comorbid conditions that may have an untoward effect on cognition.
- Older adults with a history of cancer do not appear to be at increased risk for the development of Alzheimer's disease, though AD and cancer can exist as comorbid conditions.
- Few pharmacologic interventions for cancer treatment-related cognitive impairment have been identified to date. The use of compensatory strategies is often the most effective intervention to assist individuals with cancer treatment-related cognitive decline in maximizing their daily functioning.

References

1. Altekruse SF, et al., editors. SEER Cancer Statistics Review, 1975–2007. Bethesda, MD: N.C. Institute; 2010.
2. Vincent GK, Velkoff VA. The next four decades, the older population in the United States: 2010 to 2050. Current Population Reports. Washington, DC: U.S.C. Bureau; 2010. p. P25–1138.
3. Wefel JS, et al. 'Chemobrain' in breast carcinoma? A prologue. Cancer. 2004;101(3):466–75.
4. Hermelink K, et al. Cognitive function during neoadjuvant chemotherapy for breast cancer: results of a prospective, multicenter, longitudinal study. Cancer. 2007;109(9):1905–13.
5. Schagen SB, et al. Change in cognitive function after chemotherapy: a prospective longitudinal study in breast cancer patients. J Natl Cancer Inst. 2006;98(23): 1742–5.
6. Hurria A, et al. Cognitive function of older patients receiving adjuvant chemotherapy for breast cancer: a pilot prospective longitudinal study. J Am Geriatr Soc. 2006;54(6):925–31.
7. Meyers CA, Albitar M, Estey E. Cognitive impairment, fatigue, and cytokine levels in patients with acute myelogenous leukemia or myelodysplastic syndrome. Cancer. 2005;104(4):788–93.
8. Meyers CA, Byrne KS, Komaki R. Cognitive deficits in patients with small cell lung cancer before and after chemotherapy. Lung Cancer. 1995;12(3):231–5.
9. Newman S, et al. Postoperative cognitive dysfunction after noncardiac surgery: a systematic review. Anesthesiology. 2007;106(3):572–90.
10. Sheline GE, Wara WM, Smith V. Therapeutic irradiation and brain injury. Int J Radiat Oncol Biol Phys. 1980;6(9):1215–28.
11. Crossen JR, et al. Neurobehavioral sequelae of cranial irradiation in adults: a review of radiation-induced encephalopathy. J Clin Oncol. 1994;12(3):627–42.
12. Lee AW, et al. Factors affecting risk of symptomatic temporal lobe necrosis: significance of fractional dose and treatment time. Int J Radiat Oncol Biol Phys. 2002;53(1):75–85.
13. Chang EL, et al. Neurocognition in patients with brain metastases treated with radiosurgery or radiosurgery plus whole-brain irradiation: a randomised controlled trial. Lancet Oncol. 2009;10(11):1037–44.
14. Ahles TA, et al. Neuropsychologic impact of standard-dose systemic chemotherapy in long-term survivors of breast cancer and lymphoma. J Clin Oncol. 2002;20(2):485–93.
15. Brezden CB, et al. Cognitive function in breast cancer patients receiving adjuvant chemotherapy. J Clin Oncol. 2000;18(14):2695–701.

16. Schagen SB, et al. Late effects of adjuvant chemotherapy on cognitive function: a follow-up study in breast cancer patients. Ann Oncol. 2002;13(9): 1387–97.
17. Schagen SB, et al. Cognitive deficits after postoperative adjuvant chemotherapy for breast carcinoma. Cancer. 1999;85(3):640–50.
18. Hurria A, et al. A prospective, longitudinal study of the functional status and quality of life of older patients with breast cancer receiving adjuvant chemotherapy. J Am Geriatr Soc. 2006;54(7):1119–24.
19. van Dam FS, et al. Impairment of cognitive function in women receiving adjuvant treatment for high-risk breast cancer: high-dose versus standard-dose chemotherapy. J Natl Cancer Inst. 1998;90(3):210–8.
20. Wefel JS, et al. The cognitive sequelae of standard-dose adjuvant chemotherapy in women with breast carcinoma: results of a prospective, randomized, longitudinal trial. Cancer. 2004;100(11):2292–9.
21. Wefel JS, et al. Acute and late onset cognitive dysfunction associated with chemotherapy in women with breast cancer. Cancer. 2010;116(14):3348–56.
22. Syrjala KL, et al. Neuropsychologic changes from before transplantation to 1 year in patients receiving myeloablative allogeneic hematopoietic cell transplant. Blood. 2004;104(10):3386–92.
23. Ahles TA, et al. Psychologic and neuropsychologic impact of autologous bone marrow transplantation. J Clin Oncol. 1996;14(5):1457–62.
24. Friedman MA, et al. Course of cognitive decline in hematopoietic stem cell transplantation: a within-subjects design. Arch Clin Neuropsychol. 2009;24(7): 689–98.
25. National Cancer Institute. Biological therapy. Treatments that use your immune system to fight cancer (NIH Publication No. 03-5406). 2003.
26. Clark JW. Biological response modifiers. Cancer Chemother Biol Response Modif. 1996;16:239–73.
27. Scheibel RS, et al. Cognitive dysfunction and depression during treatment with interferon-alpha and chemotherapy. J Neuropsychiatry Clin Neurosci. 2004;16(2):185–91.
28. Bender CM, et al. Cognitive function and quality of life in interferon therapy for melanoma. Clin Nurs Res. 2000;9(3):352–63.
29. Capuron L, et al. Baseline mood and psychosocial characteristics of patients developing depressive symptoms during interleukin-2 and/or interferon-alpha cancer therapy. Brain Behav Immun. 2004;18(3): 205–13.
30. Valentine AD, et al. Mood and cognitive side effects of interferon-alpha therapy. Semin Oncol. 1998;25(1 Suppl 1):39–47.
31. Valentine AD, Meyers CA. Neurobehavioral effects of interferon therapy. Curr Psychiatry Rep. 2005;7(5): 391–5.
32. Maki PM, Sundermann E. Hormone therapy and cognitive function. Hum Reprod Update. 2009;15(6): 667–81.
33. Nelson CJ, et al. Cognitive effects of hormone therapy in men with prostate cancer: a review. Cancer. 2008;113(5):1097–106.
34. Schilder CM, et al. Effects of tamoxifen and exemestane on cognitive functioning of postmenopausal patients with breast cancer: results from the neuropsychological side study of the tamoxifen and exemestane adjuvant multinational trial. J Clin Oncol. 2010;28(8):1294–300.
35. Green HJ, et al. Altered cognitive function in men treated for prostate cancer with luteinizing hormone-releasing hormone analogues and cyproterone acetate: a randomized controlled trial. BJU Int. 2002;90(4): 427–32.
36. Wefel JS, Kayl AE, Meyers CA. Neuropsychological dysfunction associated with cancer and cancer therapies: a conceptual review of an emerging target. Br J Cancer. 2004;90(9):1691–6.
37. Pallis AG, et al. EORTC elderly task force position paper: approach to the older cancer patient. Eur J Cancer. 2010;46(9):1502–13.
38. Kemeny MM, et al. Barriers to clinical trial participation by older women with breast cancer. J Clin Oncol. 2003;21(12):2268–75.
39. Taylor WC, Muss HB. Adjuvant chemotherapy of breast cancer in the older patient. Oncology (Williston Park). 2010;24(7):608–13.
40. Given B, Given CW. Older adults and cancer treatment. Cancer. 2008;113(12 Suppl):3505–11.
41. Pal SK, Hurria A. Impact of age, sex, and comorbidity on cancer therapy and disease progression. J Clin Oncol. 2010;28(26):4086–93.
42. Gállego Pérez-Larraya J. A phase II trial of temozolomide in elderly patients with glioblastoma and poor performance status (KPS < 70): preliminary results of the ANOCEF "TAG" trial. Neuro Oncol. 2010;12 Suppl 4:iv76.
43. Stummer W, et al. Favorable outcome in the elderly cohort treated by concomitant temozolomide radiochemotherapy in a multicentric phase II safety study of 5-ALA. J Neurooncol. 2011;103(2):361–70.
44. Gerstein J, et al. Postoperative radiotherapy and concomitant temozolomide for elderly patients with glioblastoma. Radiother Oncol. 2010;97(3):382–6.
45. Hurria A, Lachs M. Is cognitive dysfunction a complication of adjuvant chemotherapy in the older patient with breast cancer? Breast Cancer Res Treat. 2007;103(3):259–68.
46. Bial AK, Schilsky RL, Sachs GA. Evaluation of cognition in cancer patients: special focus on the elderly. Crit Rev Oncol Hematol. 2006;60(3):242–55.
47. Mohile SG, et al. Cognitive effects of androgen deprivation therapy in an older cohort of men with prostate cancer. Crit Rev Oncol Hematol. 2010;75(2): 152–9.
48. Ahles TA, et al. Longitudinal assessment of cognitive changes associated with adjuvant treatment for breast cancer: impact of age and cognitive reserve. J Clin Oncol. 2010;28(29):4434–40.

49. Heflin LH, et al. Cancer as a risk factor for long-term cognitive deficits and dementia. J Natl Cancer Inst. 2005;97(11):854–6.
50. Wefel JS, Meyers CA. Cancer as a risk factor for dementia: a house built on shifting sand. J Natl Cancer Inst. 2005;97(11):788–9.
51. Roe CM, et al. Cancer linked to Alzheimer disease but not vascular dementia. Neurology. 2010;74(2): 106–12.
52. Burke WJ. Cancer linked to Alzheimer disease but not vascular dementia. Neurology. 2010;75(13):1216. author reply 1216.
53. Roe CM, et al. Alzheimer disease and cancer. Neurology. 2005;64(5):895–8.
54. DeAngelis LM, Delattre JY, Posner JB. Radiation-induced dementia in patients cured of brain metastases. Neurology. 1989;39(6):789–96.
55. Levin VA, et al. Phase II study of accelerated fractionation radiation therapy with carboplatin followed by PCV chemotherapy for the treatment of anaplastic gliomas. Int J Radiat Oncol Biol Phys. 2002;53(1):58–66.
56. Castellon SA, et al. Neurocognitive performance in breast cancer survivors exposed to adjuvant chemotherapy and tamoxifen. J Clin Exp Neuropsychol. 2004;26(7):955–69.
57. Keime-Guibert F, Napolitano M, Delattre JY. Neurological complications of radiotherapy and chemotherapy. J Neurol. 1998;245(11):695–708.
58. Valentine AD. Managing the neuropsychiatric adverse effects of interferon treatment. BioDrugs. 1999;11(4): 229–37.
59. Bruera E, et al. Patient-controlled methylphenidate for the management of fatigue in patients with advanced cancer: a preliminary report. J Clin Oncol. 2003;21(23):4439–43.
60. Bruera E, et al. Patient-controlled methylphenidate for cancer fatigue: a double-blind, randomized, placebo-controlled trial. J Clin Oncol. 2006;24(13):2073–8.
61. Sarhill N, et al. Methylphenidate for fatigue in advanced cancer: a prospective open-label pilot study. Am J Hosp Palliat Care. 2001;18(3):187–92.
62. Meyers CA, et al. Methylphenidate therapy improves cognition, mood, and function of brain tumor patients. J Clin Oncol. 1998;16(7):2522–7.
63. Shaw EG, et al. Phase II study of donepezil in irradiated brain tumor patients: effect on cognitive function, mood, and quality of life. J Clin Oncol. 2006;24(9): 1415–20.
64. Chan AS, et al. Phase II study of alpha-tocopherol in improving the cognitive function of patients with temporal lobe radionecrosis. Cancer. 2004; 100(2):398–404.
65. Konat GW, et al. Cognitive dysfunction induced by chronic administration of common cancer chemotherapeutics in rats. Metab Brain Dis. 2008;23(3): 325–33.
66. Zhao W, et al. Administration of the peroxisomal proliferator-activated receptor gamma agonist pioglitazone during fractionated brain irradiation prevents radiation-induced cognitive impairment. Int J Radiat Oncol Biol Phys. 2007;67(1):6–9.
67. Acharya MM, et al. Rescue of radiation-induced cognitive impairment through cranial transplantation of human embryonic stem cells. Proc Natl Acad Sci USA. 2009;106(45):19150–5.
68. Baker LD, et al. Effects of aerobic exercise on mild cognitive impairment: a controlled trial. Arch Neurol. 2010;67(1):71–9.
69. Yaguez L, et al. The effects on cognitive functions of a movement-based intervention in patients with Alzheimer's type dementia: a pilot study. Int J Geriatr Psychiatry. 2010;26(2):173–81.
70. Korstjens I, et al. Quality of life of cancer survivors after physical and psychosocial rehabilitation. Eur J Cancer Prev. 2006;15(6):541–7.
71. Wong-Goodrich SJ, et al. Voluntary running prevents progressive memory decline and increases adult hippocampal neurogenesis and growth factor expression after whole-brain irradiation. Cancer Res. 2010; 70(22):9329–38.
72. Sherer M, Meyers CA, Bergloff P. Efficacy of post-acute brain injury rehabilitation for patients with primary malignant brain tumors. Cancer. 1997;80(2): 250–7.
73. Gehring K, et al. Cognitive rehabilitation in patients with gliomas: a randomized, controlled trial. J Clin Oncol. 2009;27(22):3712–22.

28 Evaluating Cognition in Patients with Chronic Obstructive Pulmonary Disease

Elizabeth Kozora and Karin F. Hoth

Abstract

In this chapter, we focus on the neuropsychological evaluation of patients with chronic obstructive pulmonary disease (COPD), a common adult pulmonary disorder characterized by restrictive airflow and respiratory distress. First, we will review the epidemiology and diagnostic criteria of COPD and of the most common medical comorbidities. Next, we will review the literature of cognition in patients with COPD and identify the most consistent neuropsychological deficits in the population. Multidisciplinary rehabilitation is commonly prescribed for COPD patients. We will discuss the role of the neuropsychologist within the team. Finally, to more clearly illustrate the neuropsychological evaluation in patients with COPD, we will discuss a fictional case from our center with details regarding frequent referral questions, special considerations for the clinical interview, selection of cognitive tests, interpretation of tests, and final recommendations for the patient and/or the interdisciplinary rehabilitation team.

Keywords

Pulmonary disease • COPD • Airflow limitation • Hypoxia

Chronic obstructive pulmonary disease (COPD) is a chronic progressive pulmonary disease with significant physical, cognitive, and psychological sequelae. There are several types of restrictive lung diseases (e.g., COPD, emphysema), and although conditions vary across individuals, they are all related to airflow limitation. COPD is a preventable/treatable disease; however, the "pulmonary" component, characterized by airflow limitation, is not fully reversible. The airflow limitation is usually progressive and associated with

E. Kozora, Ph.D. (✉) • K.F. Hoth, Ph.D.
Division of Psychosocial Medicine, Department of Medicine, National Jewish Health, 1400 Jackson St., Room M107G, Denver, CO 80206, USA

Departments of Psychiatry and Neurology, University of Colorado Denver, Aurora, CO, USA
e-mail: kozorae@njhealth.org; hothk@njhealth.org

L.D. Ravdin and H.L. Katzen (eds.), *Handbook on the Neuropsychology of Aging and Dementia*, Clinical Handbooks in Neuropsychology, DOI 10.1007/978-1-4614-3106-0_28,

an abnormal inflammatory response in the lung to noxious particles and gases [1]. COPD is currently recognized as the fourth leading cause of death in the United States, accounting for more than 120,000 deaths annually, and is predicted to be the third leading cause of death by 2020. Although mortality in men appears to be peaking in the USA, for women, mortality continues to rise and may exceed that among men [2]. In addition, COPD progresses with age and is more prevalent in older populations. In the USA, 15% of the total population aged 55–64 will have at least moderate COPD, which increases to over 25% for those older than 75 [3].

COPD is clinically heterogeneous and can result from several etiologies with the primary being cigarette smoke. Cigarette smoking has been clearly established as the most important risk factor, with approximately 10–15% of smokers developing COPD. Notably, smokers lose lung function in a dose-dependent matter and a majority of smokers will have reduced lung function as they age [1]. Eighty percent of individuals who have COPD, and 80% who die from COPD, are smokers [2]. Other risk factors are estimated to contribute between 27% and 60% of overall COPD mortality [4]. Several distinct mechanisms and genetic factors may alter individual responses. Factors that may contribute to accelerated loss of lung function include occupational exposures (i.e., farming or work in dusty occupations), environmental air pollution (increased particulates), and indoor air exposure (smoke from use of biomass fuels), but there are also likely genetic determinants such as mutations in the serine proteinase inhibitor alpha$_1$-protease inhibitor. Other factors include early life events such as maternal smoking and low birth weight, asthma, and mucus hypersecretion [1]. Although male gender predominance in COPD has been reported, it is primarily related to exposure to cigarettes and other toxins, and it has been suggested that COPD is equally prevalent among genders [4]. Women do appear to have different comorbidities with lower prevalence of ischemic heart disease but higher prevalence of congestive heart failure, osteoporosis, and diabetes [5]. Morbidity and mortality in COPD have also been inversely related to socioeconomic status [2].

Classification of Severity of COPD

The current gold standard for classifying COPD severity and monitoring progression is the Global Initiative for Chronic Obstructive Lung Disease (GOLD) classification system (2008), where the criteria rely on measures of airflow limitation from spirometry to stratify COPD into four stages (see Table 28.1). Spirometry measures the amount and rate of air a patient breathes in and out over a period of time. The GOLD classification criteria are based on spirometry results obtained after administration of an inhaled bronchodilator, such as albuterol. Testing before and after a bronchodilator minimizes variability in how the test is administered and provides some information about the potential responsiveness of the airways to medication. As can been seen in Table 28.1, the major difference across COPD stages is decreasing FEV$_1$, which reflects the volume of air that can be forced out in the 1 s after taking a deep breath.

The functional impact of COPD on any individual patient is due not only to degree of airflow limitation, but also to symptom severity (e.g., shortness of breath, exercise intolerance). Airflow limitation and symptom severity are associated, but do not have a one to one relationship. The authors of the GOLD criteria acknowledge this and suggest that COPD stage should be thought

Table 28.1 COPD GOLD stage classification

GOLD stage	Spirometric classification based on post-bronchodilator FEV$_1$
I Mild	FEV$_1$/FVC < 0.7 FEV$_1$ ≥ 80% predicted
II Moderate	FEV$_1$/FVC < 0.7 50% ≤ FEV$_1$ < 80% predicted
III Severe	FEV$_1$/FVC < 0.7 30% ≤ FEV$_1$ < 50% predicted
IV Very severe	FEV$_1$/FVC < 0.7 FEV$_1$ < 30% predicted or FEV$_1$ < 50% plus chronic respiratory failure

FEV$_1$ forced expiratory volume in 1 s, *FVC* forced vital capacity of as a general indication as to the initial approach to management. The GOLD statement does, however, provide general descriptors of typical presentation of patients at each stage. In stage I "mild COPD," chronic chough and sputum production may be present, but not always. At this stage, the individual is usually aware that his or her lung function is abnormal. In stage II "moderate COPD," shortness of breath typically develops on exertion, and cough and sputum production sometimes are also present. This is the stage at which patients typically seek medical attention because of chronic respiratory symptoms or an exacerbation of their disease. In stage III "severe COPD," greater shortness of breath, reduced exercise capacity, fatigue, and repeated exacerbations that almost always have an impact on patient's quality of life may be present. In stage IV "very severe COPD," respiratory failure may lead to effects on the heart such as cor pulmonale (right side heart failure). At this stage, quality of life is appreciably impaired, and exacerbations may be life threatening. The most common causes of death in COPD are from cardiovascular complications, lung cancer, and in patients with very advanced COPD, respiratory failure.

Common Medical Diagnostic Tests

Diagnosis of COPD by a physician involves a thorough medical history, physical examination, spirometry, and a chest X-ray with additional measures ordered depending upon the clinical situation. In the following section, additional information about common medical tests a neuropsychologist may encounter when reviewing the medical record of a patient with COPD will be reviewed.

Spirometry

As mentioned above, spirometry is needed to make a certain diagnosis of COPD. The test measures the volume of air exhaled during a maximal forced expiratory maneuver (i.e., blowing out as hard and fast as possible until lungs feel absolutely empty). The patient must take a deep breath and blow into a mouthpiece attached to a spirometer. A computerized sensor within the spirometer calculates and graphs the results, typically presented as volume vs. time. Of particular importance for COPD diagnosis and monitoring is the volume forced out within the first second (forced expiratory volume in 1 s, FEV1) and total volume of air forced out of the lungs (forced vital capacity, FVC).

Alpha-1 Antitrypsin Screening

Alpha-1 antitrypsin deficiency (α-1) is a genetic disorder that can cause liver disease and early-onset emphysema. α-1 antitrypsin is a protein primarily produced in the liver and released into the blood stream that protects the lungs against damage from things like infections and smoke. In addition to treatments that may be used in COPD in general (e.g., bronchodilators, corticosteroids), some individuals with α-1 antitrypsin deficiency may be candidates for α-1 augmentation therapy.

Exercise Capacity

Exercise capacity is an important component of the evaluation of COPD patients, given that limitations in exercise capacity have a significant impact on day to day functioning. Several different exercise measures are available including treadmill or cycle testing, the 6-min walk test, or shuttle walk testing. Assessment of exercise capacity is most often conducted in the context of pulmonary rehabilitation or physical therapy evaluation.

Dyspnea

Given that a patient's degree of pulmonary disease does not directly correlate with disability, it is often helpful to obtain a subjective rating from the patient on the impact of their shortness of breath. A commonly used measure of breathlessness in

COPD is the Modified Medical Research Council (MRC) dyspnea scale [6]. The scale is a five-item questionnaire on which patients rate their own disability from dyspnea, with grade 1 indicating the least impact from breathlessness (i.e., only breathless with strenuous exercise) and grade 5 indicating the most severe impact (i.e., too breathless to leave the house or breathless when dressing/undressing).

Additional tests that are often ordered for patients with COPD include arterial blood gas measurement, sleep study, cardiology evaluation, occupational medicine, and health and behavior assessment with a psychologist or psychiatrist.

Common Medical Comorbidities of COPD

COPD has traditionally been understood as a disease of the lungs characterized by chronic airflow obstruction; however, the importance of extrapulmonary effects of COPD has become increasingly recognized over the past decade [7–9]. COPD has systemic effects that can have an important impact on the patient's health including cachexia, skeletal muscle wasting, osteoporosis, anemia, cardiovascular disease, and depression. The consequences of systemic inflammation on other organ systems have been one major area of focus in understanding extrapulmonary changes in COPD [10].

Cardiovascular disease is one of the most prevalent comorbidities in COPD [11–14]. COPD is associated with a 2–3-fold increase in the risk of ischemic heart disease, stroke, and sudden death [14]. In fact, more patients with COPD are hospitalized and die from cardiovascular causes than respiratory causes [15]. Although smoking is a risk factor for both COPD and cardiovascular disease, the association between airflow obstruction (e.g., FEV_1) and cardiovascular disease exists even after adjusting for risk factors that are common to both conditions including age, sex, smoking history, cholesterol, and socioeconomic class, suggesting that there is a direct underlying relationship [13]. Additional medical comorbidities of COPD typically include anemia and osteoporosis [16].

COPD is also associated with an increased rate of psychological symptoms, particularly anxiety and depression. In a comprehensive review of 81 studies, Hynninen et al. [17] reported that the prevalence of psychiatric disorders ranged from 30% to 58%. Depression and anxiety appear to be the most commonly observed psychological problems in COPD [17–21]. The prevalence of depression has been estimated between 10% and 79.1% [17, 22–24]. Some of the discrepancies in estimates may relate to the method of assessing depression. For example, prior studies with higher levels of depression have tended to use self-report questionnaires rather than a clinically derived diagnosis of major depression [25, 26]. Eiser and colleagues [27] screened a large group of COPD patients with moderate to severe COPD using screening questionnaires followed with a psychiatric interview. They report prevalence rates of depression of 35% using the questionnaire and 21% by clinical interview. This is consistent with another study that diagnosed depression in COPD utilizing a structured psychiatric clinical interview and reported that 23% of the COPD patients had major depression [28]. The prevalence of depression in older adults in the general population has been estimated between 8% and 20%; thus, studies to date clearly indicate higher depression rates in patients with COPD [29].

The symptoms of anxiety, depression, and dyspnea are not mutually exclusive. Whereas dyspnea is a characteristic feature of panic attacks, feelings of panic and anxiety are also a frequent manifestation of pulmonary disease. In COPD, approximately one third of patients meet clinical criteria for an anxiety disorder, with panic disorder being the most common. Approximately one fourth of patients meet criteria for panic disorder, which is 10 times the rate in the general population [19]. Symptoms of depression and anxiety are important to consider as they may contribute to cognitive impairment in COPD, in addition to their impact on quality of life.

Neuropsychological Studies in COPD

Multiple studies using standardized tests have identified neuropsychological deficits in patients with COPD [30–36]. The pattern and extent of cognitive dysfunction reported in COPD varies across patients and appears to be associated with disease severity. In COPD patients with moderate to severe hypoxemia, deficits have been reported in simple motor movement and overall strength, perceptual-motor integration, abstract reasoning, attention to auditory stimuli, learning and memory, and language skills [31, 33–35, 37–39]. Some studies in COPD patients have suggested that even mild hypoxemia may be associated with impairment in higher cerebral functioning. Prigatano, et al. [33] studied 100 mildly hypoxemic COPD patients (mean age = 61.5, mean PaO_2=66.3) and reported deficits in this group compared to controls in abstract reasoning and attention to auditory stimuli. Grant et al. [31] combined data from a number of sites of a multicenter NIH trial and reported that mildly hypoxemic COPD patients (mean age=61.6, mean PaO_2=67.8) performed significantly lower than controls on a global index of cognitive functioning. Twenty-seven percent of COPD patients with mild hypoxemia showed global deficits as compared to 61% of patients with severe hypoxemia. The mildly hypoxemic group performed significantly below matched controls on measures of associate learning, immediate recall of verbal and nonverbal material, logical analysis and reasoning, sustained visual attention, and fine motor coordination. Liesker et al. [40] also reported that 30 COPD patients with mild hypoxemia showed decline in visuomotor speed and attention compared to 20 health controls. In a large review of COPD studies with and without hypoxemia, the correlations between cognitive functions and degree of hypoxemia were less impressive and thought to be inconsistent [16].

Due to the age of the COPD population, the potential for other central nervous system (CNS) disorders, including a progressive neurodegenerative disorder such as Alzheimer's disease (AD), should be considered in differential diagnosis. We compared 32 mildly hypoxic COPD patients to 32 subjects with mild Alzheimer's disease (AD) and 32 healthy controls matched on age, education, and gender [41]. Results indicated that the mild AD group performed worse than the COPD group on all measures except verbal fluency. Neuroimaging studies have reported hypoperfusion in frontal and association areas in COPD [39, 42]. In contrast to AD or another neurodegenerative process, there may be some improvement in cognition in patients with COPD, particularly memory gains following oxygen or multidisciplinary rehabilitation. Therefore, repeat neuropsychological assessment 6–12 months following treatment, as well as consultation from neurology and neuroradiology, may be useful in a complete workup in COPD patients with severe memory disorders.

Interdisciplinary Treatment of COPD

Comprehensive rehabilitation programs for treatment of COPD include a wide range of assessment procedures and educational programs, instruction on respiration, psychosocial support, and exercise training with the goal of restoring patients to the highest level of independent function [43]. There is evidence that suggests that comprehensive multidisciplinary rehabilitation programs can also improve cognitive functioning and psychological status in emphysema/COPD patients [25, 43–45]. Studies from our group have suggested improved verbal memory and visuomotor sequencing in patients with lung volume reduction surgery compared to rehabilitation at 6-month follow-up using a comprehensive battery [46]. In a later study with a much larger sample, there were no differences between the two groups on a visuomotor sequencing task over a 3-year period [47]. Notably, the first study utilized a comprehensive battery, and the second study included only the measure of visuomotor sequencing.

Role of Neuropsychologist

At hospitals such as ours (National Jewish Health (NJH) in Denver, CO), the role of the neuropsychologist in the pulmonary assessment and rehabilitation process is well established and integral to the program. Physicians board-certified in pulmonology are directly responsible for assessment, diagnosis, treatment, and evaluation. In addition, board-certified physicians in cardiology, allergy and immunology, otolaryngology, orthopedics, and other medical specialties are available to evaluate a variety of comorbid medical disorders in the COPD patients. Physical therapists and exercise physiologists formulate the plan to help individuals reach their maximal physical function, and occupational therapists teach efficient coordinated activities for daily living skills specifically designed to limit breathlessness. The team also includes a respiratory therapist to assist in diagnostic procedures, a patient education coordinator to develop and maintain educational materials, a pharmacist to assist staff and patients with medication issues and a dietitian to provide assessment and recommendations for nutritional care. A behavioral health clinician (including clinical psychologists and social workers) is available for all patients for consultation and intervention to address adjustment to illness, adherence concerns, other behavioral factors impacting illness, and mental health issues impacting medical management. In addition, there is access to a smoking cessation counselor to assist with behavioral and pharmacological interventions of tobacco cessation and a psychiatrist for patients who need medical and or pharmacological intervention to treat possible psychiatric comorbid conditions.

The neuropsychologists on the team evaluate patients who are experiencing cognitive difficulties, such as deficits in memory or attention, and work closely with the team to recognize deficits and help adapt treatment plans to the specific patient's cognitive strengths and weaknesses. In contrast to the behavioral health clinician specifically evaluating health behaviors, coping styles, depression, and emotional factors, the neuropsychologist's role in our clinic is specifically devoted to cognitive functioning and to any continued consultation for neurology, neuroradiology, etc. Specific referral questions will be reviewed below.

Common Neuropsychological Referral Questions

The referrals for neuropsychological assessment in our facility are typically initiated by the pulmonologist or the behavioral health clinician after their initial appointment with a patient. Intake documents also track patient/family concerns regarding memory and mental abilities, and some COPD patients are flagged prior to their visit for brief cognitive evaluations. All referrals essentially request information regarding (1) the presence, degree, and domains of cognitive impairment; (2) etiological factors (i.e., is cognitive dysfunction related primarily to COPD or other factors such as other CNS changes such as a progressive dementia); (3) what is the role of depression and anxiety in the cognitive dysfunction; (4) what impact do the cognitive skills have on the day to day life of the patient (i.e., patients ability to live independently given cognitive impairment); and (5) is the patient able to understand and carry out medical treatment regimens.

The neuropsychologist might address potential problems with medication adherence (i.e., whether the patient has adequate compensatory strategies), difficulties related to use of inhaler or use of oxygen, and the patient's capacity to care for themselves following surgery/major medical intervention.

Clinical Interview

When conducting a clinical neuropsychological interview with patients with COPD, there are several unique issues to consider in addition to gathering the typical background/medical history information that would be obtained during any neuropsychological evaluation. First, for patients on oxygen, it is helpful to discuss at the beginning of the appointment how much oxygen they require to last through the assessment. It is far better to determine ahead of time that more oxygen is required than to run out midway through testing. Acute drops in oxygen saturation and associated symptoms like fatigue might impact test results causing them to poorly reflect the patient's typical status. If oximetry is available in your clinical setting, it can be helpful to obtain a resting measure of SaO_2 to determine if the patient is hypoxemic on the day of testing. Asking about perceived shortness of breath and level of fatigue on the day of testing is also helpful to understand if the day is typical for the patient.

Depending upon one's clinical setting, it may be helpful to provide additional explanation of the multidisciplinary model of care, specifically the role of neuropsychology in treating patients with COPD (e.g., some common roles are described in the referral question section above). Patients with COPD may be referred by pulmonary or primary care physicians who are concerned about the patient's cognition, while the patient is primarily focused on respiratory symptoms like shortness of breath and has not raised his or her own concerns about cognition. Explaining the neuropsychological evaluation in the context of improving quality of life and daily functioning and understanding cognitive strengths and weaknesses to assist the medical team in working with the patient can be helpful in alleviating hesitance a patient may feel about seeing a neuropsychologist.

During the interview, it is helpful to ask if patients and their family members have noticed fluctuations in the patient's perceived cognitive function in association with changes in respiratory status. Patients might experience fluctuations in cognitive status depending upon their physical activity level, symptoms of COPD, on or off oxygen, or after taking medications. Many patients with COPD experience exacerbations of their symptoms that require outpatient treatment with steroids or hospitalization. Anecdotally, patients with COPD and their families often describe worsening cognition following hospitalization, as can be the case with any ICU or hospital stay, although the reasons for this in COPD specifically have not been explored in the research literature. Understanding potential fluctuations in cognitive symptoms can help with determining the degree to which cognitive symptoms are attributable to pulmonary disease and making recommendations about how patients can plan the timing of engaging in demanding cognitive tasks.

Due to the impact that physical symptoms of COPD have on activities of daily living, it is necessary to spend some time clarifying with the patient how their cognitive symptoms impact daily tasks. Patients tend to report about activities that they can and cannot do and are less likely to think about *what* aspect of the task is difficult for them. The distinction between limitations in daily tasks due to physical vs. cognitive symptoms is clearly important for diagnosing cognitive impairment and may require some additional prompting in this population.

As a part of any neuropsychological interview, information about past history that may impact brain function is obtained. In COPD, patients are more likely than the general population to have had past environmental exposure to toxins/chemicals, as this is one risk factor for subsequently developing COPD. Furthermore, since smoking is the top risk factor for COPD and nicotine use and use of other substances are common, it is important to ask about potential substance use. There is surprisingly little information regarding actual rates of substance abuse in COPD, as the few articles published to date on alcohol use in COPD have primarily examined the impact of alcohol use on pulmonary symptoms [48]. Nonetheless, in our clinic, we have observed that concerns about alcohol use are common enough in patients referred for neuropsychological testing to have incorporated expanded substance use questions as an area of focus in the interview.

Neuropsychological Testing

The neuropsychological test battery used in our COPD population emphasizes domains of processing speed and attention, learning and memory for verbal and nonverbal material, executive functions, and visuoconstructive and visuomotor skills. Intellectual testing or estimated IQ testing are also frequently assessed. Various language skills and academic abilities (i.e., math, spelling, reading comprehension) might also be considered in relation to the referral question and concerns about comprehension of oral and written information and role in day to day activities (i.e., understanding written instructions and forms, paying their own bills, etc.). As with most evaluations, considerations for test selection include the age and education of the patient, the overall health and expected stamina of the patient, and the referral question. We also recommend that patient's with prescribed oxygen have sufficient oxygen available in their tanks upon the start of the appointment. In our facility, backup oxygen is available if necessary but may require special arrangements in some outpatient facilities.

In our clinic, there may also be differences in testing based on availability of the patient. In-state patients with complex referral question (i.e., COPD vs. progressive dementia vs. depression) are typically scheduled for more in-depth evaluations whereas out-of-state patients scheduled to be in our clinic for 1–2 weeks are more likely to get a brief neuropsychological battery designed specifically for our COPD clinic (see case example below). Interpretation of tests utilizing normative data adjusting for age, education, gender, and ethnicity is always considered. In our clinical setting, the neuropsychological test results for the COPD clinic are available within 24 h and presented at the weekly team meeting in order to incorporate findings into day-to-day care and provide specific recommendations (i.e., neurology, neuroradiology) for patients who require additional evaluation of the CNS.

Case Example of Neuropsychological Screening in COPD

As an example, we will review a neuropsychological evaluation performed on a female patient participating in the COPD assessment and rehabilitation program at National Jewish Health in Denver, CO. Ms. Smith is a 69-year-old Caucasian, right-handed female who was referred by her pulmonologist for our brief out-of-state NP battery due to concerns regarding cognitive dysfunction identified in her intake forms and by the pulmonologist during his or her on-site intake. Ms. Smith reported some difficulty with her memory during our interview. Family members present during the interview indicated that she frequently forgets appointments, is slow to complete tasks, and may not be taking her medications correctly. They also reported that she has difficulty understanding complex information. Regarding the onset of her memory concerns, Ms. Smith and her family indicated that her memory difficulty began approximately 5 years ago with noticeable worsening following both of her hospitalizations for COPD exacerbations in the past year. Medical records indicate that Ms. Smith has a history of tobacco abuse, COPD GOLD stage II, and high blood pressure. She smoked an average of one pack of cigarettes from age 18–60, but has not smoked in 9 years. The patient had no history of head injury, other neurological illness, learning disability, substance abuse, psychological difficulties, or hearing/visual problems. Ms. Smith graduated from high school with average grades and later obtained training and was certified as a home nursing aid. She worked full time for 30 years and had been retired for 10 years at the time of her evaluation. Medications included ipratropium-albuterol nebulizer four times per day, lisinoprin 10 mg per day, metroprolol 200 mg per day, oxazepam 60 mg per day, oxygen 2.5 L as needed, Spiriva 18 mcg per day, and Ventolin 108 mcg every 4–6 h.

No unusual behaviors were noted during the evaluation, and the patient was fully ambulatory and taking oxygen. Her SaO_2 level at the beginning of the session was 93. She did not appear to have any difficulty understanding test instructions, and her effort appeared within normal limits. She completed the brief measure of psychological functioning (Hospital Anxiety and Depression Scale, [49]), and she endorsed mild symptoms of depression.

Impairment levels for the patient's neuropsychological tests scores (based on normative data adjusting for age, education, and when possible gender and ethnicity) are shown in Table 28.2. Overall, her neuropsychological test results indicate mild to moderate cognitive dysfunction. Based on her educational and work history, as well as her estimated premorbid IQ, these scores likely represent a decline from average premorbid functioning. As noted in Table 28.2, Ms. Smith was moderately impaired in her learning and severely impaired in her memory for verbal information and mildly impaired for visually presented material. Her recognition for verbal and visual information following a delay was intact. She was impaired in her drawing of a clock to command with difficulty noted in terms of spacing of numbers and ability to set hands to the required time. There was some evidence of mild to moderate

Table 28.2 Brief neuropsychological battery for COPD assessment: case example

Function	Measure	Performance range
Intellectual functioning		
Oral reading/estimated premorbid IQ	WTAR[a]	Average
Attention and processing speed		
Attention to numeric sequences	WAIS-IV[b] digit span	Mildly impaired
Visual scanning and tracking speed	Trailmaking Test[c] Form A	Average
Nonverbal attention and learning	WAIS-IV coding	Average
Executive functioning and problem solving		
Sequencing efficiency	Trailmaking Test Form B	Mildly to moderately impaired
Verbal abstract reasoning	WAIS-IV similarities	Average
Nonverbal reasoning	WAIS-IV matrix reasoning	Average
Learning and memory		
Verbal list acquisition	HVLT-R[d] total trials 1–3	Mildly to moderately impaired
Verbal list free recall	HVLT-R delayed recall	Severely impaired
Verbal list recognition	HVLT-R recognition	Average
Nonverbal acquisition	BVMT-R[e] total trials 1–3	Mildly impaired
Nonverbal recall	BVMT-R delayed recall	Mildly impaired
Nonverbal recognition	BVMT-R recognition	Average
Language functioning		
Naming to confrontation	BNT—Short Form[f]	Below average
Verbal fluency	COWAT[g]	Mildly impaired
Semantic fluency	Animal naming	Mildly to moderately impaired
Visuospatial functioning		
Visuoconstruction	WAIS-IV block design	Average
Drawing to command	Clock[h] drawing	Moderately impaired
Drawing to copy	Clock copy	Average

[a]WTAR = Wechsler Test of Adult Reading [50]
[b]WAIS-IV = Wechsler Adult Intelligence Scale—Fourth Edition [50]
[c]Trailmaking Test [51]
[d]HVLT-R = Hopkins Verbal Learning Test—Revised [52]
[e]BVMT-R = Brief Visuospatial Memory Test—Revised [53]
[f]BNT = Boston Naming Test—Short Form [54]
[g]COWAT = Controlled Oral Word Association Test [55]
[h]Clock Drawing Test [26, 56]

sequencing difficulty (Trails B); however, basic reasoning was intact. We would not expect her to have significant difficulty with medical decision making with careful discussion. She had mild difficulty with auditory attention. Her naming ability was generally within normal limits, but she was slow in her verbal fluency to letter and semantic cues. We concluded that her memory deficits are likely to interfere with aspects of her day-to-day function and some assistance and review of safety in her current living arrangement would be useful. The etiology of her deficits is most likely related to her medical history including COPD and prior episodes of hypoxemia. In addition, there was some evidence of a minor mood disturbance; however, it is not likely the primary cause of her cognitive difficulties. Due to the severity of her memory problems, further evaluation with a neurologist was highly recommended to further evaluate any other changes in the central nervous system and assess the potential for reversible disorders. Repeat testing following any substantial medical or multidisciplinary treatment may also be useful in identifying significant changes (improvement or decline) over time. She was diagnosed with cognitive disorder NOS from the DSM-IV nosology.

Recommendations provided to the patient, her family, and the rehabilitation team first addressed her poor verbal learning and memory and the importance of using compensation techniques. Given their concerns regarding medication use, it was recommended she use a carefully constructed checklist or a pill box for medication types and dosages by the hour. Use of a schedule or appointment book was also recommended for day-to-day activities. The patient's relative strengths were in visual learning and memory (mildly impaired vs. moderately to severely impaired); therefore, some techniques to capitalize on this were discussed with her and the rehabilitation team. Instead of verbally communicating instructions for new activities, it was recommended that she learn by watching and using visual cues. For example, instead of describing a new activity, such as getting on a treadmill to exercise, demonstrate the activity and have her practice several times. In addition, keeping written notes available for new procedures might be useful. As with other patients with COPD, visuomotor skills were slightly impaired, and additional time to complete tasks involving motor function should be considered. As noted by her family, she was a little slow to generate words, and this is likely related to her COPD, as this is a common finding in the literature. It is not likely to interfere dramatically with her day-to-day life but having additional time to express herself may be more comfortable for the patient.

Clinical Pearls

- Patients with COPD demonstrate cognitive impairment that worsens with severity of COPD and the presence of hypoxemia.
- Cognitive areas that are most commonly impaired include aspects of verbal learning and memory, visuomotor speed, and verbal fluency.
- Identification of cognitive dysfunction in COPD patients may be mediated by a number of comorbidities, including cardiovascular disease, depression, and anxiety.
- Determine at the onset of the appointment if the patient is prescribed oxygen therapy and whether sufficient oxygen is available in his or her tanks to last throughout the exam.
- Query about exposure to environmental toxins as well as smoking and substance use/history.
- It is common for patients with COPD and their families to describe worsening cognition following hospitalization, as can be the case with any ICU or hospital stay, yet this has not been systematically studied.
- Moderate to severe neuropsychological deficits may suggest the need for additional neurologic workup (i.e., neurologic exam, neuroimaging) to assess other CNS comorbidities.
- Repeat neuropsychological testing following medical therapy (i.e., oxygen or medication changes) or comprehensive rehabilitation may be useful in documenting change over time and to assess any potential for other CNS disorders.
- Identification of cognitive strengths and weaknesses in COPD patients can be utilized to propose compensation techniques for day-to-day activities and for a rehabilitation team to work effectively with the patient.

References

1. Shapiro SD, Reilly JJ, Rennard SI. Chronic bronchitis and emphysema. In: Mason RJ, editor. Murray and Nadel's textbok of respiratory medicine. 5th ed. Philadelphia: WB Saunders; 2010.
2. Mannino DM, Homa DM, Akinbami LJ, Ford ES, et al. Chronic obstructive pulmonary disease surveillance—United States, 1971–2000. MMWR Surveill Summ. 2002;51(6):1–16.
3. Stockley RA, Mannino D, Barnes PJ. Burden and pathogenesis of chronic obstructive pulmonary disease. Proc Am Thorac Soc. 2009;6(6):524–6.
4. Mannino DM, Buist AS. Global burden of COPD: risk factors, prevalence, and future trends. Lancet. 2007;370(9589):765–73.
5. Almagro P, Lopez Garcia F, Cabrera F, Montero L, et al. Comorbidity and gender-related differences in patients hospitalized for COPD. The ECCO study. Respir Med. 2010;104(2):253–9.
6. Fletcher CM, Elmes PC, Fairbairn AS, Wood CH. The significance of respiratory symptoms and the diagnosis of chronic bronchitis in a working population. Br Med J. 1959;2(5147):257–66.
7. Agusti A, Thomas A. Neff lecture. Chronic obstructive pulmonary disease: a systemic disease. Proc Am Thorac Soc. 2006;3(6):478–81.

8. Agusti A. Systemic effects of chronic obstructive pulmonary disease: what we know and what we don't know (but should). Proc Am Thorac Soc. 2007;4(7):522–5.
9. Celli BR, MacNee W. Standards for the diagnosis and treatment of patients with COPD: a summary of the ATS/ERS position paper. Eur Respir J. 2004;23(6): 932–46.
10. Gan WQ, Man SF, Senthilselvan A, Sin DD. Association between chronic obstructive pulmonary disease and systemic inflammation: a systematic review and a meta-analysis. Thorax. 2004;59(7):574–80.
11. Boussuges A, Rossi P, Gouitaa M, Nussbaum E. Alterations in the peripheral circulation in COPD patients. Clin Physiol Funct Imaging. 2007;27(5): 284–90.
12. Han MK, McLaughlin VV, Criner GJ, Martinez FJ. Pulmonary diseases and the heart. Circulation. 2007;116(25):2992–3005.
13. Maclay JD, McAllister DA, Macnee W. Cardiovascular risk in chronic obstructive pulmonary disease. Respirology. 2007;12(5):634–41.
14. Mills NL, Miller JJ, Anand A, Robinson SD, et al. Increased arterial stiffness in patients with chronic obstructive pulmonary disease: a mechanism for increased cardiovascular risk. Thorax. 2008;63(4): 306–11.
15. Anthonisen NR, Connett JE, Enright PL, Manfreda J. Hospitalizations and mortality in the Lung Health Study. Am J Respir Crit Care Med. 2002;166(3): 333–9.
16. Dodd JW, Getov SV, Jones PW. Cognitive function in COPD. Eur Respir J. 2010;35(4):913–22.
17. Hynninen KM, Breitve MH, Wiborg AB, Pallesen S, et al. Psychological characteristics of patients with chronic obstructive pulmonary disease: a review. J Psychosom Res. 2005;59(6):429–43.
18. Agle DP, Baum GL. Psychological aspects of chronic obstructive pulmonary disease. Med Clin North Am. 1977;61(4):749–58.
19. Norwood R. Prevalence and impact of depression in chronic obstructive pulmonary disease patients. Curr Opin Pulm Med. 2006;12(2):113–7.
20. Wamboldt FS. Anxiety and depression in COPD: a call (and need) for further research. COPD. 2005;2(2):199–201.
21. Weaver TE, Narsavage GL. Physiological and psychological variables related to functional status in chronic obstructive pulmonary disease. Nurs Res. 1992;41(5):286–91.
22. Gift AG, McCrone SH. Depression in patients with COPD. Heart Lung. 1993;22(4):289–97.
23. van Ede L, Yzermans CJ, Brouwer HJ. Prevalence of depression in patients with chronic obstructive pulmonary disease: a systematic review. Thorax. 1999;54(8):688–92.
24. Aydin IO, Ulusahin A. Depression, anxiety comorbidity, and disability in tuberculosis and chronic obstructive pulmonary disease patients: applicability of GHQ-12. Gen Hosp Psychiatry. 2001;23(2):77–83.
25. Agle DP, Baum GL, Chester EH, Wendt M. Multidiscipline treatment of chronic pulmonary insufficiency. 1. Psychologic aspects of rehabilitation. Psychosom Med. 1973;35(1):41–9.
26. Goodglass H, Kaplan E. The assessment of aphasia and related disorders. Philadelphia: Lea and Febiger; 1983.
27. Eiser N, Harte R, Spiros K, Phillips C, et al. Effect of treating depression on quality-of-life and exercise tolerance in severe COPD. COPD. 2005;2(2):233–41.
28. Kunik ME, Roundy K, Veazey C, Souchek J, et al. Surprisingly high prevalence of anxiety and depression in chronic breathing disorders. Chest. 2005;127(4): 1205–11.
29. Unutzer J, Patrick DL, Simon G, Grembowski D, et al. Depressive symptoms and the cost of health services in HMO patients aged 65 years and older. A 4-year prospective study. JAMA. 1997;277(20): 1618–23.
30. Fix AJ, Golden CJ, Daughton D, Kass I, et al. Neuropsychological deficits among patients with chronic obstructive pulmonary disease. Int J Neurosci. 1982;16(2):99–105.
31. Grant I, Heaton RK, McSweeny AJ, Adams KM, et al. Neuropsychologic findings in hypoxemic chronic obstructive pulmonary disease. Arch Intern Med. 1982;142(8):1470–6.
32. Krop HD, Block AJ, Cohen E. Neuropsychologic effects of continuous oxygen therapy in COPD. Chest. 1973;64(3):317–22.
33. Prigatano GP, Parsons O, Wright E, Levin DC, et al. Neuropsychological test performance in mildly hypoxemic patients with chronic obstructive pulmonary disease. J Consult Clin Psychol. 1983;51(1):108–16.
34. Incalzi RA, Gemma A, Marra C, Muzzolon R, et al. Chronic obstructive pulmonary disease. An original model of cognitive decline. Am Rev Respir Dis. 1993;148(2):418–24.
35. Stuss DT, Peterkin I, Guzman DA, Guzman C, et al. Chronic obstructive pulmonary disease: effects of hypoxia on neurological and neuropsychological measures. J Clin Exp Neuropsychol. 1997;19(4):515–24.
36. Ozge C, Ozge A, Unal O. Cognitive and functional deterioration in patients with severe COPD. Behav Neurol. 2006;17(2):121–30.
37. Krop HD, Block AJ, Cohen E. Neuropsychological effects of continuous oxygen therapy in chronic obstructive pulmonary disease. Chest. 1977;64:317–22.
38. Grant I, Prigatano GP, Heaton RK, McSweeny AJ, et al. Progressive neuropsychologic impairment and hypoxemia. Relationship in chronic obstructive pulmonary disease. Arch Gen Psychiatry. 1987;44(11): 999–1006.
39. Antonelli Incalzi R, Marra C, Giordano A, Calcagni ML, et al. Cognitive impairment in chronic obstructive pulmonary disease—a neuropsychological and spect study. J Neurol. 2003;250(3):325–32.
40. Liesker JJ, Postma DS, Beukema RJ, ten Hacken NH, et al. Cognitive performance in patients with COPD. Respir Med. 2004;98(4):351–6.

41. Kozora E, Filley CM, Julian LJ, Cullum CM. Cognitive functioning in patients with chronic obstructive pulmonary disease and mild hypoxemia compared with patients with mild Alzheimer disease and normal controls. Neuropsychiatry Neuropsychol Behav Neurol. 1999;12(3):178–83.
42. Ortapamuk H, Naldoken S. Brain perfusion abnormalities in chronic obstructive pulmonary disease: comparison with cognitive impairment. Ann Nucl Med. 2006;20(2):99–106.
43. Toshima MT, Kaplan RM, Ries AL. Experimental evaluation of rehabilitation in chronic obstructive pulmonary disease: short-term effects on exercise endurance and health status. Health Psychol. 1990;9(3):237–52.
44. Emery CF, Leatherman NE, Burker EJ, MacIntyre NR. Psychological outcomes of a pulmonary rehabilitation program. Chest. 1991;100(3):613–7.
45. Kozora E, Tran ZV, Make B. Neurobehavioral improvement after brief rehabilitation in patients with chronic obstructive pulmonary disease. J Cardiopulm Rehabil. 2002;22(6):426–30.
46. Kozora E, Emery CF, Ellison MC, Wamboldt FS, et al. Improved neurobehavioral functioning in emphysema patients following lung volume reduction surgery compared with medical therapy. Chest. 2005;128(4):2653–63.
47. Kozora E, Emery CF, Zhang L, Make B. Improved neurobehavioral functioning in emphysema patients following medical therapy. J Cardiopulm Rehabil Prev. 2010;30(4):251–9.
48. Greene CC, Bradley KA, Bryson CL, Blough DK, et al. The association between alcohol consumption and risk of COPD exacerbation in a veteran population. Chest. 2008;134(4):761–7.
49. Zigmond AS, Snaith RP. The hospital anxiety and depression scale. Acta Psychiatr Scand. 1983;67(6):361–70.
50. Wechsler D. Wechsler adult intelligence scale—Fourth edition. San Antonio, TX: Pearson Education, Inc.; 2008.
51. Reitan RM, Wolfson D. The Halstead-Reitan neuropsychology test battery. Tucson: Neuropsychological Press; 1988.
52. Brandt J, Benedict RH. Hopkins Verbal Learning Test—Revised. Lultz, FL: Psychological Assessment Resources, Inc.; 1991.
53. Benedict RH. Brief Visuospatial Memory Test—Revised. Lutz, FL: Psychological Assessment Resources, Inc.; 1997.
54. Fastenau PS, Denburg NL, Mauer BA. Parallel short forms for the Boston Naming Test: psychometric properties and norms for older adults. J Clin Exp Neuropsychol. 1998;20(6):828–34.
55. Borkowski JG, Benton AL, Spreen O. Word fluency and brain damage. Neuropsychologia. 1967;5:135–40.
56. Kozora E, Cullum CM. Qualitative features of clock drawings in normal aging and Alzheimer's disease. Assessment. 1994;1(2):179–88.

Hepatic Encephalopathy

29

Robin C. Hilsabeck and Amy L. Webb

Abstract

Hepatic encephalopathy (HE) is a metabolically-induced, usually reversible neuropsychiatric syndrome that results in significant morbidity and mortality. The incidence is unknown, but it is estimated that most individuals with cirrhosis develop some degree of HE, and advanced age is a risk factor. Cognitive, behavioral, and motor dysfunction are the characteristic features, although the pattern and severity differ among grades. Neuropsychologists are most likely to encounter HE in the context of liver transplant evaluations. The current chapter reviews the classification and pathogenesis of HE, diagnosis and treatment considerations, and also provides a clinical case example and reviews practical issues that will arise for neuropsychologists involved in the care of patietns with HE.

Keywords

Minimal hepatic encephalopathy • Portosystemic encephalopathy • End-stage liver disease • Chronic liver disease • Cirrhosis • Neuropsychological • Neuroimaging • Neurophysiological

R.C. Hilsabeck, Ph.D., ABPP (✉)
Psychology Service, South Texas Veterans Health Care System, 7400 Merton Minter Blvd., San Antonio, TX 78229, USA

Department of Psychiatry, University of Texas Health Science Center at San Antonio, San Antonio, TX, USA

Department of Psychiatry, University of California, San Diego, San Diego, CA, USA
e-mail: hilsabeck@uthscsa.edu

A.L. Webb, M.D.
Psychology Service, South Texas Veterans Health Care System, 7400 Merton Minter Blvd., San Antonio, TX 78229, USA

Hepatology Clinic, South Texas Veterans Health Care System, San Antonio, TX, USA

Department of Medicine, University of Texas Health Science Center at San Antonio, San Antonio, TX, USA
e-mail: amy.webb@va.gov

L.D. Ravdin and H.L. Katzen (eds.), *Handbook on the Neuropsychology of Aging and Dementia*, Clinical Handbooks in Neuropsychology, DOI 10.1007/978-1-4614-3106-0_29,

Hepatic encephalopathy (HE), also referred to as portosystemic encephalopathy (PSE), is a metabolically induced, usually reversible neuropsychiatric syndrome resulting from failure of the liver to perform its detoxifying function. HE is usually associated with acute and/or chronic liver dysfunction but can also be due to portosystemic shunts that divert portal blood into circulation before removal of toxins by the liver. In its mildest form, HE manifests as subtle cognitive or motor difficulties that may not be detectable upon clinical exam alone. HE is one of the most serious complications of liver dysfunction and is a feature of fulminant hepatic failure. In its most severe form, HE results in coma and death. Between one-third and one half of hospitalizations of patients with cirrhosis are due to HE, and the frequency of hospitalization for HE has doubled over the past decade, with average hospital stays between 5 and 7 days [1, 2]. HE is a marker of poor prognosis [3], resulting in death in over 75% of patients within 3 years of their first episode [4]. In patients with acute liver failure, prognosis is even grimmer, with only about half surviving hospitalization [5]. Although rare, acute liver failure is the most frequent indication for emergency liver transplantation in most countries [6].

Classification and Grading of HE

In 1998, a working party was convened at the 11th World Congress of Gastroenterology to standardize the definition and classification of HE in an effort to bring consistency to the literature for more precise study, particularly in clinical trials. Nomenclature for type and subcategories of HE was proposed and is shown in Table 29.1 [7]. The type of HE is based on underlying liver dysfunction. Type A is associated with *a*cute liver dysfunction, type B with portosystemic *b*ypass in the absence of liver disease, and type C with liver *c*irrhosis, which is the most common. The subcategories of episodic, persistent, and minimal are based partly on course and partly on severity of HE. Importantly, use of the term "subclinical" HE was discouraged due to concern that it trivialized the clinical significance of a condition with detrimental effects on ability to perform complex tasks like driving [8–13], and health-related quality of life (HRQOL) [14–17], and outcome [18–23].

Table 29.1 Nomenclature of hepatic encephalopathy (HE)

Type of HE	Subcategory of HE
A—associated with acute liver failure	Episodic—onset of delirium (without evidence of preexisting dementia) that may develop spontaneously or after a precipitating event and may be recurrent (i.e., occur more than once within a year)
B—associated with portal–systemic bypass without intrinsic liver disease	Persistent—continuing cognitive impairment that interferes with social and/or occupational functioning that may be mild (grade 1) or severe (grades 2–4) or recur soon after treatment is discontinued
C—associated with cirrhosis and portal hypertension or portal–systemic shunts	Minimal—continuing cognitive impairment without obvious mental status changes (grade 0) that may negatively affect daily activities (e.g., driving)—formerly referred to as "subclinical"

Severity of HE is graded on a scale from 0 to 4, where 0 represents a normal clinical examination and 4 is coma. Grade 0 is also known as "minimal HE," and grades 1–4 are considered "overt HE." The most widely used method of grading HE is the West Haven Criteria (WHC) [24, 25], which is determined by clinical examination and based on the subjective evaluation of the clinician (see Table 29.2). This method has been criticized for lack of sensitivity to detect subtle brain dysfunction [26]. Neuropsychological or neurophysiological measures are recommended to identify less severe stages of HE [7, 27]. It is important to remember that although specific criteria have been determined to be characteristic of each grade, clear distinctions between grades sometimes cannot be made, and patients may fluctuate from grade to grade within minutes or hours, further clouding the clinical picture.

Table 29.2 West Haven criteria for grading hepatic encephalopathy (HE)

Grade	Characteristics
0	No abnormalities
1	Trivial lack of awareness Euphoria or anxiety Shortened attention span Impairment of addition or subtraction
2	Lethargy or apathy Disorientation for time Obvious personality change Inappropriate behavior
3	Somnolence or semi-stupor Responsive to stimuli Confused, gross disorientation Bizarre behavior
4	Coma

Although the true incidence of HE is unknown, it is estimated that most, if not all, individuals with cirrhosis eventually develop some degree of HE, and advanced age is a risk factor [28]. Overt HE is estimated to affect about 10% of patients with well-compensated cirrhosis (i.e., no serious complications) and about 40% of patients with decompensated cirrhosis, [29, 30] and is considered the "hallmark" of acute liver failure [31]. Rates of minimal HE are more difficult to determine since it may be missed on clinical examination, but it has been estimated to be present in 50–80% of cirrhotic patients when appropriately sensitive methods are used for identification [32–34].

Pathogenesis

The exact mechanisms underlying HE are complex and still largely unknown, but ammonia neurotoxicity plays a major role [35–38]. A primary reason ammonia may build up in the blood stream is disruption of the urea cycle. Urea is a nitrogen-containing waste product of protein metabolism. When protein is metabolized, deamination (break down) of amino acids produces ammonia. In addition to protein metabolism, intestinal bacteria produce ammonia which is then absorbed into the portal system, the major source of blood flow to the liver. A healthy liver would quickly convert ammonia into urea, which would then be excreted primarily by the kidneys. In the presence of liver dysfunction, ammonia is synthesized more slowly into urea or not at all, allowing ammonia to accumulate in the blood stream. Healthy muscle tissue metabolizes ammonia in this manner, but individuals with cirrhosis are impaired due to muscle wasting, physician recommendations for low-protein "liver failure" diets, and an increased catabolic state (i.e., when the body is breaking down tissue). Certain medications (e.g., benzodiazepines) sensitize the central nervous system (CNS) to ammonia, even at normal levels. Natural benzodiazepines may also be important since a benzodiazepine antagonist (e.g., flumazenil) briefly improves the clinical course of some patients who were not administered pharmaceutical doses of benzodiazepines [39].

When pathologic ammonia is allowed to reach the brain, astrocytes provide the primary means to eliminate it through the synthesis of glutamine [35]. Glutamine is produced by adding one molecule of ammonia to glutamate, which is an amino acid present in over 90% of neurons where it acts as an excitatory neurotransmitter. As glutamine accumulates, its osmotic effect causes the astrocyte to take in water, resulting in brain edema and increased intracranial pressure (ICP). Thus, HE is hypothesized to occur when astrocytes are unable to maintain osmotic equilibrium in response to the ammonia-induced increase in glutamine. On autopsy, astrocytes of patients with chronic liver disease show morphologic features characteristic of Alzheimer type II astrocytosis (e.g., pale, enlarged, and frequently paired nuclei, prominent nucleole, proliferation of cytoplasmic organelles) [35].

Another by-product of the ammonia-induced increase in glutamine that may contribute to the pathogenesis of HE is oxidative stress [40–42], which results when reactive oxygen species (ROS) such as free radicals and peroxides cannot be removed efficiently, causing significant damage to cell structures and even cell death. Ammonia has been shown to generate ROS when added to astrocyte cultures [43, 44], and glutamine increases free radical production [45]. Ammonia also induces oxidative and nitrosative stress in mitochondria after being carried in and released by glutamine [46–48].

Other neurotransmitter systems also are affected by ammonia both directly and indirectly through alteration of transmitter synthesis and recirculation [35, 49]. Altered serotonergic and dopaminergic transmission has been described [50–52], as has activation of glutamatergic NMDA receptors and modulation of γ-aminobutyric acid (GABA) receptors by elevated levels of neurosteroids and endogenous benzodiazepines [53, 54]. Overstimulation of excitatory NMDA receptors by ammonia has been shown to induce neuromodulation, neurodegeneration, and neuronal apoptosis [53].

Inflammatory mediators, such as pro-inflammatory cytokines like tumor necrosis factor-alpha (TNF-α), interleukin-(IL)-1, and IL-6, whether produced in the brain as a result of edema and/or ICP or in the periphery in response to infection, also have been implicated in the pathogenesis of HE [40, 42, 55]. This hypothesis is supported by a more rapid progression to severe HE in the presence of infection in patients with acute liver failure [56, 57], as well as astrocyte swelling induced by cytokine exposure in cell cultures [58].

Table 29.3 Common precipitating factors of hepatic encephalopathy (HE)

Electrolyte imbalance
Hyponatremia—abnormally low levels of sodium in the blood
Hypokalemia—abnormally low levels of potassium in the blood
Metabolic alkalosis—pH or acidity of tissue is elevated above normal levels
Increased nitrogen load
Gastrointestinal bleeding
Excess dietary protein
Azotemia—abnormally high levels of nitrogen-containing compounds (e.g., urea) in the blood
Constipation
Central nervous system-acting drugs (especially narcotics, tranquilizers, and sedatives)
Infection (particularly bacterial peritonitis, urinary tract, skin, or pulmonary)
Surgery
Dehydration
Urinary obstruction
Renal failure
Transjugular intrahepatic portosystemic shunt (TIPS), particularly in patients aged 60 and older
Superimposed liver injury from acute hepatitis, drug-induced liver injury, etc.
Hepatocellular carcinoma
Terminal liver disease

Clinical Presentation

Cognitive, behavioral, and motor dysfunction are the characteristic features of HE, although the pattern and severity differ among grades. Patients with overt HE display changes in mental status over the course of hours or days consistent with the diagnostic criteria for delirium detailed in the Diagnostic and Statistical Manual of Mental Disorders, Fourth Edition—Text Revision (DSM-IV-TR) [59]. Overt HE can develop spontaneously, but is often precipitated by electrolyte imbalances, increased nitrogen load, medications, infection, and/or a host of other factors (see Table 29.3). Once HE and any precipitating factors are identified and treated, patients usually return to baseline functioning within a few days (i.e., episodic HE). In cases of persistent HE, which is less common, the patient's mental status continues to fluctuate for more than 4 weeks without returning to baseline and this is an indication for liver transplantation [60].

The most severe grade of HE, grade 4, is the easiest to recognize, as patients are usually in a coma. Although patients may respond to pain, there often is no response to voice or gentle physical prodding and no spontaneous speech. Patients may open their eyes, but this is not done on command or in conjunction with any purposeful behavior. Decerebrate or decorticate posturing may be seen, even without sternal pressure [61] and may be a sign of raised ICP. Increased ICP is associated with poor outcome, including high rates of mortality, if not controlled [62].

Hallmarks of grade 3 are somnolence and confusion, including disorientation to place [63]. Patients in grade 3 are difficult to rouse and keep awake and may not orient to the clinician. Once awakened, they have trouble paying attention and participating in conversation. They may act strangely and laugh inappropriately, display paranoia, or become easily agitated. Motor findings may include clonus (i.e., rapid involuntary muscle contraction and relaxation after forced extension or stretching), Babinski's sign (i.e., toes splay out instead of curve inward when sole of foot is rubbed with a blunt instrument), or nystagmus (i.e., rapid involuntary eye movements that are usually side to side but can be up and down).

In grade 2, patients are often lethargic but easy to arouse and engage in conversation. Their movements and thinking are slow. Their speech tends to be slow and monotonous and also may be soft and dysarthric. They typically are aware of their location (i.e., setting and city) but usually are not oriented to time (i.e., month or day of the week). Although most can obey simple commands and recognize common objects, they typically cannot perform simple addition and subtraction and have trouble remembering recent events. Cranial nerves are usually intact, but patients in grade 2 may display either decreased or increased tone and/or deep tendon reflexes, reduced speed or clumsiness of rapid alternating movements, ataxia, tremor, and/or asterixis (i.e., "flapping" of the wrist when arms are held straight out with wrists flexed and fingers outstretched and widely separated). Patients too lethargic to lift their arms can be instructed to grasp the examiner's hands or extend the tongue since sustained movement in patients with asterixis oscillates between tense and relaxed (i.e., never constant) [34]. They may have fetor hepaticus, a uniquely pungent, sweet odor of the breath.

Patients in grade 1 HE are usually alert and typically oriented to place and generally to time. They may sometimes appear lethargic, but they more often report that they are tired, and their sleep–wake cycle is off. They may be sleeping more than usual or have reversal in their sleep–wake cycle, so they sleep more during the day and need medication to sleep at night. These patients often can perform simple arithmetic but have trouble with multiplication or division. Handwriting may be small and difficult to read. Similar to patients in grade 2, memory for recent events is impaired. Motor abnormalities are similar to those displayed by patients in grade 2, as well, although dysarthria, tremor, and hyperreflexia are the most common in grade 1 [63, 64]. It is important to remember, however, that motor abnormalities in overt HE can be transient and do not always align with a particular grade of HE. The possible exception to this is asterixis, which, when present, is usually an indicator of grade 2 [60].

As noted above, patients with minimal HE, or grade 0, usually display no obvious abnormalities on clinical exam. However, they sometimes exhibit subtle motor dysfunction, with motor akinesia (i.e., difficulty initiating motor movements), tremor, and rigidity being most common [65]. They or their family members may complain of cognitive problems, disturbances in sleep, appetite, and sexuality, and reduced efficiency in performing work and home activities. Ability to perform basic activities of daily living, such as bathing and dressing, are often not affected. Cognitive testing displays a frontal–subcortical pattern of deficits, with impairments most often seen in psychomotor speed, attention/concentration, visuospatial/constructional skills, and executive functions [66–68]. Poor performances on measures of learning and memory may be found but usually are secondary to attentional and visuospatial/perceptual difficulties rather than deficits in memory per se [69, 70]. Intellectual functioning and language abilities typically are preserved.

Differential Diagnosis

Because the symptoms of HE are not specific, it should be considered only in patients with known or suspected liver disease or other portosystemic shunts. The clinician must additionally rule out

Table 29.4 Hepatic encephalopathy differential diagnosis

Intracranial bleeding
Subdural hematoma
Intracranial hemorrhage
Metabolic encephalopathies caused by
Uremia
Sepsis
Hypoglycemia
Hypoxia
Ketoacidosis
Hypercapnea
Thyroid dysfunction
Cerebral edema
Ischemic brain disease
Ischemic stroke
Transient ischemic attack
Central nervous system abscess, encephalitis, or meningitis
Central nervous system neoplasm
Wilson's disease
Substance-induced intoxication or withdrawal
Postictal state

other causes of mental status change with neurological symptoms, including intracranial bleeding, metabolic abnormalities, ischemic brain disease, CNS infection or neoplasm, Wilson's disease, substance-induced delirium, and postictal state (see Table 29.4). Seizures and focal neurological signs, such as hemiparesis and hemiplegia, are uncommon [71] and may suggest another etiology. If HE does not resolve within 72 h of treatment, another cause of encephalopathy or unresolved precipitating factor should be considered.

Treatment

Given the primary role of ammonia neurotoxicity in the pathogenesis of HE, management strategies focus on reduction and/or elimination of ammonia, in addition to treatment of precipitating factors, when identified [72, 73]. The most commonly administered treatment for HE is lactulose, which is a nonabsorbable disaccharide that remains undigested until it reaches the colon. It reduces plasma ammonia levels by inhibiting ammonia production of bacteria and increasing fecal nitrogen excretion. It is usually administered orally, but in the more severe grades of HE or in patients with ascites (i.e., fluid retention in the abdominal cavity) or peritonitis (i.e., inflammation of visceral or abdominal lining), administration via retention enema is preferred [34, 60].

In spite of its long-standing and widespread use, the efficacy of lactulose has been questioned [74], and patients are often noncompliant due to unpleasant side effects, such as increased intestinal gas, abdominal distention and cramping, and diarrhea [60]. Therefore, alternative treatments for HE are a topic of intense study [75]. Nonabsorbable antibiotics, such as neomycin and vancomycin, have been suggested with the goal of reducing bacteria-producing ammonia in the gut. However, their efficacy has not been well established, and prolonged use can result in significant adverse effects (e.g., inner ear and/or kidney problems, bacterial resistance, or fungal colonization). A recent and more promising alternative or adjunct to lactulose is rifaximin, a semisynthetic derivative of rifamycin, which has been shown to reduce the number and length of hospitalizations for HE [76, 77]. Because of the expense of rifaximin, it has been recommended only for patients who are lactulose refractory or intolerant [1, 78].

Due to the lack of effective treatments for HE, prevention is the goal [7, 34], particularly given evidence of increased severity of cognitive impairment with each additional episode of overt HE [79]. Along with diligent management of underlying liver disease and its complications, close monitoring of dietary protein intake is recommended in patients with a history of HE, as large amounts of protein can increase plasma ammonia levels and possibly precipitate HE while too little protein correlates with mortality and development of complications [80, 81]. Findings on dietary supplementation with branched-chain amino acids have been mixed, with some studies showing positive effects on cognitive functioning [82, 83], particularly in patients with persistent HE [84], and prolonged event-free survival [85], and others showing no effect at all [86]. Liver transplantation is indicated for patients with recurrent episodic or persisting HE due to increased mortality rates [87], with extracorporeal albumin dialysis serving as a potential bridge to liver transplantation [88, 89].

Clinical Evaluation

Although the core manifestations of HE have been recognized and agreed upon for years, a "gold standard" for the diagnosis of HE remains elusive. Definition and classification of even the basic behavioral and motor alterations needs further refinement to distinguish among grades of HE, particularly the less severe grades. Therefore, diagnosis must be based on multiple approaches, including clinical examination, laboratory findings, neuroimaging, neurophysiological measures, and neuropsychological assessment.

Clinical Examination

The clinical interview and physical and neurological exams are the mainstays for assessing HE. The clinician must ensure a history of known or suspected liver disease or the presence of a portosystemic shunt and exclude other potential causes of encephalopathy. Early identification of HE is crucial as delays in diagnosis may result in death. A thorough review of possible precipitating factors also is critical so that appropriate treatment can be initiated promptly. For inpatients with HE, examination of mental status should be performed at least 2–3 times a day [34].

In determining grade of HE, the WHC (Table 29.2) can be employed quickly and easily and provides a useful "ballpark" of the patient's clinical status [27]. In more severe grades of HE, the Glasgow Coma Scale (GCS) [90] may be a useful adjunct, supplying additional information about ocular and motor responses and thus allowing for wider separation among patients in grades 3 and 4 [63]. In less severe grades, and particularly in minimal HE, neurocognitive tests and neurophysiological measures are recommended [7].

Because some of the items in the WHC are not operationally defined and do not correspond well to the progression of HE, Ortiz and colleagues [91] developed the Clinical Hepatic Encephalopathy Staging Scale (CHESS). The CHESS consists of nine manifestations of HE that can be easily recognized and categorized into dichotomous groups (see Table 29.5) and was designed to

Table 29.5 Clinical Hepatic Encephalopathy Staging Scale (CHESS)

1. Does the patient know which month he/she is in (i.e., January, February)?	
0. Yes	1. No, or he/she does not talk
2. Does the patient know which day of the week he/she is in (i.e., Thursday, Friday, Sunday…)?	
0. Yes	1. No, or he/she does not talk
3. Can he/she count backwards from 10 to 1 without making mistakes or stopping?	
0. Yes	1. No, or he/she does not talk
4. If asked to do so, does he/she raise his/her arms?	
0. Yes	1. No
5. Does he/she understand what you are saying to him/her? (based on the answers to questions 1–4)	
0. Yes	1. No, or he/she does not talk
6. Is the patient awake and alert?	
0. Yes	1. No, he/she is sleepy or fast asleep
7. Is the patient fast asleep, and is it difficult to wake him/her up?	
0. Yes	1. No
8. Can he/she talk?	
0. Yes	1. He/she does not talk
9. Can he/she talk correctly? In other words, can you understand everything he/she says, and he/she doesn't stammer?	
0. Yes	1. No, he/she does not talk or does not talk correctly

provide a means to monitor the severity of HE. The CHESS provides a score from 0 (low) to 9 (high), which reflects the severity of HE, not the grade. Factor analysis supported two factors corresponding to "mild" and "severe" HE, which is consistent with recent proposals to classify HE into more clinically meaningful categories of "low-" (grades 1 and 2) or "high-grade" (grades 3 and 4) rather than trying to make fine-grained differentiations among grades 0–4. Like the WHC, the CHESS should be augmented with the GCS for more severe HE and with neurocognitive and/or neurophysiological measures for less severe grades.

A modified version of the WHC, the Hepatic Encephalopathy Scoring Algorithm (HESA), was developed by Hassanein and colleagues [64] in an attempt to improve its objectivity and sensitivity. The HESA combines the clinical exam with neuropsychological tests to determine HE grade, relying heavily on subjective clinical evaluation in the more severe grades where neuropsychological testing is not possible and more heavily on objective testing in the less severe grades where dysfunction may not be as evident on clinical exam (see Table 29.6). Initial findings confirm increased sensitivity and accuracy of the HESA compared to the WHC in grading HE [64].

Laboratory Findings

Blood ammonia levels are often elevated in patients with overt HE but do not always correlate with HE grade [92, 93]. However, significantly elevated blood ammonia levels (>150–200 μmol/l) in a comatose patient without a history of recent seizures are strongly suggestive of HE [60]. It is important to perform the assay within 30 min of drawing blood, or levels may be artificially inflated [94].

Neuroimaging

The primary role of neuroimaging in evaluation of HE is to rule out other possible etiologies of neurobehavioral changes [95] and to establish the presence of cerebral edema, particularly in acute liver failure. Because clinical symptoms of increased ICP (e.g., hypertension, bradycardia) may not be present, ICP monitoring devices may be helpful to identify cerebral edema early and prevent herniation until liver transplantation can be performed [96]. Typical neuroimaging findings in HE include hyperintensities in the globus pallidus on magnetic resonance imaging (MRI) T1-weighted images (see Fig. 29.1), elevated glutamine/glutamate peaks and decreased myo-inositol and choline signals on proton magnetic resonance spectroscopy (^{1}H MRS), and white matter abnormalities on MRI fast fluid-attenuated inversion recovery sequences (FLAIR) and diffusion-weighted images (DWI) [97]. In cirrhotic patients with minimal HE, T2 hyperintensities along the corticospinal tract (see Fig. 29.2) are suggestive of mild edema [98, 99] and have been found to relate to abnormalities in central motor pathways that resolve (as do some cognitive difficulties) after liver transplantation [100]. In patients with HE due to portosystemic shunt and no liver disease, MRI can be especially helpful as dietary manganese that is not cleared by the liver accumulates in the basal ganglia and is detected as hyperintensities on T1-weighted images when exam may have found mild Parkinson-like movement changes only [94].

Neurophysiological Measures

Advantages of neurophysiological measures are that they are not influenced by demographic variables, such as gender, education, or cultural background, and they are easy to administer by staff without extensive training. Electroencephalogram (EEG) has been used to diagnose HE since the 1950s [101]. However, because findings are not specific to HE, EEG and other neurophysiological measures are most useful in the comatose patient [102], when the diagnosis is uncertain (i.e., focal neurological signs or seizure activity is present or the patient has "normal" mental status) or when evidence of worsening HE is needed [103]. The most common EEG findings in HE are slowed mean dominant frequencies, and in minimal HE,

Table 29.6 Hepatic Encephalopathy Scoring Algorithm (HESA)

	Time | | |: | | 24 Hour Clock
4	○ No eyes opening ○ No verbal/voice response ○ No reaction to simple commands
	All applicable ⇒ Grade 4 ○ otherwise continue examination
3	○ Somnolence ○ Confusion ○ Disoriented to place ○ Bizarre Behavior / Anger/Rage ○ Clonus/Rigidity / Nysatgmus / Babinsky ☐ Mental Control = 0
	3 or more applicable⇒Grade 3 ○ otherwise continue examination
2	○ Lethargy ○ Loss of time ○ Slurred Speech ○ Hyperactive Reflexes ○ Inappropriate Behavior ☐ Slow Responses ☐ Amnesia of recent events ☐ Anxiety ☐ Impaired Simple Computations
	2 or more ○ and 3 or more ☐ applicable ⇒ Grade 2 ○ otherwise continue
1	○ Sleep disorder / Impaired Sleep Pattern ○ Tremor ☐ Impaired complex computations ☐ Shortened attention span ☐ Impaired Construction ability ☐ Euphoria or Depression
	4 or more applicable ⇒ Grade 1 ○ otherwise Grade 0
HE Grade	|__|

Note: ○ indicates symptoms assessed using clinical judgment, and ☐ indicates symptoms assessed using neuropsychological measures

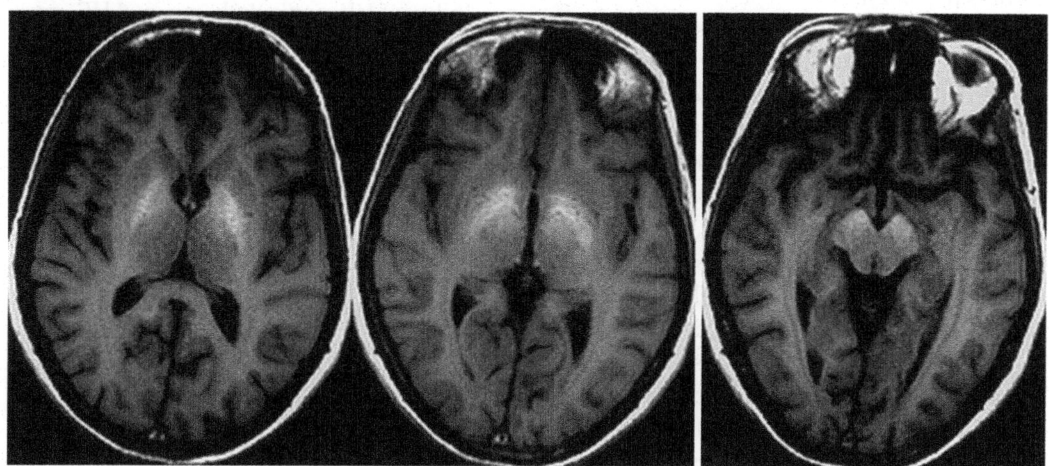

Fig. 29.1 Hyperintensities in the globus pallidus secondary to hepatic encephalopathy. Transverse T1-weighted MR images of the brain in a patient with chronic liver failure and parkinsonism. Observe the bilateral and symmetric high T1 signal-intensity change involving the globus pallidus and the anterior midbrain

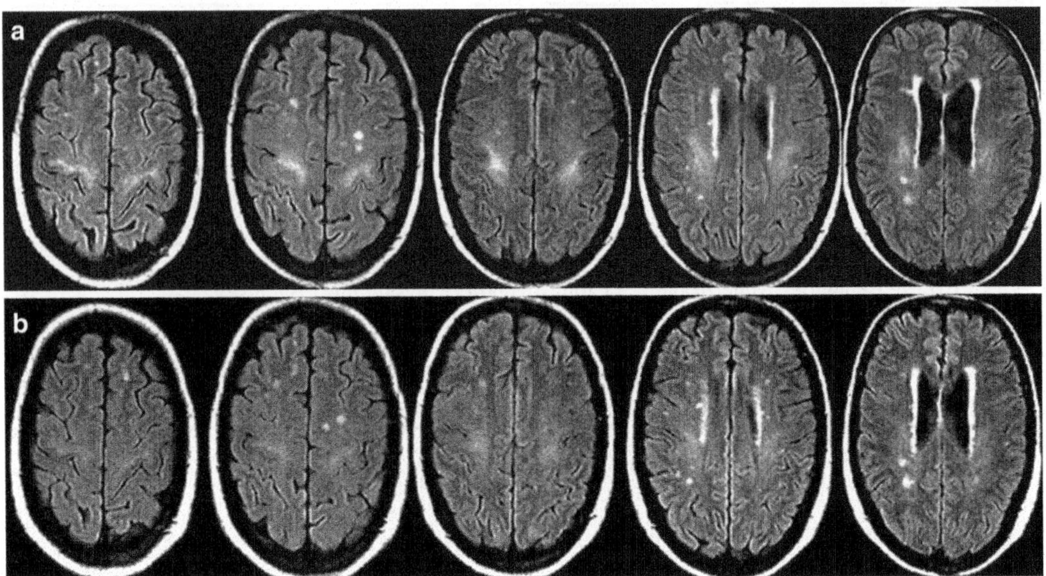

Fig. 29.2 Hyperintensities in the corticospinal tract secondary to hepatic encephalopathy. (**a**) Transverse T2-weighted fast FLAIR images obtained in a patient with liver cirrhosis during an episode of hepatic encephalopathy. Observe the symmetric areas of increased signal intensity along the corticospinal tract in both cerebral hemispheres. (**b**) This signal-intensity abnormality almost completely reverses on a follow-up study obtained few months later, when the patient showed no signs of overt hepatic encephalopathy

you may see relatively slowed activity within the δ (delta) and θ (theta) frequency bands [104]. In patients with minimal HE, changes in EEG have been shown to be predictive of developing overt HE and thus may have prognostic utility [23]. EEG has been criticized for use in detecting HE because it measures cortical rather than subcortical activity, which is where most of the pathology in HE is hypothesized to exist.

Other neurophysiological measures that have been used to identify HE include evoked potentials (EPs) and critical flicker frequency (CFF). EPs, the latency between presentation and detection of a stimulus, may be slightly delayed in patients with minimal HE, shown most often using P300 oddball paradigms [22, 105–107], but findings are not specific and often confounded by alcohol use or diabetes, which also delay EPs, and are frequently found in patients with cirrhosis [108]. In CFF, the patient is asked to press a button when a steady light has changed into a flicker and when a flickering light has become a steady, fused light. Patients with minimal and lower grades of HE have shown reduced ability to detect the light flickering or fusing [109–111].

Neuropsychological Assessment

Neuropsychologists are most likely to encounter HE in the context of liver transplant evaluations. Pre-transplant evaluations usually are conducted on an outpatient basis, but occasionally they must be performed while the patient is hospitalized and awaiting transplantation. Of course, the possibility of HE, particularly minimal HE, must always be considered in patients with cirrhosis, regardless of reason for referral or inpatient versus outpatient status. Neuropsychologists also are called upon to assess for HE in the context of clinical trials for management of HE and when insertion of a transjugular intrahepatic portosystemic shunt (TIPS) for management of portal hypertension is planned [112]. Onset or worsening of HE is common after placement of TIPS, occurring in 35–55% of patients within the first year [113]. Baseline assessment and subsequent monitoring is important for identifying and treating HE before it escalates and the patient's status becomes critical, particularly in the first 3 months, since 90% of post-TIPS HE occurs in this time frame [113, 114]. The level of neuropsychological assessment will depend on the severity of HE, with more comprehensive testing reserved for those with grades 0 or 1. It often is difficult for patients with grades 2 and 3 to participate reliably for more than 10–15 min. Fatigue is also frequently a factor, even in patients with no or minimal HE, so full day evaluations are not routinely employed.

Clinical Interview

Changes in cognitive and motor functioning secondary to minimal HE are often subtle and result in cognitive inefficiencies rather than frank impairment, but still significantly affect daily functioning, including ability to work and drive. With regard to driving, patients with minimal HE report more traffic violations and motor vehicle accidents than those without cognitive dysfunction [11–13]. Common cognitive complaints include trouble paying attention, concentrating, remembering, and completing tasks. Aphasia, significant memory problems such as repeating stories or forgetting recent events even when reminded, and lateralized motor problems (i.e., weakness or motor abnormality on one side only) are uncommon and usually indicate another etiology. Patients often have difficulty pinpointing when the symptoms began, but usually indicate that they are not worsening significantly over time. Report of gradual cognitive decline over time in the absence of recurrent episodic HE is suggestive of possible neurodegenerative disease process, psychological factors, or medical conditions other than minimal HE contributing to cognitive complaints.

Additional complaints often include fatigue and changes in appetite, sleep, energy, and activity levels. Patients with minimal HE report reduced HRQOL, such as limited social interactions and recreational pastimes and difficulties managing home and work duties [14–17]. Although the patient may endorse affective symptoms, it is important to establish that these changes do not occur in conjunction with increasingly depressed or anxious mood.

As with any patient referred for neuropsychological assessment, ruling out other possible causes of cognitive impairment, including stroke, seizure disorder, traumatic brain injury, or other neuromedical condition, is necessary. Gathering information about psychiatric and substance use histories, academic and social functioning, and family medical history also is important for differential diagnosis. Information from a collateral source is helpful when assessing patients with minimal HE due to the possibility of poor insight and/or awareness [115] and essential when assessing patients with overt HE who often cannot report reliably.

Test Selection

Selection of measures will depend on the setting (inpatient vs. outpatient), severity of HE, and reason for evaluation (e.g., pre-transplant, monitoring of HE in clinical trials or following TIPS). In the case of pre-transplant outpatient evaluations, most patients are either unimpaired or have minimal HE, so comprehensive neuropsychological evaluation is appropriate. Assessment of current intellectual and/or estimated premorbid functioning, language, visuospatial/constructional skills, attention and processing speed, executive functioning, learning and memory, emotional status, and HRQOL is recommended. Because one of the purposes of the pre-transplant evaluation is to rule out neurodegenerative diseases, such as Alzheimer's disease, it is important to include tests that can distinguish cortical from subcortical patterns of deficits. A couple of studies have found support for the utility of the Repeatable Battery for the Assessment of Neuropsychological Status (RBANS) [116] in pre-transplant evaluations [117, 118], with one study confirming the expected subcortical pattern of deficits using the Randolph Cortical-Subcortical Deviation Score detailed in the RBANS manual [118]. When pre-transplant evaluations must be conducted on an inpatient basis and the patient can tolerate more detailed assessment (i.e., is at grade 2 HE or less), the RBANS may be a good choice since it taps multiple cognitive domains, can be administered in less than 30 min, and is easy to transport.

With regard to emotional status, brief self-report measures rather than longer measures of psychopathology (e.g., Minnesota Multiphasic Personality Inventory—2) [119] are used to minimize fatigue. Of course, if there are concerns about significant psychopathology, particularly in the context of pre-transplant evaluation, use of a more comprehensive measure of psychological functioning may be warranted. For HRQOL, the Medical Outcomes Study Short Form (SF-36) [120] is commonly used and enables comparisons to other chronic diseases, but disease specific measures also are available, including the Chronic Liver Disease Questionnaire [121], the National Institute of Diabetes and Digestive and Kidney Disease (NIDDK)—Quality Assessment [122], and Liver Disease Quality of Life Instrument [123]. Recently, a measure of HRQOL for use specifically with minimal HE patients showed promising initial validity [124]. Table 29.7 displays a sample outpatient pre-transplant battery and suggested modifications for inpatient status.

When monitoring HE in the course of clinical trials, you want to select measures that can be completed by patients with more severe HE but also are sensitive enough to detect subtle changes in cognition in the less severe grades. This was one of the goals of the HESA [64], which allows one to measure changes in HE severity across all grades and is now required in Federal Drug Administration (FDA)-sponsored studies. Although more validation of the HESA is needed, particularly in the lower grades, it is a viable option for clinical trials, as the neuropsychological measures administered are well known and widely used with modifications to ensure feasibility of administration and scoring in the inpatient setting while maintaining sensitivity for detecting impairment.

Table 29.7 Sample neuropsychological battery for pre-transplant evaluation

Wechsler Test of Adult Reading [137]
Repeatable Battery for the Assessment of Neuropsychological Status [116]
Trail Making Test [125]
Stroop Color and Word Test [138]
Boston Naming Test [139]
Controlled Oral Word Association Test [140]
Animal Naming [140]
Wisconsin Card Sorting Test—64-Card Version [141]
Finger Tapping Test [125]
Grooved Pegboard [142]
Beck Depression Inventory-II [143]
Beck Anxiety Inventory [144]
Chronic Liver Disease Questionnaire [121]

Note: For inpatient evaluations, suggest administration of the first three tests only

When the goal is to identify the presence of minimal HE outside the context of pre-transplant evaluation or clinical trials, such as when conducting evaluations pre- and post-TIPS insertion or for monitoring risk of developing overt HE during clinic visits, a comprehensive battery may not be necessary or appropriate. The consensus statement generated by the 1998 working group mentioned previously [7] recommended at least two of the following four measures be used to assess for minimal HE: Parts A and B of the Trail Making Test (TMT) [125] (also known as the Number Connection Test), block design test, and digit symbol test. Also recommended was the Psychometric Hepatic Encephalopathy Score (PHES) [126], which has been validated in several languages across several countries, including Germany, Italy, and Spain [127]. The PHES is a composite score based on demographic-adjusted z-scores from Parts A and B of the TMT, digit symbol, line tracing, and serial dotting (see Fig. 2 in Chap. 23 for a picture of the latter two measures). Scores ≤ -4 are considered to reflect minimal HE.

The PHES, along with the RBANS, also was recommended recently by a group of experts convened by the International Society for Hepatic Encephalopathy and Nitrogen Metabolism (ISHEN) for use in patients at risk for developing minimal HE [128]. One limitation of the PHES for use in the United States is that line tracing and serial dotting have not yet been normed in the United States. A limitation of the RBANS is that it has not been systematically studied as a method for detecting or monitoring HE [129]. Computerized cognitive measures are another method beginning to be used, with the Inhibitory

Control Task (ICT), a computerized variant of the continuous performance test, showing good initial validity [130–132], including ability to predict future car crashes and traffic violations [13].

Case Example: Characterization of Overt and Minimal HE [133]

Following is a case example of a 46-year-old non-Hispanic White man with end-stage liver disease (ESLD) secondary to hepatitis C virus and alcoholic hepatitis. Mr. J graduated from high school and worked primarily as a machinist until he became disabled from ESLD. He was being followed in a hepatology clinic at a university hospital and agreed to participant in a research study examining quality of life in persons with chronic liver disease. As part of this research protocol, a brief neurocognitive battery consisting of a modified version of the Rey Complex Figure Test (RCF) [134], Digit Cancellation (DC) [134], Trail Making Test (TMT), and the written version of the Symbol Digit Modalities Test (SDMT) [135] was administered during a routine clinic visit. Mr. J completed this battery on three occasions: once during an episode of overt HE judged to be grade 1, once during minimal HE, and once 5 months post-transplant. His raw scores on these measures at each of the three time points are presented in Table 29.8.

Cognitive performance on all measures during Mr. J's episode of overt HE was more than three standard deviations below the normative mean, and he evidenced a mild tremor while performing tasks. He exhibited significant difficulty copying this version of the RCF, which was modified to be more simplistic than the original figure. Even after having viewed the figure three times, his learning score (i.e., raw score = 5) revealed that he did not encode much additional information beyond that encoded on the initial (copy) trial (i.e., raw score = 3.5). Moreover, he forgot half of the details of the figure after a 20-min delay. On a measure of selective attention, Digit Cancellation, he required a long time to complete the task and made a significant number of errors (both omission and commission). He was able to complete the TMT, albeit very slowly, and he made several cognitive-switching errors on Part B. On the SDMT, he performed very slowly and made a few errors. His cognitive and motor findings during this episode of overt HE are typical of those seen in patients with grade 1 HE [136].

A couple of months later, after his episode of overt HE had resolved, Mr. J's performance on this brief battery was significantly improved. His action tremor was gone, and his test scores were essentially within normal limits, except for SDMT, which was approximately 1.5 standard deviations below the normative mean. Five months post-transplant, Mr. J exhibited continued improvement, particularly on measures relying on executive function (i.e., RCF learning, TMT Part B, and SDMT). Although some of these

Table 29.8 Mr. J's cognitive test performances over time

	Pre-transplant 7 months Grade 1 HE	Pre-transplant 5 months Grade 0 (Minimal) HE	Post-transplant 5 months
Modified RCF copy	3.5	20	19
Modified RCF learning	5	16	19
Modified RCF% forgotten	50.0	6.3	5.6
DC total time (s)	278	225	200
DC total errors	31	9	9
TMT-A (s)	85	40	34
TMT-B (s)	>300	110	60
SDMT	18	31	44

Note: *RCF* Rey Complex Figure, *DC* Digit Cancellation, *TMT* Trail Making Test, *SDMT* Symbol Digit Modalities Test (written version)

improvements may have been due to practice effects, others were too significant to be attributed to practice effects alone. The contrast between test performances during minimal HE and post-transplant suggests that although Mr. J generally performed within normal limits on all but one task (i.e., SDMT) pre-transplant, he was still performing below his baseline. The pattern of findings also is consistent with the literature showing compromised frontal–subcortical circuits.

Clinical Pearls

- HE is associated with impaired abilities to perform complex tasks (e.g., driving), reduced HRQOL, and poor outcome, including death.
- Severity of HE is usually graded on a scale from 0 (minimal) to 4 (coma), and sometimes distinctions among grades are difficult to determine due to fluctuations in a patient's status or limitations in the methods available for grading HE.
- Overt HE typically requires hospitalization and quick identification and treatment of precipitating events to prevent continued deterioration and death.
- Blood ammonia levels may not correspond to clinical severity of HE and have little clinical significance if serially followed.
- Minimal HE is present in 50–80% of cirrhotic patients and usually undetected unless tested with neuropsychological or neurophysiological measures.
- Although HE should be high on the list of diagnostic possibilities in delirious patients with cirrhosis, other causes of mental status change, such as alcohol withdrawal, occult gastrointestinal bleed, infection, and dehydration, must be ruled out since they are also common in patients with cirrhosis.
- In patients with worsening of HE but no clear precipitating factor, check for noncompliance with lactulose or other HE treatments since patients sometimes are not compliant due to unpleasant drug side effects or poor memory.
- In patients with minimal HE, a frontal–subcortical pattern of deficits and cognitive inefficiencies are characteristic; aphasia, significant forgetting such as that seen in Alzheimer's disease, and lateralized deficits suggest another etiology.
- Traffic violations and motor vehicle accidents are more common in cirrhotic patients with minimal HE than those without, so careful inquiry about driving is needed, and physician recommendation for the patient to stop driving may be advised.

References

1. Leevy C, Phillips J. Hospitalizations during the use of rifaximin versus lactulose for the treatment of hepatic encephalopathy. Dig Dis Sci. 2007;52:737–41.
2. Poordad FF. Review article: the burden of hepatic encephalopathy. Aliment Pharmacol Ther. 2007;25(S1):3–9.
3. Stewart C, Malinchoc M, Kim W, Kamath PS. Hepatic encephalopathy as a predictor of survival in patients with end stage liver disease. Liver Transpl. 2007;13:1366–71.
4. Bustamante J, Rimola A, Ventura PJ, Navasa M, Ciera I, Reggiardo V, et al. Prognostic significance of hepatic encephalopathy in patients with cirrhosis. J Hepatol. 1999;30:890–5.
5. Bernuau J, Durand F. Early prediction of encephalopathy in hospitalized patients with severe acute liver disease: the narrow window of opportunity for transplant-free survival. J Hepatol. 2009;51:977–80.
6. Bernal W, Auzinger G, Dhawan A, Wendon J. Acute liver failure. Lancet. 2010;376:190–201.
7. Ferenci P, Lockwood A, Mullen K, Tarter R, Weissenborn K, Blei AT. Hepatic encephalopathy—definition, nomenclature, diagnosis, and quantification: final report of the working party at the 11th World Congresses of Gastroenterology, Vienna, 1998. Hepatology. 2002;35:716–21.
8. Schomerus H, Hamster W, Blunck H, Reinhard U, Mayer K, Dolle W. Latent portasystemic encephalopathy. I. Nature of cerebral functional defects and their effect on fitness to drive. Dig Dis Sci. 1981;26:622–30.
9. Watanabe A, Tuchida T, Yata Y, Kuwabara Y. Evaluation of neuropsychological function in patients with liver cirrhosis with special reference to their driving ability. Metab Brain Dis. 1995;10:239–48.
10. Wein C, Koch H, Popp B, Oehler G, Schauder P. Minimal hepatic encephalopathy impairs fitness to drive. Hepatology. 2004;39:739–45.
11. Bajaj JS, Hafeezullah M, Hoffmann RG, Saeian K. Minimal hepatic encephalopathy: a vehicle for accidents and traffic violations. Am J Gastroenterol. 2007;102:1903–9.

12. Bajaj JS, Hafeezullah M, Hoffmann RG, Varma RR, Franco J, Binion DG, et al. Navigation skill impairment: dimension of the driving difficulties in minimal hepatic encephalopathy. Hepatology. 2008;47:596–604.
13. Bajaj JS, Saeian K, Schubert CM, Hafeezullah M, Franco J, Varma RR, et al. Minimal hepatic encephalopathy is associated with motor vehicle crashes: the reality beyond the driving test. Hepatology. 2009;50:1175–83.
14. Groeneweg M, Quero JC, De Bruijn I, Hartmann IJ, Essink-bot ML, Hop WC, et al. Subclinical hepatic encephalopathy impairs daily functioning. Hepatology. 1998;28:45–9.
15. Schomerus H, Hamster W. Quality of life in cirrhotics with minimal hepatic encephalopathy. Metab Brain Dis. 2001;16:37–41.
16. Arguedas MR, DeLawrence TG, McGuire BM. Influence of hepatic encephalopathy on health-related quality of life in patients with cirrhosis. Dig Dis Sci. 2003;48:1622–6.
17. Prasad S, Dhiman RK, Duseja A, Chawla YK, Sharma A, Agarwal R. Lactulose improves cognitive functions and health-related quality of life in patients with cirrhosis who have minimal hepatic encephalopathy. Hepatology. 2007;45:549–59.
18. Amodio P, Del Piccolo F, Marchetti P, Angeli P, Iemmolo R, Caregaro L, et al. Clinical features and survival of cirrhotic patients with subclinical cognitive alterations detected by the number connection test and computerized psychometric tests. Hepatology. 1999;29:1662–7.
19. Amodio P, Del Piccolo F, Petteno E, Mapelli D, Angeli P, Iemmolo R, et al. Prevalence and prognostic value of quantified electroencephalogram (EEG) alterations in cirrhotic patients. J Hepatol. 2001;35:37–45.
20. Das A, Dhiman RK, Saraswat VA, Verma M, Naik SR. Prevalence and natural history of subclinical hepatic encephalopathy in cirrhosis. J Gastroenterol Hepatol. 2001;16:531–5.
21. Romero-Gomez M, Boza F, Garcia-Valdecasas MS, García E, Aguilar-Reina J. Subclinical hepatic encephalopathy predicts the development of overt hepatic encephalopathy. Am J Gastroenterol. 2001;96:2718–23.
22. Saxena N, Bhatia M, Joshi YK, Garg PK, Tandon RK. Auditory P300 event-related potentials and number connection test for evaluation of subclinical hepatic encephalopathy in patients with cirrhosis of the liver: a follow-up study. J Gastroenterol Hepatol. 2001;16:322–7.
23. Saxena N, Bhatia M, Joshi YK, Garg PK, Dwivedi SN, Tandon RK. Electrophysiological and neuropsychological tests for the diagnosis of subclinical hepatic encephalopathy and prediction of overt encephalopathy. Liver. 2002;22:190–7.
24. Conn HO, Leevy CM, Vlahcevic ZR, Rodgers JB, Maddrey WC, Seeff L, et al. Comparison of lactulose and neomycin in the treatment of chronic portal-systemic encephalopathy. Gastroenterology. 1977;72:573–83.
25. Atterbury CE, Maddrey WC, Conn HO. Neomycin-sorbitol and lactulose in the treatment of acute portal-systemic encephalopathy. A controlled, double-blind clinical trial. Am J Dig Dis. 1978;23:398–406.
26. Citro V, Milan G, Tripodi FS, Gennari A, Sorrentino P, Gallotta G, et al. Mental status impairment in patients with West Haven grade zero hepatic encephalopathy: the role of HCV infection. J Gastroenterol. 2007;42:79–82.
27. Dhiman RK, Saraswat VA, Sharma BK, Sarin SK, Chawla YK, Butterworth R, et al. Minimal hepatic encephalopathy: consensus statement of a working party of the Indian Association for Study of the Liver. J Gastroenterol Hepatol. 2010;25:1029–41.
28. Riggio O, Angeloni S, Salvatori FM, De Santis A, Cerini F. Incidence, natural history, and risk factors of hepatic encephalopathy after transjugular intrahepatic portosystemic shunt with polytetrafluoroethylene-covered stent grafts. Am J Gastroenterol. 2008;103: 2738–46.
29. D'Amico G, Morabito A, Pagliaro L, Marubini E. Survival and prognostic indicators in compensated and decompensated cirrhosis. Dig Dis Sci. 1986;31:468–75.
30. Ginés P, Quintero E, Arroyo V, Teres J, Bruguera M, Rimola A, et al. Compensated cirrhosis: natural history and prognostic factors. Hepatology. 1987;7:122–8.
31. O'Grady JG, Schalm SW, Williams R. Acute liver failure: redefining the syndromes. Lancet. 1993;342:273–5.
32. Kim WR, Brown RS, Terrault NA, El-Serag H. Burden of liver disease in the United State: Summary of a workshop. Hepatology. 2002;36:227–42.
33. Cash WJ, McConville P, McDermott E, McCormick PA, Callender ME, McDougall NI. Current concepts in the assessment and treatment of hepatic encephalopathy. Q J Med. 2010;103:9–16.
34. Bajaj JS. Review article: the modern management of hepatic encephalopathy. Aliment Pharmacol Ther. 2010;31:537–47.
35. Butterworth RF. Effects of hyperammonaemia on brain function. J Inherit Metab Dis. 1998;21(S1):6–20.
36. Shawcross DL, Jalan R. The pathophysiologic basis of hepatic encephalopathy: central role for ammonia and inflammation. Cell Mol Life Sci. 2005;62:2295–304.
37. Cordoba J, Minguez B. Hepatic encephalopathy. Semin Liver Dis. 2008;28:70–80.
38. Bjerring PN, Eefsen M, Hansen BA, Larsen FS. The brain in acute liver failure. A tortuous path from hyperammonemia to cerebral edema. Metab Brain Dis. 2009;24:5–14.
39. Barbaro G, Di Lorenzo G, Soldinui N, Giancaspro G, Bellomo G, Belloni G, et al. Flumazenil for hepatic encephalopathy grade III and IVa in patients with cirrhosis: an Italian multicentre double-blind, placebo-controlled, cross-over study. Hepatology. 1998;28:374–8.
40. Haussinger D, Schliess F. Pathogenetic mechanisms of hepatic encephalopathy. Gut. 2008;57:1156–65.
41. Butterworth RF. Thiamine deficiency-related brain dysfunction in chronic liver failure. Metab Brain Dis. 2009;24:189–96.

42. Seyan AS, Hughes RD, Shawcross DL. Changing face of hepatic encephalopathy: role of inflammation and oxidative stress. World J Gastroenterol. 2010;16:3347–57.
43. Master S, Gottstein J, Blei AT. Cerebral blood flow and the development of ammonia-induced brain edema in rats after portacaval anastomosis. Hepatology. 1999;30: 876–80.
44. Kosenko E, Venediktova N, Kaminsky Y, Montoliu C, Felipo V. Sources of oxygen radicals in brain in acute ammonia intoxication in vivo. Brain Res. 2003;981:193–200.
45. Norenberg MD. Oxidative and nitrosative stress in ammonia neurotoxicity. Hepatology. 2003;37:245–8.
46. Rama Rao KV, Jayakumar AR, Norenberg MD. Role of oxidative stress in the ammonia-induced mitochondrial permeability transition in cultured astrocytes. Neurochem Int. 2005;47:31–8.
47. Albrecht J, Norenberg MD. Glutamine: a Trojan horse in ammonia neurotoxicity. Hepatology. 2006;44: 788–94.
48. Bjerring PN, Hauerberg J, Frederiksen HJ, Jorgensen L, Hansen BA, Tofteng F, et al. Cerebral glutamine concentration and lactate-pyruvate ratio in patients with acute liver failure. Neurocrit Care. 2008;9:3–7.
49. Butterworth RF. Hepatic encephalopathy: a neuropsychiatric disorder involving multiple neurotransmitter systems. Curr Opin Neurol. 2000;13:721–7.
50. Lozeva V, Montgomery JA, Tuomisto L, Rocheleau B, Pannunzio M, Huet PM, et al. Increased brain serotonin turnover correlates with the degree of shunting and hyperammonemia in rats following variable portal vein stenosis. J Hepatol. 2004;40:742–8.
51. Lozeva-Thomas V. Serotonin brain circuits with a focus on hepatic encephalopathy. Metab Brain Dis. 2004;19:413–20.
52. Pidoplichko VI, Dani JA. Acid-sensitive ionic channels in midbrain dopamine neurons are sensitive to ammonium, which may contribute to hyperammonemia damage. Proc Natl Acad Sci USA. 2006;103:11376–80.
53. Albrecht J, Bender AS, Norenberg MD. Potassium-stimulated GABA release is a chloride-dependent but sodium- and calcium-independent process in cultured astrocytes. Acta Neurobiol Exp (Wars). 1998;58:169–75.
54. Ahboucha S, Butterworth RF. Pathophysiology of hepatic encephalopathy: a new look at GABA from the molecular standpoint. Metab Brain Dis. 2004;19:331–43.
55. Odeh M. Pathogenesis of hepatic encephalopathy: the tumor necrosis factor-α theory. Eur J Clin Invest. 2007;37:291–304.
56. Rolando N, Wade J, Davalos M, Wendon J, Philpott-Howard J, Williams R. The systemic inflammatory response syndrome in acute liver failure. Hepatology. 2000;32:734–9.
57. Vaquero J, Polson J, Chung C, Helenowski I, Schiodt FV, Reisch J, et al. Infection and the progression of hepatic encephalopathy in acute liver failure. Gastroenterology. 2003;125:755–64.
58. Haussinger D, Schliess F. Astrocyte swelling and protein tyrosine nitration in hepatic encephalopathy. Neurochem Int. 2005;47:64–70.
59. American Psychiatric Association. Diagnostic and statistical manual of mental disorders. 4 (text revision)th ed. Washington, DC: American Psychiatric Association; 2000.
60. Munoz SJ. Hepatic encephalopathy. Med Clin North Am. 2008;92:795–812.
61. Wehbe E, Saad D, Delgado F, Ta H, Antoun SA. Reversible hepatic decerebration: a case report and review of the literature. Eur J Gastroenterol Hepatol. 2010;22:759–60.
62. Mukherjee KK, Chhabra R, Khosla VK. Raised intracranial pressure in hepatic encephalopathy. Indian J Gastroenterol. 2003;22(S2):62–565.
63. Hassanein T, Blei AT, Perry W, Hilsabeck R, Stange J, Larsen FS, et al. Performance of the Hepatic Encephalopathy Scoring Algorithm in a clinical trial of patients with cirrhosis and severe hepatic encephalopathy. Am J Gastroenterol. 2009;104:1392–400.
64. Hassanein TI, Hilsabeck RC, Perry W. Introduction to the Hepatic Encephalopathy Scoring Algorithm (HESA). Dig Dis Sci. 2008;53:529–38.
65. Jover R, Company L, Gutierrez A, Zapater P, Perez-Serra J, Girona E, et al. Minimal hepatic encephalopathy and extrapyramidal signs in patients with cirrhosis. Am J Gastroenterol. 2003;98:1599–604.
66. McCrea M, Cordoba J, Vessey G, Blei AT, Randolph C. Neuropsychological characterization and detection of subclinical hepatic encephalopathy. Arch Neurol. 1996;53:758–63.
67. Weissenborn K, Ennen JC, Schomerus H, Ruckert N, Hecker H. Neuropsychological characterization of hepatic encephalopathy. J Hepatol. 2001;34:768–73.
68. Mooney S, Hassanein TI, Hilsabeck RC, Ziegler EA, Carlson MD, Maron LM, et al. Utility of the Repeatable Battery for the Assessment of Neuropsychological Status (RBANS) in patients with end stage liver disease awaiting liver transplant. Arch Clin Neuropsychol. 2007;22:175–86.
69. Weissenborn K, Heidenreich S, Giewekemeyer K, Ruckert N, Hecker H. Memory function in early hepatic encephalopathy. J Hepatol. 2003;39:320–5.
70. Ortiz M, Cordoba J, Jacas C, Flavia M, Esteban R, Guardia J. Neuropsychological abnormalities in cirrhosis include learning impairment. J Hepatol. 2006;44:104–10.
71. Cadranel JF, Lebietz E, De Martino V, Bernard B, El Koury S, Tourbah A, et al. Focal neurological signs in hepatic encephalopathy in cirrhotic patients: underestimated entity? Am J Gastroenterol. 2001;96: 515–8.
72. Morgan MY, Blei A, Grungreiff K, Jalan R, Kircheis G, Marchesini G, et al. The treatment of hepatic encephalopathy. Metab Brain Dis. 2007;22:389–405.
73. Phongsamran PV, Kim JM, Abbott JC, Rosenblatt A. Pharmacotherapy for hepatic encephalopathy. Drugs. 2010;70:1131–48.
74. Als-Nielsen B, Gluud LL, Gluud C. Non-absorbable disaccharides for hepatic encephalopathy: systematic review of randomised trials. Br Med J. 2004;328:1046.

75. Mullen KD, Amodio P, Morgan MY. Therapeutic studies in hepatic encephalopathy. Metab Brain Dis. 2007;22:407–23.
76. Neff GW, Kemmer N, Zacharias V, Kaiser T, Duncan C, McHenry R, et al. Analysis of hospitalizations comparing rifaximin versus lactulose in the management of hepatic encephalopathy. Transplant Proc. 2006;38:3552–5.
77. Huang E, Esrailian E, Spiegel BMR. The cost effectiveness and budget impact of competing therapies in hepatic encephalopathy—a decision analysis. Aliment Pharmacol Ther. 2007;26:1147–61.
78. Maclayton DO, Eaton-Maxwell A. Rifaximin for treatment of hepatic encephalopathy. Gastroenterology. 2009;43:77–84.
79. Bajaj JS, Schubert CM, Heuman DM, Wade JB, Gibson DP, Topaz A, et al. Persistence of cognitive impairment after resolution of overt hepatic encephalopathy. Gastroenterology. 2010;138:2332–40.
80. Kondrup J, Muller MJ. Energy and protein requirements of patients with chronic liver disease. J Hepatol. 1997;27:239–47.
81. Merli M, Riggio O. Dietary and nutritional indications in hepatic encephalopathy. Metab Brain Dis. 2009;24:211–21.
82. Egberts EH, Schomerus H, Hamster W, Jurgens P. Branched chain amino acids in the treatment of latent portosystemic encephalopathy. A double-blind placebo-controlled cross-over study. Gastroenterology. 1985;88: 887–95.
83. Plauth M, Egberts EH, Hamster W. Long-term treatment of latent portosystemic encephalopathy with branched-chain amino acids: a double-blind placebo-controlled crossover study. J Hepatol. 1993; 17:308–14.
84. Marchesini G, Dioguardi FS, Bianchi GP. The Italian multicenter study group. Long-term oral branched-chain amino acids in advanced cirrhosis: a double-blind casein-controlled trial. J Hepatol. 1990;11: 92–101.
85. Muto Y, Sato S, Watanabe A. Effects of oral branched-chain amino acid granules on event-free survival in patients with liver cirrhosis. Clin Gastroenterol Hepatol. 2005;3:705–13.
86. Schulz GJ, Campos ACL, Coelho JCU. The role of nutrition in hepatic encephalopathy. Curr Opin Clin Nutr Metab Care. 2008;11:275–80; Carithers R. Liver transplantation. American Association for the Study of Liver Diseases. Liver Transpl. 2000; 6:122–35.
87. Cordoba J, Minguez B. Hepatic Encephalopathy. Sem Liver Dis. 2008;28:70–80.
88. Stange J, Mitzner SR, Klammt S, et al. Liver support by extracorporeal blood purification: a clinical observation. Liver Transpl. 2000;6:603–13.
89. Stadlbauer V, Wright AK, Jalan R. Role of artificial liver support in hepatic encephalopathy. Metab Brain Dis. 2009;24:15–26.
90. Teasdale G, Jennett B. Assessment of coma and impaired consciousness. A practical scale. Lancet. 1974;2:81–4.
91. Ortiz M, Cordoba J, Dovals E, Jacas D, Pujadas F, Esteban R, et al. Development of a clinical hepatic encephalopathy staging scale. Aliment Pharmacol Ther. 2007;26:859–67.
92. Bass NM. Review article: the current pharmacological therapies for hepatic encephalopathy. Aliment Pharmacol Ther. 2007;25(S1):23–31.
93. Sotil EU, Gottstein J, Ayala E, Randolph C, Blei AT. Impact of preoperative overt hepatic encephalopathy on neurocognitive function after liver transplantation. Liver Transpl. 2009;15:184–92.
94. Eroglu Y, Byrne WJ. Hepatic encephalopathy. Emerg Med Clin North Am. 2009;27:401–14.
95. Mullen K. Review of the final report of the 1998 Working Party on definition, nomenclature and diagnosis of hepatic encephalopathy. Aliment Pharmacol Ther. 2007;25(S1):11–6.
96. Jalan R. Pathophysiological basis of therapy of raised intracranial pressure in acute liver failure. Neurochem Int. 2005;47:78–83.
97. Rovira A, Alonso J, Cordoba J. MR Imaging findings in hepatic encephalopathy. Am J Neuroradiol. 2008;29:1612–21.
98. Cordoba J, Alonso J, Rovira A, Jacas C, Sanpedro F, Castells L, et al. The development of low-grade cerebral edema in cirrhosis is supported by the evolution of 1 H-magnetic resonance abnormalities after liver transplantation. J Hepatol. 2001;35:598–604.
99. Rovira A, Cordoba J, Sanpedro F, Grive E, Rovira-Gols A, Alonso J. Normalization of T2 signal abnormalities in hemispheric white matter with liver transplant. Neurology. 2002;59:335–41.
100. Cordoba J, Raguer N, Flavia M, Vargas V, Jacas C, Alonso J, et al. T2 hyperintensity along the cortico-spinal tract in cirrhosis relates to functional abnormalities. Hepatology. 2003;38:1026–33.
101. Foley JM, Watson CW, Adams RD. Significance of the electroencephalographic changes in hepatic coma. Trans Am Neurol Assoc. 1950;75:161–5.
102. Guerit JM, Amantini A, Amodio P, Andersen KV, Butler S, de Weerd A, et al. Consensus on the use of neurophysiological tests in the intensive care unit (ICU): electroencephalogram (EEG), evoked potentials (EP), and electroneuromyography (ENMG). Clin Neurophysiol. 2009;39:71–83.
103. Guerit JM, Amantini A, Fischer C, Kaplan PW, Mecarelli O, Schnitzler A, et al. Neurophysiological investigations of hepatic encephalopathy: ISHEN practice guidelines. Liver Int. 2009;29:789–96.
104. Amodio P, Marchetti P, Del Piccolo F, de Tourtchaninoff M, Varghese P, Zuliani C, et al. Spectral versus visual EEG analysis in mild hepatic encephalopathy. Clin Neurophysiol. 1999; 110:1334–44.
105. Weissenborn K, Scholz M, Hinrichs H, Wiltfang J, Schmidt FW, Kunkel H. Neurophysiological assessment of early hepatic encephalopathy. Electroencephalogr Clin Neurophysiol. 1990;75:289–95.
106. Kugler CF, Lotterer E, Petter J, Wensing G, Taghavy A, Hahn EG, et al. Visual event-related

P300 potentials in early portosystemic encephalopathy. Gastroenterology. 1992;103:302–10.
107. Kugler CF, Petter J, Taghavy A, Lotterer E, Wensing G, Hahn EG, et al. Dynamics of cognitive brain dysfunction in patients with cirrhotic liver disease: an event-related P300 potential perspective. Electroencephalogr Clin Neurophysiol. 1994;91:33–41.
108. Amodio P, Montagnese S, Gatta A, Morgan MY. Characteristics of minimal hepatic encephalopathy. Metab Brain Dis. 2004;19:253–67.
109. Kircheis G, Wettstein M, Timmermann L, Schnitzler A, Haussinger D. Critical flicker frequency for quantification of low-grade hepatic encephalopathy. Hepatology. 2002;35:357–66.
110. Romero-Gomez M, Cordoba J, Jover R, del Olmo JA, Ramirez M, Rey R, et al. Value of the critical flicker frequency in patients with minimal hepatic encephalopathy. Hepatology. 2007;45:879–85.
111. Sharma P, Sharma BC, Puri V, Sarin SK. Critical flicker frequency: diagnostic tool for minimal hepatic encephalopathy. J Hepatol. 2007;47:67–73.
112. O'Carroll RE. Neuropsychological aspects of liver disease and its treatment. Neurochem Res. 2008;33: 683–90.
113. Colombato L. The role of transjugular intrahepatic portosystemic shunt (TIPS) in the management of portal hypertension. J Clin Gastroenterol. 2007;41(S3):344–51.
114. Montagnese S, Schiff S, Catta A, Riggio O, Morgan MY, Amodio P. Hepatic encephalopathy: you should only comment on what you have actually measured. J Gastroenterol. 2010;45:342–3.
115. Bajaj JS, Saeian K, Hafeezullah M, Hoffmann RG, Hammeke TA. Patients with minimal hepatic encephalopathy have poor insight into their driving skills. Clin Gastroenterol Hepatol. 2008;61:1135–9.
116. Randolph C. Repeatable Battery for the Assessment of Neuropsychological Status manual. San Antonio, TX: The Psychological Corporation; 1998.
117. Sorrell JH, Zolnikov BJ, Sharma A, Jinnai I. Cognitive impairment in people diagnosed with end-stage liver disease evaluated for liver transplantation. Psychiatry Clin Neurosci. 2006;60:174–81.
118. Mooney S, Hasssanein TI, Hilsabeck RC, Ziegler EA, Carlson M, Maron LM, et al. Utility of the Repeatable Battery for the Assessment of Neuropsychological Status (RBANS) in patients with end-stage liver disease awaiting liver transplant. Arch Clin Neuropsychol. 2007;22:175–86.
119. Butcher JN, Dahlstrom WG, Graham JR, Tellegen A, Kaemmer B. MMPI-2 (Minnesota Multiphasic Personality Inventory-2): manual for administration and scoring. Minneapolis: University of Minnesota Press; 1989.
120. Ware JE, Sherbourne CD. The MOS 36-item short-form health survey (SF-36). Conceptual framework and item selection. Med Care. 1992;30:473–83.
121. Younossi ZM, Guyatt G, Kiwi M, Boparai N, King D. Development of a disease specific questionnaire to measure health related quality of life in patients with chronic liver disease. Gut. 1999;45:295–300.
122. Kim WR, Lindor KD, Malinchoc M, Petz JL, Jorgensen R, Dickson ER. Reliability and validity of the NIDDK-QA instrument in the assessment of quality of life in ambulatory patients with cholestatic liver disease. Hepatology. 2000;32:924–9.
123. Gralnek IM, Hays RD, Kilbourne A, Rosen HR, Keeffe EB, Artinian L, et al. Development and evaluation of the liver disease quality of life instrument in persons with advanced, chronic liver disease-the LDQOL1.0. Am J Gastroenterol. 2000;95: 3552–65.
124. Zhou Y, Chen S, Jiang L, Guo C, Shen Z, Huang P, et al. Development and evaluation of the quality of life instrument in chronic liver disease patients with minimal hepatic encephalopathy. J Gastroenterol Hepatol. 2008;24:408–15.
125. Reitan RM, Wolfson D. The Halstead-Reitan neuropsychological test battery: theory and clinical interpretation. 2nd ed. Tuscon, AZ: Neuropsychology Press; 1993.
126. Weissenborn K, Heidenreich S, Ennen J, Ruckert N, Hecker H. Attention deficits in minimal hepatic encephalopathy. Metab Brain Dis. 2001;16:13–9.
127. Amodio P, Campagna F, Olianas S, Iannizzi P, Mapelli D, Penzo M, et al. Detection of minimal hepatic encephalopathy: normalization and optimization of the Psychometric Hepatic Encephalopathy Score. A neuropsychological and quantified EEG study. J Hepatol. 2008;49:346–53.
128. Randolph C, Weissenborn K, Hilsabeck R, Kato A, Kharbanda P, Li Y, et al. Neuropsychological assessment of hepatic encephalopathy: International Society on Hepatic Encephalopathy and Nitrogen Metabolism (ISHEN) practice guidelines. Liver Int. 2009;29:629–35.
129. Bajaj JS. Current and future diagnosis of hepatic encephalopathy. Metab Brain Dis. 2010;25:107–10.
130. Bajaj JS, Saeian K, Verber MD, Hischke D, Hoffmann RG, Franco J, et al. Inhibitory control test is a simple method to diagnose minimal hepatic encephalopathy and predict development of overt hepatic encephalopathy. Am J Gastroenterol. 2007; 102:754–60.
131. Bajaj JS, Hafeezullah M, Franco J, Varma RR, Hoffmann RG, Knox JF, et al. Inhibitory control test for the diagnosis of minimal hepatic encephalopathy. Gastroenterology. 2008;135:1591–600.
132. Amodio P, Ridola L, Schiff S, Montagnese S, Pasquale C, Nardelli S, et al. Improving the inhibitory control task to detect minimal hepatic encephalopathy. Gastroenterology. 2010;139:510–8.
133. Ziegler EA, Hilsabeck RC, Carlson MD, Hassanein TI, Perry W. Resolution of cognitive impairment after liver transplantation: a case study [abstract]. Arch Clin Neuropsychol. 2001;16:738.
134. Franklin GM, Heaton RK, Nelson LM, Filley CM, Seibert C. Correlation of neuropsychological and

MRI findings in chronic/progressive multiple sclerosis. Neurology. 1988;38:1826–9.
135. Smith A. Symbol Digit Modalities Test (SDMT): manual (revised). Los Angeles, CA: Western Psychological Services; 1982.
136. Mattarozzi K, Campi C, Guarino M, Stracciari A. Distinguishing between clinical and minimal hepatic encephalopathy on the basis of specific cognitive impairment. Metab Brain Dis. 2005;20:243–9.
137. Wechsler D. Wechsler Test of Adult Reading. San Antonio, TX: The Psychological Corporation; 2001.
138. Golden CJ, Freshwater SM. Stroop color and word test: revised examiner's manual. Wood Dale, IL: Stoelting Co.; 2002.
139. Kaplan EF, Goodglass H, Weintraub S. The Boston Naming Test. 2nd ed. Philadelphia: Lippincott Williams & Wilkins; 1983.
140. Benton AL. Development of a multilingual aphasia battery: progress and problems. J Neurol Sci. 1969;9:39–48.
141. Kongs SK, Thompson LL, Iverson GL, Heaton RK. Wisconsin Card Sorting Test-64 Card Version. Lutz, FL: Psychological Assessment Resources; 2000.
142. Matthews CG, Klove H. Instruction manual for the Adult Neuropsychology Test Battery. Madison, WI: University of Wisconsin Medical School; 1964.
143. Beck AT, Steer RA, Brown G. Beck Depression Inventory-II Manual. San Antonio, TX: Psychological Corporation; 1996.
144. Beck AT, Steer RA. Beck Anxiety Inventory: manual. San Antonio, TX: The Psychological Corporation; 1990.

Late-Onset Schizophrenia

30

Tracy D. Vannorsdall and David J. Schretlen

Abstract

Given that psychotic symptoms are relatively common in the older adults and can accompany a variety of conditions, correctly identifying the etiology of psychosis in older patients is essential for developing the most effective treatment plan. Here we focus on the identification and management of late-onset schizophrenia and schizophrenia-like psychosis.

Keywords

Psychosis • Schizophrenia • Late-onset schizophrenia • Very-late-onset schizophrenia-like psychosis • Geriatrics • Older adults • Assessment • Cognition

Symptoms of psychosis, including delusions, hallucinations, loosening of associations, and thought disorder, are prevalent in geriatric populations. In a Swedish community sample of 347 nondemented adults who were 85 years old at study entry, 10.1% were found to have at least one psychotic-type symptom. The most common of these were hallucinations (6.9%), paranoid ideation (6.9%), and delusions (5.5%) [1]. Earlier studies reported that psychosis was present in more than 25% of older patients admitted to inpatient geropsychiatric units [2] and more than 33% of older adults admitted to a hospital for psychiatric treatment for the first time [3]. Psychosis can occur in a variety of conditions and disorders of late life with etiologies including acute conditions such as delirium, or the effects of substance use or withdrawal. Alternatively, psychotic symptoms may arise from chronic degenerative

T.D. Vannorsdall, Ph.D., ABPP (✉)
Department of Psychiatry and Behavioral Sciences, Johns Hopkins University School of Medicine, 600 North Wolfe Street, Meyer 218, Baltimore, MD 21287-7218, USA
e-mail: tvannor1@jhmi.edu

D.J. Schretlen, Ph.D., ABPP
Department of Psychiatry and Behavioral Sciences, Johns Hopkins University School of Medicine, 600 North Wolfe Street, Meyer 218, Baltimore, MD 21287-7218, USA

Russell H. Morgan Department of Radiology and Radiological Science, Johns Hopkins University School of Medicine, 600 North Wolfe Street, Meyer 218, Baltimore, MD 21287-7218, USA
e-mail: dschret@jhmi.edu

L.D. Ravdin and H.L. Katzen (eds.), *Handbook on the Neuropsychology of Aging and Dementia*, Clinical Handbooks in Neuropsychology, DOI 10.1007/978-1-4614-3106-0_30,

conditions such as moderate to severe Alzheimer's disease or Lewy body dementia. Finally, a variety of late-life psychiatric illnesses including delusional disorder, mood disorder with psychotic features, bipolar disorder, and both early- and late-onset schizophrenia (LOS) can also be accompanied by prominent psychotic features.

History and Terminology

Most individuals with schizophrenia develop symptoms of psychosis in late adolescence or early adulthood. As a result, our understanding of thought disorders primarily stems from these early-onset patients. However, it has long been recognized that such symptoms can emerge for the first time later in life. Unfortunately, late-life psychosis has historically been inconsistently described, imprecisely defined, and understudied. Manfred Bleuler, who first brought attention to the study of late-life psychosis, crystallized these difficulties with an often-cited quote [4, 5]:

> One can hardly deal with late onset schizophrenic pictures without being reminded again and again how right Kraepelin was when he called the science of psychoses of old age 'the darkest area of psychiatry'. Indeed, today as in earlier times the ground seems to shake under our feet, and our basic psychiatric terms seem to lose their meaning, when one grapples with late onset schizophrenias (p. 259).

In fact, the rigorous study of late-onset psychotic symptoms started with M. Bleuler who, in 1943, observed that 15% of the schizophrenia patients he examined had an onset of symptoms after 40 years of age and another 4% developed symptoms after age 60 [5]. Noting that nearly half of his late-onset cases evidenced symptoms that were consistent with those seen in the early-onset schizophrenia, Bleuler coined the term "late-onset schizophrenia" to reflect a disorder with an onset of schizophrenia-like symptoms occurring at age 40 years or later. However, this classification did not immediately take hold in the USA or Great Britain. Rather, the term "late paraphrenia" was more commonly used to reference onset of all schizophrenia-like symptoms and delusional disorders with onset after age 55 or 60 [6, 7].

Late paraphrenia was included as a diagnosis in ICD-9, and in ICD-10, the term was included as a part of the diagnosis of delusional disorder. Despite the lack of data to support an age cutoff, in the DSM-III, schizophrenia was defined as having an onset *before* age 45, thus reflecting the "praecox" view of Kraepelin with typical disease onset in late adolescence and early adulthood. As evidence that schizophrenia can emerge after age 44 accumulated, the age cutoff was eliminated and replaced with a late-onset specifier in the DSM-III-R. Subsequent revisions removed the late-onset specifier, and the most recent edition (DSM-IV-TR) simply notes that an onset after age 45 is both possible and associated with certain characteristics including female preponderance, better premorbid functioning, more paranoid delusions and hallucinations, and less disorganization and negative symptoms than are characteristic of early-onset schizophrenia.

An International Late-Onset Schizophrenia Group met in 1998 in order to encourage greater consistency in the recognition, classification, and treatment of late-life schizophrenia. Although there were still no data to justify specific age cut points for diagnostic classification, it was felt that some delineation of age groups was necessary in order to stimulate further research in this area. In the resulting consensus statement [8], it was concluded that there was sufficient evidence to justify the adoption of two illness classifications: LOS and very-late-onset schizophrenia-like psychosis (VLOSLP). The former was conceptualized as a subtype of schizophrenia with an onset occurring after age 40 years. VLOSLP was defined as having an onset after age 60 and applies when the symptoms cannot be attributed to an affective disorder or a progressive structural brain abnormality. It was so named in order to reflect the relative diagnostic uncertainty that arises when attempting to identify a primary psychotic disorder at an age in which the risk for dementia-related psychoses begins to rise.

Epidemiology

Despite the findings and age cutoffs recommended by the consensus conference statement, the terms LOS and VLOSLP have yet to be uniformly adopted and the ages used to define "late-onset" still vary across studies. Not surprisingly, gaining an accurate estimate of the incidence of LOS and VLOSLP has proven difficult. The issue is further complicated by the fact that many studies assessing the epidemiology of schizophrenia do not include older adults, and those that do make varying levels of effort to exclude individuals whose psychotic symptoms might be due to such causes as dementias or delirium.

The available evidence suggests that the 1-year prevalence rate of schizophrenia, irrespective of age of onset, in people ages 45–64 is 0.6% [9]. The proportion of individuals with schizophrenia whose symptoms emerge after age 40 (i.e., LOS) is estimated to be 23.5%, with only 3% developing symptoms after age 60 (i.e., VLOSLP) [10]. The community prevalence estimates for those age 65 and older range from 0.1 to 0.5% [11–13], and the incidence of VLOSLP is estimated to be in the range of 17–24 per 100,000 [14]. Greater age tends to confer greater risk for the disorder, as data from first admission reports for patients age 60 and above indicate the annual incidence of schizophrenia-like psychosis increases by 11% with each 5-year increase in age [15]. Further, while most individuals with LOS or VLOSLP first develop symptoms in their 50s, 60s, and 70s, Cervantes, Rabins, and Slavney [16] reported a woman who, after detailed examination, was found to have developed LOS at the age of 100. Thus, it appears that LOS/VLOSLP can develop at any age in late adulthood.

Clinical Features

The symptom of schizophrenia, regardless of the age of onset, can include the positive symptoms of delusions, hallucinations, and disorganized speech and behavior, along with negative symptoms such as affective flattening, alogia, and avolition. According to DSM criteria, in order to justify the diagnosis of schizophrenia, these symptoms must disrupt a person's ability to function in major life roles, not be accompanied by prominent mood symptoms, and not be due to substance use. Numerous similarities have been noted between the clinical presentation of LOS/VLOSLP and early-onset schizophrenia. In fact, they are often described as being more similar than different, particularly with respect to their positive symptom presentation [8]. On the other hand, evidence suggests that early- and late-onset cases are not identical conditions in terms of their clinical phenomenology (see Table 30.1).

Table 30.1 Comparison of patient characteristics by age of onset

Characteristic	Early-onset schizophrenia	Late-onset schizophrenia	Very-late-onset schizophrenia-like psychosis
Age	<40	41–59	60+
Sex differences	M>W	W>M	W>M
Negative symptoms	Prominent	Less prominent	Uncommon
Positive symptoms	Prominent	Prominent	Prominent
Thought disorder	Prominent	Uncommon	Uncommon
Partition delusion	Uncommon	Less common	Common
Family history of schizophrenia	Common	Less common	Uncommon
Early-life maladjustment	Common	Less severe	Uncommon
Cognitive decline over time	Absent	Uncommon	Uncommon
Efficacious antipsychotic dose	Greater	Lower	Lower

Adopted from Reeves and Brister [63] and Palmer and colleagues [21]

Late-Onset Schizophrenia

There are a number of relative, and sometimes subtle, differences in symptom presentation that differentiate early- and late-onset schizophrenia. One of the most notable and reliably reported differences is the relative paucity of classic negative symptoms such as affective flattening or blunting in persons with LOS [17–19]. Almeida and colleagues [20] found that only 8.5% of participants in their cohort evinced negative symptoms, and those that did appeared only mildly affected. In contrast, more recent investigations of large numbers of well-characterized subjects suggests that while those with LOS experience relatively fewer negative symptoms than those with early onset of the disease, individuals with LOS still show greater negative symptoms than age-matched healthy controls [21].

Individuals with LOS are also markedly less likely to experience formal thought disorder (e.g., loosening associations, circumstantiality, etc.) than those who develop schizophrenia in adolescence or early adulthood [17, 19]. For example, Pearlson and colleagues [17] looked at individuals who had an onset of symptoms after age 45 and found that formal thought disorder was present in only 5.6% of cases. In contrast, thought disorder was present in 51.9% of young adults with early-onset schizophrenia and in 54.5% of older early-onset cases. Pearlson et al. also found that the overall occurrence of formal thought disorder decreased as age of onset increased, such that individuals with the latest onset (i.e., VLOSLP) showed markedly lower rates of disordered thinking.

With respect to positive symptoms, patients with LOS are more likely to report visual, tactile, and olfactory hallucinations than are those with early-onset schizophrenia [17, 22], Alzheimer-type dementia with psychosis, or major depression [23]. When auditory hallucinations are present in LOS, they are more likely to consist of a third-person, running commentary and accusatory or abusive content [19]. The content of the delusions in early- and late-onset schizophrenia may also differ, with LOS patients being more likely to experience persecutory and partition delusions (i.e., the belief that people, objects, or radiation can pass through what would normally constitute a barrier to such passage) [17, 19]. Such delusions frequently involve the belief that people or animals invade one's residence at night. For example, we had one patient with VLOSLP who was convinced that the light on a distant power line actually was a device being used to monitor her behavior at home. It has also been reported that some Schneiderian first-rank symptoms, such as delusions of control and thought insertion, thought withdrawal, or thought broadcasting, are far more likely to occur in LOS than in dementia-related psychosis [23].

Very-Late-Onset Schizophrenia-Like Psychosis

Relatively few studies have focused on the presentation of patients who develop psychoses for the first time in very late life and whose symptoms meet criteria for VLOSLP. Nonetheless, available evidence does suggest some unique and identifying symptoms in these patients. For example, there is a high prevalence of sensory deficits including a notable preponderance of conduction deafness [7, 24] and social isolation in those with VLOSLP [7].

Perhaps even more so than in LOS, formal thought disorder and negative symptoms are extremely rare in those with onset at age 60 or later [4, 20, 25]. Nevertheless, most, if not all, positive symptoms of early-onset schizophrenia can also appear in those with VLOSLP. Helping to differentiate VLOSLP from psychotic symptoms arising due to other etiologies are the partition delusions that occur in up to 70% of VLOSLP cases [17, 26, 27] but are less common in early-onset schizophrenia. The nature and pattern of positive symptoms of schizophrenia seen in VLOSLP also tends to be rather unlike the psychotic symptoms seen in the so-called *organic* psychoses of aging such as Alzheimer's disease and Lewy body dementia. A more characteristic delusion of patients with Alzheimer-type dementia is that others are stealing personal effects that the patient actually has misplaced or hidden and forgotten. That is, unlike dementing conditions wherein delusions and hallucinations tend to be less organized and persistent, the psychotic symptoms of VLOSLP tend to be more organized, fully formed, and stable features of the condition. As is discussed below, also unlike psychoses in dementia, the psychotic symptoms of VLOSLP are not invariably associated with a decline in cognition over time.

When considering the positive symptoms of schizophrenia evident in VLOSLP, there is a high prevalence of visual hallucinations [19, 25, 28]. Multimodal hallucinations are also quite common in this group. In a well-characterized cohort of persons with VLOSLP from south London, Howard [4] found visual hallucinations in 40% of the sample, with 32% experiencing these as well-formed visual hallucinations. Further, approximately 20% had what were described as Charles Bonnet-type complex recurrent visual hallucinations (sometimes described as "Charles Bonnet syndrome plus" [29]). Also common, reported in 59.4% of the sample, were visual misinterpretations and misidentifications.

In comparison to the prominent visual disturbances, auditory hallucinations were even more common in the London cohort, as 70% of those with VLOSLP were noted to have nonverbal auditory hallucinations. Another sizable proportion of participants (49.5%) endorsed auditory hallucinations consisting of third-person voices or voices speaking directly to the patient. Hallucinations in other modalities were common as well, with 30–32% reporting olfactory, gustatory, or tactile hallucinations with delusional elaboration. Finally, equally notable were the high rates of delusions of persecution (84.2%) and reference (76.3%) seen in VLOSLP.

Risk Factors and Associated Features

A number of studies have examined risk factors for the development of LOS and VLOSLP including gender, age, premorbid functioning, family history of schizophrenia and dementia, APOE genotype, pharmacological treatment response, and brain morphometry.

Gender

Perhaps the most consistent risk factor for the development of schizophrenia or psychotic symptoms in late life is gender. Unlike early-onset schizophrenia in which there is a male predominance, considerable evidence indicates that a disproportionate number of individuals diagnosed with LOS and VLOSLP are female [13, 20, 25, 26, 30]. In one early study of gender differences in schizophrenia onset across the lifespan, Castle and Murray [13] found a male to female ratio of 1.56:1 in the 16–25-year age group. The ratio was roughly equal among those with onset around age 30. However, for those whose psychosis emerged for the first time between 66 and 75 years of age, the male to female ratio declined to just 0.38:1.0. Further, this difference appears to persist even after accounting for gender differences in social role expectations and care-seeking behavior [31, 32].

Age

Age also appears to be a risk factor, particularly for developing VLOSLP. The risk of developing schizophrenia is highest in adolescence and early adulthood. It declines during mid-adulthood but then increases again after age 60, at which time very LOS-like psychoses occur with increasing frequency. VLOSLP has been found to occur in 10 individuals per 100,000 adults in the 60–65 age bracket. Thereafter, the rates rise steadily to 25 per 100,000 among adults aged 90 and above [15].

Premorbid Functioning

Although some studies suggest poor childhood adjustment in both early- and late-onset schizophrenia [33], many investigations have found notable differences in rates of successful social and role functioning between early- and late-onset cases. Generally, individuals who develop psychosis late in life tend to have better premorbid educational attainment, greater occupational success, and less impaired psychosocial functioning than is seen in early-onset schizophrenia

[18, 34, 35]. For example, in one study [13], half of those with early-onset schizophrenia were judged to have poor premorbid work adjustment as compared to only 15% of the LOS group. Similarly, while 43% of early-onset subjects were rated as showing poor premorbid social adjustment, only 22% of those with LOS were rated as such. Rates of marriage were also twice as high among LOS compared to early-onset cases (66% vs. 33%).

While later onset of schizophrenia and psychosis may be associated with better psychosocial functioning and perhaps a less severe form of the disease, evidence suggests that those who do develop schizophrenia/VLOSLP in late life are more likely to have a history of mild premorbid schizoid or paranoid personality traits that do not meet criteria for a personality disorder [7, 17, 18]. Further, evidence suggests that while their psychosocial deficits are not as severe as those with early-onset schizophrenia, they still have greater rates of general psychopathology and functional disability than healthy normal controls [30].

Family History

Family studies of LOS and VLOSLP tend to be small and have methodological shortcomings. There is some evidence that those with LOS may have higher rates of schizophrenia among relatives than unaffected individuals [34]. However, studies also have found lower rates of schizophrenia among relatives of those with late- compared to early-onset schizophrenia [17, 36]. There does not appear to be an increased rate of schizophrenia among relatives of patients with VLOSLP [21], nor does there appear to be an increased prevalence of family history of Alzheimer's disease, vascular dementia, Lewy body dementia, or APOE ε4 alleles in LOS or VLOSLP [37]. Consistent with this, LOS patients do not show the hallmark neuropathological indicators associated with neurodegenerative dementias on autopsy [38].

Pharmacological Treatment Response

Although there tends to be a lack of well-controlled, double-blind trials, and overreliance on case reports or series, available evidence indicates that LOS and VLOSLP often respond well to antipsychotic medications. Further, effective treatment can often be reached at doses that are a fraction of those used for early-onset cases. Based on open-label observations, Howard [8] found that LOS can often be effectively managed on antipsychotic doses that are approximately 40% as high as that needed for younger patients. Similarly, Barak [35] reported that 71.4% of individuals with VLOSLP reached a favorable response to an atypical antipsychotic (risperidone) as compared to just 57.1% of older patients with early-onset schizophrenia. As in all populations, antipsychotic side effects can include sedation, anticholinergic effects, extrapyramidal effects, weight gain/diabetes, hyperglycemia, tardive dyskinesia, and neuroleptic malignant syndrome.

Neuroanatomy

Neuroanatomic investigations of individuals with schizophrenia have generally failed to detect major changes that differentiate LOS cases from early-onset schizophrenia. Anatomic brain imaging studies of individuals with LOS have found increased ventricle-to-brain ratios in LOS/VLOSLP compared to matched healthy controls [35, 39, 40]. Semiquantitative analyses of brain MRI scans have demonstrated larger thalamic volume in LOS compared to early-onset schizophrenia [41] and smaller third ventricle volumes compared to age-matched controls [42]. Focal changes, such as reduced volumes of the left temporal lobe and superior temporal gyrus, are also similar to those found in early-onset cases [40, 43]. With respect to white matter abnormalities, some early studies reported that large subcortical white matter hyperintensities were common in LOS [44]. However, subsequent studies that carefully controlled for organic cerebral disorders failed to replicate these earlier findings among late-onset cases [35, 45, 46]. More recent diffusion tensor imaging findings also failed to find significant differences in fractional anisotropy or mean diffusivity between those with VLOSLP and age-matched unaffected adults, arguing further against structural white matter abnormalities as a potential etiology for psychotic symptoms late in life [47].

Cognitive Profile and Course

Contrary to Kraepelin's notion that schizophrenia involves a progressive "dementia praecox," there is now compelling evidence that early-onset schizophrenia is a neurodevelopmental disorder that rarely involves progressive dementia. While the development of schizophrenia in early life certainly is associated with widespread cognitive dysfunction, it does not predict worsening cognitive decline in late life relative to age-matched controls [48, 49]. Some experts have suggested that the emergence of psychotic symptoms late in life may signal the onset of a neurodegenerative process [50]. Further, given that LOS/VLOSLP arises at a time in which rates of dementia begin to rise, differentiating the cognitive pattern of a primary psychiatric disease from the psychoses that can accompany dementia is important from a treatment planning perspective.

Persons with early-onset schizophrenia show severe and pervasive deficits across virtually all domains of cognitive functioning. The most pronounced impairments typically appear to involve psychomotor speed, verbal memory, and attention [51, 52]. Beginning in the mid-1990s, studies began finding that both early- and late-onset schizophrenia involve cognitive dysfunction [18, 48] and that early- and late-onset groups tended to perform quite similarly to one another on cognitive testing. In these early studies, the primary differences seen between the early- and late-onset groups tended to occur on tests of learning/memory and abstraction/mental flexibility, with later age of onset being associated with better performance on these tasks. Vahia and colleagues [30] recently replicated the finding that outpatients with both early- and late-onset schizophrenia performed more poorly than healthy controls on most cognitive tests, but that those with LOS showed less severe dysfunction on most measures, and these differences in cognitive impairment were accompanied by notable functional differences. Their early- and late-onset groups were equivalent in terms of crystallized verbal abilities and working memory as assessed by Wechsler subtests (Wechsler Information, Vocabulary, Similarities, and Arithmetic subtests). However, the LOS patients showed less severe impairment than early-onset cases on tests of processing speed (Digit Symbol), visuoconstruction (Block Design), executive functioning (WCST perseverative responses), and verbal memory as assessed by CVLT long-delay free recall (when adjusted for Trial 5 learning). In addition to showing less severe cognitive deficits, the LOS group performed better than early-onset patients on performance-based measures of functional capacities, social skills, and health-related quality of life. Interestingly, in this sample, patients with LOS showed less severe positive but equally severe negative symptoms when compared to early-onset cases. The groups did not differ in severity of depression.

Most studies examining the cognitive profile of schizophrenia emerging in late life have combined patients with LOS and VLOSLP. As a result, less is known about whether there are any unique VLOSLP-related cognitive deficits. Those studies that do address this issue have found that the cognitive deficits associated with VLOSLP are widespread, with no pronounced differences in cognition between LOS and VLOSLP [8].

Of critical importance is determining whether the onset of psychosis late in life signals the presence or onset of a dementing condition. Available evidence suggests that the pattern of cognitive deficits seen in early- and late-onset schizophrenia differ from those seen in Alzheimer's disease, with schizophrenia of any age of onset showing a pattern of deficient learning coupled with intact retention [18, 48, 53, 54]. This lies in contrast to the impairments seen in Alzheimer's disease, wherein there are deficits in both learning and retention skills.

Several longitudinal studies have sought to determine whether LOS/VLOSLP might herald the development of a progressive dementia syndrome, but most of these [49, 55, 56] have found a pattern of stable cognition over a period of several years. For example, one longitudinal [57] study of patients with early- or late-onset schizophrenia, mild Alzheimer's disease, Alzheimer's disease with psychotic features, and healthy controls found that both dementia groups showed steep cognitive declines over a 2-year period whereas both schizophrenia groups and the normal controls remained cognitively stable over the same interval. However, the finding of stable cognitive functioning over time in LOS is not uniform. A few studies with longer follow-up periods have reported that some patients decline over time. For example, Holden [14] conducted a retrospective chart review and found that 35% of people with LOS developed dementia within a 3-year follow-up period. Brodaty and colleagues [50] reported that 9 of 19 (47%) older adults with LOS subjects developed dementia over a period of 5 years, whereas none of the 24 healthy controls developed dementia over the same period. In a longitudinal study of psychogeriatric clinic patients, Rabins and Lavrisha [23] examined the rates of conversion to dementia (as indicated by declines in MMSE of ≥4 points and fulfillment of DSM-IV criteria for dementia) in 28 cognitively intact, nondepressed patients with LOS; 48 patients with depression but not dementia or psychosis; and 47 patients with dementia and psychosis. While approximately half the LOS cases developed dementia by 10-year follow-up, those with LOS were no more likely to develop dementia than those with late-life major depression. Further, those with dementia plus psychosis had shorter life expectancies than those with LOS or major depression alone.

Taken together, cross-sectional and longitudinal studies suggest that while individuals with LOS may perform more poorly than normal controls on tests of learning and memory, they can be differentiated from those with primary dementing conditions by the relative preservation of retention and recognition skills. Further, the psychosis of LOS and VLOSLP is not invariably associated with deteriorating cognitive abilities, and many patients remain cognitively stable over time. Given the variability in cognitive outcomes, a progressive dementia syndrome does not appear to be the underlying etiology of LOS/VLOSLP.

Assessment

Given the age of the population in question, when a patient presents with symptoms of psychosis late in life, the referral question tends to focus on differentiating between late-life psychosis and a primary dementing illness. However, psychosis in late life can stem from several etiologies including acute conditions such as a delirium, degenerative conditions like moderate to severe dementia, or any of several psychiatric illnesses, including delusional disorder, mood disorder with psychotic features, bipolar disorder, and either early- or late-onset schizophrenia (see Table 30.2). In light of the differential course and survival rates for these various etiologies, an accurate diagnostic formulation is crucial to formulating the most effective treatment plan.

Clinical Interview and Symptom Assessment

As described above, the cognitive deficits of LOS/VLOSLP are relatively nonspecific and usually milder than those seen in older adults with early-onset schizophrenia. Thus, evaluation and proper diagnosis of these patients rely heavily on taking a thorough history of the patient's premorbid functioning and the nature and course of the psychotic symptoms. We have found that a knowledgeable informant can provide critically important data. This is particularly the case if a patient is experiencing intrusive psychotic symptoms at the time of the evaluation. However, the

Table 30.2 Common differential diagnoses

Delirium
Substance use or withdrawal
Alzheimer's disease, moderate to severe
Lewy body dementia
Delusional disorder
Mood disorder with psychotic features
Bipolar disorder
Schizophrenia (early onset)

absence of an identifiable family member, friend, or caregiver who knows the patient well enough to provide such input suggests a level of social isolation that is fairly common in LOS patients. Determining the duration of symptoms can itself be a challenge given that these patients often lead relatively solitary lives. In fact, many such individuals only come to the attention of care providers after a neighbor becomes concerned about paranoid or other floridly psychotic behavior. For example, one of our patients repeatedly and angrily confronted the neighbor that she believed was breaking in and stealing money from her home. It was only after repeated unsuccessful attempts to convince the patient otherwise that the neighbor contacted the local police, which prompted the patient's admission to our geriatric psychiatry service.

As LOS and VLOSLP are associated with various premorbid characteristics, when taking a clinical history, particular attention should be paid to the individual's occupational and social functioning during mid-life. Did the patient achieve a reasonable degree of occupational success by mid-adulthood, or is their work history characterized by difficulty maintaining employment, "underemployment" (working at jobs for which they are clearly overqualified), or recurrent problems working with others so that they quit jobs or were terminated? Since LOS and VLOSLP are associated with the presence of mild premorbid schizoid or paranoid personality traits, it can also be helpful to determine whether an individual has a full and socially connected existence or gravitated toward solitary activities in their adulthood. Similarly, it is helpful to determine whether an individual's history suggests a lack of interest or success in forming romantic relationships or a general lack of relationships that could be characterized as close or warm. It is helpful to determine if the patient is described as mistrustful of others, quick to perceive slights or threats, or frankly suspicious. Although this is informative, the paranoia that often characterizes LOS/VLOSLP makes it difficult to obtain these details directly from the patient and sometimes from others as well. Rather, these individuals are often suspicious of the assessment procedures, reticent to disclose personal information, or unwilling to allow a knowledgeable informant to speak to the neuropsychologist or treatment team.

As was outlined above, LOS and VLOSLP are associated with common but not pathognomonic clinical features. These include prominent positive symptoms, such as auditory hallucinations of accusatory or abusive voices, visual hallucinations, and paranoid, persecutory, or partition delusions. Negative symptoms (i.e., alogia, avolition, and affective blunting) tend to be less prominent, and formal thought disorder is relatively rare. In our clinic, we augment our clinical interview with the Scale for the Assessment of Negative Symptoms (SANS) and Scale for the Assessment of Positive Symptoms (SAPS). These semistructured interview/observation rating scales [58] can help quantify the severity of positive and negative symptoms. The SANS is a 25-item scale with five subscales: affective flattening, alogia, avolition/apathy, anhedonia/asociality, and inattention. The SAPS consists of 35 items and four subscales: hallucinations, delusions, bizarreness, and formal thought disorder. Both scales include a global rating, and symptoms are rated as they occurred over the preceding month.

Differentiating LOS/VLOSLP from Other Psychiatric Disorders

A thorough review of a patient's clinical and psychiatric history is essential to diagnosis, as the symptom presentation and cognitive deficits can be similar to other disorders. Affective disorders, including bipolar disorder and unipolar depression, also are common in older adults and can be accompanied by frank psychosis. The symptoms of LOS/VLOSLP do not couple tightly with fluctuations in a patient's mood. If psychotic symptoms resolve with return to a euthymic state or a patient exhibits mood-congruent psychotic features in manic and depressed states, LOS/VLOSLP should not be diagnosed, and consideration should be given to a diagnosis of depression with psychotic features or bipolar disorder. In our clinic, we routinely administer the 15-item Geriatric Depression Scale [59]. The diagnostic validity and reliability of this version are comparable to those of the original 30-item version [60, 61], and this appears to be the case for middle-aged adults as well [62]. Finally, although delusions can be a feature of LOS and VLOSLP, they differ from a late-life delusional disorder in that the latter is characterized by the presence of a nonbizarre delusion that occurs in the absence of prominent auditory or visual hallucinations. Further, delusional disorders are often associated with preserved premorbid personality, intact intelligence, and intact functioning in matters that are unrelated to the content of the delusion. This contrasts with the symptoms of LOS and VLOSLP in that the delusions may be bizarre, multimodal hallucinations are common, and both cognitive and functional deficits may be present.

Differentiating LOS/VLOSLP from Dementia Syndromes

Psychosis can occur in a variety of dementia syndromes such Alzheimer's disease, Lewy body dementia, Parkinson's disease, and vascular dementia. However, there are several means of differentiating a primary psychiatric disorder from a primary degenerative cognitive disorder in an older patient. Because of the high rates of sensory deficits in LOS/VLOSLP, we often find it helpful to begin by evaluating the patient's auditory and basic visuoperceptual abilities. Hearing can be informally assessed during the clinical interview by performing basic comprehension and repetition tasks or by having the patient close his or her eyes and indicate in which ear they hear the examiner's fingers rubbing lightly. If auditory deficits are present but mild to moderate, we often use a microphone and amplifier worn in the ear during cognitive assessment. More severe deficits may warrant delaying neuropsychological testing until after an audiology consultation. A pocket vision screener can be used to screen for problems with near visual acuity. We find it useful to keep a selection of magnifying reading glasses in various strengths for patients with decreased near visual acuity to use during testing. Finally, we often rely on the Judgment of Line Orientation, Hooper Visual Organization Test, and Boston Naming Test to detect the presence of visual misperceptions, which are common in LOS and VLOSLP.

Differentiating the psychosis of late-life schizophrenia from the psychosis that can accompany dementia should include a characterization of the initial symptoms and the temporal course of the condition. Hallucinations and delusions are rarely an initial symptom of dementia. Rather, in primary dementia syndromes, early cognitive decline is often the first indication of a disorder. These cognitive impairments tend to be at least moderately severe by the time psychotic symptoms emerge in patients with a primary dementing illness. In contrast, the psychotic symptoms of LOS and VLOSLP are often the first and most prominent manifestations of these conditions. While cognitive deficits often co-occur with the hallucinations and delusions, these deficits are usually not severe enough by themselves to bring a patient to clinical attention. Qualitatively, the hallucinations and delusions of LOS and VLOSLP tend to be more organized, elaborate, and stable than those seen in dementia. Finally, while not an essential feature of dementing illnesses, it is helpful to assess whether the patient has experienced a decline in cognition and if so, over what period of time. A decline in cognition and functioning over a period of months to years is often a sign of dementia. The cognitive weaknesses seen in LOS and VLOSLP, in contrast, tend to be stable features of the disorder and generally do not worsen over time, particularly when symptoms emerge between age 40 and 60 (i.e., LOS).

When attempting to diagnose an older patient with psychosis, it is also important to assess the presence of other symptoms that are characteristic of particular dementia syndromes, as their presence decreases the likelihood that the patient has LOS. Both LOS and VLOSLP are associated with a broad, generalized pattern of mild cognitive dysfunction. However, some features are generally not seen in these patients. Apraxia and naming deficits are not typical of LOS/VLOSLP, whereas they are prominent in Alzheimer's disease. Similarly, in a patient with visual hallucinations, the presence of axial rigidity, disproportionate impairment on tests of visual-perceptual or visual-constructional ability, and other Parkinsonian features would raise the suspicion for a Lewy body dementia and reduce the likelihood of LOS in the differential diagnosis. Several studies have found that patients with LOS or VLOSLP also be differentiated from those with dementia by their relatively preserved retention of newly acquired information as demonstrated by tests such as the HVLT-R or CVLT-II.

Medical Rule Outs and Recommendations

As with many conditions warranting a clinical neuropsychological evaluation in older adults, particular care must be taken to rule out the presence of delirium or another organic cause of psychosis when LOS/VLOSLP is in the differential. Learning about the course of the patient's symptoms can be illuminating. Unlike delirium in which hallucinations and delusions appear to wax and wane, the psychotic symptoms of LOS/VLOSLP tend to be stable and persistent. They rarely show marked fluctuations over time. We often recommend the patient undergo standard laboratory blood studies (e.g., complete blood count, glucose, TSH, electrolytes, BUN, creatinine, liver function, B12, folate, RPR, etc.) in order to rule out thyroid conditions, infections, glucose or electrolyte abnormalities, vitamin deficiencies, and other metabolic abnormalities. A toxicology screen should be considered, particularly if there is a suspected history of substance abuse. Any recent changes in drug use should also be considered, as older adults can be particularly vulnerable to drug withdrawal. Similarly, it can be helpful to review the patient's medication history to assess for the potential effects of anticholinergic medications and adverse drug interactions. Brain imaging can be informative in determining whether any strokes, tumors, or other cerebral abnormalities might account for the late-onset of psychotic symptoms. Finally, given the increased rates of sensory deficits in patients with LOS/VLOSLP relative to older patients with affective disorder, early-onset schizophrenia, and age-matched controls [4, 17], recommendations for formal audiology and ophthalmology workups are often helpful to assess the extent to which sensory deficits might contribute to misinterpretations in older patients with psychosis. See Table 30.2 for common considerations in the differential diagnosis.

Treatment Recommendations

As outlined above, a substantial proportion of patients with LOS/VLOSLP show effective treatment response to relatively low-dose neuroleptics. For some patients, such treatment can limit their experience to a single acute episode. We have found that a geriatric psychiatrist is the most appropriate person to manage a patient's psychotropic medications. Further, if sensory impairments are present, attempts should be made to remedy these as well as possible, as they might contribute to perceptual aberrations. Even if full correction of sensory impairments is not possible, it can be helpful to educate patients about the potential contribution of hearing or vision impairments to their symptoms and difficulties with everyday functioning.

There are also a number of psychosocial interventions and recommendations appropriate in this population. These include supportive and cognitive-behavioral therapies. Aguera-Ortiz and Renese-Prieto [4] outlined a number of "tips and tricks" for the psychological management of patients with late-life schizophrenia. Even though patients may have difficulty forming an initial attachment to their treatment providers, attempts should be made to establish a good therapeutic relationship and a supportive atmosphere. It is not necessary to agree with a patient's delusional system, but rather to be empathic and understanding. Listening to psychotic complaints in a nonjudgmental manner may lessen the likelihood that they will act on their agitation (e.g., by confronting neighbors). It can also help address a patient's social isolation, especially if it leads to entry into a larger social sphere. More generally, we have found it important to educate family members and caregivers and to help create a network of persons (e.g., family members, friends, neighbors, church members) who can help ensure a patient's ongoing safety. In some instances, the establishment of a conservatorship or guardianship may be in the patient's best interest.

Clinical Pearls

- LOS/VLOSLP is associated with female gender, increased age, premorbid schizoid or paranoid personality traits, poor premorbid social and occupational functioning, social isolation, and sensory deficits.
- Symptoms tend to consist primarily of positive symptoms such as auditory or visual hallucinations or paranoid delusions. Partition delusions are particularly common and are fairly unique to LOS/VLOSLP. There is also often a notable lack of negative symptoms and formal thought disorder.
- Similar to early-onset schizophrenia, LOS/VLOSLP is associated with a generalized, nonspecific pattern of cognitive dysfunction. However, the cognitive impairment tends to be less severe than early-onset schizophrenia. It differs from that seen in patients with dementia with psychosis by virtue of the relative sparing of memory abilities and the absence of cortical features and extrapyramidal signs. LOS and VLOSLP are primarily nondementing disorders.
- When an older patient presents with psychotic symptoms, it is important to first rule out delirium, identifiable medical etiologies, and the effects of medications or toxins, as well as prominent mood symptoms.
- Treatment, both psychosocial and pharmacological, can be successful in helping affected individuals maintain maximal functional independence and remain safe.

References

1. Ostling S, Skoog I. Psychotic symptoms and paranoid ideation in a nondemented population-based sample of the very old. Arch Gen Psychiatry. 2002;59(1):53–9.
2. Champagne LL, et al. Psychosis in geropsychiatric inpatients with and without dementia. Int J Geriatr Psychiatry. 1996;11(6):523–7.
3. Burke WJ, Roccaforte WH, Wengel SP. Characteristics of elderly patients admitted for the first time to a psychiatric facility. J Geriatr Psychiatry Neurol. 1988;1(3):159–62.
4. Howard R, Rabins PV, Castle DJ. Late onset schizophrenia. Philadelphia: Wrightson Biomedical; 1999. p. 278.
5. Bleuler M. Die spatschizophrenen Krankheitsbilder. Fortschr Neurol Psychiatr. 1943;15:259–90.
6. Roth M, Morrissey JD. Problems in the diagnosis and classification of mental disorder in old age; with a study of case material. J Ment Sci. 1952;98(410):66–80.
7. Kay DW, Roth M. Environmental and hereditary factors in the schizophrenias of age ("late paraphrenia") and their bearing on the general problem of causation in schizophrenia. J Ment Sci. 1961;107:649–86.
8. Howard R, et al. Late-onset schizophrenia and very-late-onset schizophrenia-like psychosis: an international consensus. The International Late-Onset Schizophrenia Group. Am J Psychiatry. 2000;157(2): 172–8.
9. Keith SJ, Regier AM, Rae DS. Schizophrenic disorders. In: Robins LN, Regier DA, editors. Psychiatric disorders in America: the epidemiologic catchment area study. New York: Free Press; 1991. p. 449.
10. Harris MJ, Jeste DV. Late-onset schizophrenia: an overview. Schizophr Bull. 1988;14(1):39–55.
11. Copeland JR, et al. Alzheimer's disease, other dementias, depression and pseudodementia: prevalence, incidence and three-year outcome in Liverpool. Br J Psychiatry. 1992;161:230–9.
12. Copeland JR, et al. Schizophrenia and delusional disorder in older age: community prevalence, incidence, comorbidity, and outcome. Schizophr Bull. 1998;24(1):153–61.
13. Castle DJ, Murray RM. The epidemiology of late-onset schizophrenia. Schizophr Bull. 1993;19(4):691–700.
14. Holden NL. Late paraphrenia or the paraphrenias? A descriptive study with a 10-year follow-up. Br J Psychiatry. 1987;150:635–9.
15. van Os J, et al. Increasing age is a risk factor for psychosis in the elderly. Soc Psychiatry Psychiatr Epidemiol. 1995;30(4):161–4.
16. Cervantes AN, Rabins PV, Slavney PR. Onset of schizophrenia at age 100. Psychosomatics. 2006;47(4):356–9.
17. Pearlson GD, et al. A chart review study of late-onset and early-onset schizophrenia. Am J Psychiatry. 1989;146(12):1568–74.

18. Jeste DV, et al. Clinical and neuropsychological characteristics of patients with late-onset schizophrenia. Am J Psychiatry. 1995;152(5):722–30.
19. Howard R, et al. A comparative study of 470 cases of early-onset and late-onset schizophrenia. Br J Psychiatry. 1993;163:352–7.
20. Almeida OP, et al. Psychotic states arising in late life (late paraphrenia) psychopathology and nosology. Br J Psychiatry. 1995;166(2):205–14.
21. Palmer BW, McClure FS, Jeste DV. Schizophrenia in late life: findings challenge traditional concepts. Harv Rev Psychiatry. 2001;9(2):51–8.
22. Huber G, Gross G, Schuttler R. Late schizophrenia (author's transl). Arch Psychiatr Nervenkr. 1975;221(1):53–66.
23. Rabins PV, Lavrisha M. Long-term follow-up and phenomenologic differences distinguish among late-onset schizophrenia, late-life depression, and progressive dementia. Am J Geriatr Psychiatry. 2003;11(6): 589–94.
24. Cooper AF. Deafness and psychiatric illness. Br J Psychiatry. 1976;129:216–26.
25. Howard R, Almeida O, Levy R. Phenomenology, demography and diagnosis in late paraphrenia. Psychol Med. 1994;24(2):397–410.
26. Herbert ME, Jacobson S. Late paraphrenia. Br J Psychiatry. 1967;113(498):461–9.
27. Howard R, et al. Permeable walls, floors, ceilings and doors. Partition delusions in late paraphrenia. Int J Geriatr Psychiatry. 1992;7(10):719–24.
28. Rabins P, Pauker S, Thomas J. Can schizophrenia begin after age 44? Compr Psychiatry. 1984;25(3): 290–3.
29. Howard R, Levy R. Charles Bonnet syndrome plus: complex visual hallucinations of Charles Bonnet syndrome type in late paraphrenia. Int J Geriatr Psychiatry. 1994;9(5):399–404.
30. Vahia IV, et al. Is late-onset schizophrenia a subtype of schizophrenia? Acta Psychiatr Scand. 2010;122(5):414–26.
31. Angermeyer MC, Kuhn L. Gender differences in age at onset of schizophrenia. An overview. Eur Arch Psychiatry Neurol Sci. 1988;237(6):351–64.
32. Hambrecht M, et al. Transnational stability of gender differences in schizophrenia? An analysis based on the WHO study on determinants of outcome of severe mental disorders. Eur Arch Psychiatry Clin Neurosci. 1992;242(1):6–12.
33. Lohr JB, et al. Minor physical anomalies in older patients with late-onset schizophrenia, early-onset schizophrenia, depression, and Alzheimer's disease. Am J Geriatr Psychiatry. 1997; 5(4):318–23.
34. Castle DJ, et al. Schizophrenia with onset at the extremes of adult life. Int J Geriatr Psychiatry. 1997;12(7):712–7.
35. Barak Y, et al. Very late-onset schizophrenia-like psychosis: clinical and imaging characteristics in comparison with elderly patients with schizophrenia. J Nerv Ment Dis. 2002;190(11):733–6.
36. Howard RJ, et al. A controlled family study of late-onset non-affective psychosis (late paraphrenia). Br J Psychiatry. 1997;170:511–4.
37. Howard R, et al. Apolipoprotein e genotype and late paraphrenia. Int J Geriatr Psychiatry. 1995;10(2): 147–50.
38. Purohit DP, et al. Alzheimer disease and related neurodegenerative diseases in elderly patients with schizophrenia: a postmortem neuropathologic study of 100 cases. Arch Gen Psychiatry. 1998;55(3):205–11.
39. Jeste DV, et al. Relationship of neuropsychological and MRI measures to age of onset of schizophrenia. Acta Psychiatr Scand. 1998;98(2):156–64.
40. Pearlson GD, et al. Quantitative D2 dopamine receptor PET and structural MRI changes in late-onset schizophrenia. Schizophr Bull. 1993;19(4):783–95.
41. Corey-Bloom J, et al. Quantitative magnetic resonance imaging of the brain in late-life schizophrenia. Am J Psychiatry. 1995;152(3):447–9.
42. Rabins PV, et al. MRI findings differentiate between late-onset schizophrenia and late-life mood disorder. Int J Geriatr Psychiatry. 2000;15(10):954–60.
43. Howard R, et al. Magnetic resonance imaging volumetric measurements of the superior temporal gyrus, hippocampus, parahippocampal gyrus, frontal and temporal lobes in late paraphrenia. Psychol Med. 1995;25(3):495–503.
44. Tonkonogy JM, Geller JL. Late-onset paranoid psychosis as a distinct clinicopathologic entity: magnetic resonance imaging data in elderly patients with paranoid psychosis of late onset and schizophrenia of early onset. Neuropsychiatry Neuropsychol Behav Neurol. 1999;12(4):230–5.
45. Howard R, et al. White matter signal hyperintensities in the brains of patients with late paraphrenia and the normal, community-living elderly. Biol Psychiatry. 1995;38(2):86–91.
46. Symonds LL, et al. Lack of clinically significant gross structural abnormalities in MRIs of older patients with schizophrenia and related psychoses. J Neuropsychiatry Clin Neurosci. 1997;9(2):251–8.
47. Jones DK, et al. A diffusion tensor magnetic resonance imaging study of frontal cortex connections in very-late-onset schizophrenia-like psychosis. Am J Geriatr Psychiatry. 2005;13(12):1092–9.
48. Heaton R, et al. Neuropsychological deficits in schizophrenics. Relationship to age, chronicity, and dementia. Arch Gen Psychiatry. 1994;51(6):469–76.
49. Heaton RK, et al. Stability and course of neuropsychological deficits in schizophrenia. Arch Gen Psychiatry. 2001;58(1):24–32.
50. Brodaty H, et al. Long-term outcome of late-onset schizophrenia: 5-year follow-up study. Br J Psychiatry. 2003;183:213–9.
51. Schretlen DJ, et al. Neuropsychological functioning in bipolar disorder and schizophrenia. Biol Psychiatry. 2007;62(2):179–86.
52. Heinrichs RW, Zakzanis KK. Neurocognitive deficit in schizophrenia: a quantitative review of the evidence. Neuropsychology. 1998;12(3):426–45.

53. Miller BL, et al. Brain lesions and cognitive function in late-life psychosis. Br J Psychiatry. 1991;158: 76–82.
54. Almeida OP, et al. Cognitive features of psychotic states arising in late life (late paraphrenia). Psychol Med. 1995;25(4):685–98.
55. Laks J, et al. Absence of dementia in late-onset schizophrenia: a one year follow-up of a Brazilian case series. Arq Neuropsiquiatr. 2006;64(4):946–9.
56. Rajji TK, Mulsant BH. Nature and course of cognitive function in late-life schizophrenia: a systematic review. Schizophr Res. 2008;102(1–3):122–40.
57. Palmer BW, et al. Are late-onset schizophrenia spectrum disorders neurodegenerative conditions? Annual rates of change on two dementia measures. J Neuropsychiatry Clin Neurosci. 2003;15(1):45–52.
58. Andreasen NC, et al. Correlational studies of the Scale for the Assessment of Negative Symptoms and the Scale for the Assessment of Positive Symptoms: an overview and update. Psychopathology. 1995;28(1):7–17.
59. Sheikh JI, Yesavage JA. Geriatric Depression Scale (GDS): recent evidence and development of a shorter version. Clin Gerontologist. 1986;5(1–2):165–73.
60. Almeida OP, Almeida SA. Short versions of the geriatric depression scale: a study of their validity for the diagnosis of a major depressive episode according to ICD-10 and DSM-IV. Int J Geriatr Psychiatry. 1999;14(10):858–65.
61. Mitchell AJ, et al. Which version of the geriatric depression scale is most useful in medical settings and nursing homes? Diagnostic validity meta-analysis. Am J Geriatr Psychiatry. 2010;18(12): 1066–77.
62. Fieldstone SC, et al. Validation of the 15-item Geriatric Depression Scale for clinical use with young and middle-aged adults. J Int Neuropsychol Soc. 2010;16(S1):41.
63. Reeves RR, Brister JC. Psychosis in late life: emerging issues. J Psychosoc Nurs Ment Health Serv. 2008;46(11):45–52.

Capacity Evaluations in Older Adults: Neuropsychological Perspectives

31

Joel E. Morgan and Bernice A. Marcopulos

Abstract

Aging necessarily brings with it changes in one's functional abilities, and this often occurs in the setting of declining cognition. Changes in mental capacities may be subtle, even almost imperceptible, or they may be so glaringly apparent that no one can deny their presence. Older adults with cognitive decline are clearly vulnerable, and this places them at greater risk for abuse and exploitation. Neuropsychologists are becomingly increasingly called upon to consult about such mental capacities in the elderly, to provide opinions to families and courts of law regarding one's abilities to care for themselves as well as make decisions about their health care, finances and other important matters. In this chapter we discuss the role of the neuropsychologist in such capacity evaluations and provide an assessment framework for professionals who may be new to this interesting aspect of practice.

Keywords

Elderly decision-making capacity • Competency • Guardianship • Financial • Health care • Individual freedom

Few would disagree that older adults are among the most vulnerable members of society. Scientific research and technological advances over the last half-century have led to improvements in medicine and health-care delivery, resulting in greater numbers of the older adults living to advanced years. For many, late life typically brings age-related changes in health that often affect physical status, cognitive functions, or emotional and social adjustment. Consequently, changes in cognition

J.E. Morgan, Ph.D. (✉)
Department of Neurology and Neurosciences, UMDNJ—New Jersey Medical School, Madison, NJ 07940, USA
e-mail: joelmor@comcast.net

B.A. Marcopulos, Ph.D.
Department of Graduate Psychology, James Madison University, MSC 7401, 70 Alumnae Drive, Harrisonburg, VA 22807, USA
e-mail: marcopba@jmu.edu

L.D. Ravdin and H.L. Katzen (eds.), *Handbook on the Neuropsychology of Aging and Dementia*, Clinical Handbooks in Neuropsychology, DOI 10.1007/978-1-4614-3106-0_31,

and mental status often have significant bearing on an individual's capacity to make informed decisions about important aspects of their life, including their health care, living status, finances, beneficiaries, and other personal matters [1]. While some older individuals are fortunate enough to remain cognitively intact well into their 80s or 90s, many are not, and they may therefore be vulnerable to exploitation by others or unknowingly victimized by their own poor judgment and delimited cognitive capacity.

Neuropsychological consultation in forensic (legal) contexts is growing at exponential rates [2] where neuropsychologists lend their expertise to a wide range of services to the trier of facts [3]. Among the various roles pursued by neuropsychologists in forensic contexts is the assessment of an individual's competencies [4]. In this chapter, we discuss the issues regarding the assessment of competency in older adults, that is, that aspect of mental ability recognized in law as sufficient for the making of decisions [5], such as for giving informed consent to one's health care, the making of a will (i.e., "testamentary capacity"), and the management of one's finances [6], among others. We will discuss the general principles of law as they pertain to such issues of these capacities, the common disorders affecting older adults that may impede cognition and decisional capacity, and suggest appropriate assessment methodologies and assessment instruments in a variety of such competency evaluations. Case examples from the authors' practices are utilized to illustrate these issues and methods.

The Legal Perspective

Capacity refers to *mental capacity*, or mental ability, that is, competency. The concept may be expressed by the question, "Does this person have the requisite mental abilities to perform this specific task?" From the legal vantage point, the presence of a mental disorder or disability does not necessarily equate with or imply an inability to perform a given task, that is, incompetency. Although necessary, the presence of a disorder or disease affecting cognition is insufficient by itself to form a judgment of incompetency. One must demonstrate specific functional impairment on tasks necessary to meet minimal standards for that particular capacity as a consequence of the disorder. Civil competency, similar to competency in criminal contexts, refers to a person's functional ability to make a particular kind of decision or to perform a particular kind of task [7]. The context of the decision at issue is critical to the determination of competency, not merely the examinee's mental status.

In matters involving criminal competency, questions arise concerning a defendant's capacity or ability to proceed to trial (e.g., does he have the presence of mind to know the principal players in the court setting, that he is in a court of law, the ability to assist his attorney, etc.), to waive rights, make a plea, be sentenced, be executed, and the like [4]. Civil competency is similar conceptually, most generally expressed by the question: Does the person have the competency, the mental capacity, to make a certain decision (i.e., to consent to health-care treatment, to care for oneself and one's property, to control their own finances, to make a will, etc.). Both criminal and civil competency questions entail the mental status of the individual—that is, does one have the ability, the capacity; that is, is one *competent*?

Ingrained within the American psyche and reflected throughout the American jurisprudence system is the concept that people have the right to self-determination. Self-determination extends to individuals with mental disorders as well, except when significant harm to others results from their actions or if they are considered incompetent to make the *particular* decision in question. Thus, the right to self-determination "is not absolute" [7]. The precise meaning of competence may differ depending on the specific question and the context; there is no single legal criterion that applies to all questions of civil competency [8]. Jurisdictional differences or subtleties in statutes must also be considered, and the reader is cautioned to be familiar with individual state laws.

Neuropsychological assessment should take into account not only the cognitive status of the examinee but the nature of the capacity issue or question with which the examinee is expected to comprehend and act on in a reasonable, rational, and informed manner. As the reader will see in later sections of this chapter, the mere presence of cognitive impairment, psychiatric disorder, or mental status abnormality by itself is insufficient to declare someone incompetent. In a similar vein, an individual may be considered competent for a particular task or decision but not for another. Therefore, the legal standard of competency may be said to vary as a function of the issue or question at hand, and the neuropsychological assessment of competence must consider general cognitive functions as well as case-specific abilities. Because of their expertise in general clinical skills, knowledge of the effects of aging and disease on cognition and behavior, and their diagnostic acumen, neuropsychologists are well suited for such evaluations [9]. Formal psychometric assessment is just one of two prongs of necessary assessment methodology; the other prong of assessment requires detailed questioning of the examinee relative to his understanding of the issues and decisions involved, their ramifications, potential effects on self and pertinent others, reasoning behind one's choice, and in all, a comprehensive assessment of the examinee's judgment. Thus, even though a neuropsychologist might find deficits in those cognitive abilities that are most salient for a particular capacity evaluation, this does not mean the respondent lacks capacity. The specific tasks must be directly assessed.

The neuropsychologist may be consulted to evaluate persons in a number of different types of civil competencies. The ABA–APA Working Group on the Assessment of Capacity in Older Adults prepared a handbook to guide psychologists evaluating civil capacities of older adults which covers six civil capacities: medical consent capacity, sexual consent capacity, financial capacity, testamentary capacity, capacity to drive, and capacity to live independently. The most common of these include the need for guardianship in making health-care decisions and the management of one's finances, and testamentary capacity, that is, the competency to make a will, among others. Grisso [8], as has the American Bar Association [11] as well as Moye and Braun [10], have proposed conceptual models for the assessment of capacity. The current chapter discusses some of these methodologies, but the interested reader is referred to these sources for greater details concerning those models.

Guardianship is a legal determination where the state delegates authority over a person's estate (property) or decisional capacity (for instance financial management or health care) to another individual. Decisions regarding guardianship typically emanate from family after concern arises about the elder person's decisional abilities, often after an "incident" occurs that raises such concerns. Depending on the jurisdiction, guardianship may be specific to a particular issue, such as in the management of one's finances or in making decisions regarding one's health care. Conversely, some jurisdictions provide for more general as opposed to specific guardianship.

In matters concerning the management of one's finances, the neuropsychologist examiner will need to probe into the examinee's financial background, monetary expenditures, and other related matters that are typically thought of as quite personal. As the subject of such legal determinations, the elder will of course be required to disclose such information, traditional privacy concerns notwithstanding. Assessment of financial capacity necessarily entails addressing abilities and judgments beyond those ordinarily assessed in a neuropsychological evaluation, such as knowledge of one's assets and liabilities, income, expenses, savings, math skills involving money, and knowledge of reasonable costs of goods and services. Older adults are particularly prone to exploitation by unscrupulous individuals regarding monetary matters.

Assessment of one's judgment regarding health-care decisions is multidimensional, as is true of all of the capacity decisions in this chapter. Beyond traditional psychometric assessment, the examiner will need to probe the examinee's understanding of the health-care issue(s) in question. Does the elder understand the pros and cons of the decision? Does the elder know what to expect with agreement or disagreement of the medical issue? Does the examinee have sufficient reasoning capacity to weigh the decision, and its consequences, to a reasonable extent? Is the elder emotionally prepared to make such a decision, or will he/she be prepared with treatment? These and other pertinent health-care decisions must be comprehensively addressed in an assessment.

Testamentary capacity is an issue that most typically arises after the will has been prepared. That is, questions concerning an individual's judgment at the time the will was executed commonly arise after the will's execution and often after the death of the testator (the person preparing the will) [7]. In the latter instance, postmortem analyses of the testator's capacity and judgment is required of the neuropsychologist, a process involving a good deal of research, review of documentation, and collateral interviews [6, 12]. Executive functions are particularly important for testamentary competence [1]. Questions concerning the vulnerability of the testator to undue influence necessarily arise in many of these assessments, as well [13], what with the growth of blended families and transfer of enormous intergenerational wealth [14].

Cognitive and Behavior Change in Older Adults

Cognitive change is generally thought to be an inevitable part of aging, most commonly affecting speed of cognitive processing that typically affects attention, language, memory, and executive functions. These changes are referred to as "cognitive aging" and are thought to be normal and expected [15]. Researchers characterize the age-related changes in cognition as either "benign" or "malignant" [16]. Benign cognitive change, or cognitive aging, is sometimes also referred to as "age-related cognitive decline" (ARCD) and is thought to be the hallmark of generally healthy aging. Contemporary practice indicates that ARCD is typically used interchangeably with normal aging [16, 17]. Normative studies have determined performance/ability levels for older adults on many neuropsychological instruments [18–20]. Neuropsychologists retained in this type of referral context should be familiar with norms for older adults and expectations of both normal and pathological cognitive change.

Contrasted with ARCD, or normal aging, is abnormal or malignant cognitive aging, where greater cognitive impairment is present (i.e., dementia). An "in-between" state has also been identified, mild cognitive impairment (MCI; [16, 21]), characterized by the presence of a memory complaint, normal activities of daily living, normal global cognitive functions, and abnormal memory functions when compared to age and education norms [22]. Clinically, MCI patients manifest memory impairment to a similar extent to patients with mild Alzheimer's disease (AD) type, but unlike MCI patients whose other cognitive functions are relatively unimpaired, AD patients show more impairment in other cognitive domains as well [15, 16, 22]. The concept of MCI, however, is not without some controversy. This controversy concerns the accuracy and utility of the concept of MCI and essentially whether or not MCI, the putative "in-between" state, represents an independent entity thought to be largely nonprogressive or simply represents the earliest stages of AD and progressive decline [23, 24]. Conceptual and diagnostic issues aside, the major concern relative to the present chapter has to do with the examinee's cognitive abilities in the real world, particularly as they relate to concerns about ability to make informed decisions, that is, capacity/competency.

There are numerous neuropathological processes of a neurodegenerative nature that occur in older adults. Research suggests that nearly 70% of the dementias seen in older adults are accounted for by Alzheimer's disease (AD), Parkinson's disease dementias (PD-D), Lewy body dementia (LBD), and frontotemporal dementia (FTD) [25]. Vascular dementia (VaD) and other forms of dementia make up the rest, with VaD thought to be the second most prevalent dementia after AD [26]. Each of these dementias may present somewhat differently and have a different course over time, but with progression, all usually result in severe global impairment [27]. These disorders typically impair many aspects of cognitive functioning, eventually rendering patients incapable of managing their affairs and providing for normal activities of daily living. Depending on the severity of their symptoms, these patients may be unable to form reasonable judgments or make informed decisions. They therefore may be vulnerable to undue influence by others and be in need of guardianship to protect their interests.

Changes in personality, behavior, and/or social comportment are not uncommon in older adults. These may be the essential features of an emerging FTD, exacerbation of chronic psychiatric disorder, behavioral sequelae of cerebral neoplasm (e.g., glioma), vascular process (e.g., Binswanger's disease), delirium, or paraneoplastic syndrome, among others. Some alterations in behavior or cognition may be reversible with treatment or static in nature, while others are inexorably progressive. The examining neuropsychologist will need a complete medical history and recognition as to the nature of the disorder, its typical course, and prognosis.

Some disorders affecting older adults may result in changes of cognition or behavior, but as previously noted, these changes may not rise to a level for a determination of definite incompetency. In the case of decreased cognition, mild attention, memory, executive functioning, verbal comprehension, conceptualization, and processing, speed decrements may not have a deleterious effect on one's capacity to render appropriately reasoned decisions regarding finances, health care, and so forth [28–32].

Case Example: Refusing Medical Care

Although such mild cognitive loss may not demonstrably affect decisional capacity, changes in mood, behavior, or personality may render decision making quite impaired. Take for example the case of a hospitalized elderly female who refused treatment/surgery of her gangrenous foot. Surgeons said that unless amputated, her foot would eventually lead to widespread infection throughout her body and her death. The physicians making the referral for competency to refuse medical treatment believed she had dementia, likely Alzheimer's. She was uncooperative, spoke little, remained in bed, ate very little, and had no living family. She was brought to the hospital by her landlord, from whom she rented a small apartment, paid for with her social security and small teacher's pension. The landlord became concerned when neighbors reported they had not seen her come or go in weeks. Upon entering her apartment, the landlord found her in bed, unkempt with poor hygiene, in an apartment that obviously had not been cleaned in some time. Concerned about her condition, he brought her to the hospital.

On examination, the patient was only marginally cooperative at first, refusing to be interviewed. After meeting with her briefly several times, she became more cooperative and testing was completed. It was clear that her generally normal psychometric test results were not consistent with deficiencies of cognition; she was certainly not demented. But her mood, behavior, lack of hygiene, and collateral contact with neighbors were consistent with severe depressive illness. A psychiatric consult was requested, and the patient agreed to a trial of antidepressant medication. With eventual improvements in her depression, she did agree to the surgery. Interestingly, on interview, she noted, "…looking back it really didn't matter to me about my foot or my life… I thought I didn't have much life left anyway… so why bother?" It is worth noting, however, that in some instances where a mentally ill patient refuses life-saving treatment, the examining psychiatrist or hospital administrator may be appointed as a temporary guardian. This is most common in cases originating in hospitals or nursing homes when patients refuse to have treatment that physicians recommend, especially life-saving treatment. Refusal of life-saving treatment by patients is almost always questioned by their physicians, raising the specter of diminished mental capacity [33].

This case is illustrative of two important considerations: (1) factors other than cognitive impairment due to neurologic disease (e.g., dementia) may affect decision-making capacity, depression in this case, and (2) some conditions that adversely affect judgment are reversible with treatment (but many are not).

Case Example: Financial Guardian

Do persons with mental retardation necessarily lack the capacity to manage their financial affairs? Most readers would probably agree that the answer is "not necessarily." Although the right to self-determination for persons with intellectual disability has come under the scrutiny of the law for some time, the central issue and related questions are far from resolved [34]. The following case presentation highlights some of these concerns.

At the time of the referral, Ms. M.W. was a 73-year-old, single never married, female living semi-independently in a home willed to her by her parents. She had a male boarder who assisted with chores and related matters and a bookkeeper who came every 2 weeks to pay bills and handle such record keeping. She had a long history of documented intellectual impairment, having attended a private school for the disabled where a Stanford–Binet test administered at age 14 indicated her Full Scale IQ to be 63. M.W. completed high school and afterward "helped" in her father's office but had never had gainful employment. She lived at home with her parents and after their deaths, remained in the house. Her father had arranged for several trust funds for her that paid a monthly annuity on which she lived. She had an older brother who was the executor of his parents' estate. He lived out of state but was nonetheless in good contact with M.W. and provided appropriate support.

M.W. used a credit card for purchases of clothes, groceries, and other items and provided purchases to the bookkeeper. But M.W. could also write checks, and although she did this very infrequently, concern arose after a number of very large expenditures were noted by the bookkeeper. It seemed that M.W. had been exploited by a number of unscrupulous individuals and had paid for a new roof, appliances, and other high-ticket items when she was approached by a phone call or "knock on the door." It is common for older adults and the disabled to be exploited in this manner.

When her brother found out about these unnecessary expenditures, totaling many thousands of dollars, he sought financial guardianship, claiming that his sister's judgment in financial matters was seriously deficient. M.W. had not consulted with him, the bookkeeper, her boarder, or *anyone* about the necessity of replacing the roof and purchasing these expensive items but had made the decision to do so on her own. She had apparently not remembered that the roof had been replaced 3 years previously at a cost of $12,000.00 and would be good for at least another 25 years!

The examination methodology included a review of many records, collateral interviews with M.W.'s brother and bookkeeper, and neuropsychological evaluation. Neuropsychological assessment was supplemented with many questions concerning money, arithmetic, and related concerns. It hardly needs to be noted, but the reader will know that ethically, it matters little what side in a forensic context retains your services, simply call it like it is.

Interestingly, M.W.'s IQ (Wechsler) was now 58, yet she drove her car around town and maintained social activities in her church and bingo club. In fact, she seemed to function quite well within her very predictable and structured lifestyle, that is, with the exception of her judgment and awareness of monetary matters. M.W. had little knowledge of her annuity, monies spent, bills, and other obligations, and even worse, she had extremely impaired basic arithmetic skills. In fact, she was observed leaving a ten-dollar bill as a tip in a restaurant for a lunch that was less than $6.00!

Ultimately, M.W. was judged to be "financially incompetent" and her brother was awarded financial guardianship. The assessment report was very clear, however, that in the opinion of the neuropsychologist, none of M.W.'s other independent activities needed monitoring.

This case illustrates the fact that sometimes guardianship is appropriate, particularly in a well-documented, circumscribed, and specific domain. The reader will note the importance of amending standard neuropsychological assessment methodology with appropriate, detailed questions, observations, and interviews. Professional tests and psychometric considerations are obviously important, but so are in vivo assessment techniques.

Case Example: Dementing Illness and the Will

In a case in which one of the authors was involved, a wealthy, prominent gentleman was sued by his son-in-law for changing his will and cutting out his now deceased daughter and her heirs. The man had progressive supranuclear palsy (PSP) and was quite physically and cognitively impaired. He had hypophonia, limited visual gaze, impaired swallowing, other physical limitations, and was thought to be demented, thus providing a rationate for the suit. Had the man's ne'er-do-well son talked his father out of leaving part of his fortune to his sister's child after her death? The reader may think this scenario is right out of a bad B movie of the 1940s, but it is not fictional.

In this case, the testator's condition made assessment almost impossible since he was physically limited and speech was barely intelligible. Assessment methodology had to utilize as much multiple choice questioning as possible, limiting the assessment considerably. In addition to neuropsychologists, both sides of the legal challenge called neurologist experts as well. Because of the gentleman's condition, greater retrospective analysis needed to be utilized, as well as interviews with many family members. The essential question was, did the gentleman's condition cause cognitive impairment to a sufficient extent that he was vulnerable to the purported undue influence of his son?

Expert's for the testator opined that despite his medical condition, he was competent to have changed his will, that he was aware of the pertinent facts and issues, and that the new will was made free of any outside influence. However, ultimately, the man's condition made it impossible for plaintiff expert (representing the daughter's estate, the granddaughter) to obtain enough reliable and valid information from him to adequately and competently assess his status at the time the will was changed. In such instances, the court usually responds in a conservative fashion, siding with the testator in that plaintiff failed to document beyond a reasonable doubt that the gentleman was so impaired at the time the new will was executed that he did not know what he was doing. In this case, the examinee's condition had no doubt worsened since the execution of the will, given the progressive nature of PSP.

The reader will note that it is not uncommon that competency evaluations present difficult clinical and methodological issues. Sometimes, providing a scientifically informed, competent examination and forensic opinion is extremely challenging. The reader will want to use best neuropsychological practices [35], appropriate norms, and collateral interviews, all supplemented with comprehensive and specific questioning concerning the examinee's understanding of the issues involved. It is important to remember that the presence of cognitive impairment is insufficient by itself to warrant a determination of incapacity and that ultimately it is one's clinical judgment that must take precedence.

Clinical Pearls

- Just because someone has a diagnosis of dementia does not mean that they lack capacity, although this greatly increases the likelihood. Capacity must be assessed by directly examining the skills needed to meet the particular legal standard.
- Lacking capacity in one area (such as testamentary) does not automatically render a person incompetent in others (such as medical treatment).
- Lacking capacity at one point in time does not mean that the person will lack capacity in the future, unless the cause for incapacity is due to a known progressive illness such as Alzheimer's disease. Capacity may need to be reassessed in the future.
- Capacity involves both execution of tasks and decision making about the issue.
- Impairment on neuropsychologist tests does not equate to lack of capacity. The clinical neuropsychologist needs to augment neuropsychological test results with specific task information to make a recommendation about capacity.

References

1. Marson DC, Huthwaite J, Hebert T. Testamentary capacity and undue influence in the elderly: a jurisprudent therapy perspective. Law Psychol Rev. 2004;28:71–96.
2. Kaufmann PM. Cases, controversies, and legal authority in neuropsychological practice. Clin Neuropsychol. 2009;23(4):556 [CE Workshop presented at the 7th Annual AACN Conference, San Diego, CA.].
3. Greiffenstein MF. Basics of forensic neuropsychology. In: Morgan JE, Ricker JH, editors. Textbook of clinical neuropsychology. New York: Psychology Press; 2008. p. 905–41.
4. Marcopulos BA, Morgan JE, Denney RL. Neuropsychological evaluation of competency to proceed. In: Denney RL, Sullivan JP, editors. Clinical neuropsychology in the criminal forensic setting. New York: Guilford Press; 2008. p. 176–203.
5. Marson DC. Loss of financial capacity in dementia: conceptual and empirical approaches. Aging Neuropsychol Cogn. 2001;8:164–81.
6. Greiffenstein MF. Testamentary competence: antemortem and postmortem neuropsychological analysis. Newsletter. 2003;40(21):7–36.
7. Melton GB, Petrila J, Poythress NG, Slobogin C. Psychological evaluations for the courts: a handbook for mental health professionals and lawyers. 3rd ed. New York: Guilford; 2007.
8. Grisso T. Evaluating competencies: forensic assessments and instruments. 2nd ed. New York: Springer Science; 2003.
9. Heilbronner RL, Sweet JJ, Morgan JE, Larrabee GJ, Millis SR. American Academy of Clinical Neuropsychology Consensus Conference Statement on the neuropsychological assessment of effort, response bias, and malingering. Clin Neuropsychol. 2009;23: 1093–129.
10. Moye J, Braun M. Assessment of capacity. In: Lichtenberg PA, editor. Handbook of assessment in clinical gerontology. Amsterdam: Elsevier; 2010. p. 581–618.
11. American Bar Association and American Psychological Association Assessment of Capacity in Older Adults Project Working Group. Assessment of older adults with diminished capacity: a handbook for psychologists. Washington, DC: American Bar Association and American Psychological Association; 2008.
12. Shulman KI, Cohen CA, Hull I. Psychiatric issues in retrospective challenges of testamentary capacity. Int J Geriatr Psychiatry. 2005;20:63–9.
13. Shulman KI, Cohen CA, Kirsh FC, Hull IA, Champine JD. Assessment of testamentary capacity and vulnerability to undue influence. Am J Psychiatry. 2007;164: 722–7.
14. Moye J, Marson DC. Assessment of decision-making capacity in older adults: an emerging area of practice and research. J Gerontol B Psychol Sci Soc Sci. 2007;62:3–11.
15. Smith GE, Bondi MW. Normal aging, mild cognitive impairment and Alzheimer's disease. In: Morgan JE, Ricker JH, editors. Textbook of clinical neuropsychology. New York: Psychology Press; 2008; 768–780.
16. Smith G, Rush BK. Normal aging and mild cognitive impairment. In: Attix DK, Welsh-Bohmer KA, editors. Geriatric neuropsychology: assessment and intervention. New York: Guilford Press; 2006;27–55.
17. Caccappolo-Van Vliet E, Manly J, Tang MX, Marder K, Bell K, Stern Y. The neuropsychological profiles of mild Alzheimer's disease and questionable dementia as compared to age-related cognitive decline. J Int Neuropsychol Society. 2003;9:720–32.
18. Smith GE, Ivnik RJ, Lucas J. Assessment techniques: tests, test batteries, norms and methodological approaches. In: Morgan JE, Ricker JH, editors. Textbook of clinical neuropsychology. New York: Psychology Press; 2008;38–57.
19. Ivnik RJ, Malec JF, Smith GE, Tangalos EG, Petersen RC, Kokmen E, et al. Mayo's older American normative studies: WAIS-R, WMS-R, and AVLT norms for ages 56 through 97. Clin Neuropsychol. 1992;6(Suppl): 1–104.
20. Heaton R, Grant I, Matthews C. Comprehensive norm s for an expanded Halstead reitan neuropsychological battery: demographic corrections, research findings, and clinical applications. Odessa, FL: Psychological Assessment Resources, Inc.; 1991.
21. Flicker C, Ferris SH, Reisberg B. Mild cognitive impairment in the elderly: predictors of dementia. Neurology. 1991;41:1006–9.
22. Petersen RC, Smith GE, Waring S, Ivnik RJ, Tangalos EG, Kokmen E. Mild cognitive impairment: clinical characterization and outcome. Arch Neurol. 1999;56:303–8.
23. Andrikopoulos J. Looking into the crystal ball of mild cognitive impairment: what I see is Alzheimer's disease. In: Morgan JE, Baron IS, Ricker JH, editors. Casebook of clinical neuropsychology. New York: Oxford University Press; 2011;540–559.
24. Whitehouse P, Brodaty H. Mild cognitive impairment. Lancet. 2006;17:367.
25. Welsh-Bohmer KA, Warren LH. Neurodegenerative dementias. In: Attix DK, Welsh-Bohmer KA, editors. Geriatric neuropsychology: assessment and intervention. New York: Guilford Press; 2006;56–88.
26. Haaland KA, Swanda RM. Vascular dementia. In: Morgan JE, Ricker JH, editors. Textbook of clinical neuropsychology. New York: Psychology Press; 2008;384–91.
27. Lezak MD, Howieson DB, Loring DW. Neuropsychological assessment. 4th ed. New York: Oxford; 2004.
28. Gurrera RJ, Moye J, Karel MJ, Azar AR, Armesto JC. Cognitive performance predicts treatment decisional abilities in mild to moderate dementia. Neurology. 2006;66:1367–72.
29. Marson DC, Cody HA, Ingram KK, Harrell LE. Neuropsychological predictors of competency in

Alzheimer's disease using a rational reasons legal standard. Arch Neurol. 1995;52:955–9.
30. Marson DC, Chatterjee A, Ingram KK, Harrell LE. Toward a neurologic model of competency: cognitive predictors of capacity to consent in Alzheimer's disease using three different legal standards. Neurology. 1996;46:666–72.
31. Marson DC, Sawrie SM, McInturff B, Snyder S, Chatterjee A, Stalvey T, et al. Assessing financial capacity in patients with Alzheimer's disease: a conceptual model and prototype instrument. Arch Neurol. 2000;57:877–84.
32. Okonkwo OC, Griffith HR, Belue K, Lanza S, Zamrini EY, Harrell LE, Brockington JC, Clark D, Raman R, Marson DC. Cognitive models of medical decision-making capacity in patients with mild cognitive impairment. J Int Neuropsychol Soc. 2008;14:297–308.
33. Wettstein RM, Roth LH. The psychiatrist as legal guardian. Am J Psychiatry. 1988;145:600–4.
34. Carey A. On the margins of citizenship: intellectual disability and civil rights in twentieth century America. Philadelphia, PA: Temple University Press; 2009.
35. American Academy of Clinical Neuropsychology (AACN). American Academy of Clinical Neuropsychology (AACN) practice guidelines for neuropsychological assessment and consultation. Clin Neuropsychol. 2007;21:209–31.

Index

L.D. Ravdin and H.L. Katzen (eds.), *Handbook on the Neuropsychology of Aging and Dementia*,
Clinical Handbooks in Neuropsychology, DOI 10.1007/978-1-4614-3106-0,